Third Edition

HOME CARE
NURSING PRACTICE

CONCEPTS AND APPLICATION

Third Edition

HOME CARE NURSING PRACTICE

CONCEPTS AND APPLICATION

ROBYN RICE, MSN-R, PhD(C), RN-C
Clinical Associate Professor
Barnes College of Nursing
The University of Missouri—St. Louis
St. Louis, Missouri

Home Care Clinical Nurse Specialist
American Nursing Development
Maryville, Illinois

with 169 illustrations

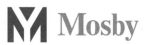 Mosby

A Harcourt Health Sciences Company

St. Louis   London   Philadelphia   Sydney   Toronto

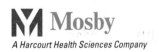

Mosby

A Harcourt Health Sciences Company

Vice President, Nursing Editorial Director: Sally Schrefer
Senior Editor: Loren Wilson
Developmental Editor: Nancy L. O'Brien
Project Manager: John Rogers
Project Specialist: Cheryl A. Abbott
Designer and Cover Art: Kathi Gosche

NOTICE
Pharmacology is an ever-changing field. Standard safety precautions must be followed, but as new research and clinical experience broaden our knowledge, changes in treatment and drug therapy may become necessary or appropriate. Readers are advised to check the most current product information provided by the manufacturer of each drug to be administered to verify the recommended dose, the method and duration of administration, and contraindications. It is the responsibility of the licensed prescriber, relying on experience and knowledge of the patient, to determine dosages and the best treatment for each individual patient. Neither the publisher nor the editor assumes any liability for any injury and/or damage to persons or property arising from this publication.

Mosby, Inc.
A Harcourt Health Sciences Company
11830 Westline Industrial Drive
St. Louis, Missouri 63146

Printed in the United States of America

International Standard Book Number 0-323-01107-1

00   01   02   03   04   CL/FF   9 8 7 6 5 4 3 2 1

CONTRIBUTORS

SALLY C. ADAMS, BSN, RN
Manager
BJC Home Infusion Services
St. Louis, Missouri

KAREN BALAKAS, PhD, RN
Associate Professor
Maryville University
St. Louis, Missouri

ELLEN BARKER, MSN, RN, CNRN
President
Neuroscience Nursing Consultants
Greenville, Delaware

VIRGINIA K. DRAKE, DNSc, RN, CS, APN
Legal Nurse Consultants, Inc.
Private Practice
St. Louis, Missouri

PATRICIA E. FREED, MSN, EdD, RN
Associate Professor
Jewish College of Nursing and Allied Health
St. Louis, Missouri

SUSAN HEADY, PhD, RN
Associate Professor
Department of Nursing
Webster University
St. Louis, Missouri

KATHRYN A. HOUSTON, MSN, RN, CS, GNP
Geriatric Nurse Practitioner and Continence
  Consultant in Long Term Care
St. Louis, Missouri

RUTH LAUNIUS JENKINS, PhD, RN
Associate Professor
Barnes College of Nursing
The University of Missouri—St. Louis
St. Louis, Missouri

ROBERTA A. KORDISH, MSN, RN, CNS
Director of Sales and Marketing
Professional Nurse Associates
A Health Design Plus Company
Hudson, Ohio

GAIL B. LEWIS-REA, MSN, PhD(c), RN
Clinical Associate Professor
Barnes College of Nursing
The University of Missouri—St. Louis
St. Louis, Missouri

SANDRA LINDQUIST, PhD, RN
Clinical Associate Professor
Barnes College of Nursing
The University of Missouri—St. Louis
St. Louis, Missouri

ANNETTE M. LYNCH, MSN, RN, CNS
Director, Quality Management and Compliance
Professional Nurse Associates
A Health Design Plus Company
Hudson, Ohio

S. TROY MCMULLIN, PharmD, BCPS
Clinical Pharmacist, Critical Care
Barnes-Jewish Hospital
St. Louis, Missouri

DONNA BRIDGMAN MUSSER, PhD(c), RN
Assistant Clinical Professor and Coordinator of
  Technology
Barnes College of Nursing
The University of Missouri—St. Louis
St. Louis, Missouri

GAIL NICHOLS, MFA, RN
Quality Improvement Coordinator and Educator
BJC Hospice and Supportive Care
St. Louis, Missouri

DAVID J. RITCHIE, PharmD, BCPS
Professor of Pharmacy Practice
St. Louis College of Pharmacy
Clinical Pharmacist, Infectious Diseases
Barnes-Jewish Hospital
St. Louis, Missouri

ANNE CAHILL SCHAPPE, PhD, RN
Associate Professor
Webster University
St. Louis, Missouri

JOANNE P. SHEEHAN, BSN, JD, RN
Principal in Law Firm of Friedman, Newman,
  Levy, Sheehan, and Carolan
Fairfield, Connecticut

MARLAINE C. SMITH, PhD, RN
Associate Professor and MSN Program Director
University of Colorado Health Sciences Center
  School of Nursing
Denver, Colorado

GAYLE H. SULLIVAN, BSN, JD, RN
Medical Liability Consultant
Quality Assurance Associates, Inc.
Fairfield, Connecticut

SAUNDRA J. TRIPLETT, MSN, RN
Director, Clinical Quality Resources
SSM Home Care
St. Louis, Missouri

JEAN WATSON, PhD, RN, FAAN, HNC
Distinguished Professor of Nursing
Endowed Chair, Caring Science
University of Colorado Health Sciences Center
  School of Nursing
Denver, Colorado

GAIL F. WILKERSON, MSN, RN, CS
Gerontological Clinical Nurse Specialist
Regional Director of Wellness Services
Sunrise Assisted Living
St. Louis, Missouri

LENORE R. WILLIAMS, MSN, RN, CNS
Director of Operations
Professional Nurse Associates
A Health Design Plus Company
Hudson, Ohio

For Jack

ABOUT THE AUTHOR

Clinician, educator, author, and nurse advocate, Robyn Rice has worked in home care for more than 15 years. Robyn serves as the Home Care Column Editor for the *Journal of Geriatric Nursing* and is the author of several nursing references, including *Manual of Home Health Nursing Procedures, 2/e; Handbook of Home Health Nursing Procedures, 2/e; Manual of Pediatric and Postpartum Home Care Procedures;* and *Handbook of Pediatric and Postpartum Home Care Procedures.* In addition, Robyn has presented many workshops and seminars at the state, national, and international levels; contributed chapters and articles to a number of nursing books and journals; and served as an item writer for the ANCC's Home Health Nurse Certification examination and the NCLEX-RN examination.

Robyn is a Clinical Associate Professor in the Barnes College of Nursing at the University of Missouri—St. Louis. She teaches adult health, home, and community nursing care and is currently developing a home care nursing Internet course for CEUs/elective credit. She is also a certified home health nurse and serves as a home care clinical nurse specialist for American Nursing Development in Maryville, Illinois. Currently Robyn is a doctorate of philosophy candidate in nursing at the Health Sciences Center at the University of Colorado in Denver. Robyn was voted Who's Who in Professional Nursing in 1993 and was named Southern Illinois University's Alumnus of the Year in 1996.

PREFACE

With shortened hospital stays and an expansion of community-based health care services, it is my belief that a person's health primarily resides in, and is influenced by, his or her own home environment. Therefore as a practice profession, it is imperative that all nurses have a clear understanding of the issues and considerations involving patient care in the home setting. Fundamental to this is an understanding of the purposes and goals of home care, as well as how nurses care for patients at home. Moreover, I would like to suggest that what we nurses do in the home is not home health, rather home *care*. To me this represents an essential movement away from the technical and toward a holistic focus of practice that includes the patient, the patient's family and/or caregiver, and home environment. It reflects an appreciation of health from the patient's perspective to include all the patient is and wants to be—hence, the title change of this third edition from home health to home *CARE* nursing practice.

The third edition of *Home Care Nursing Practice: Concepts & Application* is designed to present a grand overview of contemporary home care and community-based nursing practice. Theoretical and clinical perspectives are given. The special challenges of the home setting call for nurses to be self-directed professionals with a concern for cost-effective and quality patient care. Such a balance in caring is not always easy to achieve. This book was written to give such guidance and vision in practice to those nurses choosing to work in home care.

The material in the third edition of *Home Care Nursing Practice* is completely updated with many new chapters added to reflect the ever-expanding knowledge base in home care. Practicing home care nurses will find that this new edition certainly meets their current learning needs. Discharge planning nurses, case managers, and registered nurses considering entering home care, can all benefit from this text. Nurses involved in the administrative and educational aspects of home care agency operation will find this book to be a useful resource for orientation and clinical support purposes. In that *Home Care Nursing Practice* has such a strong academic focus, student nurses at the undergraduate and graduate levels will find this text to be a valuable resource they can carry from the classroom into the home care setting.

Home Care Nursing Practice is organized into four major parts. Part I, Concepts of Home Care Nursing, reviews concepts pertinent to general nursing practice within the home setting. Discussions include role preparation and orientation; staff safety concerns; recommendations for working with student nurses; developing the plan of care; Medicare-based documentation guidelines, including tips for working with OASIS; infection control measures; and quality care concerns.

Nurses who can articulate their role drive clinical policy; therefore, Chapter 2, Understanding Home Care Nursing: Applying Theory to Clinical Practice, has been structured to illuminate a working definition of health, as well as to address the purpose and goals of home care. A new chapter, Caring for Families in the Home (Chapter 4), has been added to complete the theoretical circle of knowing in home care. Of importance, this chapter offers family role theory and interventions for working with families in crisis. Chapter 7, Patient Education in the Home, discusses issues of health teaching for patients across the life span. Chapter 8, Legal and Ethical Issues in Home Care, provides sound clinical practice guidelines for nurses working in the sometimes unpredictable environment of the home milieu. Chapter 9, Case Management and Leadership Strategies for Home Care Nurses, discusses issues such as caseload organization; collaborating with the multidisciplinary team; clinical leadership strategies, such as committee work; and care path development.

Part II, Clinical Application, discusses patients typically visited in the home. Nursing interventions for patients with chronic obstructive pulmonary disease, congestive heart failure, diabetes, bowel and bladder dysfunction, and AIDS are discussed, as well as caregiving concerns related to wound care and home rehabilitation. High-technology care, such as mechanical ventilation and IV therapy, are also included. Chapter 19, The Patient with Neurological Dysfunction, provides clinical guidelines for patients with Alzheimer's disease, cerebral vascular accident, and multiple sclerosis. Part II also provides a detailed discussion of the role of the home medical equipment vendor, as well as the equipment and products available for home use. Descriptions of commonly used home care products and equipment will assist the reader to use them appropriately and effectively. (Please note that any descriptions of specific products or equipment is not intended to be an endorsement on the part of the author or publisher.) To reinforce the importance of patient teaching, I have highlighted patient education guidelines throughout the clinical chapters.

Part III, Special Clinical and Community Issues, addresses special patient populations and home environment issues the home care nurse is likely to encounter. Individual chapters deal with maternal-child and postpartum patients; patients with mental health disorders; elderly patients; and patients receiving hospice care. Topics include clinical recommendations for patients experiencing schizophrenia or acute depression, physiological changes and nursing interventions associated with aging patients, and spiritual and palliative care issues. Chapter 25, Managing Environmental Threats in the Home, is a new chapter that highlights the impact the environment can have on an individual's health and offers recommendations for environmental care.

Part IV, Future Trends, is composed of all new chapters that offer insights into what patients and nurses can expect to encounter in our new century. Chapter 26, From Telehealth to Telecare, presents current information on how telecommunications is

used in home care, with suggestions for further research and practice. Chapter 27, Complementary Therapies and Home Care Nursing Practice, presents a very holistic overview of nontraditional therapies such as therapeutic touch, aromatherapy, storytelling, poetry, and many others used for fostering the best levels of health. Finally, in a fitting Epilogue to this new edition, we are honored to have Dr. Jean Watson share her philosophical perspectives of caring in the home.

Two points about this new edition should be noted. First, the term *caregiver* is sued throughout the book to denote the patient's family, friend, or significant other, who may assist the patient and the nurse in carrying out the plan of care. Although most patients live at home with their families, some patients receive care and support from other sources. For this reason, I chose to use the term *caregiver* to encompass the services of all who provide assistance. Second, as a primary component of patient education, clean technique is commonly taught in the home setting today. As a standard of practice, home care nurses should perform procedures using aseptic technique whenever possible. Infection control precautions should provide safety for the patient, the caregiver, and the home care team.

The information in this book will assist all nurses to care for patients with different educational, social, economic, and cultural backgrounds. In addition, my intent is that the book be used to increase the nurse's understanding of clinical issues and high technology related to patient care, the importance of working with caregivers or family members, the purpose and use of a multidisciplinary approach, the impact of patient education in fostering self-care management, and the basics of Medicare regulations governing reimbursement for services rendered. I wrote the book to inspire autonomy of nursing practice and creative, new ways of thinking. I sincerely hope that the information and recommendations in this book be integrated with a sensitivity to the special concerns and special privileges that home care nursing practice provides.

Robyn Rice

ACKNOWLEDGMENTS

I want to thank my husband Jack for all his love and support. I could not do this work without him. *Jack, I love you very much!*

Since this book first published in 1992 there have been several people who have been very helpful to me in work, career, and writing issues. I am here and giving you this book largely because of their support. I would like to say thank you to:

- Dr. Jerry Durham, Dean at Barnes College of Nursing at The University of Missouri—St. Louis. Dr. Durham is a most excellent Dean and a very *good* man.
- Dr. Ruth O'Brien at the University of Colorado's School of Nursing for her caring and mentorship in helping me complete my PhD.
- Jackie Washington of St. Louis, Missouri for as-sisting me with student placement and clinicals at a time when I really needed the help.
- The home care and hospice departments of BJC Health Services of St. Louis, Missouri (Ruth Castellano, Director); St. Anthony's Health Center in Alton, Illinois (Paula Bull, Director); and SSM Health Services of St. Louis, Missouri (Saundra J. Triplett, Director).
- Mosby editors, Loren Wilson and Nancy O'Brien, who have never-ending patience and understanding. Also, Cheryl Abbott, who was a great help with production issues.

Last, I wish to thank my friends, colleagues, and loved ones . . . our chapter contributors who have tried so hard to share all they know with all of you. They are the *caring kind.*

KNOWING IN NURSING

I stepped outside of myself so that I could know
So that I could know the meaning of the earth
Its green springs and quiet winter nights
So that I could know the depths
of the great, blue ocean
A place from which we all came.

I stepped outside of myself so that I could know
that there was more than the moon,
and the sun, and the stars . . .
And that when I looked upon the earth
so that I could know the meaning of life and
appreciate its continuance in death.

I stepped outside of myself so that I could know
how to raise my arms in loving, caring ways
And say to those who would listen
Let me share myself with you and all that I know . . .

From Rice R: A little art in home care: poetry and storytelling for the soul, *J Geriatr Nurs* 20(3):165, 1999.

CONTENTS

Part I Concepts of Home Care Nursing, 1

1 HOME CARE NURSING PRACTICE: HISTORICAL PERSPECTIVES AND PHILOSOPHY OF CARE, 3
Robyn Rice

Historical Perspectives, 3
Social Perspectives, 4
The Impact of Government Regulations and Policy on Home Care, 7
The Impact of Technology on Home Care, 12
Contemporary Home Care Nursing: A Philosophy of Practice, 13
Summary, 14

2 UNDERSTANDING HOME CARE NURSING: APPLYING THEORY TO CLINICAL PRACTICE, 15
Robyn Rice

Theory Development and Its Importance to Nursing, 16
Nursing Theory Relevant to Home Care Nursing Practice, 16
The Concept of Health in Home Care, 18
A Theoretical Framework for Home Care: The Rice Model of Dynamic Self-Determination for Self-Care, 19
Summary, 22

3 THE ROLE OF THE HOME CARE NURSE AND ORIENTATION STRATEGIES, 24
Sandra Lindquist, Donna Bridgman Musser, Robyn Rice

Understanding Caring in the Home, 24
Understanding the Role of the Home Care Nurse, 25
Skills to Support Role Implementation, 25
Nurse Profile, 26
Role Preparation and Orientation, 27
Advanced Practice Nurses, 30
Implementing Student Learning in Home Care, 33
Summary, 35
Appendix III-I: Internet Resources for Home Care Nurses, 37

4 CARING FOR FAMILIES IN THE HOME, 47
Ruth Launius Jenkins

Definition of Family, 47
Philosophical Perspectives of Family-Focused Care, 47
Home Care Applications, 50
Summary, 56

5 DEVELOPING THE PLAN OF CARE AND DOCUMENTATION, *58*
Robyn Rice

Preparing for the Home Visit, *58*
Conducting the Home Visit, *58*
Medicare Documentation Guidelines for Reimbursement of Home Care Services, *64*
Summary, *74*
Appendix V-I: Medical Nutrition Therapy: Assessment of Patient's Nutrient Requirements, *75*

6 INFECTION CONTROL IN THE HOME, *81*
Robyn Rice, Gail B. Lewis-Rea

From Past to Present: Understanding the Need for Infection Control, *81*
Epidemiology, *83*
Mechanism of Infection, *88*
Home Care Application, *89*
Administrative Considerations, *96*
Summary, *97*
Appendix VI-1: Patient Education Guidelines to Reduce the Risk of Transmitting a Communicable Disease, *100*

7 PATIENT EDUCATION IN THE HOME, *102*
Robyn Rice, Karen Balakas, Virginia K. Drake, Patricia E. Freed, Anne Cahill Schappe

Teaching and Learning, *102*
Conceptual Basis, *103*
Motivational Factors for Learning and Self-Determination for Self-Care, *105*
Principles of Adult Learning, *106*
Patient Education and the Nursing Process, *108*
Teaching Strategies and Tools, *109*
Teaching Strategies for Special Patient Groups in Home Care, *110*
Summary, *122*

8 LEGAL AND ETHICAL ISSUES IN HOME CARE, *124*
Gayle H. Sullivan, Joanne P. Sheehan, Robyn Rice

Understanding Our Legal System, *124*
Understanding More About Malpractice, *125*
What All Home Care Nurses Should Know Before Accepting Employment, *127*
Documentation Issues, *129*
Advance Directives, *133*
Informed Consent, *134*
Right to Confidentiality in Medical Records, *135*
Telecare, *135*
Common Areas of Liability and How to Avoid Them, *135*
Summary, *139*

9 CASE MANAGEMENT AND LEADERSHIP STRATEGIES FOR HOME CARE NURSES, *140*
Robyn Rice

Management and Leadership Strategies, *140*
Trends in Management: Case Management, *141*
Clinical Applications of Case Management in the Home, *143*
Trends in Leadership: Empowerment, *149*
Clinical Applications of Leadership: Committee Work, *149*
Summary, *151*

Appendix IX-I: Care Path (CP)
    Standard: Skin/Integumentary
    System, *153*
Appendix IX-II: Patient/Caregiver
    Care Path: Home Guide, *157*

**10 QUALITY PATIENT
    CARE,** *161*
Saundra J. Triplett, Robyn Rice

Philosophy of Quality
    Improvement, *162*
Quality Improvement Team, *162*
Theoretical Framework, *164*
QI Program Components, *166*
Measuring Quality, *167*
Quality Improvement Tools, *168*
Cost Versus Benefit Is the
    Future, *170*
Summary, *171*

**Part II Clinical
    Application,** *173*

**11 THE PATIENT WITH
    CHRONIC OBSTRUCTIVE
    PULMONARY DISEASE,** *175*
Robyn Rice

Description, *175*
Epidemiology, *176*
Etiology and Pathophysiology, *176*
Home Oxygen Therapy, *178*
Humidification and Aerosol
    Therapy, *183*
Infection Control Issues, *185*
Screening for Chronic Obstructive
    Pulmonary Disease, *186*
Home Care Application, *186*
Patient Education, *190*
Pulmonary Rehabilitation, *191*
Summary, *191*
Appendix XI-I: Medical Nutrition
    Therapy: Chronic Obstructive
    Pulmonary Disease, *194*
Appendix XI-II: Chest
    Physiotherapy at Home, *198*

**12 THE PATIENT WITH
    CONGESTIVE HEART
    FAILURE,** *200*
Robyn Rice, S. Troy McMullin

Significance and Prevalence, *200*
Pathophysiology, *200*
Classification of Congestive Heart
    Failure, *202*
Home Care Application, *202*
Summary, *210*
Appendix XII-I: Medical
    Nutrition Therapy: Congestive
    Heart Failure, *211*

**13 THE VENTILATOR-
    DEPENDENT PATIENT,** *215*
Robyn Rice

Pathophysiology, *216*
Principle Equipment Used for
    Home Respiratory Support, *217*
Home Discharge Planning, *219*
Home Care Application, *223*
Pediatric Issues, *230*
Summary, *230*
Appendix XIII-I: Home Ventilator
    Management, *232*

**14 THE PATIENT WITH
    CHRONIC WOUNDS,** *239*
Robyn Rice

Etiology and Pathophysiology of
    Chronic Wounds, *239*
Classification of Chronic
    Wounds, *242*
Mechanisms of Wound
    Healing, *243*
Home Care Application, *244*
Summary, *256*
Appendix XIV-I: Medical
    Nutrition Therapy: Pressure
    Ulcers, *258*
Appendix XIV-II: Dermal Wound
    Care Products, *262*

15 THE PATIENT WITH DIABETES, *265*
Susan Heady

Pathophysiology and
   Classification of Diabetes, *265*
Acute Complications, *266*
Chronic Complications, *267*
Home Care Application, *267*
Summary, *276*

16 THE PATIENT WITH BLADDER DYSFUNCTION, *278*
Kathryn A. Houston

Definition of the Problem, *278*
Prevalence, *278*
Physiology of the Lower Urinary
   Tract, *278*
Abnormalities of Micturition, *279*
Classification of Urinary
   Incontinence, *279*
Effects of Aging on Bladder
   Function, *280*
Home Care Application, *280*
Summary, *294*
Appendix XVI-I: Drugs Used to
   Treat Urinary Incontinence, *296*

17 THE PATIENT RECEIVING HOME CARE REHABILITATION SERVICES, *297*
Robyn Rice

Indications for Rehabilitation
   Services, *298*
Home Care Application, *299*
Summary, *306*
Appendix XVII-I: Seating Tips for
   the Chairbound Patient, *307*
Appendix XVII-II: Adaptive
   Equipment Commonly Used in
   the Home, *309*

18 THE PATIENT RECEIVING HOME INFUSION THERAPIES, *310*
Sally C. Adams

Overview, *310*
Administrative Issues, *311*
Home Care Application, *313*
Summary, *329*

19 THE PATIENT WITH NEUROLOGICAL DYSFUNCTION, *330*
Ellen Barker, Robyn Rice

Cerebrovascular Accident (CVA),
   330
Home Care Application, *332*
Multiple Sclerosis (MS), *344*
Home Care Application, *346*
Dementia: Alzheimer's Type, *348*
Home Care Application, *349*
Summary, *353*
Appendix XIX-I: Stroke Risk
   Screening, *354*

20 THE PATIENT WITH AIDS, *356*
Robyn Rice, David J. Ritchie

Pathophysiology, *357*
HIV Presentation and Clinical
   Course of AIDS, *358*
Mechanism of Transmission, *358*
Epidemiology, *359*
Occupational and Casual
   Transmission, *360*
Screening, *360*
Home Care Application, *360*
Living at Home With Aids, *372*
Summary, *374*

Part III **Special Clinical and Community Issues,** *377*

21 **MATERNAL-CHILD NURSING: POSTPARTUM HOME CARE,** *379*
Annette M. Lynch, Roberta A. Kordish, Lenore R. Williams

Historical Perspectives, *379*
Philosophy of Care, *380*
Scope of Services, *380*
Home Care Application, *381*
Summary and Implications for the Future, *398*

22 **THE MENTAL HEALTH PATIENT,** *401*
Patricia E. Freed

Philosophy of Mental Health Home Care Services, *402*
Home Care Applications for Depression, *405*
Home Care Applications for Schizophrenia, *409*
Summary, *415*

23 **THE ELDERLY PATIENT,** *417*
Gail F. Wilkerson

Demographics, *417*
Physiology of Aging, *418*
The Elderly Home Care Patient, *420*
Patient Care Issues in the Home Setting, *420*
Home Care Application, *425*
Summary, *428*

24 **THE HOSPICE AND PALLIATIVE CARE PATIENT,** *430*
Gail Nichols, Robyn Rice

History and Development of Hospice, *430*

The Medicare Hospice Benefit, *431*
Admission to a Hospice Program, *431*
Patient Profiles, *432*
The Hospice Team: A Multidisciplinary Approach, *432*
Home Care Application, *434*
Understanding Emotional Reactions to Death, *442*
Caregivers' Concerns and Bereavement Support, *444*
Pediatric Hospice, *446*
Summary, *448*
Appendix XXIV-I: Dosing Data for Acetaminophen (APAP) and NSAID, *451*
Appendix XXIV-II: Dose Equivalents for Opioid Analgesics in Opioid-Naive Children and Adults ≥50 kg Body Weight, *452*
Appendix XXIV-III: Commonly Used Adjuvant Analgesics, *453*

25 **MANAGING ENVIRONMENTAL THREATS IN THE HOME,** *457*
Robyn Rice

Environmental Threats in the Home: Problem Identification, *457*
Contextual Issues, *459*
Analysis of the Problem: Home Care Nursing Perspectives, *460*
Recommendations, *461*
Summary, *462*
Appendix XXV-I: Making Your Home Toxin Free, *464*

Part IV   **Future Trends,** *467*

26   **FROM TELEHEALTH
TO TELECARE:
IMPLICATIONS FOR
CLINICAL PRACTICE,** *469*
Robyn Rice

Historical Perspectives, *469*
Telehealth and the Discipline of
   Nursing, *470*
Implementation of Telehealth in
   Home Care, *470*
Critical Underlying Issues in the
   Literature, *471*
Research on Telehealth, *472*
Implications for Home Care
   Nursing Practice, Education,
   and Research, *476*
Areas for Future Research, *477*
Summary, *478*

27   **COMPLEMENTARY
THERAPIES AND HOME
CARE NURSING
PRACTICE,** *480*
Marlaine C. Smith

History and Background, *480*
Theoretical Foundations, *482*

Survey of Alternative/
   Complementary Therapies, *483*
Implications for Home Care
   Nursing Practice, *496*
Summary, *496*
Appendix XXVII-I: Resources for
   Information on Alternative
   Therapies, *498*

Epilogue

**RECONSIDERING CARING
IN THE HOME,** *500*
Jean Watson

Relationship-Centered Caring as a
   Starting Point and Basis for
   Professional Nursing in the
   Home, *500*
Professional Home Care Nursing
   Is Not Defined as Doing, *501*
Some Elements of a Mature
   Nursing Paradigm for Home
   Care Nursing, *501*

Appendix

LABORATORY VALUES, *503*

PART I

CONCEPTS OF HOME CARE NURSING

HOME CARE NURSING PRACTICE: HISTORICAL PERSPECTIVES AND PHILOSOPHY OF CARE

Robyn Rice

The advent and growth of the home care industry has resulted from public demand for quality health care, societal pressure for cost containment of health care services, and advances in medical and communication technologies that transcend traditional boundaries of care. Diagnostic-related groups (DRGs) were legislated in the 1980s to control cost inflation in the health care system. As a result many patients are now discharged from the hospital into the home "sicker and quicker." Home care nursing continues to evolve within this multicultural milieu, providing care for patients with complex and diverse health care needs.

Home care nursing consists of principles of nursing practice that are both old and new. Although intricately bound to government and health care provider policy regulating reimbursement of visits, home care nursing blends concepts of community health nursing with disease-focused care that is holistic in manifestation. This text explores the evolution and continued development of home care nursing and describes historical, societal, and governmental regulatory events that have shaped this special kind of nursing practice. In addition, the implications of advances in medical and communication technologies in home care are discussed. Last, a philosophy of home care nursing with recommendations for practice is given.

HISTORICAL PERSPECTIVES

The following chronology outlines significant events in understanding the history of home care. Home care services have their roots in visits made to the sick poor by religious orders during the late 1700s. In 1796 the Boston Dispensary was one of the first to provide home care in the United States. A founding principle of the Boston Dispensary reveals its philosophy of care:[3] "The sick, without being pained by separation from their families, may be attended and relieved at home."

The American concept of home care was founded by visiting nurses. The first visiting nurses in America were called *district nurses,* a British term credited to Florence Nightingale (1820-1910) for nurses who cared for the sick at home (Figure 1-1). In the late 1800s home nursing services were organized and administered by laypersons. These agencies provided unlicensed, skilled nursing care and taught cleanliness and home care techniques to the ill and their families. In 1877 the Women's Branch of the New York City Mission was the first group to employ a graduate nurse to care for the sick at home.[10]

A voluntary agency was established in 1885 in Buffalo, New York, to provide home nursing care. In 1886 other voluntary agencies that provided patients with similar home health care services emerged in Boston and Philadelphia. These would later become Visiting Nurse Associations (VNAs).

In 1893 the Henry Street Settlement House in New York City was established by Lillian Wald and

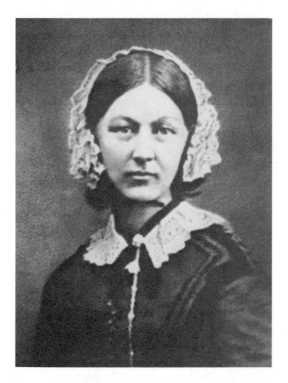

Figure 1-1 Florence Nightingale. (Copyright Hulton Getty, Chicago, Ill.)

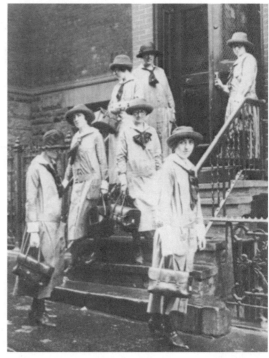

Figure 1-2 Nurses at the Henry Street Settlement House, early 1900s. (Copyright Bettmann/Corbis, Tacoma, Wash.)

Mary Brewster to provide care for the sick and poor.[10] Home care nurses were employed to tend the health needs of tenement residents (Figure 1-2).

In 1898 graduate nurses were hired by the Los Angeles County Health Department to make visits to the sick poor. This was the first governmental health department to set up such services. The term *public health nurse* was subsequently coined.

By 1890 there were 21 VNAs in the United States, most of which employed only one nurse. Late in the nineteenth century, VNAs increased in number. The growing social consciousness and the increasing wealth of the United States to fund such services were contributing factors.[8] In 1908 some home care services were covered for policyholders of Metropolitan Life Insurance in New York City.[10] By 1909 approximately 565 organizations across the country employed a total of 1416 visiting nurses.[3]

With the dawn of the 1900s the Frontier Nursing Services was established in rural Kentucky by

Mary Breckinridge. Its purpose was to provide home care to rural mountain people (Figure 1-3). Home care nursing continued to serve urban needs as well (Figure 1-4).

The number of home care agencies grew during World War II as home visits by physicians began to decline. After World War II home care services developed at an ever-increasing rate, with tremendous growth experienced by nonprofit or "voluntary" home health agencies such as the VNAs, as well as public health departments.[8] Today the home care industry continues to thrive as the delivery of patient care and scope of services reflect societal demands for cost-effective, quality health care available to all people in the United States.

SOCIAL PERSPECTIVES

The following chronology describes social factors that have influenced home care. Before the 1960s home care was viewed as a community service.

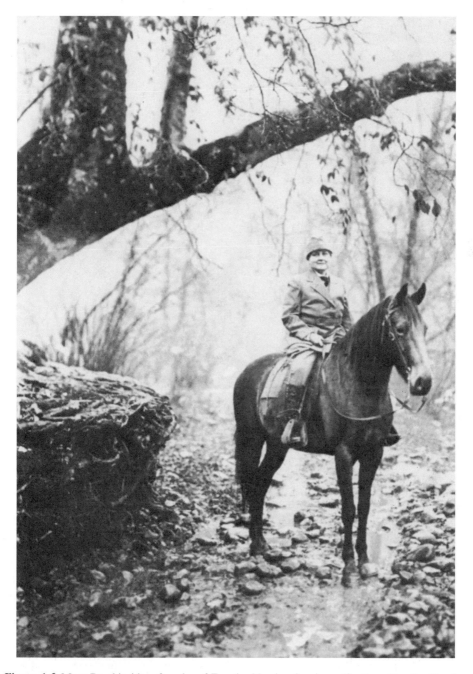

Figure 1-3 Mary Breckinridge, founder of Frontier Nursing Services. (Courtesy Frontier Nursing Services, Wendover, Ky.)

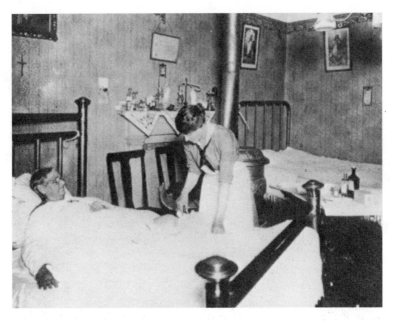

Figure 1-4 The visiting nurse in the patient's home. (Courtesy Visiting Nurse Association of Greater St. Louis, St. Louis, Mo.)

Although the focus of community and public health nursing was one of health promotion, home care nursing in particular focused on health restoration and caring for the sick. Agencies such as the VNAs established the fundamentals of bringing health care services into homes. The essential mission of these agencies was to provide quality home care to all patients without regard for their ability to pay for services. Government intervention, private foundations and endowments, and other organizations such as the United Way made agency operation possible.

In the mid-1960s a growing elderly population, advances in medical technology, and public demand for universal access to the health care system had tremendous influence on the home care industry. There were more patients to be seen and fewer resources to cover the cost of visits.

Medicare and Medicaid, public managed care systems, were legislated in 1965 in response to societal pressures that demanded easily accessible health care for the elderly, poor, and mentally ill. Medicare is a federal program; Medicaid is a state program.

Under Medicare, home care programs were established in 1966. Since the enactment of Medicare, Medicare-certified home care agencies have generated a significant portion of their income from care provided to Medicare beneficiaries. Today Medicare remains the largest single payer of home care services, hence its significance to home care nursing practice.

Medicare is Title XVIII of the Social Security Act. Although eligibility requirements continue to broaden, it ensures federally financed health insurance for those over age 65 as covered by Social Security or the Railroad System. Administered initially by the Bureau of Insurance in the Department of Health, Education, and Welfare (DHEW), Medicare has been managed by the Health Care Financing Administration (HCFA) in the Department of Health and Human Services (DHHS) since 1978. Medicare has two parts: A and B. Part A reimburses hospital or posthospital costs (including home health care) and is funded by Social Security revenues. Part B is primarily funded by the insured's monthly premiums and covers physician services, laboratory services, medical equipment and supplies, speech and physical therapy, and a variety of other health services and supplies.[7]

Medicare eligibility criteria for coverage are reviewed in Chapter 5. Most home care services under Medicare are subject to claims reviews by intermediaries, which are private insurance companies approved by Medicare as claims processors. Intermediaries, located in certain geographical regions across the country, are under contract to the government. Their purpose is to ensure appropriate disbursement of Medicare monies to home care agencies operating within their geographical region. Intermediaries accomplish this purpose by reviewing the delivery of home care services using government guidelines such as those outlined in the Home Health Insurance Manual, Publication Number 11 (HIM-11). A major intermediary is Blue Cross.

Medicaid and other government sources along with third-party payers provide additional coverage for home care services. Medicaid was legislated by Title XIX of the Social Security Act, providing health care to low-income populations. Medicare provides coverage for elderly adults, whereas Medicaid frequently subsidizes health care of needy children.

Administered by the states, Medicaid monies are subsidized by state and federal governments. Medicaid covers skilled and unskilled home care services as directed by a physician. Medicaid limits some of the home care services normally provided under Medicare. It becomes the primary payment source when the patient is no longer eligible for Medicare. Medicaid coverage of home care services varies from state to state.

Title III of the Older American Act (OAA) and Title XX (Grant-In-Aid), legislated in the 1960s and 1970s, also subsidize home care services but to a more limited degree than Medicare and Medicaid. Title III of the OAA and Title XX are designed to subsidize home care services for the elderly and for low-income populations. Both of these programs are directed toward health restoration and self-care management at home.[3]

Cost savings in home care as compared with hospital care is still unclear.[9,17] The problem is that the real costs of providing home care go beyond direct financial costs. Real costs include human and indirect costs of home care. The human costs include the psychosocial, physical, and health burden borne by patients/caregivers who utilize home care services.[9] Indirect costs include medications, respite services, health of the caregiver, family stability, and the psychosocial burden of providing home care. More research should be done in this area. However, all things considered, the overall savings in keeping the patient at home appears greater and more beneficial to society than unnecessary and preventable hospitalizations.[5,10,17] In addition and key to public policy making, it appears to be a patient-preferred way of receiving care.

Along with government monies came regulations and policies that changed the nature of the home care industry. As the following sections demonstrate, this also influenced home care nursing practice.

THE IMPACT OF GOVERNMENT REGULATIONS AND POLICY ON HOME CARE

The following chronology describes government regulatory and public policy issues that influenced home care and nursing practice. Historically, home care has been synonymous with nursing. As a result patient care outside the hospital was strongly influenced, managed, and controlled by nurses. Before the enactment of the Medicare program, the emphasis of care was focused on health promotion and restoration therapies. During the 1960s this changed.

Although home care needs are viewed as primarily "nursing" in nature, the American Medical Association insisted on a medical framework that directed home care services in return for lending support to the Medicare program.[10] As a result the U.S. government mandated physician certification as a requirement for all Medicare services, including home care. Therefore home care beneficiaries (patients) were assigned to the care of a physician, with the plan of care established and reviewed by the physician. Disease and disability, with an increasing emphasis on home technology in service delivery, became fundamental to the plan of care. Consequently, traditional home care nursing was brought under the auspices of medicine. As a result the primary focus of home care nursing practice is presently directed toward restorative, rehabilitative, and palliative (hospice) therapies. At present, health promotional behaviors are primarily viewed as a consequence of care as influenced by government and private provider regulations for reimbursement of visits.

Government regulation of health care continues to be felt throughout the home care industry. In 1985 new summary forms appeared from Medicare—HCFA 485, 486, 487, and 488—as a means of providing documentation guidelines for reimbursement and quality control. Reorganization and restructuring of home care agencies such as the development of quality patient care programs consequently occurred.

The arrival of DRGs in the 1980s had far-reaching effects on the growth of the home care industry. DRGs are determined by medical diagnosis, extent of illness, and average length of stay for a specified illness, along with other statistical data.[2] As a result of the hospital prospective payment system (PPS) for DRGs, hospitals were awarded predetermined amounts of money for patient care. In terms of financial gain, it remained in the hospital's interest to facilitate early discharge. Increased referrals to home care services resulted. In response to this growing home care population, home care agencies expanded staff, resources, and technological services. Home care—traditionally nonproprietary—was now becoming a big business,[10] a growing and very competitive business.

In the mid-1980s major growth in the home care industry was experienced by proprietary (for profit) agencies and hospital-based home care departments that could provide a vast array of services, such as respiratory, home medical equipment, and pharmacy departments, and whose financial resources could withstand Medicare regulations and public policy making.[10] Traditional home care agencies such as the VNAs that provided many free visits continued to inherit the indigent patient population, while experiencing a loss of "paying" patients to these proprietary and hospital-based agencies. It is believed that the decline in voluntary or nonprofit agencies seen in the 1980s was related to an inability to compete with the tremendous resources and facilities of hospital-based agencies, along with difficulties in adhering to the numerous HCFA and state regulations.[10] However, the quality of VNA services and their dedication to their communities continue to be well respected and much emulated.

Federal regulations in the late 1980s and early 1990s mandated new requirements for quality control and expanded the coverage of home care services. Home care aide training and competency requirements, the establishment of a state home care hotline for patient complaints, and an increase in Medicare hospice (Figure 1-5) and home intravenous therapy programs (Figure 1-6) resulted. Physicians received reimbursement for care-plan oversight. A federal requirement for advance directives that specify patient/caregiver wishes regarding durable power of attorney for health care, as well as living will requests, occurred.

The majority of patients seen in home care are older adults (Figure 1-7). In a study by Dey (1996) elderly home care patients were predominately women (70%), 75 to 84 years of age (43%), white (70%), living in a private residence (93%), and living with family members (55%). For both elderly men and women, the most frequent primary admission diagnosis was heart disease, followed by essential hypertension, malignant neoplasms, diabetes, and chronic obstructive pulmonary disease. Such information gives insight as to the type of care home care nurses will likely provide.[6]

By the early 1990s postpartum and pediatric home care services increased (Figure 1-8). Mental health services, assisted living programs, homemaker services, maternal-child programs, and related community and traditional public health services are current trends in marketing strategies. In addition, increasing numbers of Health Maintenance Organizations (HMOs) were now beginning to provide home visits[4] (see Chapter 9).

Future focuses of home care services will likely involve pain management programs, as well as chronic and palliative care programs.[5] Because patients are increasingly becoming empowered and informed consumers of care, as well as voting taxpayers, their role in determining what kinds of care they receive will likely supersede the traditional patient-nurse-physician relationship, which gave the physician sole authority for decision making. Finally, because the public is reaching for innovative approaches to health care, the home care industry will likely experience a boom in complementary therapies for healing, such as therapeutic touch[12] (see Chapter 27).

Government regulation and public policy since the early 1990s continue to affect the home care industry and, ultimately, home care nursing practice. Home care has become a principle target for cost

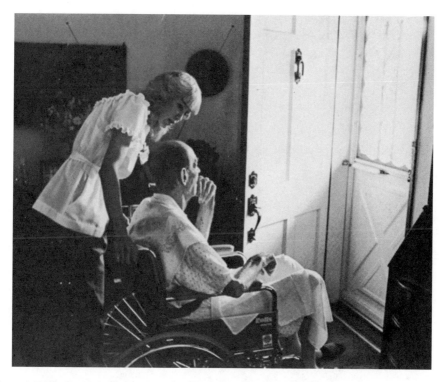

Figure 1-5 The hospice nurse offers a ray of sunshine. (Courtesy Anne Allen, St. Louis, Mo.)

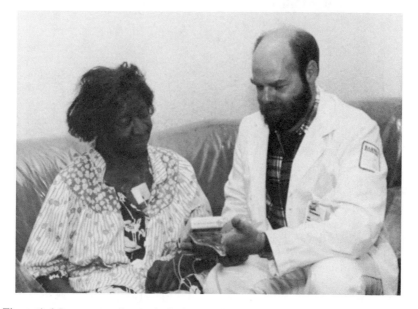

Figure 1-6 Intravenous therapy in the home. (Courtesy Barnes Hospital, St. Louis, Mo.)

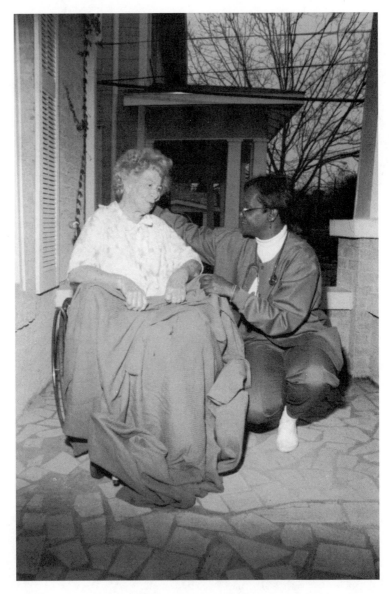

Figure 1-7 Caring for the older adult. (Courtesy Ruth Constant and Associates, Beaumont Home Health Services, Inc., Beaumont, Tex.)

cutting by the federal government as a result of Medicare expenditures rising from $3.9 billion to an estimated $20.5 billion during the period from 1990 to 1997.[19] To compound matters, talk of financial fraud and abuse abounds. To control the rapid growth and costs of home care, as well as to promote some consistent standards of care, the federal gov- ernment has made two major policy moves. First, HCFA called for the development of a national data base that would help demonstrate the outcomes or effects of patient care, and improve the quality process (outcome-based quality improvement or OBQI).[15] This is known as the Outcomes and As- sessment and Information Set (OASIS), which was

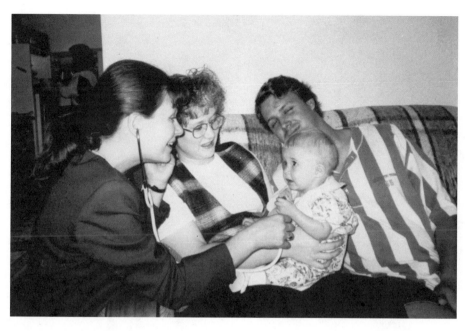

Figure 1-8 Pediatric nurse caring for the family. (Courtesy Family Services and Visiting Nurse Association of Alton, Ill.)

developed at the Centers for Health Policy and Services Research, University of Colorado[15,16] (see Chapter 10). Second, as part of the 1997 Balanced Budget Act, OASIS data are to be used to develop and define PPS for Medicare-certified home care services.

Prospective payment in home care will entail setting a rate or a set of rates for a specific amount of service (e.g., a skilled nursing visit or an entire episode of home health care) that is known "before" the service is provided. HMOs began doing this in the early 1990s. Potential advantages of a PPS include incentives for providing services efficiently. The potential for fraud and abuse should be minimized. In addition, a PPS allows the home care agency to retain profits generated by increases in efficiency. From a nursing standpoint, a PPS eliminates wasted services and has the potential to allow nurses to concentrate on patients with complex health care needs.

However, as a profession home care nurses should pay close attention to the implementation of any form of capitation (e.g., prorated monies for

care based on patient diagnosis or case mix) to ensure quality standards. A potential disadvantage that a PPS may have for patients is an underutilization of services as home care agencies are driven to maximize profit. In short, and of concern to home care nurses, capitation radically changes the motivation of the Medicare-certified home care agency from providing as much care as possible, which existed with the old retrospective or "fee-for-service" payment systems, to providing less care . . . the bare minimum necessary to still turn a profit. In addition, under a PPS, less qualified ancillary or paraprofessionals may be utilized rather than more competent, expensive professional staff. For example, an agency may decide to use minimally trained home care aides and assistants instead of registered nurses. The PPS is supposed to be in place by October 2000, but many experts believe it will be deferred until some of the previously discussed issues are resolved. PPS and interim payment regulations have certainly had an influence on the home care industry. According to the National Association of Home Care, from 1997

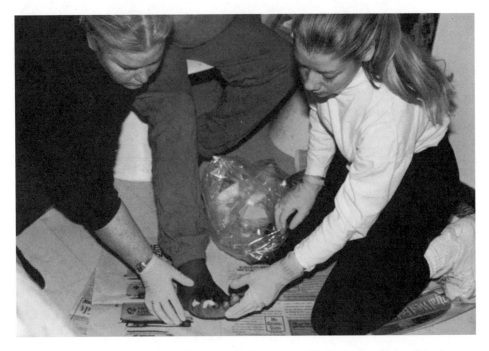

Figure 1-9 Working with student nurses in home care. (Photo courtesy Robyn Rice.)

to 1999 the number of Medicare-certified home care agencies fell by 24.5%.[11] Of concern to home care nurses is that patients in rural and less populated areas who were historically seen by smaller home care agencies, which have since closed as a result of the inability to keep up with the regulations, are no longer receiving home care services.

The 1990s also reflect changes in the fundamentals of home care nursing practice. Although there is lively debate in academia regarding where home care fits into nursing curriculum, schools of nursing are increasing their emphasis on home visits in curriculum planning. This is viewed as important in preparing students for the realities of nursing practice in our new century (Figure 1-9). In addition, in 1993 the American Nurse's Credentialing Center (ANCC) administered the first examination recognizing home care nursing as a specialty practice—a specialty practice that blends with, yet is distinct from, community and public health nursing. The American Nurses Association (ANA) has also established standards of care for home care nursing practice.[1]

THE IMPACT OF TECHNOLOGY ON HOME CARE

Advancing technology in home care represents a future market for telehealth services. Telehealth is broadly defined as using telecommunications to provide patient care (see Chapter 26). Telecommunications in the home can take the form of access to Internet services, telemonitoring and medical devices, and personal emergency response systems.[18] To date, the most common type of telehealth service is via the telephone. Now, equipment such as cellular phones and portable computers are increasing the nurse's connectivity to the patient (Figure 1-10). For many home care nurses, "deliberately" assisting patients to achieve outcomes of care via telecommunication will be a new perspective on what constitutes caring and will begin a philosophical dialogue on what telecaring in the home really means.

Many factors have resulted in a renaissance of nursing care within the patient's home environment. It is also clear that home care nursing practice will continue to evolve and be shaped by (1) increased patient acuity levels, as well as chronic care needs at

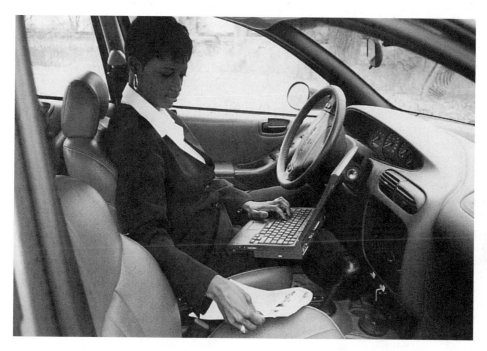

Figure 1-10 Considering the impact of technology in home care. (Photo courtesy Robyn Rice.)

home; (2) advances in medical technology and telecommunication services that transcend physical and financial boundaries; (3) social and economic restructuring of health care services; (4) the tremendous variation of patient problems and concerns when health care needs are managed at home; and (5) home care nurses, endeavors to maximize quality improvement (QI) in the home milieu.

CONTEMPORARY HOME CARE NURSING: A PHILOSOPHY OF PRACTICE

Home care nursing is the delivery of quality nursing care to patients in their home environment; it is provided on an intermittent or part-time basis. As discussed in Chapter 2, a fundamental purpose of care is to foster patient self-care management. Of consequence, the patient's caregiver or family and home environment (which includes community resources) are viewed as critical elements of a successful plan of care. It is recognized that patient/caregiver cooperation and self-determination for optimal health or best level of functioning are important to achieving successful self-care management at home. Therefore a holis-

tic focus of care is emphasized. Within this description, home care nurses recognize that health is not solely determined by physiological measurements or dollars for care but represents all the patient is and *wants* to be.[13] Likewise, as discussed in the epilogue, it is recognized that the healing and caring tradition of home care nursing is nested within a relationship-centered ethic.

Furthermore, home care nursing practice should reflect the current state of knowledge in the field of patient care. Individual state Nurse Practice Acts dictate the activities that nurses may legally carry out in the home. Ethics in practice will reflect beneficence (to do good for the patient) and nonmaleficence (to do no harm to the patient).[13,14] Agency policy and procedures and standards of care will also influence the delivery of care, as will the availability of resources such as equipment, supplies, funding, and patient family systems as discussed in Chapter 4.[5]

Quality patient care is accomplished through a multidisciplinary approach, whereby home care nurses, functioning as case managers, orchestrate the plan of care. The plan of care, based on the nursing process of assessing, diagnosing, planning, implementing, and evaluating, is directed as follows:

- Providing health restorative, rehabilitative, and palliative (hospice) therapies. Health promotional behaviors are viewed as a very important consequence of these therapies.
- Educating the patient/caregiver about the illness or disability and mutually identified health care needs. Recommendations to promote optimal health or best level of functioning and self-care management follow.
- Developing patient/caregiver competence, decision making, and judgment in self-care management at home.
- Fostering positive patient/caregiver adjustment to and coping mechanisms for changes in lifestyle, role, and self-concept as a result of illness or disability.
- Reintegrating the patient/caregiver back into the family, community, and social support systems.

Home care nursing is an art and a science and dedicated to providing quality patient care in the home and community setting. Such a philosophy reflects a commitment to ongoing educational programs that advance knowledge and clinical expertise, to research that validates home care as a preferred alternative to hospitalization, to driving home care agency clinical policy and decision making that best serves the interest of the public, to ethically viewing nursing practice as more than dollars for care, and to fostering political strength and solidarity of the nursing profession in order to provide for the health care needs of our nation today and tomorrow.

SUMMARY

Home care will continue to be a growth industry shaped by government regulations and social pressures for economically viable alternatives in health care. As the "eyes" and "ears" of the physician; as the implementors of health care policy that emphasizes cost-effective, quality care; as the ones who are most intimately connected to the public . . . it is key that home care nurses recognize and value their pivotal role in determining what home care is and what it will become. Such a realization allows

nursing to demonstrate its true value to society and opens portals of professional autonomy and caring that we have yet to imagine. As described in subsequent chapters in this book, such responsibilities will require home care nurses to be expert clinicians, creative thinkers, and articulate leaders in health care.

REFERENCES

1. American Nurses Association: *Standards of home health nursing practice,* Kansas City, Mo, 1986, The Association.
2. Balinsky W, Starkman J: The impact of DRGs on the health care industry, *Health Care Manage Rev* 12:61, 1987.
3. Buhler-Wilkerson K: Left carrying the bag: experiments in visiting nursing, *Nurs Res* 36(1):42, 1986.
4. Dee-Kelly P and others: Managed care: an opportunity for home care agencies, *Nurs Clin North Am* 29(3):471, 1994.
5. Dennis LI and others: The relationship between hospital readmissions and of medicare beneficiaries with chronic illnesses and home care nursing interventions, *Home Healthcare Nurse* 14(4):303, 1996.
6. Dey AN: Characteristics of elderly home health care users. In *Vital and health statistics of the Centers for Disease Control and Prevention,* Washington, DC, 1996, U.S. Department of Health and Human Services.
7. Health Care Financing Administration: *Home health insurance manual* (Pub No. 11), Washington, DC, 1995, U.S. Department of Health and Human Services.
8. Kilbane IK: The demise of free care, *Nurs Clin North Am* 23(2):435, 1988.
9. Morton K: Family caregiving: who provides the care, and at what cost? *Nurs Econ* 15(5):243, 1997.
10. Mundinger M: *Home care controversy: too little, too late, too costly,* Rockville, Md, 1983, Aspen Systems.
11. National Association for Home Care: *Basic statistics about home care,* Washington, DC, 2000, The Association.
12. Peck S: The efficacy of therapeutic touch for improving functional ability in elders with degenerative arthritis, *Nurs Sci Q* 11(3):123, 1998.
13. Rice R: Ethics in home health: dollars for care, *Geriatr Nurs* 17(6):348, 1998.
14. Rooney A: Everyday ethics and home health care challenges, *Home Health Care Manage Prac* 9(6):31, 1997.
15. Shaughnessy PW, Crisler KS: *Outcome-based quality improvement: a manual for home care agencies on how to use outcomes,* Washington, DC, 1995, National Association for Home Care.
16. Shaughnessy P and others: Outcome-based quality improvement in the information age, *Home Health Care Manage Prac* 10(2):11, 1998.
17. Varricchio C: Human and indirect costs of home care, *Nurs Outlook* 42(4):151, 1994.
18. Warner I: Telemedicine in home health care: the current status of practice, *Home Health Care Manage Prac* 10(2):62, 1998.
19. Wilson A, Twiss A: Using outcomes and OASIS as strategic tools, *Home Healthcare Nurse Manager* 3(1):19, 1999.

UNDERSTANDING HOME CARE: APPLYING THEORY TO CLINICAL PRACTICE

Robyn Rice

Every discipline faces the challenges of how to implement professional responsibilities. We ask ourselves, "How should the job be done?" "What direction or focus should be taken to accomplish goals of work?" "What are these goals and how should they be determined?" For nursing these questions are complicated by the fact that quality patient care and professional standards of practice are significantly influenced by political, social, and economic factors within this country. Likewise, differences among nurses in their level of educational preparation, work experience, and personal world view are additional variables that also affect how nurses care for patients.

As health care continues to move away from traditional hospital settings and into the community, home care nurses will probably face great demands for change and innovation. For these nurses the challenges of providing quality patient care will likely involve caring for increased numbers of sicker patients and their families across the life span. For example, in today's economic climate the frequency of home visits and the time allocated to care for the patient will likely be compressed. As a cost effective measure, home care nurses will likely use evolving forms of electronic communication to supplement physical visits. They will understand and define telecaring. In addition, home care nurses will likely experience an expansion of their role, reflecting increased responsibilities for assisted living programs, personal care homes, palliative care programs, and a variety of alternative health care delivery systems in the community. Yet

in the community these nurses will continue to attend to the very real and enormous health care needs of our multicultural society, (i.e., health care needs that are not always matched by adequate patient and environmental resources). Nurses who work in the challenging milieu of home care should consider the following questions: "What is the purpose of home care?" "What responsibilities do home care nurses have to their patients?" "What, if any, are the patients' responsibilities for their own health?" "How is care to be determined, implemented, and evaluated?" With the changing regulatory and economic restructuring of health care in this country, "How can home care nurses ensure quality patient care yet maintain professional standards of practice?" Finally, because nursing is defined as the science of human caring, "How do nurses provide care in such a complex milieu as the home setting?"

There are no simple answers to these questions. However, it is clear that the spectrum of illness and health care is so broad and expansive that responsibilities for home care must be shared by nurses, patients, and family members or caregivers as needed. It is also clear that innovations in health care must be cost effective yet maintain professional standards of practice, lest finances become the one and only consideration in the plan of care.

A financial model of health care, so valued by many of today's health care organizations, treats diseases and not people.[14] It is the author's position that people (and not body parts) experience healing, and such models are not cost effective in

15

the long run because they waste the most precious resource of all, which is "ourselves." The public, as educated consumers of care and voting taxpayers, is increasingly demanding holistic approaches to care that are not only accessible in terms of dollars but also bring a sense of well-being and balance into their lives.[14] Moreover, the public is insisting on health care models that enable it to have a voice in it's own care. It is important for nurses to conceptualize their role in this process. For, nurses who can articulate their role (e.g., "who" they are, "what" they do, and "why" what they do is an invaluable service to the public) have a basis from which to maintain professional standards of practice and *to contribute to the growth of nursing as a professional discipline.*

The purpose of this chapter is to provide home care nurses with a theoretical basis for caring in the home. A brief overview of major nursing theory relevant to home care is discussed. Health, as a concept, is briefly reviewed. An original theoretical framework to support home care nursing practice is presented at the end of this chapter. There are many theories useful in understanding home care, and to cover all of them is beyond the scope of a single chapter. Refer to the reference list at the end of this chapter for further resources in nursing theory.

THEORY DEVELOPMENT AND ITS IMPORTANCE TO NURSING

Theories begin with assumptions about nature and human behavior.[3,4,5,17] They are derived from many ways of knowing, including life reflection, work experiences, and quantitative, as well as qualitative, forms of research.[2,5,20] Often theories are derived within conceptual frameworks, systems, or models that seek to explain relationships or phenomena of concern. Such frameworks or models allow the user to visualize diagrammatically how the concepts of a theory are linked to one another. In addition, such frameworks or models may generate hypotheses and empirical methods to evaluate the proposed linkages.[4,10]

Theories and conceptual frameworks or models are important to nursing because they define and guide the boundaries of professional practice and identify key nurse-patient-caregiver relationships that emerge with caring. Moreover, nursing theories may build on each other and contribute to each nurse's thinking on the human experiences of life

and death. They promote insights into professional practice and serve as a basis for inquiry and research. Most important, awareness of nursing theory enables nurses to define their role in health care (e.g., stand their ground) and, on a broader scope, to crusade for health care policy that benefits both the public and the profession.

NURSING THEORY RELEVANT TO HOME CARE NURSING PRACTICE

Many nursing theorists have had a tremendous impact on nursing practice. The following section highlights those nursing theorists that are particularly helpful in understanding home care.

Our earliest theoretical legacy

In her book, *Notes on Nursing,* Florence Nightingale describes disease as a reparative process not necessarily accompanied by suffering.[12] Nightingale, the first nursing and environmental theorist, considered disease to be an effort of nature to remedy a process of poisoning or decay. She believed that nurses should primarily focus their interventions on causes and symptoms of suffering, not on the symptoms of the disease.

Nightingale emphasizes the impact of environment and sanitation on patient recovery. She cites five essential points in securing "the health of houses": pure air, pure water, efficient drainage, cleanliness, and light.[12]

To this day Nightingale's beliefs are reflected in basic infection control practices such as handwashing and infectious waste disposal and are key nursing interventions in home care. Moreover, her conviction that nurses should focus not only on disease manifestation but also examine disease causality was a beginning step in understanding the concept of health.

Science of unitary human beings

Martha Rogers' science of unitary human beings theory proposes that the study of nursing is the study of human and environmental fields (forms of energy).[20] Integral to the human-environmental field process are concepts of patterning and continuous change. Human and environment are viewed as irreducible, pandimensional energy fields characterized by patterning. Pattern flows in higher and lower frequencies (consider the movement of a slinky toy), continuously changing in creative and unpredictable ways. In this regard patient and nurse come together in a process involving mutual choice, mutual participation, mutual awareness, and caring.[21] Groups and communities also represent energy fields.

A key concept in Rogers' work is her thinking on healing modalities. Rogers believed that the focus of shared, noninvasive healing modalities is the human-environmental field rather than that of direct physical care.[18,19] These modalities continue to evolve as our awareness (reflecting greater diversity, faster rhythms, motions, and ways of knowing) transcends time and space, allowing individuals to get in touch with their integral nature of unbroken wholeness. Such modalities include therapeutic touch, imagery, meditation, light, color, music, sound, movement, chanting, drumming, humor, laughter, affirmations, storytelling, poetry, art, dreaming, dance, and other healing rituals that are becoming more popular in home care today. Such modalities are often referred to as *alternative* or *complementary therapies* and have a long history in Eastern medicine.

Rogers' thoughts on people as everchanging energy fields that interact with other fields have special relevance in home care, especially with hospice and palliative care applications. Feelings such as faith, hope, and love are not easily measured but certainly exist. When traditional therapies fail or death approaches, patients may seek alternate forms of care and comfort such as complementary therapies, as well as intense intrapersonal exchanges. It may well be that such interactions represent human movement in dimensions where we come to know each other beyond what we can physically taste, touch, smell, hear, and see. Rogers called this knowing *pattern recognition and appreciation.* Although very much grounded in physics, home care nurses should recognize that Rogers' theory also offers an explanation as to how aesthetic nurse and patient interactions happen and why they are meaningful.

Transcultural nursing

Madeleine Leininger's transcultural nursing theory proposes that cultural care provides the broadest and most important means that nurses can use to promote health and well-being.[8] Leininger suggests that nursing is an inherently transcultural profession. Transcultural care knowledge is essential if nurses are to give competent and necessary care to people from different cultures.

Leininger views care as the essence of nursing.[5,8] Care is regarded as the means to help patients recover from illness or unfavorable life conditions. Leininger links care with culture and proposes that they should not be separated in nursing actions and decisions. Regardless of cultural background, all people are seen as dependent on human care for growth and survival (e.g., regardless of culture diversity all individuals share universal care needs for survival, comfort, and growth). Leininger suggests that the ultimate goal of cultural care nursing is for nurses to assist, support, or enable all individuals to maintain well-being, improve life, or face death.[8,18] To accomplish this goal, nurses must be prepared to experience and know culture.

Home care nurses move through a variety of communities and often care for patients from different cultural backgrounds. Therefore Leininger's work has a good fit with home care because home care nursing practice is very culturally focused. A key application of Leininger's theory in home care is for nurses to know the patient from the patient's perspective. Such knowing implies understanding the patient's definition and perspective of health. This certainly includes recognizing that the concept of health and care is individually and culturally defined.

Self-care deficit theory

Dorothea Orem's self-care deficit theory of nursing describes three concepts that are basic to nursing practice: self-care, self-care deficits (dependent-care deficit), and nursing systems.[13] The health focus of Orem's self-care theory is for individuals and families to maintain a state of wellness. Self-care encompasses the basic activities that aid health promotion, well-being, and health maintenance.

Self-care deficits occur when individuals can no longer meet their self-care requisites. Self-care requisites include the need for food, air, rest, social interaction, and other components of human function. They are categorized by Orem as universal, developmental, or health deviation self-care requisites. These self-care requisites are the focus of health-related behaviors of individuals, families, and communities.

Nursing systems, the third concept of Orem's theory, are multidimensional and viewed as wholly compensatory, partly compensatory, or supportive-educative systems.[13,18] If the patient requires complete nursing care and is unable to assist with health needs, care is categorized as wholly compensatory. In home care this might translate into a dependent patient role. Care that can be performed by both patient and nurse is termed partly compensatory. In home care this might translate into an interdependant role between the patient and nurse. Care is categorized as supportive-educative when nurses are able to assist patients to make their own decisions and take actions to fulfill self-care requisites. In home care this could be translated into patient home independence, whereby the services of the nurse are not (or rarely) needed.

Orem's theory views care as something to be performed by both nurses and patients.[13] The role of the nurse is to provide education and support that help patients acquire the necessary abilities to perform self-care. Orem's theory is foundational to home care because it begins to truly acknowledge the role of the patient in managing his or her own health, which is referred to as *self-care*. Moreover, the abundance of literature on self-care practices in the home today has largely evolved from Orem's work.

Health as expanding consciousness

The central thesis of Margaret Newman's theory of health as expanding consciousness is that health is the expansion of consciousness.[11] Consciousness is viewed as coexistent with the universe and residing in all matter. Persons are identified by their patterns of consciousness—the person "is" consciousness. Within this context Newman views the highest form of knowing as loving.

Health and illness are viewed by Newman as a single process and moves through varying degrees of organization and disorganization as one unitary process. Building on Rogers' work, Neuman believes that health encompasses disease and reflects an underlying pattern of person-environment interaction.[5,11] According to Neuman, a pattern can be something the person does (consciously or unconsciously) that affects his or her health. For example, a habit or regular activity that affects the person's health is a pattern. The nurse engages the patient in pattern recognition and appreciation; energy is shared. During this process, new insights emerge for the patient that may lead to new levels of thinking and different ways of living and being.

Neuman's theory is fairly radical because it moves nursing away from traditional western viewpoints that expound "good" and "bad" dichotomies of health. A key application of Neuman's work to home care is for nurses to understand that health and illness do not necessarily exist at opposite ends of a continuum.

Theory of human caring

Jean Watson's theory of human caring in nursing proposes human caring as the moral ideal of nursing.[3,23] Nurses participate in human caring to protect, enhance, and preserve humanity by assisting individuals to find meaning in illness, pain, and existence and to help others gain self-knowledge, self-control, and self-healing.[3,23]

Illness is not a disease but rather disharmony within a person's inner self. Watson views health as unity and harmony within the body, mind, and soul. Attainment of such harmony generates self-knowledge, self-reverence, self-healing, and self-care processes. Moreover, when nurses assist patients to find meaning in their existence, patients gain self-knowledge, self-control, self-love, choice, and self-determination in health decisions and lifestyle management.[23] Watson articulates a holistic viewpoint of patient care that is fundamental to home care. Most important, Watson's conceptualizations of caring embody the essence of professional nursing practice (e.g., who nurses are and what they do).

In rethinking the previous material toward some understanding of home care, nurses should begin to recognize linkages among the different nursing theorists. For example, what Rogers called *pattern recognition and appreciation* would most likely be referred to by Watson as *caring moments*. Such thinking lends richness to theory development, as well as clinical practice in home care.

THE CONCEPT OF HEALTH IN HOME CARE

One's health evolves from many things, including physical health, mental health, spiritual-aesthetic health, and relational health to name a few. Health does not represent a being free of disease or habits. People are not perfect. Within this context, connotations or labeling of "good" and "bad" health have very little meaning as people cogitate both in life. Rather, consider viewing health in terms of quality of life or best level of functioning. This means that even if the patient has disease, disability, or is dying, if he or she is at his or her best level of functioning, then this probably represents optimal health for that patient.[11]

In order to achieve successful and realistic working relationships with the public, home care nurses should learn to appreciate health in holistic terms and on the patient's own ground.[6] This means knowing health as a dynamic (active) process that encompasses everything about the patient and the patient's life.[1,2,7] This also means understanding that health is not solely determined by particulate values such as weight or blood cholesterol levels but evolves from all the patient can be and *wants* to be. In this regard, home care nurses offer their services to assist patients to realize their own potentials for optimal health.

A THEORETICAL FRAMEWORK FOR HOME CARE: THE RICE MODEL OF DYNAMIC SELF-DETERMINATION FOR SELF-CARE

Home care nurses can offer extensive support, education, and resources, but unless patients actively manage their health care needs, the plan of care is likely to be unsuccessful. Consider the high-tech home care patient standing on the corner of a busy street trying to sell the battery from his intravenous pump for illicit drug money. Consider the elderly home care patient with congestive heart failure who tells the nurse, "I don't care what you or the doctor say, I am going to eat my salt!" Consider the postpartum home care patient who tells the nurse, "I want to breast-feed my baby girl, but I am just afraid I will do something that won't be good for her." Consider the eight-year-old pediatric home care patient who runs and tries to hide when the nurse visits to change his or her burn dressing. These examples are realities for nurses who work in home care across this country. They call for a shift in theoretical thinking for nurses who, for too long, have focused on doing things "to" patients instead of working "with" them. They call for nursing strategies that facilitate patient participation with a mutually determined plan of care. This relates to the fundamental purpose of home care.

The purpose of home care is not to make patients well. Wellness is certainly a desirable consequence of nursing actions in the home milieu, but it is not guaranteed. In fact, some patients such as those in hospice programs go home to die. Rather, *the purpose of home care is to provide patients (and caregivers) with the understanding, support, treatment, information, and caring they need to successfully manage their health care needs at home.* For out of active self-care management optimal health will arise.

Building on the previously mentioned nursing theories, the author proposes a nursing theory called the *Rice Model of Dynamic Self-Determination for Self-Care.* Simply stated, dynamic self-determination for self-care refers to patient *choice* regarding what balances his or her health. It is derived from numerous patient (and caregiver) motivational factors for self-care, which include interpersonal perceptions of health beliefs, sociocultural influences, locus of control, support systems, available resources, and disease processes. It is achieved through numerous self-care strategies that meet holistic needs for health (e.g., everything the patient is and wants to be).[15] It is a dynamic process (one subject to change) in which the goal is optimal health. Optimal health arises from best level of functioning and may be evaluated by numerous indicators, including physiological stability, intrapersonal harmony, resonance, patient satisfaction with his or her health care, and quality of life to name a few.

The home care nurse's role is that of *facilitator* of patient self-determination for self-care through numerous strategies, including patient education, patient advocacy, spiritual-aesthetic communion, and case management. The Rice model of Dynamic Self-Determination for Self-Care is shown in Figure 2-1.

Patients (and caregivers) are viewed as holistic entities of care. Health care needs (and nursing interventions) are mutually decided on by the patient and nurse. Patients' perceptions of health care needs are reflected in a lifetime continuum of seeking and knowing optimal health. Such balance is achieved when mind, body, and spirit are without need and resonate with nature.

Dynamic self-determination for self-care allows patients to bridge the gap between need and goal attainment. The caring relationship among nurse-

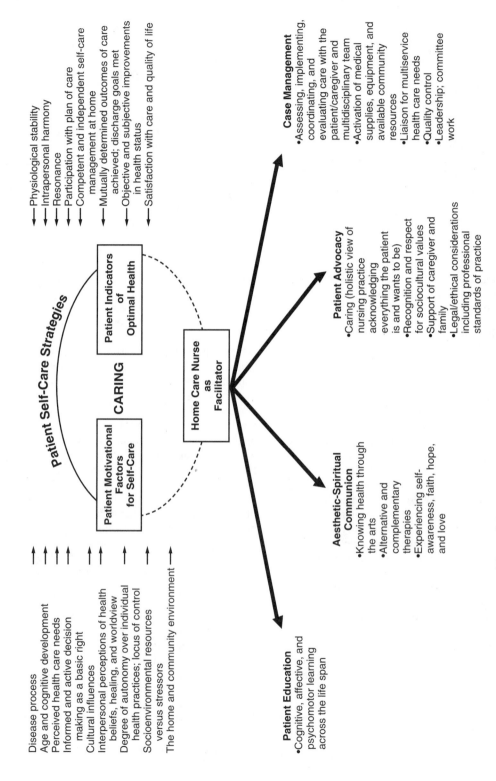

Figure 2-1 The Rice model of Dynamic Self-Determination for Self-Care.

Patient Self-Care Strategies

Patient Motivational Factors for Self-Care

CARING

Patient Indicators of Optimal Health

Home Care Nurse as Facilitator

Disease process
Age and cognitive development
Perceived health care needs
Informed and active decision making as a basic right
Cultural influences
Interpersonal perceptions of health beliefs, healing, and worldview
Degree of autonomy over individual health practices; locus of control
Socioenvironmental resources versus stressors
The home and community environment

→ Physiological stability
→ Intrapersonal harmony
→ Resonance
→ Participation with plan of care
→ Competent and independent self-care management at home
→ Mutually determined outcomes of care achieved; discharge goals met
→ Objective and subjective improvements in health status
→ Satisfaction with care and quality of life

Patient Education
• Cognitive, affective, and psychomotor learning across the life span

Aesthetic-Spiritual Communion
• Knowing health through the arts
• Alternative and complementary therapies
• Experiencing self-awareness, faith, hope, and love

Patient Advocacy
• Caring (holistic view of nursing practice acknowledging everything the patient is and wants to be)
• Recognition and respect for sociocultural values
• Support of caregiver and family
• Legal/ethical considerations including professional standards of practice

Case Management
• Assessing, implementing, coordinating, and evaluating care with the patient/caregiver and multidisciplinary team
• Activation of medical supplies, equipment, and available community resources
• Liaison for multiservice health care needs
• Quality control
• Leadership; committee work

patient-caregiver moves through stages of dependence, interdependence, and independence. Exacerbation of illness or disability may cause patient regression to a previous phase. Likewise, disease process, disability, or cognitive development may predispose the patient to a certain phase. The three phases of the nurse-patient-caregiver caring relationship are as follows:

1. *Dependence.* Initially the home care nurse performs the majority of care and begins to facilitate self-care by understanding and working with patient/caregiver motivational factors for optimal health.
2. *Interdependence.* As skills, knowledge, and confidence are gained, the patient/caregiver performs the majority of care, which is reinforced and supported by the home care nurse as needed.
3. *Independence.* The patient/caregiver is able to perform self-care activities and achieves a state of optimal health with minimal or no intervention by the home care nurse.

Dynamic self-determination for self-care has the following premises[16]:

- Each person has a great deal of influence over his or her health, and it is our intrinsic nature to seek (through motivational factors) some measure of optimal health.
- Optimal health refers to best level of functioning and is multidimensional.
- The processes of medical treatment and health education do not guarantee optimal health because home care is administered by nurses and other health professionals on an intermittent basis and optimal health reflects patients' entire life processes, including who they are and what they want to be.
- The patient is regarded as a holistic entity across the life span.
- Patient participation with the plan of care and successful management of health care needs at home result from dynamic self-determination for self-care, which is manifested by self-care strategies that foster optimal health.
- Participation occurs by nurse-patient-caregiver collaboration with the multidisciplinary team in goal setting, decision making, and knowing.

The patient/caregiver role is an active role and will primarily determine health outcomes.
- The patient/caregiver shares responsibility for the patient's care, which is facilitated by the home care nurse.
- The role of the home care nurse is that of *facilitator* of patient self-determination for self-care and involves many facets of caring (educator, advocate, case manager, and spiritual-aesthetic communer).
- The caregiver (or family) is viewed as an extension of the patient and the patient's needs. The role of the caregiver is to care for the patient, therefore the caregiver is cared for much as if he or she were the patient.
- The caring relationship between the nurse-patient-caregiver must reflect a trusting and safe working environment for all involved.

Dynamic self-determination for self-care is an ongoing, very personal, and contemplative process. It arises from patient motivation for optimal health and will involve patient-nurse-environment interaction that reflects forms of pattern appreciation and caring that simply move beyond three-dimensional thinking.

It is recognized that some patients are not ideal candidates for home care because they exhibit little or no cooperation with the nurse. However, dynamic self-determination for self-care is *not* intended to be an automatic avenue for premature patient discharge from home care services when nurses are faced with problems of patient/caregiver nonparticipation with the plan of care. Rather, motivational factors for self-care can be reassessed by home care nurses in order to identify any patient/caregiver lack of information, misunderstandings, insecurities, or concerns with the plan of care.

Dynamic self-determination for self-care can be useful to home care nurses in a variety of ways. As a research tool it can be reflected in the interview process when the home care nurse asks the following questions:

What do you want to learn or know about your health?

What kinds of things do you think you need to feel your best?

Are you willing to work with me to get as healthy as you believe you can be?

Furthermore, the model can be incorporated into an admission assessment tool in assisting staff to organize and develop the plan of care. For example, after the initial assessment the following questions can be asked:

• What are the patient/caregiver's health care needs (immediate medical referral needs)?
• What kinds of services or care does the patient/caregiver want? *Prioritize and implement nursing interventions based on patient/caregiver self-perceived survival needs for self-care.*
• Is the patient willing and able to participate in the plan of care? If the patient is unable to learn health teaching or manage self-care, is there a caregiver or family member who can assume some of these responsibilities? Does the home environment support safe delivery of services (e.g., adequate housing, trust, resources, and neighborhood issues)? If the answer is an absolute "no" to the three previous questions, consider alternate methods of health care service delivery and approaches. The patient may not be an appropriate candidate for home care. This is particularly true for high-tech home care services such as home ventilator management, which will require a great deal of active patient/caregiver involvement and much environmental support.

The model can be used as a theoretical framework for developing clinical pathways or plans of care. For example, wound care or diabetic teaching may well be assessed from patient/caregiver self-determined needs for care. As optimal health is achieved, discharge from home care services is appropriate.

The model would be particularly helpful as an orientation tool for staff new to home care. It could also be used to familiarize student nurses with their role expectations in home care. The model provides concepts for testing and further theory development in home care. Its acknowledgment of the importance of multidimensional patient and nurse interactions lays groundwork for things we have yet to imagine. Finally, the model's greatest strength is that it offers a commonsense approach to home care and many forms of community nursing care.

Evidence supporting the Dynamic Self-Determination for Self-Care model is qualitative in nature and derived from 16 years of practical working experience in home care. Theoretical support has occurred by anecdotal evidence.[22] The model has been supported by both verbal and written communication from home care nurses and educators on both a national and an international level who report that the model is consistent with practice needs in the home.[15,17,22] Also, quantitative and qualitative research supporting motivational factors for self-care and indicators of optimal health abound in the literature.

Dynamic self-determination for self-care emphasizes *shared* responsibility for optimal health among the nurse, patient, and caregiver. It is proposed as a clinical practice theory specifically aimed at home and community care—a theory that will continue to be shaped by government and political and social reforms for health care, as well as endeavors to engage others in the sacred dance of knowing and caring.[9]

SUMMARY

As home care continues to evolve within the social and economic restructuring of this country, its purpose and implementation will continue to reflect the health care needs of our nation and home care nurses' endeavors to provide quality patient care. This chapter has presented ideas and concepts that give home care nurses direction and guidance to achieve the complex tasks they face. Theories, questions, and ideas serve to generate thinking.[24] And therein lie the real answers to our many challenges.

REFERENCES

1. Boykin A: Aesthetic knowing grounded in an explicit conception of nursing, *Nurs Sci Q* 7(4):158, 1994.
2. Carper B: Fundamental patterns of knowing in nursing, *Adv Nurs Sci* 1(1):13, 1978.
3. Chinn P, Kramer M: *Theory and nursing,* ed 5, St. Louis, 1999, Mosby.
4. Fawcett J: *Analysis and evaluation of nursing theories,* Philadelphia, 1993, FA Davis.
5. Fawcett J: *Conceptual models of nursing,* ed 4, Philadelphia, 1999, FA Davis.
6. Gadow S: Existential advocacy: philosophical foundations of nursing. In: Spicker S, Gadow S, editors: *Nursing images and ideals,* New York, 1980, Springer.
7. Hess J: The ethics of compliance: a dialectic, *Adv Nurs Sci* 19(1):18, 1996.
8. Leininger M: *Transcultural nursing: concepts, theories, and practices,* ed 3, Philadelphia, 1999, FA Davis.

9. Liehr P, Smith M: Middle range theory-spinning research and practice to create knowledge for the new millennium, *Adv Nurs Sci* 2(4):81, 1999.

10. Monti E, Tingen M: Multiple paradigms of nursing science, *Adv Nurs Sci* 21(4):64, 1999.

11. Newman M: *Health as expanding consciousness,* New York, 1994, National League for Nursing Press.

12. Nightingale F: *Notes on nursing: what it is and what it is not,* New York, 1969, Dover, Appleton.

13. Orem D: *Nursing: concepts and practice,* ed 6, St. Louis, 1999, Mosby.

14. Peters R: The negative effect of the clinical model of "health": implications for health care policy, *J Healthcare Finance* 25(1):78, 1998.

15. Rice R: Dynamic self-determination for self-care. Presentation at the Indiana State Home Care Conference in Indianapolis, May, 1995.

16. Rice R: Key concepts of self-care in the home, *J Geriatr Nurs* 19(1):52, 1998.

17. Rice R: Dynamic self-determination for self-care. Presentation at the National Association for Home Care, San Diego, Calif, October, 1999.

18. Riehl-Sisca J: Conceptual models for nursing practice, ed 5, Norwalk, Conn, 1998, Appleton & Lange.

19. Rogers M: The science of unitary human beings: current perspectives, *Nurs Sci Q* 7(1):33, 1994.

20. Silva M and others: From carper's patterns of knowing to ways of being: an ontological philosophical shift in nursing, *Adv Nurs Sci* 18(1):1, 1985.

21. Smith M: Caring and the science of unitary human beings, *Adv Nurs Sci* 21(4):14, 1999.

22. Universite' De Moncton in New Brunswick, Canada: Communication with Assistant Professor Cormeir-Daigle regarding implementing Dynamic Self-Determination for Self-Care in their home care assessment tool, 1994.

23. Watson J: *Human and human care: a theory of nursing,* New York, 1988, National League for Nursing Press.

24. Watson J: Postmodernism and knowledge development in nursing, *Nurs Sci Q* 8(2):60, 1993.

THE ROLE OF THE HOME CARE NURSE AND ORIENTATION STRATEGIES

3

Sandra Lindquist, Donna Bridgman Musser, and Robyn Rice

Virtually every aspect of nursing offers certain attractions to professionals who wish to work in that specialty area. Why would one choose home care nursing? Most nurses who elect to practice in this specialty do so because they enjoy working within the community. Compared with traditional hospital settings, practice in the home environment offers nurses an expanded role associated with autonomy of practice. Community networking and socialization, independent time management, and more "normal" working hours are additional incentives (although home care agencies operate 24 hours a day, 7 days a week, the majority of working hours are weekdays with periodic on-call and weekend duties). For others, the work is simply a calling.

This chapter describes role preparation and implementation for home care nurses. Some key concepts presented in this chapter include issues influencing responsibilities of home care nurses, home care agency guidelines for orienting new nurses, key elements of the role of the nurse, and utilization of advanced practice nurses in home care. This chapter concludes with a section on working with student nurses in home care, because they represent our professional future.

UNDERSTANDING CARING IN THE HOME

Home care nurses work with a variety of patients across the life span. Nurses will encounter elderly patients with chronic disease, mothers and their newborn babies, patients who have elected to go home to die, and numerous others. A key focus of practice will involve strategies that foster patient and family self-care, as well as interventions for best level of health[1,10] (see Chapter 2). Self-care can simply be defined as the patient picking and choosing what self-care actions balance him or her. It reflects a great deal of personal interaction between the patient and nurse as a means to enhance independent living and quality of life.[10] Forbes reports that a sensitivity to patient needs and the interpersonal skills of the nurse appear to be the most important dimensions of patient satisfaction with home care services.[5] In addition, patient involvement and active participation with the plan of care also reflect increased patient satisfaction with care. Characteristics such as listening to the patient, appearing to be interested in the patient, being sensitive to the patient's needs, having a cheerful manner, and communicating well are all identified as positive aspects of caring in the home.[5] Of consequence, home care nursing is relationship centered and has a holistic rather than technical focus of care. Hence, nursing interventions in the home will often involve the entire household and address health teaching and psychologic, sociologic, spiritual, and physical care.[10,13] Finally, because care is provided directly in the home, the issue of patient trust is more salient than in most other professional relationships.[4] Therefore, caring in the home charges the nurse to honor the patient's uniqueness, to foster a trusting relationship based on mutual respect and participation with the plan of care, and to inspire the patient to engage in life as fully as possible.

UNDERSTANDING THE ROLE
OF THE HOME CARE NURSE

In fostering patient and caregiver self-care and best level of health, home care nurses function in multiple roles. They must be expert clinicians and educators who are comfortable working in the home milieu. They must recognize that meaningful forms of caring are also found in the arts. Role expectations will also require individuals to function as case managers who are willing to assume leadership responsibilities for an autonomous nursing practice that directs multidisciplinary care. Nurses fulfill several key roles in home care, which include those of educator, advocate, case manager, and spiritual-aesthetic communer.

Patient educator

By definition, home care nurses visit the patient on a part-time and intermittent basis. Because the nurse's contact with the patient and caregiver is limited, it is important that the nurse teaches patients how to manage their health care needs at home. Part of this process will involve making information available to patients and assisting them to take those health actions that work the best for them (see Chapter 7).

Patient advocate

The essence of advocacy is to care for the patient.[6] This implies not only that procedural care is done correctly (nurse as hands on technical caregiver) but also that the patient's dignity and rights as a human being are respected in the process. Moreover, caring within the context of advocacy represents a holistic view of home care nursing practice that acknowledges health from the patient's perspective. In other words, health is all the patient is and *wants* to be. This requires a respect for sociocultural values and an appreciation of the impact of the family and home environment on the health of the patient. Advocacy in caring will certainly reflect professional standards and ethics of practice (see Chapters 8 and 23).

Case manager

Case management involves assessing, implementing, coordinating, and evaluating outcomes of care (see Chapter 9). At present, home care nurses are expected to provide cost-effective, quality care.

Such expectations require nurses to have a definite plan of care with realistic goals and outcomes of care that are derived from the patient, family or caregiver, and multidisciplinary team, which includes the physician. Such expectations require the nurse to be cognizant of regulations affecting reimbursement for services, as well as an awareness of what services in the community are available to the patient. Home care nurses as case managers are expected to play a primary role in quality improvement (QI) strategies, which may include benchmarking clinical practices for evaluation of effectiveness (see Chapter 10).

Spiritual-aesthetic communer

For many home care nurses there comes a realization that expressions of faith, hope, and love provide a spiritual care that deeply nurtures the patient. This suggests a movement away from a biomedical model of care that emphasizes the technical cure of body parts and toward an appreciation of health and healing within the arts (see Chapter 27). Spiritual-aesthetic communion represents multidimensional caring whereby the nurse and patient resonate to higher levels of understanding and self-awareness.[14] Such a process provides patients with new insights regarding how they will care for themselves (even if this means coming to terms with how they will experience their own deaths). Spiritual-aesthetic communion reflects those caring moments between patient and nurse when words are not always necessary to convey feelings and meaning.[15] Such experiences reside in the heart of nursing.

SKILLS TO SUPPORT ROLE
IMPLEMENTATION

As discussed in the following, qualities and characteristics that address home care nurse role implementation include advanced assessment and evaluation skills, effective communication skills, sound judgment, effective documentation skills, flexibility and critical/creative thinking, and self-direction.

Advanced assessment and evaluation skills

The home care nurse must be able to perform an in-depth holistic assessment of the patient, family, and home environment. An assessment of available community services as a source of referral for patient/caregiver needs is also important. This is followed by an ongoing evaluation that determines the patient's progress (or lack of progress) in meeting outcomes of care. The home care nurse's assessment and evaluation provides guidelines for changes in the plan of care or the frequency of visits. Most important, assessment and evaluation are the basis for offering patients/caregivers choices in their health care such as changes in the plan of care, referral to specialty services, placement in a long-term care facility or hospice, homemaker or assisted living services, rehospitalization, or discharge from home care services.

Effective communication skills

Since the patient, the physician, and the home care agency are separated by distance, nurses must maintain open communication channels to implement the plan of care and coordinate the services of the multidisciplinary team. Effective communication skills are also essential for case conferencing with the multidisciplinary team. Furthermore, in the home milieu, nurses will teach patients who have unique ways of doing things and personal convictions. Effective communication fosters good working relationships with the patient/caregiver despite differences in educational levels and religious and/or ethnic backgrounds. Moreover, communication is the basis for aesthetics in home care nursing practice.

Sound judgment

Moving away from the institutional setting and working in the patient's home affords certain freedoms in practice and entails different responsibilities. Although the physician is just a phone call away, the plan of care and number of visits are frequently adjusted by the home care nurse. If the nurse determines that the patient needs immediate medical attention, a trip to the emergency room or physician's office may be necessary. Home care nurses must use sound judgment and decision-making skills when determining what actions to take. For example, sound judgment is also required when differentiating between a safe housing area or situation and an unsafe one. Home care nurses must know when to proceed and when to stop and confer with their patient service managers regarding questionable, possibly unsafe, situations for both patient and nurse.

Effective documentation skills

Whether working for a Medicare-certified home care agency or other provider, home care nurses must have an accurate knowledge of any regulatory documentation guidelines for care. Such documentation is often the basis for provider coverage of home visits and serves as a marker for agency accreditation (see Chapters 1 and 5).

Flexibility and critical/creative thinking

Some nurses feel comfortable practicing home care and view visiting various neighborhoods and working in the patient's home as both challenging and rewarding. Other nurses may have difficulty adjusting to home environments that differ from their own. Home care does not take place in a controlled environment. Improvisation of supplies, equipment, or therapies in the home setting is necessary and requires flexibility and critical/creative thinking. Critical/creative thinking is also needed for essential committee work that directly influences clinical practice issues.

Self-direction

Home care nurses are largely self-directed. They set up their own daily and weekly schedules, adding patients to their caseload as requested and adjusting their schedules accordingly. They must familiarize themselves with the patient service area and orient themselves to the location of each patient's home. In addition, changes in the plan of care and the frequency of visits are typically initiated by the home care nurse as part of case management.

NURSE PROFILE

Home care nurses are not merely critical care or hospital-based nurses who "just run into the home to do a procedure." Such an attitude is disparaging to those nurses who work closely with patients and their families, sometimes in environments with few resources. Like other specialty areas of practice, nursing care in the home setting requires special preparation and knowledge.

Ideally, nurses entering home care should be educated at the baccalaureate level.[8] This background provides a basis for nursing practice that involves management skills, family and community concepts, and expanded clinical experiences in community health settings. In addition, baccalaureate graduates have an in-depth exposure to the nursing process with an emphasis on critical/creative thinking and decision making.

Home care nursing practice is very complex and requires independent decision making and precise assessment. A minimum of 1 year of postgraduate medical-surgical experience is recommended as a basis for entry into home care. Specialty assignments such as pediatric or high-tech home care should be reflected in the nurse's work experience. In addition to education and work history, individual nurse characteristics such as ability to work in the home and community, knowledge base, and maturity level are key factors that will determine if home care is a good fit for the nurse.

ROLE PREPARATION AND ORIENTATION

When nurses become employed by a home care agency, they should receive an orientation to the agency that prepares them to work in home care. This preparation is usually done by staff development through a formal orientation schedule and periodic in-service programs.

Home care agency orientation

Visits by the home care nurse are based on patient needs for self-care and best level of health. Universal factors influencing patient care in the home include the following:

Age-related and cultural factors (specific patient needs that may vary with the age and cultural preference of the patient)

Psychobiological factors (mental, emotional, spiritual, and physiological needs)

Specific disease manifestation (chronic, congenital, short-term, or terminal)

Socioeconomic and environmental factors (availability of family support systems to assist with the plan of care, availability of medical supplies, adequate food and housing, and access to the medical system)

It is important to remember that orientation will assist most nurses to transition from hospital to community-based practice. As the eyes and ears of the physician, many nurses will be moving from a world of "Nurse do this" to one of "Nurse, what do we do?" Therefore orientation should begin by acquainting nurses with the universal factors as a means to help them conceptualize what home care nursing is all about and how practice differs from that in the more controlled environment of the hospital.[9] The formal orientation should include (but not be limited to) the following preparatory exercises.

Review of documents stating the home care agency's philosophy of care, scope of services, and program evaluation. These documents indicate how the agency regards home care nursing practice, patient care, its place within the community, and standards of care. An organizational structure should be reviewed at this time. The purpose and function of the various agency committees, as well as the QI program, should also be discussed. The patient care plan or care path can serve as an orientation tool to the QI program and outline nursing care for patient groups frequently encountered in the home.

Review of the home care agency's policy and procedure manual. The agency should have a manual, updated yearly, that provides guidelines for all aspects of patient care, including infection control.[12] This manual should be reviewed with nurses during orientation. Policies regarding reporting issues or concerns through the chain of command and on-call, as well as weekend, service delivery should also be discussed.

Review of documentation forms and procedures; orientation to computers. The use of all agency forms, including the visit report, patient care plan or care path, time cards, daily and weekly itinerary logs, and the travel chart, should be explained during orientation. If the agency is using laptop computers, nurses should receive extensive orientation until they are comfortable operating such equipment.

Introduction to the multidisciplinary team and ancillary services. It should be emphasized that attending multidisciplinary conferences and referring patients to specialty services strengthen the plan of care and will be expected of nurses as case managers. The purpose and roles of the multidisciplinary team and ancillary services should be explained. New nurses should learn when and how to refer patients to specialists such as the home care aide; registered dietitian; physical, occupational, or speech language pathologist; hospice nurse; social

---

Box 3-1   CLINICAL INDICATORS FOR MULTIDISCIPLINARY REFERRALS

Clinical Indicators for Advanced Practice Nurse (APN) Referral

Complex patient care issues

Lack of patient response to the medical treatment plan

Staff needs for support, advocacy, and encouragement

Clinical Indicators for Home Care Aide Referral

Assisted or complete personal care services are needed, including:

Bathing

Grooming

Preparing meals

Eating

Oral hygiene

Skin and/or nail care

Toileting and elimination

Ambulating

Exercises

Light housekeeping

Washing clothes

Grocery shopping

Procedural care within the auspices of the job description

Clinical Indicators for Hospice Referral

Palliative care needs

Respite care needs for the patient/caregiver

Patient care needs are "stable," but the patient/caregiver has ongoing needs (e.g., counseling, coping mechanisms), not covered by "routine home care benefits"

Extensive patient care needs not met by usual home care coverage (e.g., extensive pain management or psychological or spiritual care needs)

Patient/caregiver's need for extra assistance from volunteers (e.g., picking up medications, groceries, or other supplies; talking to and being with someone)

The home care agency or organization is unable to provide the extent of services needed or requested by the patient/caregiver

Request by patient/caregiver in preparation for what to expect at the time of death and after

Clinical Indicators for Nutritional Therapist

Special diet orders

Failure to thrive; pediatric growth and development issues

Certain disease processes such as chronic obstructive pulmonary disease, diabetes, congestive heart failure, complicated wounds

Obesity

Anorexia

Clinical Indicators for Psychiatric Home Care Nurse Referral

Unrelieved stress or high-anxiety states

Continued nonparticipation with the plan of care

Depression

Hallucinations

Delusions

Dementia

Unrealistic or unreasonable thought patterns

Thoughts of suicide

Prolonged grief

Maladaptive coping

Manipulative patients

Chronic, debilitating illnesses

Inability to sleep, rest, or eat

Bizarre dress or behavior

Sexually seductive patients

Patient abuse and/or neglect

Confusion or emotional lability

No physical limitations but unsafe outside of the home as a result of mental/emotional state

Active psychiatric diagnosis

Management and evaluation of a patient care plan

Clinical Indicators for Skilled Nursing (RN or LPN Under RN Supervision)

Observation and assessment of the patient's condition when only the specialized skills of a medical professional can determine the patient's status

Teaching and training activities

Administration of medications

Tube feedings

Nasopharyngeal and tracheostomy aspiration

Catheter care

Wound care

Ostomy care

Nutritional needs

Medical gases

Rehabilitation nursing (includes bowel and bladder programs)

Venipuncture

Management and evaluation of a patient care plan

Box 3-1   CLINICAL INDICATORS FOR MULTIDISCIPLINARY REFERRALS—cont'd

Clinical Indicators for Rehabilitation Referral
Physical Therapy

Decreased ability to roll, move about, or come to a
    sitting position in bed
Decreased ability to transfer
Impaired balance and/or coordination
Decreased gait ability or special devices or gait aids;
    unable to ascend or descend stairs or enter and
    exit the home
Functional loss of range of motion or strength in any
    extremity
Therapeutic intervention for pain or edema control
Caregiver instruction in methods of assisting pa-
    tients with any of the above losses or in the estab-
    lishment of a home exercise program
Equipment recommendations to enhance the func-
    tional abilities of patients or increase the ease of
    caring for patients
Management and evaluation of a patient care plan

Occupational Therapy

Decreased ability to perform the activities of daily
    living (ADL) (e.g., bathing, dressing, toileting,
    cooking, eating)
Instruction in one-handed techniques (e.g., fine
    motor treatment)
Impaired cognition, perception, or awareness of
    body parts (e.g., sensory, perceptual, and neurode-
    velopmental treatment)
Joint protection techniques, pain or edema control,
    and/or splinting
Instruction in energy conservation techniques
Equipment recommendations or adaptations to pa-
    tients' environment to enhance functional ability

Speech Language Pathologist

Decreased ability to express and/or receive commu-
    nication
Impaired cognition and/or memory

Impaired ability to phonate
Dysphagia with need for swallowing instructions
Apraxic

Clinical Indicators for Social Service Referral

Discord or miscommunication between the patient-
    caregiver-family-home care team
Family fighting
Severely impaired vision and/or hearing
Living alone with the diagnosis of functional or
    organic brain syndrome (dementia or Alzheimer's)
Malnutrition
Terminal conditions
Suspected or observed child or dependent elder abuse
    or neglect
Depression, manic depression, anxiety reaction, or
    schizophrenia for basic counseling (refer to the psy-
    chiatric home care nurse for problems with thought
    disorders)
Recent amputees
Newly diagnosed diabetics
Multiple sclerosis (MS)
Stroke or paralysis
High-tech home care services
Acquired immunodeficiency syndrome (AIDS)
Counseling for long-range planning and decision
    making
Inadequate housing conditions (e.g., the need for air
    conditioning or other assistance with heating and
    cooling)
Stress management
Patient/caregiver nonparticipation with the plan of
    care
Need for long-term care placement
Inadequate financial resources
Inadequate caregivers or caregivers who are "over-
    whelmed" with the patient's multiple health care
    needs
Community resource planning

---

worker; or advanced practice nurse. Documentation guidelines for reimbursement of specialty services and requirements when making the referral
should be reviewed.[7]

  If individuals from each specialty service can
personally participate in the orientation, new nurses
can begin to place a name with a face. Box 3-1 describes clinical indicators for multidisciplinary re-

ferrals. In addition, familiarity with local medical
suppliers, wound-care vendors, and commodity
representatives in the community enhances home
care nurses' abilities to recommend products and
community services to the patient and caregiver. In-
teragency networking on a local, regional, and national level via the Internet should also be encouraged (see Appendix III-I).

Instruction on community safety and map reading. Commuting to patients' homes in a safe manner is a concern for all nurses working within the community. Some areas may be unsafe and declared off-limits. Safety precautions should be reviewed (Box 3-2). The local police department may be willing to give a yearly "safety in the community" in-service for nurses. A street guide or road map is recommended. A car or cellular phone is also recommended to enhance communication when nurses are out in the field.

Although perspectives on wearing a uniform in the field vary, nurses should be taught to view uniforms and name badges as important forms of identification to the public. From the author's past experience as a Visiting Nurse Association (VNA) nurse, the traditional navy uniform worn by many VNA and public health nurses is a recognized symbol of respect and professionalism within the neighborhood.

Introduction to the home milieu. During orientation, it is also important to discuss the concept of home milieu. *Home milieu* refers to working in the patient's home environment, which may include family and/or caregivers, pets, friends, farms, and communities.

In the home milieu, home care nurses may work in cities or in the countryside (Figure 3-1). Patient populations, practice needs, and transportation issues will vary in these areas. As applicable, orientation should support role implementation in both urban and rural settings.

In addressing the home milieu it should be emphasized that the patient's home environment, within a sociocultural context, may be drastically different from that of the nurse. Although professional standards of practice should be maintained, new nurses should be reminded that when going into a patient's home "they are the guest," and they should behave accordingly. Although healthy sanitation and health practices are to be encouraged, nurses must realize that roaches and dirty dishes are a way of life for certain families. As opposed to hospital practice, clean rather than sterile technique is commonly used. Consequently, it is important that home care nurses leave their personal prejudices and convictions at home.

Finally, when working in the home milieu, sensitivity to ethnicity and the fact that people ultimately have the right to "live their own lives" should be stressed.

Instruction on home improvisation. Creative intervention is often a part of home care nursing. Inadequate supplies need not prevent delivery of needed care. Home improvisations such as using a coat hanger attached to a door hook for an IV pole, making a robe by pinning a blanket, preparing homemade normal saline or acetic acid for irrigation fluids, and using newspapers covered with cheesecloth for a bed pad should be reviewed.

Special training and certification. Home care nurses who are expected to perform certain speciality services may require special training and certification. For example, nurses who are entering home IV therapy may be required to become chemotherapy certified as part of their conditions for employment. Likewise, nurses entering hospice may be given special training and certification in therapeutic touch.

Ethical considerations. Ethical issues arise in the many stressful patient/caregiver situations that home care nurses encounter. In addition to neglect and abuse issues, ethical concerns with which home care nurses will be involved include patients with insufficient or inadequate food, housing, or medical supplies; patients who lack proper support systems; and patients who choose to die at home.

It is important to support new nurses coming into home care by reviewing some of the legal and ethical concerns they may encounter, along with suggestions for resolution. It is important to identify home care agency staff that nurses can turn to should they experience problems in the field. Chapter 8 discusses the nurse's responsibilities when working in the sometimes overwhelming home milieu.

In addition to in-house orientation, patient service managers or supervisors should plan for joint field visits as a part of the orientation program. This allows new nurses to observe their peers coordinating and giving care in the home. Staff expertise is also fostered by ongoing in-service training that reviews pharmacology, medical-surgical and psychosocial issues, quality improvement, and any regulations that influence the delivery of patient care.

ADVANCED PRACTICE NURSES

In home care, advanced practice nurses such as clinical nurse specialists (CNSs) serve as educators, consultants, caregivers, patient and staff advocates, speaker bureaus, and community liaisons.

Box 3-2   SAFETY IN THE COMMUNITY

Precautions to Take Prior to Visits

- Wear a name badge and uniform that clearly identifies you as a representative of the home health agency.
- Wear shoes that you can run in if necessary.
- Call patients in advance and alert them to the approximate time of your visit.
- Confirm directions to their residence. Always carry a map or local street guide in case you get lost.
- Request that unruly or overfriendly pets be properly secured before making visits.
- Keep change for a phone call in your shoe or pocket. Do not carry a purse. Before leaving the agency, lock your purse or other valuable belongings in the trunk or cover your purse with a blanket if it will be visible.

Precautions When Traveling in the Car

- Keep your car in good working order with plenty of gas. Obtain an automobile club membership for possible car problems.
- Consider use of a personal cellular phone to maximize communication.
- Store a blanket in the car in the winter and a thermos of cool water in the summer. Keep a snack in the glove compartment.
- If your car fails, turn on emergency flashers, put a CALL POLICE sign in the window, and wait for the police. Do not accept rides from strangers.
- Keep your car locked when parked or driving. Keep windows rolled up if possible.
- Park in full view of the patient's residence (avoid parking in alleys or deserted side streets).

Precautions When Traveling on Foot

- Have nursing bag and equipment ready when exiting from the car. Keep one arm free to maneuver when walking.
- Walk directly to the patient's residence in a professional, businesslike manner.
- When passing a group of strangers, cross to the other side of the street, as appropriate.
- Back away, never run from a dog. Walk slowly around farm animals to prevent frightening them.
- When leaving the patient's residence, carry car keys in your hand (pointed ends of keys between fingers may make an effective weapon).

- Avoid using subway or bus routes known to be frequented by gangs.

Precautions During Visits

- Use common walkways in buildings; avoid isolated stairs or darkened (unlit) areas.
- Always knock on the door before entering a patient's home.
- Do not make the visit if firearms are visible; contact your supervisor with concerns or problems.
- Do not make the visit if drugs or illegal substances are noted; contact your supervisor with concerns or problems.
- Do not make the visit if the patient (or family members) are verbally or physically abusive; contact your supervisor with concerns or problems. If relatives or neighbors become a safety problem, consider the following:
  - Discuss the problem with the patient, and schedule a visit time when the relative or neighborhood is quiet (e.g., early morning).
  - Make joint visits with another home care nurse or arrange for escort service.
  - Close the case for unresolved safety issues.

Defense Strategies

Run, scream, or yell "fire" or "stranger"; kick shins, instep, or groin; bite or scratch.

Use a whistle attached to your key ring, chemical sprays, or nursing bag for defense.

Throw your nursing bag at your assailant and run away in the opposite direction (never hesitate to hand over a nursing bag or anything else, but do so in a manner that enables you to escape).

Arrange a "check out" phone call with your supervisor at the end of your day.

At all costs, avoid being tied up or taken somewhere else. These scenarios have a high incidence of rape and murder.

NURSING CONSIDERATIONS The best safety recommendation is to just use good common sense. Nurses should never go into or stay in a home if they feel unsafe. They should always use good assessment skills to check their surroundings and respect and *listen* to their gut feelings.

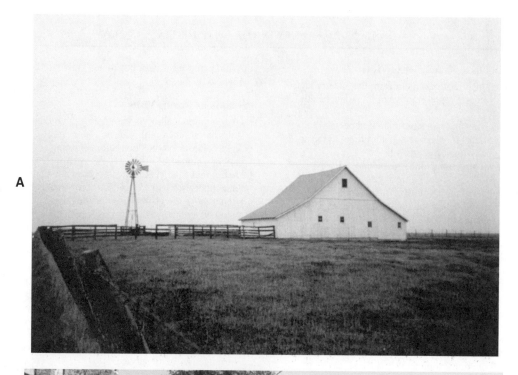

A

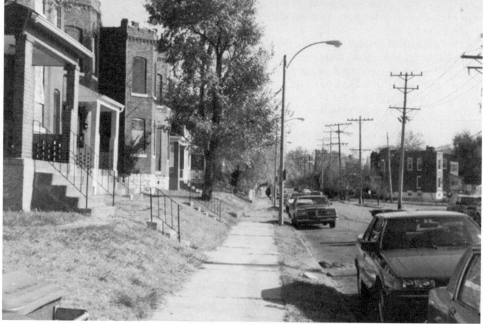

B

Figure 3-1 Rural (**A**) versus urban (**B**) areas of practice. (Photos courtesy Robyn Rice).

Although CNSs may have many duties (e.g., writing policies and procedures or serving on product evaluation, quality assurance, or forms committees), their primary focus should be patients and staff. In addition, nurse practitioners (NPs) can assist physicians and nurses with care plan oversight issues, which may include ordering medications and treatments. Of note, both CNSs and NPs serve as valuable consultants to home care nurses.

The art of consultation is "to help." Therefore in order to be available to staff on an as-needed basis, advanced practice nurses should avoid taking on a large caseload or being assigned to administrative desk duties that could consume the majority of their time. The multidimensional nature of home care demands that advanced practice nurses focus on a holistic nursing practice that encompasses patients, caregivers, and the home environment. This viewpoint moves the nurse from task-oriented to outcome-oriented care. Instead of "What are we doing?" the question becomes "Where are we going?" and "How are we getting there?"

Advanced practice nurses should assist staff with difficult clinical and ethical decisions by jointly assessing patient problems, formulating the interventions, and evaluating the outcomes. Co-visits with nurses provide an arena where information is exchanged and working relationships are defined. This establishes patterns of problem solving that home care nurses can recall for use in meeting future patient needs. As a result, confidence in assessment and decision-making abilities of the nurse are enhanced.

Resources in home care are often scarce. Home care nurses, when working with their patients and families, may find themselves in some very stressful situations. Consequently, when consulting with staff, advanced practice nurses should present a very supportive persona.

IMPLEMENTING STUDENT LEARNING IN HOME CARE

Home care agencies provide an excellent clinical practicum for educating undergraduate nursing students about home care (Figure 3-2). Through home care, students learn the basic concepts of case management and how to work with patients and their families in the home setting. It is important that faculty and home care nursing staff clarify up front exactly what their responsibilities are toward the students and exactly what the students will be doing for the patients (Box 3-3).

Student learning in home care can be fostered in many ways. Students at any level of a nursing program can do a 1-day observation in which they essentially follow home care nurses as a means to enhance their awareness of numerous forms of nursing. A log describing what they see and how it compares with hospital-based nursing is recommended.

Independent senior home visits with periodic instructor co-visits to guide learning is another way to teach home care. Students are typically assigned a simple dressing change or cardiovascular assessment. This not only fosters students' responsibility to learn but also enhances their self-direction for time management and accountability for patient care—the realities of nursing practice. Initially students will require a lot of contact with their instructor. However, as skills and confidence are gained, students will become more comfortable when making home visits without their instructor right there looking over their shoulder.

In addition, as part of a senior synthesis or a capstone course, students may follow up with patients at home at 1 and 5 weeks after discharge from the hospital and interview them to conceptualize human needs across time frames and environments. This experience provides information for a very interesting paper and directs students to look at contextual issues of care.

Finally, home care agencies may be used as clinical placement for community health nursing if they are supplemented with aggregate population experiences.[2,11]

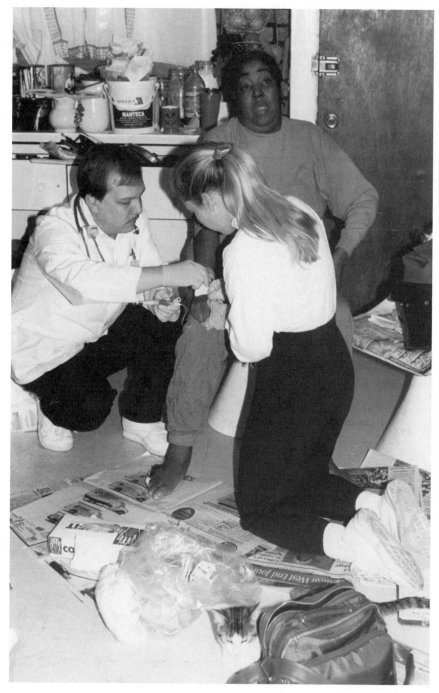

Figure 3-2 Student nurse performing venipuncture in the home. (Photos courtesy Robyn Rice).

Box 3-3   TIPS FOR HOME CARE NURSES WHO ARE WORKING WITH STUDENTS

Meet with the nursing instructor. Ask for a copy of the students' course syllabus and clinical schedule.

Key Questions to Ask

1. What days of the week will the students be in clinical? What are their clinical hours? How long will the students be with you?
2. What will the students be doing in clinical? What are their learning objectives? How does home care fit into their learning objectives?
3. Will the students be doing procedural care? If so, how will they be supervised? Who is responsible for supervising the students?
4. How is the paperwork going to be handled? Who is going to be responsible for processing the students' paperwork and ensuring its accuracy?
5. Who will be responsible for notifying the physician of changes in the patient's status? Who will be responsible for taking physician orders?
6. What will the procedure be for the school of nursing if the weather should get bad? (How will the instructor let you know if clinical is canceled?)
7. If students are merely following you and observing, ask if they are writing a log and what they are supposed to note.

Tips for Staff

1. Exchange beeper and/or cellular phone numbers with the nursing instructor. In addition, obtain the instructor's office or work number.
2. Request that the nursing instructor and/or students call or page you with any concerns. As a backup, encourage students to ask your supervisor or the desk manager for assistance in decision making.
3. Request that the home care agency have a bulletin board or mailbox where you can leave notes or information for the nursing instructor and students.
4. Assign students to patients who are challenging yet not overwhelming for the student; consult the nursing instructor about the appropriateness of the assignment. Wound care and blood draws provide good learning experiences. *Don't be stingy with patients!*
5. Conference with students when possible. Be friendly; find out how things are going. Ask the students to tell you how they are assisting their patients to meet their outcomes of care. Quiz the students on assessment findings. This is a good time to build assessment skills. Often students want to report to the physician everything they find that deviates from the norm. Explain that patients in home care often have wide variances in vital signs. Tell them to immediately report abnormal vital signs and findings to you and/or their instructor; stress that you and/or their instructor will be available to assist them in further decision making.
6. Remember that students usually go by the book. As realities set in, home care can be scary for them at first. Be supportive of the students and nursing instructor. When the students and/or nursing instructor tell you something about a patient's condition, *listen* to what they have to say. It may be necessary to make an extra home visit to evaluate the nursing instructor's and/or students' concerns.
7. Address any concerns directly to the nursing instructor. Let the nursing instructor work out problems with students. Consult your supervisor regarding unresolved problems with nursing instructors and/or students.

Don't forget to give praise when it is deserved. Remember, we were all in nursing school once.

SUMMARY

The role of the home care nurse clearly encompasses elements that are outside the realm of traditional views of nursing. Confidence, competence, and a sensitivity to the home milieu are essential qualities that are required when working in home care. In preparing nurses for this role, it is clear that these qualities should be fostered early on with our undergraduate nursing students, who represent our professional future.

Home care nurses function with a high degree of independence and personal accountability for multidisciplinary service. Their influence over the quality of patient care is *significant*. Consequently, home care nurses have an intriguing opportunity to enhance the vision of what nursing really can be.

REFERENCES

1. Bohny B: A time for self-care: role of the home healthcare nurse, *Home Healthcare Nurse* 15(4):281, 1997.
2. Bradley P: Students practice essential components of community health nursing in home health care, *J Nurs Educ* 35(9):394, 1996.
3. Dellasega C, King L: The psychogeriatric nurse in home health care: use of research to develop the role, *Clin Nurse Specialist* 10(2):64, 1996.
4. Eustis NN, Fisher LR: Relationships between home care clients and their workers: implications for quality of care, *Gerontologist* 31:447, 1991.
5. Forbes D: Clarification of the constructs of satisfaction and dissatisfaction with home care, *Public Health Nurs* 13(6):377, 1996.
6. Gadow S: Existential advocacy: philosophical foundations of nursing. In Spicker S, Gadow S, editors: *Nursing: images and ideals-opening dialogue with the humanities,* New York, 1980, Springer.
7. Health Care Financing Administration: *Home health insurance manual* (Pub No. 11), Washington, DC, 1995, U.S. Department of Health and Human Services.
8. Moore S and others: Home health nurse: stress, self-esteem, social intimacy, and job satisfaction, *Home Health Care Manage Prac* 2(3):135, 1997.
9. Osborn C, Townsend C: Analysis of telephone communication between hospice nurses and a nurse practitioneer group, *Home Health Care Manage Prac* 9(5):52, 1997.
10. Rice R: Key concepts of self-care in the home: implications for home care nurses, *Geriatr Nurs* 19(1):52, 1998.
11. Rice R: Implementing undergraduate student learning in home care, *Geriatr Nurs* 19(2):106, 1998.
12. Rice R, editor: *Manual of home health nursing procedures,* ed 2, St. Louis, 2000, Mosby.
13. Robinson K: The family's role in long-term care, *J Gerontol Nurs* 232(9):7, 1997.
14. Rogers ME: The science of unitary human beings: current perspectives, *Nurs Sci Q* 7:33, 1994.
15. Watson J: *Human science and human care—a theory of nursing,* New York, 1988, National League for Nursing.

Internet Resources for Home Care Nurses

Aging Organizations and Agencies
http://www.aoa.dhhs.gov/aoa/webres/
home-org.htm

AIDs Action Council
1875 Connecticut Avenue NW #700
Washington, DC 20009-5740
202-986-1300

Al-Anon Family Group Headquarters, Inc.
1600 Corporate Landing Parkway
Virginia Beach, VA 23454-5617
888-4AL-ANON
E-mail: WSO@al-anon.org
For meeting information in the United States and
Canada, call 888-4AL-ANON (between 8 AM and
6 PM ET Monday-Friday). You can also use this
number to locate electronic meetings.
http://www.al-anon.alateen.org/ (main homepage)
http://www.al-anon.alateen.org/alalist__usa.html
(links to state organizations)

Alcoholics Anonymous
World Services, Inc.
PO Box 459
New York, NY 10163
212-870-3400
http://www.alcoholics-anonymous.org/
http://www.alcoholics-anonymous.org/ectroff.html
(main offices by state)

Allergy and Asthma Network/Mothers of
Asthmatics, Inc.
2751 Prosperity Avenue, Suite 150
Fairfax, VA 22031
800-878-4403
703-641-9595
Fax: 703-573-7794
E-mail: aanma@aol.com
http://www.aanma.org

Alliance of Genetic Support Groups
4301 Connecticut Avenue NW
Suite 404
Washington, DC 20008
800-336-GENE
202-966-5557
Fax: 202-966-8553
E-mail: info@geneticalliance.org
http://www.geneticalliance.org

The Alzheimer's Association National
Headquarters
919 N Michigan Avenue, Suite 1000
Chicago, IL 60611-1676
800-272-3900
312-335-8700
Fax: 312-335-1110
E-mail: info@alz.org
http://www.alz.org/us/index.htm
http://www.alz.org/chapters/index.htm (local
chapters in all states)

American Academy of Allergy, Asthma, and
Immunology
Online Communications Department
611 E Wells Street
Milwaukee, WI 53202
800-822-2762
http://www.aaaai.org/

American Association for Continuity of Care
638 Prospect Avenue
Hartford, CT 06105
860-586-7525
Fax: 860-586-7550
http://www.continuityofcare.com/

American Association of Diabetes Educators
100 W Monroe Street
4th Floor
Chicago, IL 60603-1901
312-424-2426
E-mail: aade/aade@aadenet.org
http://www.aadenet.org/

American Association of Retired Persons (AARP)
National Headquarters
601 E NW Street
Washington, DC 20049
800-424-3410
http://www.aarp.org/ (main homepage)
http://www.aarp.org/statepages/ (regional and state homepages)

American Cancer Society
271 W 125th Street
New York, NY 10027-4424
800-ACS-2345
212-663-8800
http://www.cancer.org/
http://www.cancer.org/bottomdivisions.html
(to locate local chapters)

American Diabetes Association
National Office
1660 Duke Street
Alexandria, VA 22314
800-DIABETES (800-342-2383)
http://www.diabetes.org/
http://www.diabetes.org/ada/States.asp (to locate local information)

American Foundation for AIDS Research
120 Wall Street
13th Floor
New York, NY 10005
212-806-1600
Fax: 212-806-1601
http://www.amfar.org/

American Heart Association
National Center
7272 Greenville Avenue
Dallas, TX 75231
800-AHA-USA1
Women's Health Information: 888-MY-HEART
http://www.americanheart.org/

http://www.americanheart.org/affili/ (to locate local chapter)

American Juvenile Arthritis Organization
1330 W Peachtree Street
Atlanta, GA 30309
404-872-7100
Arthritis Answers: 800-283-7800
http://www.arthritis.org/ajao/

American Lung Association
800-LUNG-USA (800-586-4872)
http://www.lungusa.org/index.html

American Nurses Association
600 Maryland Avenue SW
Suite 100 West
Washington, DC 20024
800-274-4ANA
202-651-7000
Fax: 202-651-7001
http://www.nursingworld.org
http://www.nursingworld.org/affil/index.htm (links to numerous affiliated nursing organizations)

American Paralysis Association
500 Morris Avenue
Springfield, NJ 07081
800-225-0292
973-379-2690
Fax: 973-912-9433
E-mail: Paralysis@aol.com
http://www.apacure.com/

The American Parkinson Disease Association, Inc.
1250 Hylan Blvd., Suite 4B
Staten Island, NY 10305-1946
800-223-2732
Referral Center: 888-400-2732
E-mail: apda@admin.con2.com
http://www.apdaparkinson.com/
http://www.apdaparkinson.com/I&ctr.htm (for referrals)
http://www.apdaparkinson.com/chaploc.htm (to locate referrals)

American Red Cross National Headquarters
Attn: Public Inquiry Office
11th Floor
1621 N Kent Street
Arlington, VA 22209
703-248-4222
E-mail: info@usa.redcross.org
http://www.redcross.org
http://www.redcross.org/where/where.html
(to locate services near you)

American Tinnitus Association
PO Box 5
Portland, OR 97207-0005
503-248-9985
Fax: 503-248-0024
http://www.ata.org/

Anxiety Disorders Association of America
11900 Parklawn Drive, Suite 100
Rockville, MD 20852
301-231-9350
http://www.adaa.org/

Arthritis Foundation
National Office
1330 W Peachtree Street
Atlanta, GA 30309
404-872-7100
Arthritis Answers: 800-283-7800
http://www.arthritis.org
http://www.arthritis.org/offices/ (to locate local
chapters/offices)

Arthritis National Research Foundation
200 Oceangate, Suite 44
Long Beach, CA 90802
800-588-CURE (2873)
http://www.curearthritis.org/

Assisted Living Federation of America
10300 Eaton Place, Suite 400
Fairfax, VA 22030
703-691-8100
Fax: 703-691-8106
E-mail: lc@alfa.org
http://www.alfa.org/

Asthma and Allergy Foundation of America
1125 15th Street NW, Suite 502
Washington, DC 20005
202-466-7643
Fax: 202-466-8940
E-mail: info@aafa.org
http://www.aafa.org/
http://www.aafa.org/chap__sg.html (to locate local
chapters)

Cancer Information Services
National Cancer Institute
800-4-CANCER (800-422-6237)
http://cis.nci.nih.gov/

Centers for Disease Control and Prevention
1600 Clifton Road NE
Atlanta, GA 30333
404-639-3311
E-mail: netinfo@cdc.gov
http://www.cdc.gov/

Center for Disease Control NPIN
PO Box 6003
Rockville, MD 20849-6003
800-458-5231
TTY: 800-243-7012
International: 301-562-1098
International TTY: 301-588-1589
Fax: 888-282-7681
International Fax: 301-562-1050
E-mail: pubs@cdcnpin.org
http://www.cdcnpin.org/

Children's Hospice International
2202 Mt Vernon Avenue, Suite 3C
Alexandria, VA 22301
703-684-0330
Fax: 703-684-0026
http://www.chionline.org/

Children of Aging Parents
1609 Woodbourne Road, #302A
Levittown, PA 19057
800-227-7294
http://www.careguide.net/careguide.cgi/caps/
capshome.html/

Choices in Dying
National Office
1035 30th Street NW
Washington, DC 20007
800-989-WILL (9455)
202-338-9790
Fax: 202-338-0242
http://www.choices.org/

The Cooley's Anemia Foundation, Inc.
129-09 26th Avenue, #203
Flushing, NY 11354
800-522-7222
718-321-CURE (2873)
Fax: 718-321-3340
E-mail: ncaf@aol.com
http://www.thalassemia.org/

Crohn's and Colitis Foundation of America, Inc.
386 Park Avenue South
17th Floor
New York, NY 10016-8804
800-932-2423
212-685-3440
Fax: 212-779-4098
E-mail: info@ccfa.org
http://www.ccfa.org/

Cystic Fibrosis Foundation
6931 Arlington Road
Bethesda, MD 20814
800-FIGHT-CF
301-951-4422
Fax: 301-951-6378
E-mail: info@cff.org
http://www.cff.org/

Dystonia Medical Research Foundation
One E Wacker Drive
Chicago, IL 60601-1905
800-377-DYST
312-755-0198
Fax: 312-803-0138
E-mail: dystonia@dystonia-foundation.org
http://www.dystonia-foundation.org/

Easter Seals Society
230 W Monroe Street
Suite 1800
Chicago, IL 60606
800-221-6827
312-726-6200
TDD: 312-726-4258
Fax: 312-726-1494
E-mail: info@easter-seals.org
http://www.easter-seals.org/
http://www.easter-seals.org/cservices2/home.html
(to find in-home services near you)
http://www.easter-seals.org/html/services.html
(to locate any services near you)

Environmental Protection Agency
401 M Street SW
Washington, DC 20460-0003
202-260-2090
http://www.epa.gov

Endometriosis Association International
Headquarters
8585 N 76th Place
Milwaukee, WI 53223
800-992-3636
414-355-2200
Fax: 414-355-6065
E-mail: endo@endometriosisassn.org
http://www.endometriosisassn.org/

Epilepsy Foundation
4351 Garden City Drive
Landover, MD 20785
800-EFA-1000
301-459-3700
Fax: 301-577-4941
E-mail: info@efa.org
http://www.efa.org/

Family Caregiver Alliance
425 Bush Street, Suite 500
San Francisco, CA 94108
415-434-3388
Fax: 415-434-3508
E-mail: info@caregiver.org
http://www.caregiver.org

The Foundation Fighting Blindness
Executive Plaza I, Suite 800
11350 McCormick Road
Hunt Valley, MD 21031-1014
888-394-3937
800-683-5551
410-785-1414
410-785-9687
http://www.blindness.org/

Health Care Financing Administration (HCFA)
7500 Security Boulevard
Baltimore, MD 21244
410-786-3000
http://www.hcfa.org (information on Medicare,
Medicaid, and Managed Care)

Health Information (on just about anything with
multiple links)
http://www.healthfinder.org

The Hemlock Society
PO Box 101810
Denver, CO 80250-1810
800-247-7421
303-639-1202
Fax: 303-639-1224
E-mail: hemlock@privatei.com
http://www2.privatei.com/hemlock/index.html

The Hepatitis Information Network
http://www.hepnet.com

Home Medical Equipment Information
Consumer Fraud Pamphlet
Medicare and Home Medical Equipment
Information Provided by:
U.S. Department of Health and Human Services
Health Care Financing Administration
U.S. Government Printing Office: 1992-332-525
October, 1996
http://www.medicare.gov/consumerfraud.html

Hospice Association of America
228 7th Street SE
Washington, DC 20003
202-546-4759
Fax: 202-547-9559
http://www.nahc.org/HAA/home.html

Huntington's Disease Society of America
158 W 29th Street, 7th Floor
New York, NY 10001-5300
800-345-HDSA
212-242-1968
E-mail: curehd@idt.net
http://www.hdsa.mgh.harvard.edu.hdsamain.nclk/

Joint Commission on Accreditation of Healthcare
Organizations
One Renaissance Boulevard
Oakbrook Terrace, IL 60181
630-792-5000
Fax: 630-792-5005
http://www.jcaho.org/

Juvenile Diabetes Foundation International
120 Wall Street
New York, NY 10005-4001
800-JDF-CURE
212-785-9500
Fax: 212-785-9595
E-mail: info@jcfcure.org
http://www.jdfcure.org/
http://www.jdfcure.org/chapters/index.html
(to find a local chapter)

Leukemia Society of America
600 3rd Avenue
New York, NY 10016
212-573-8484
Information Resource Center: 800-955-4LSA
http://www.leukemia.org/
http://www.leukemia.org/docs/aboutlsa/
chap__docs/fs__finder.html (to locate local
chapters)

Lupus Foundation of America
1300 Piccard Drive, Suite 200
Rockville, MD 20850-4303
800-558-0121
301-670-9292
E-mail: LupusInfo@aol.com
http://www.internet-plaza.net/lupus (main
homepage)
http://www.internet-plaza.net/lupus/info/help.html
(to locate local chapter)

March of Dimes
Birth Defects Foundation
National Office
1275 Mamaroneck Avenue
White Plains, NY 10605
914-428-7100
http://www.modimes.org

The Mended Hearts, Inc.
7272 Greenville Avenue
Dallas, TX 75231-4596
800-AHAUSA1 (ask for Mended Hearts)
Fax: 214-706-5231
E-mail: dbonham@heart.org
http://www.mendedhearts.org/
http://www.mendedhearts.org/localchapters.html
(to locate local chapter)

Mental Health Net
570 Metro Place N
Dublin, OH 43017
614-764-0143
Fax: 614-764-0362
E-mail: webmaster@cmhc.com
http://www.cmhc.com

Muscular Dystrophy Association
National Headquarters
3300 E Sunrise Drive
Tuscon, AZ 85718
800-572-1717
mda@mdausa.org
http://www.mdausa.org/

Multiple Sclerosis Association of America
National Headquarters
706 Haddonfield Road
Cherry Hills, NJ 08002
800-LEARN-MS (800-532-7667)
Fax: 609-661-9797
E-mail: msaa@msaa.com
http://www.msaa.com/

Myasthenia Gravis Foundation of America
222 S Riverside Plaza
Suite 1540
Chicago, IL 60606
800-541-5454
312-258-0522
Fax: 312-258-0461
E-mail: myastheniagravis@msn.com
http://www.med.unc.edu/mgfa/welcome.htm

National Alliance for the Mentally Ill
200 N Glebe Road, Suite 1015
Arlington, VA 22203-3754
Helpline: 800-950-NAMI (6264)
Front Desk: 703-524-7600
Fax: 703-524-9094
TDD: 703-516-7991
http://www.nami.org

National Arthritis and Musculoskeletal and Skin
Diseases Information Clearinghouse
National Institutes of Health
1 AMS Circle
Bethesda, MD 20892-3675
301-495-4484
TTY: 301-565-2966
Fax: 301-718-6366
E-mail: namsic@mail.nih.gov
http://www.nih.gov/niams/healthinfo/info.htm

National Association for Down Syndrome
PO Box 4542
Oak Brook, IL 60522
http://www.nads.org/

National Association for Home Care
228 7th Street SE
Washington, DC 20003
202-547-7424
Fax: 202-547-3540
http://www.nahc.org/ (may be a members only
site)

National Association for Sickle Cell Disease
3345 Wilshire Boulevard, Suite 1106
Los Angeles, CA 90010-1880
800-421-8453
213-736-5455

National Center for Chronic Disease Prevention
and Health Promotion
Centers for Disease Control and Prevention
1600 Clifton Road NE
Atlanta, GA 30333
E-mail: ccdinfo@cdc.gov
http://www.cdc.gov/nccdphp/nccdhome.htm

The National Clearinghouse for Alcohol and Drug
Information
PO Box 2345
Rockville, MD 20847-2345
800-729-6686
Fax: 301-468-6433
E-mail: info@health.org
http://www.health.org/

National Clearinghouse on Child Abuse and
Neglect Information, National Center on Child
Abuse and Neglect
300 C Street SW
Washington, DC 20447
800-394-3366
703-385-7565
BBS: 800-877-8800
Fax: 703-385-3206
E-mail: nccanch@calib.com
http://www.calib.com/nccanch/

National Committee to Prevent Child Abuse
200 S Michigan Avenue, 17th Floor
Chicago, IL 60604-4357
800-55-NCPCA (800-835-2671)
312-663-3520
Fax: 312-939-8962
http://www.childabuse.org/

The National Council on the Aging, Inc.
409 3rd Street, SE, Suite 200
Washington, DC 20024
202-479-6653
202-479-6654
202-479-6674
Fax: 202-479-0735
http://www.ncoa.org/

National Depressive and Manic-Depressive
Association
730 N Franklin Street, Suite 501
Chicago, IL 60610-3526
800-826-3632
Fax: 312-642-7243
E-mail: myrtis@aol.com
http://www.ndmda.org/
http://www.ndmda.org/chapdir.htm (to locate a
chapter near you)

National Diabetes Information Clearinghouse
(NDIC)
1 Information Way
Bethesda, MD 20892-3560
E-mail: ndic@info.niddk.nih.gov
http://www.niddk.nih.gov/health/diabetes/ndic.htm

The National Down Syndrome Society
666 Broadway, 8th Floor
New York, NY 10012-2317
800-221-4602
212-460-9330
http://www.ndss/org/

National Headache Foundation
428 W St. James Place, 2nd Floor
Chicago, IL 60614
800-843-2256
http://www.headaches.org/

National Hemophilia Foundation
116 W 32nd Street, 11th Floor
New York, NY 10001
212-328-3700
Fax: 212-328-3777
HANDI Phone: 800-42-HANDI
HANDI Fax: 212-328-3799
E-mail: info@hemophilia.org
HANDI E-mail: handi@hemophilia.org
http://www.hemophilia.org/

National Information Center on Deafness
Gallaudet University
800 Florida Avenue NE
Washington, DC 20002-3695
202-651-5051
TTY: 202-651-5052
Fax: 202-651-5054
E-mail: nicd@gallux.gallaudet.edu
http://www.gallaudet.edu/~nicd/

National Institute of Mental Health
5600 Fishers Lane, Room 7C-02, MSC 8030
Bethesda, MD 20892-8030
E-mail: nimhinfo@mail.nih.gov
http://www.nimh.nih.gov/home.htm

National Institute of Neurological Disorders and
Stroke
PO Box 5801
Bethesda, MD 20824
http://www.ninds.nih.gov/

National Heart, Lung, and Blood Institute
NHLBI Information Center
PO Box 30105
Bethesda, MD 20824-0105
301-251-1223
E-mail: NHLBIIC@dgsys.com
http://www.nhlbi.nih.gov/nhlbi/infcntr/
infocent.htm

National Hospice Association
1901 N Moore Street, Suite 901
Arlington, VA 22209-1714
703-243-5900
Fax: 703-525-5762
E-mail: http://www.nho.org/
http://www.nho.org/database.htm (to find a
hospice)

National Kidney Foundation
30 E 33rd Street
New York, NY 10016
800-622-9010
http://www.kidney.org/

National Marfan Foundation
382 Main Street
Port Washington, NY 11050
E-mail: staff@marfan.org
800-8-MARFAN
516-883-8712
Fax: 516-883-8040
http://www.marfan.org/

National Neurofibromatosis Foundation
95 Pine Street, 16th Floor
New York, NY 10005
212-344-NNFF
http://www.nf.org/

National Organization for Rare Disorders
PO Box 8923
New Fairfield, CT 06812-8923
203-746-6518
Fax: 203-746-6481
http://www.nord-rdb.com/~orphan/

National Osteoporosis Foundation
1150 17th Street NW, Suite 500
Washington, DC 20036-4603
http://www.nof.org/

National Parkinson Foundation, Inc.
Bob Hope Parkinson Research Center
1501 NW 9th Avenue
Bob Hope Road
Miami, FL 33136-1494
800-327-4545
305-547-6666
Fax: (305) 243-4403
E-mail: mailbox@npf.med.miami.edu
http://www.parkinson.org
http://www.parkinson.org/chapters.htm (to locate
local chapters)

National Reye's Syndrome Foundation
PO Box 829
Bryan, OH 43506-0829
800-233-7393 (U.S. Only)
http://www.bright.net/~reyessyn/index.html

National Spinal Cord Injury Association
8300 Colesville Road
Suite #551
Silver Spring, MD 20910
800-962-9629
301-588-9414
http://www.spinalcord.org/

National Stroke Association
96 Inverness Drive E, Suite I
Englewood, CO 80112-5112;
303-649-9299
Fax: 303-649-1328; 20036-4603
http://www.stroke.org/

National Tuberous Sclerosis Association
8181 Professional Place, Suite 110
Landover, MD 20785-2226
800-225-6872
Fax: 301-459-0394
http://www.ntsa@ntsa.org/

National Voluntary Health Agencies
1925 K Street NW, Suite 510
Washington, DC 20006
800-654-0845
202-467-5913
Fax: 202-467-4280
http://www.nvha.org/

Obsessive-Compulsive Foundation, Inc.
PO Box 70
Milford, CT 06460-0070
203-878-5669
Fax: 203-874-2826
E-mail: info@ocfoundation.org
http://www.ocfoundation.org/

Occupational Safety and Health Administration
(OSHA)
U.S. Department of Labor
200 Constitution Avenue NW
Washington, DC 20210
http://www.osha.gov/

Outcome and Assessment Information Set
(OASIS) provides information on:
• Core items of a comprehensive assessment for
an adult home care patient
• Forming the basis for measuring patient
outcomes for purposes of outcome-based quality
improvement (OBQI)
http://www.hcfa.gov/medicare/hsqub/oasis/
hhoview.htm

Paralyzed Veterans of America
Communication Program
801 18th Street NW
Washington, DC 20006
800-424-8200
202-872-1300
http://www.pva.org/

Parkinson's Disease Foundation
William Black Medical Building
Columbia-Presbyterian Medical Center
710 W 168th Street
New York, NY 10032-9982
800-457-6676
212-923-4700
Fax: 212-923-4778
E-mail: info@pdf.org
http:www.parkinsons-foundation.org/

Prevent Blindness America
500 E Remington Road
Schaumburg, IL 60173
800-331-2020
847-843-2020
E-mail: info@preventblindness.org
http://www.preventblindness.org/

Shriner's Hospitals for Crippled Children
2900 Rocky Point Drive
Tampa, FL 33607
813-281-0300
Fax: 813-281-8113
http://shriners.com/hospitals/index.html

Sickle Cell Disease Association of America
4601 Market Street
Philadelphia, PA 19139
215-471-8686
Fax: 215-471-7441
http://www.sickle.qpg.com/

Sudden Infant Death Syndrome Alliance
1314 Bedford Avenue, Suite 210
Baltimore, MD 21208
410-653-8226
Fax: 410-653-8709

The Society for Ambulatory Care Professionals
(SACP)
One N Franklin
Chicago, IL 60606
312-422-3900
Fax: 312-422-4577
E-mail: sacpinfo@aha.org
http://www.sacp-net.org/

United Cerebral Palsy Associations
1660 L Street NW, Suite 700
Washington, DC 20036
800-872-5827
Fax: 800-776-0414
E-mail: ucpnatl@ucpa.org
http://www.ucpa.org/

United Ostomy Association
19772 MacArthur Boulevard
Suite 200
Irvine, CA 92612-2405
800-826-0826
714-660-8624
Fax: 714-660-9262
E-mail: uoa@deltanet.com
http://www.uoa.org/

The Wound Care Institute, Inc.
1541 NE 167th Street
North Miami Beach, FL 33162
305-919-9192
Fax: 305-944-6260
E-mail: Tamara@Woundcare.org
WCI is a tax exempt, non-profit organization
involved in the advancement of wound healing
and diabetic foot care.
http://woundcare.org/

CARING FOR FAMILIES IN THE HOME

Ruth Launius Jenkins

Home care nurses will encounter a variety of families who experience many different kinds of health care concerns at home. Traumatic injury, chronic illness, use of home medical equipment and advancing social technologies, environmental concerns, child rearing, dependent elders or a sick elderly member living alone, abuse and neglect, death and dying, and relational and financial concerns are just a few of the issues that families face at home. In addition, nurses involved in home care know that family dynamics may have either a positive or negative influence in care planning. Hence, the question arises, "How do nurses care for families at home?" Specifically, "What are important nursing interventions in family-focused care?" Moreover, "How should goals or outcomes of care be determined for families, who may become patients' primary caregivers at home and in many respects assume the persona of "patients' themselves?"

The purpose of this chapter is to address these questions and to enhance home care nurses' awareness of family dynamics as a means to improve care planning. Nursing interventions for family-focused care are provided. Communication strategies for fostering family decision making and home independence are offered. Because an extensive analysis of family dynamics and care is beyond the scope of a single chapter, references are provided for further information on family-focused care.

DEFINITION OF FAMILY

Definitions of "family" reflect our ever-changing society. The traditional definition of a family is father, mother, and children (nuclear family). However, home care nurses should be aware that family can also mean cohabitation; single-parent families; reconstituted or stepfamilies; extended families, which include any number and types of lineal or collateral relatives; and alternative structures, such as communal or same sex families.

For the purposes of this chapter the family will be referred to as the family unit. A broad definition of a family unit is a group of people living together or in close contact who take care of one another and who provide care, support, nurturing, and guidance for their dependent members and each other.[6,9,22] Of note, *the family unit is whatever the patient considers it to be.* The family unit can be viewed as functioning to support developmental and life changes in its members from birth until death.[10,19,23]

When defining family, home care nurses should identify key member(s) or the family spokesperson, who is often the person that will be primarily responsible for the care of the patient.[4,7,12,13] This family spokesperson is critical in assisting the home care nurse to work with the rest of the family, as well as to direct specifics of patient care at home after the nurse has left. Therefore in defining family it is also important to identify key family leaders or caregivers and to begin caring strategies with them, as well as with the patient. This is particularly true if the patient has limited ability to care for his or her self at home.

PHILOSOPHICAL PERSPECTIVES OF FAMILY-FOCUSED CARE

When I reflect on my own experiences in home care, I am reminded of the powerful task it is for the home care nurse to come to know the patient and the family when care planning. The burden of 24-hour care, once known only to the hospital nurse, is now transferred to a family member, who frequently will not be prepared for the responsibility of caregiving and decision making. For the home care nurse to be effective, he or she must empower patients with abilities for self-care and the confidence to make decisions (Box 4-1). To do this the nurse must learn a great deal about the family's group dynamics in a short period of time. I'm reminded of a passage from W. Somerset Maugham's, *The Razor's Edge,*[18] that for me expresses so clearly what nurses must recognize when giving the totality of professional care in what frequently seems like six home visits or less.

It is difficult to know people and countrymen. For men and women are not only themselves; they are also the region in which they were born, the city apartment or the farm in which they learnt to walk, the games they played as children, the old wives' tales they overheard, the food they ate, the schools they attended, the sports they followed, the poets they read, and the God they believed in. It is all these things that have made them what they are, and these are the things that you can't come to know by hearsay, you can only know them if you have lived them. You can only know them if you are them.

When applied to home care, Maugham's passage represents core elements (e.g., person, family, and environment) that must be assessed by the home care nurse when caring for families. Hence, whereas the standard home care nursing assessment will diagnose patient needs, the essence of family-focused care is best understood within the theoretical framework of systems theory.

Box 4-1   GOALS OF FAMILY-FOCUSED CARE

Be empowered for self-care.
Recognize that the illness affects all family members.
Define the problem(s) and identify the solution(s).
Mutually plan care as a priority; have alternate plans.
Improve confidence in decision making.
Participate in positive self-care activities.
Utilize available community resources for care.
Achieve maximal balance and home independence.
Evaluate progress and modify behaviors as needed.

Systems theory: a theoretical approach to family-focused care

Systems theory provides a means by which the dynamics of family interaction may be organized and assessed in the home care setting. When applying a systems theory approach, nursing practice in home care reflects constant interaction between the nurse, the environment in which care is provided, and the person (either patient or family unit who receives care).[5] The nursing focus of such interaction is to help the patient and family unit achieve optimal health and increased independence with self-care (see Chapter 2).

Systems theory overview. Von Bertalanffy and others originally introduced general system theory (GST) as a means of understanding and explaining human biological processes.[28] Systems theory offers a basic theoretical framework that emphasizes a holistic worldview and can provide direction for the implementation of a wellness-oriented approach to health care.[21,24,28] Conceptual categories in systems theory, which are of particular interest in the study of families, include *system structure,* referring to family organization and the pattern of relationships and *system functions* or *control,* referring to the purposes or goals of the family unit as a system. System functions may also be defined as the result or outcome of the structure. Key concepts for system structure (family-unit organization) are wholeness, boundaries, and hierarchies. Key concepts for system function (family-unit defined goals or health outcomes) include resources, energy, feedback (input, process, output), and homeostasis.[2,3]

Home care nurses should meld these points of view and construct care for family units that help adjust a family dynamic that may be unbalanced by illness or other stressors. The goal of such interventions is to help family units to define the problems they face and identify their own solutions. In this process, home care nurses offer their perspectives in family decision making through listening, asking questions, redirecting, and guiding patterns of helpful interactions.[26,30]

System structure (family-unit organization). In systems theory, *structure* refers to the parts that make up the whole system, which include subunits. The system in this case is the family (persons); the subunits are the individual members of the family. Subsystems can also include the spouse/significant other, parent/child, sibling/sibling or other internal or extended family member subsystems. Nurses should recognize that there is a family perceived hierarchy of interaction between these subsystems, with movement often going from the top down. For example, in the family it is customary for the parents to be in charge of the sibling subunits; sometimes older siblings may be in charge of younger siblings. The direction of responsibility or communication moves downward from those who are in charge to those who are not in charge of a particular situation. This concept does not necessarily always identify the person who will be responsible for the sick family member; that person may be an elder member outside of the family unit, thus the downward direction comes from another interaction within the family. Any unit outside of the family is called the *suprasystem,* which reflects environmental influences on the family. Suprasystems include sociocultural groups and other agencies with which the family member might have interaction with. They are also viewed as fixed constraints (e.g., the law, church, and schools) that have a definite impact on the health of the family.[2,11,15,24] There are invisible permeable boundaries that separate the family system from these suprasystems. The family unit will set the limits of those boundaries.

Systems function (family-unit defined goals or outcomes of care). Systems theory concepts that are used in analyzing family control or functions include allocation of resources; feedback (defined as some form of energy); and adaptations leading to homeostasis, self-regulation or equilibrium, and self-care. Differentiation is viewed as the family's capability and willingness to advance progressively and serially to a higher order of complexity and organization. In social terms the family unit has a tendency to grow, which is counterbalanced by a tendency to stabilize. Change is necessary for a system to grow or differentiate, using energy units such as information or knowledge.[8,24]

Feedback is the process by which the family system monitors the internal and external environmental responses to its behavior. *Input* refers to things such as energy, matter, or information that the family unit receives and processes. Each member of the family-unit subsets will process and transform the energy or information differently. Some input is used immediately, through the concepts of flow and transformation. Whatever the degree of process, the family unit as a system will demonstrate output and outcome in the form of *behavior.* Of consequence, the family is seen to adjust itself and is in some way changed. Finally, the subsystems are modified as these adjustments occur. In this process the family unit continually adapts to feedback from the outer environment. Adaptation takes one of two forms: (1) acceptance or rejection of incoming information without change, or (2) accommodation, in which a modification response changes the family unit and its structure and, thus, its function. This change is achieved by the family unit's intrinsic need as a system to achieve balance and self-regulation. When the system is in balance, there is homeostasis, steady state, or equilibrium. At this point positive family self-care activities can occur. Home care nurses should be aware that this balance is dynamic, always changing, and never static.[2,3]

The home care nurse can qualitatively assess family-unit adaptation by assessing the input/output feedback loop and by determining the state of family equilibrium. It may take time to evaluate family-unit growth and behavioral change because numerous family members may be involved in this process. However, even small changes are good.

Once a trusting relationship has been established, the home care nurse can begin to instill in the family unit the self-confidence to believe that they can meet the challenges of lay home care. Clearly, no one can make another person change. The home care nurse should assess family-unit interaction and ask, "Of the things we can to do together to take care of the sick family member, which one will you choose now?" This assisted decision-making approach ultimately encourages responsibility for decision making with the family unit, which, by virtue of the nature of home care itself, is where it should be.

In its simplest terms, systems theory shows that a system is greater than the sum of its parts. This is called *synergy* or *nonsummativity.* It means that family relationships are the catalyst to change, as well as being the most empowering and the most unifying aspects of working with families. The essence of synergy is to value family differences, to build on family strengths, and to compensate for family weaknesses. Through this process the nurse helps to create an environment that nurtures the self-esteem of each member of the family unit and creates opportunities for them to achieve a maximal degree of independence in managing their health care needs at home. This process will require not only enormous personal security and openness on the part of nurse and family but also a spirit of adventure and a sense of maturity and stability to successfully work together.[7,24]

HOME CARE APPLICATIONS
Nursing interventions

Assessing the family-unit and pertinent relationships. The first step in understanding family interactions, roles, and conflicts is to identify the primary family members or significant others who can be possible sources of assistance with the health care problem. The genogram is a means to chart the family system structure.[30] The skeleton of the genogram follows conventional genetic and genealogical charts (Figure 4-1). The focus is on the family unit in need of health care; the significant adult pair in the home is considered the *primary system;* other family members are considered the *subunits.* Typically the genogram depicts three generations of the family on horizontal lines, with children depicted on vertical lines. For example, the family unit is outlined on the middle horizontal line, with their grandparents on the top horizontal line. The children, ranked left to right and beginning with the eldest child, are on vertical lines that connect children from both generations to the family unit.

This picture can be easily drawn on a sheet of plain paper. Assessment interview data such as birth dates; marriage or commitment date; death; separation and/or divorce dates; pregnancies, miscarriages or abortions, or adoptions; health/illness history for each family member; and occupations or current activity status can be added to the diagram. During the interview, the patient or family unit may offer descriptive statements that can give insights into interpersonal relations or perceptions about individuals in the household.[4,17,27] Home care nurses should be aware that these statements are often emotional or value laden and provide clues to household interaction and power.

Authors differ slightly in the symbols used to denote the details of the genogram.[30] Generally, a square depicts a male and a circle represents a female. Miscarriage or abortion is denoted by a triangle, which includes the sex of the child if known. Separation is denoted by a single slash mark on the line connecting partners; a double slash mark denotes divorce but is also used to signify an adoption. The same data are collected on stepfamilies, with the exception of the depth of health/illness history, unless there are genetic factors in the offspring that require attention.

Home care nurses should assess who currently lives in the house and the location of extended family members. This data will assist in determining who is available to help care for the patient. In a health care milieu of early discharge, the patient is often too sick to provide his or her own care. If the patient is elderly, he or she may live alone and rely heavily on the community for health care needs, or his or her partner may be similarly disabled and have limited ability to care for the patient. Frequently the interview process and creation of the picture can help the patient and nurse identify possible resources for assistance. Moreover, the completed genogram allows the home care nurse to assess the family dynamic through the identification of the family unit and subunits, boundaries, and family hierarchy.

The genogram can also be used to assess family-unit role function. *Role* is referred to as a more or less homogeneous set of behaviors that are normatively defined and expected of a person in a given

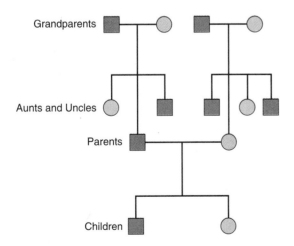

Figure 4-1 Genogram: typical nuclear family.

social setting or position. Individuals occupy multiple positions or statuses in the family. Therefore the terms *role behavior, performance,* or *enactment* are used interchangeably, since all are used to describe what a person actually does within a defined position.[16] Roles can also be culturally defined.

Since individuals maintain many roles in the family unit, there are different expectations for the various roles. The greater the degree of role enactment and role expectation, the greater the role stress or conflict, which leads to ambiguity. Knowing what role individuals perform in the family unit is essential for the home care nurse to assess for care planning. Typically the home care nurse can assess the degree of involvement of family-unit caregiver roles in such areas as financial contribution, housekeeping, childcare, child socialization, recreation, kinship (maintaining contact with family members), and therapeutic administration (meeting family member affective needs). When a family member becomes ill, role functions change. This introduces a greater chance for role stress, strain, and conflict to develop. In this case the home care nurse's responsibility may include assisting a family member to train for a caregiver role such as learning wound care or providing support as family members learn how to cope with role transitions.[1,11,14]

Assessing suprasystem support groups. As stated previously, groups or systems outside the family are referred to as the suprasystem. For the most part, the family interaction with these suprasystems may not have a daily impact on the existing home care situation. However, there is an implied influence on the resources available to the family through these suprasystems.

An ecomap may provide a clearer picture of the family unit's connection to and interaction with the greater environment of community. Ecomaps also assist in identifying community resources available to the family unit. Similar to the genogram, the primary value of the ecomap is in its visual impact[30] (Figure 4-2). The ecomap provides an overview of the family situation, including important sources of nurturing or conflict-laden connections between the family and the environment. It demonstrates the flow of resources, as well as resource deprivations. A resource is any form of support, including knowledge, money, or materials. This mapping procedure helps to highlight the

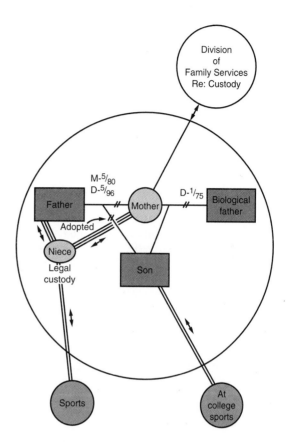

Figure 4-2 Ecomap: blended family.

nature of the interfaces between the family unit and community and points to conflicts, as well as resources to be sought.

The family-unit genogram is placed in the center of a plain sheet of paper. Circles are placed outside the family to represent people, agencies, and institutions with which the family interacts, including the extended family, work, church, and the health care system. Straight lines indicate strong connections, dotted lines indicate tenuous connections, and slashed lines indicate stressful relations. The wider the line, the stronger the tie. Arrows can be drawn alongside the lines to indicate the flow of energy and resources.[30] This picture helps the family unit gain insight into the use of energy, resources, and the type of interactions that dominate the family.[27] The ecomap can be used to increase the home care nurse's awareness of the whole family and the family unit's interaction within the larger system.[14,20,27]

The interactions of the family unit with subsystems and the greater suprasystems can create stress for the family. For example, stressed sibling subsystems may skip school, break the law by speeding, or exhibit other acting-out behavior, forcing the family to deal with these suprasystems in a way different from that in nonstressed times (e.g., law enforcement). These interactions may affect the patient's health state and require nursing intervention. In addition, the home care nurse may have to consider alternate methods of handling the family unit's health care needs, based on the suprasystem involved.

Assessing energy, information, and boundaries. An interaction system can be open or closed, which is defined by the ways in which energy flows within and through boundaries. An open system exchanges energy and matter (information) with the environment and evolves toward greater order and increased complexity, which is called *negentropy*.[2] An open system is characterized by major developmental ability. A closed system is isolated from the environment and moves toward increasing disorder and disintegration, which is called *entropy*. An open system is able to maintain a steady state by several different means of interaction.

The home care nurse will have to identify the sources of energy within the family in order to meet the health care needs of the sick member. The function of the permeable boundary, which is invisible, is to actively expand and retract, thus regulating the amount of input from the environment and output back to the environment that is allowed by the family unit. This is done to cope with stressors and achieve adaptation. In other words, input is screened so that the family can take in what is needed to promote its own survival. Open systems provide for change. An open system offers choices to successfully meet the challenges of reality. However, home care nurses should recognize that indiscriminately open families tend to become disorganized and chaotic as a result of receiving too much information. It is also important to note that the nature of the boundary depends on the family's usual ways of functioning.[8,24] Some topics may engender very closed boundaries with little information allowed in or out, whereas other topics are very open and debatable.

A closed system depends on edict and law and order and operates through the application of physical and/or psychological force. Closed family systems view change as threatening and resist it. Little information is taken from or given back to the environment.[2] People are perceived as evil or not to be trusted. Territoriality, self-protection, extreme privacy, secretiveness, scrutiny of strangers, and parental control behaviors that seem in excess of normal cautions can be observed in closed boundaries.[11] These families are rigid, and relationships are regulated by force. Control of family matters is not relinquished to outsiders or to anyone within the family unit who is not specifically assigned to a responsibility. In this case the family unit may exhibit dysfunctional behaviors.

Smilkstein's Family APGAR assessment is one means of measuring family dysfunction[25] (Box 4-2). APGAR consists of five statements about family interaction. The response choices are: "almost always" (2 points), "some of the time" (1 point), and "hardly ever" (0 points). The scores for each of the five answers are totaled. A score of 7 to 10 points suggests a highly functional family. A score of 4 to 6 points suggests a moderately dysfunctional family. A score of 0 to 3 points suggests a severely dysfunctional family.

The five statements are as follows:

1. I am satisfied with the help that I receive from my family* when something is troubling me.
2. I am satisfied with the way my family* discusses items of common interest and shares problem solving.
3. I find that my family* accepts my wishes to take on new activities or make changes in my lifestyle.
4. I am satisfied with the way my family* expresses affection and responds to my feelings such anger, sorrow, and love.
5. I am satisfied with the amount of time my family* and I spend together.

Extreme rigidity in families limits the resources made available to the family unit. Members may be deprived of necessary information and support, as well as basic physical resources. In this situation the home care nurse may have to take on a patient

---

*According to which member of the family is being interviewed, the interviewer may substitute for the word "family" either spouse, significant other, parents, or children.

Box 4-2	COMPONENTS AND DEFINITIONS OF FAMILY APGAR
Adaptation	Use of intrafamilial and extrafamilial resources for problem solving when family equilibrium is under stress
Partnership	Sharing of decision making and nurturing responsibilities by family members
Growth	Physical and emotional maturation and self-fulfillment achieved by family members through mutual support and guidance
Affection	Caring or loving relationship among family members
Resolve	Commitment to devote time to other members of the family for physical and emotional nurturing; also usually involves a decision to share wealth and space

advocacy role as a means to ensure that the patient's needs are met in caring and ethical ways (see Chapter 8).

Using emphatic communication

Seek first to understand, then to be understood. Principles of interpersonal relations have long been taught as an effective nursing assessment technique. However, if a nursing communication "technique," is sensed by the family unit as duplicity or manipulation, nothing will be achieved.[7]

Empathetic listening involves a philosophical mindset to "hear" the other. The home care nurse must listen without the intent to answer or to filter everything through his or her own perspectives. It is important for the nurse to avoid perceiving the patient's experience through the nurse's frame of reference. Instead, the nurse must deeply understand the patient's frame of reference, see the world through the patient's eyes, and understand how the patient feels. In contrast to sympathy, which can be viewed as a form of agreement, empathetic listening requires the home care nurse to know the patient and the family unit both intellectually and emotionally.

Home care nurses can assess their own empathic communication by checking their language, per-

sonal feelings, and body position. In empathetic listening, you listen not only with your ears but also with your eyes and with your heart. You listen for feeling, meaning, and behavior. You sense, you intuit, and you feel. Empathetic listening is a powerful tool that gives home care nurses accurate data with which to work. Instead of projecting their own life experiences, nurses acknowledge the realities of the other person and strive to understand what is in the patient's head and heart.

Applying this basic communication principle, home care nurses can effectively identify the patient's need and assist with problem resolution. However, it is important to note that patient motivation does not flow from satisfied needs but from those that are unsatisfied. Nurses should recognize that next to physical survival, the greatest need of a human being is psychological survival: to be understood, to be affirmed, to be validated, and to be appreciated.[7] Home care nurses must determine those unsatisfied needs in a very short time and move the patient and the family unit toward their own healing path. For the nurse the goal is to facilitate positive patient and family-unit self-care activities so that optimal health and home independence can be achieved.

Begin with the end in mind. What does the outcome look like for the family unit as a result of nursing care? The home care nurse leads the family unit in change activities, but the family unit must take ownership of the change activities. Such an approach leads to better health habits for wellness because it positions the family unit to learn to manage their lives in healthy ways. Hence families should be encouraged to think about necessary changes that will help them achieve their needs. Thus the nurse must seek to first understand the family unit's interpretation of the problem, and the family must understand the need for change and how that change will take place. The change has to be within the conceptual abilities of the patient and family unit. Thus both should be encouraged to create an image or picture of what it is they need to change and how that change will look once it is completed.[7] Moreover, home care nurses should reinforce that it is not enough to picture the outcome; rather, it is necessary to daily visualize and practice the behaviors in order to become that image. This perspective has to be one the patient and family unit can visualize, as guided by the home care nurse. Home care nurses should be aware that when you begin with the end in mind, you gain a different perspective. For the family unit, this represents a form of expanding consciousness or new awareness.

People routinely worry over past situations, as well as current situations over which they have no control. Time and imagination spent worrying can be channeled into positive activities such as building a new response, forming a new picture, and new self-care planning for health. Teaching relaxation techniques to the patient and family unit may be useful here. Complementary therapies may also be tried (see Chapter 28). Although some may not be receptive to what may sound like "new age" care, simple deep breathing can take the edge off of stress and gives everyone a moment to refocus on the task at hand. The patient and family unit must be guided from the tendency to live in the past to a perspective wherein new values and new plans can provide limitless potential.[7]

Put first things first. Putting first things first refers to the day-to-day management of life and time and to those things that must be done to achieve desired health outcomes. They represent activities that empower the family unit to use self-awareness. Empowerment comes from learning how to use imagination and strong independent will to make everyday decisions. A patient-centered plan is put into place, and the patient answers the question, "What one thing could I do that, if done on a regular basis, would make a positive difference in my life?"

The key to success is not to prioritize the change in health behavior but to schedule the change in behavior as a priority. This priority should have flexibility so that it is not an all-or-nothing event. For example, if there is an interference with a scheduled activity, then there should also be an alternate plan for the activity. Owning the responsibility of the health change is referred to as *stewardship delegation,* which involves making the patient and family unit responsible for their own outcomes.

Stewardship delegation involves clear, up-front family understanding and commitment regarding expectations in five areas as follows:

Desired results. Create a clear understanding of what should be accomplished, focusing on "what" not "how," and "results," not "methods." Clearly state how the results will be measured and when they will be accomplished.

Guidelines. Identify the parameters within which the patient should operate. There should be as few guidelines as possible to avoid the sense of delegating a method and to avoid overload.

Resources. Identify the human, financial, technical, or organizational resources on which the person can draw to accomplish the desired results.

Accountability. Set up the standards of performance that will be used to evaluate the results and the specific times when reporting and evaluation will take place.

Consequences. Specify what will happen, both good and bad, as a result of the performance or lack of performance.[7]

Providing culturally sensitive family care. The human experience within the broader context of the sociocultural milieu in which the family unit resides cannot be overlooked. *Culture* refers to existing and operating values, conceptions, norms, targets, and expectations in society that are collectively shared by people. The home care nurse should ask, "What, if any, are cultural influences on this particular family unit's health condition, and what accommodations do I need to make in order to create an effective plan of care?"

Lafaille reminds us that the relationship between culture and its affects on the health of the individuals in the family unit is significant.[16] The relationship between culture on the one hand and health and illness on the other is complex and multidimensional. Cultural influences the family unit's definitions of health and illness, as well as the life situations in which these terms are applied.

Home care nurses should be aware that the concept of what is "normal" varies not only with different cultures but also within the same culture over the course of time. The nurse must assess families within a cultural context. What is considered to be a symptom; how pain or symptoms are communicated; beliefs about illness that affect wellness; attitudes about receiving help from nurses, doctors and other professionals; and what treatment is desired or expected all carry cultural overtones.

Each cultural group's way of relating to an illness and therapy situation may reflect different attitudes toward family, group identity, and outsiders. Home care nurses should be sensitive to these cultural differences and may find that a systems theory approach will help them to discovery boundaries of which they were not previously aware (see Chapter 7).

Assisting decision making for families. Earlier we noted that empathetic listening is risky. It takes a great deal of security to go into a deep listening experience because you open yourself up—you become vulnerable. It is a paradox, in a sense, because in order to have influence you have to be influenced and you have to really understand.[7] The following counseling technique developed by the author, called *ENUFF* (empathetic, nonjudgmental, unconditional, feeling focus), can be used when the family is having trouble moving toward productive behavior.[15] It is especially helpful to assist family units identify and solve their own problems.

The ENUFF process depends as much on the behavior and demeanor of the home care nurse as it does on the family's ability to identify solutions to health-related plans of care. The nurse must assume an empathetic attitude, allowing the other persons to grow emotionally and psychologically. The nurse must feel a deep respect for the significance and worth of the other persons in order to be empathetic.[15]

The home care nurse must not judge the behavior or action of the family unit but rather accept them for who they are. This constitutes the nonjudgmental focus of the intervention. The nurse will have feelings about the family's action or lack thereof, but those feelings must not be acted on during the ENUFF process.

The term "unconditional" suggests that the nurse does not expect the family members to behave in any preconceived manner.[29] Feelings, behaviors, and reactions will be accepted at face value. To place a condition on the family's acceptance is to impose the nurse's own attitudes and belief system. This will not promote growth during a stressful event. Unconditional acceptance means saying to yourself, "The family unit is demonstrating *a*, *b*, or *c* behavior at this time, and that is just the way it is."

The *feeling focus* refers to the home care nurse's ability to identify and validate what the family is feeling about the change or health problem event. The focus of the process, the intervention, leads the patient and family unit to explore feelings in the communication session. To validate feelings is to allow their expression and thus to explore what they mean to the family unit.

The sequence of ENUFF actions is outlined in Table 4-1. The home care nurse assumes an open, caring attitude that is free of judgment and is focused without becoming distracted and without breaking eye contact. The nurse must feel for the family's struggle and express empathy through a quiet, concerned, and caring voice. The nurse should make no assumption about who the individuals are or what the individuals feel, think, believe, or want. The family unit may not be able to articulate the need, the action, the direction, or the solution at the beginning of the process, but the nurse's unconditional support will allow the family unit to find a workable solution.

The home care nurse should offer no advice at this stage. If the family's feelings are obvious, the nurse should simply and empathetically state, "You

Table 4-1 Key nursing actions in the ENUFF process

Principles	Behaviors
Offer no opinions and no advice.	Use active listening skills.
Identify feelings.	Have open body language.
Validate feelings.	Maintain good eye contact.
Ask:	Give uninterrupted attention.
Is there anything else?	Listen for unspoken needs.
Tell me more.	
What do you want?	Use facial expressions that communicate "I care."
How can that be done?	Talk softly; use a firm voice.
Press on:	Put the plan in writing.
Which would work for you?	
Which will you do?	
Offer:	
How can I help?	
Make a contract.	
State specifically:	
Who?	
What?	
When?	
Where?	
How?	
Follow up without fail.	

are really frustrated." If the feelings are not obvious, the most helpful and leading statements are: "You really have strong feelings about that. Tell me about it." This allows family members to say what they are ready to share. Identifying the emotional state is finding the feeling focus. Expressing the emotion aloud validates each individual's feelings. Moreover, it allows the feelings and begins the process of family problem solving.

Further validation of the feeling focus is necessary to make the family unit comfortable about reacting to the stress/illness event. The home care nurse might say, "That must be very difficult for you," or "I had no idea; no wonder you feel so strongly about this." Any reasonable, supportive remark is appropriate, as long as it validates the family unit's feelings. When it seems that the family unit knows that these feelings have been accepted, the nurse should ask whether they want to say anything else about the situation.

The next step is to find a solution for the problem. Ask the family unit what they want to do, to happen, to feel, or to change. In this step, both patient and family unit identifies what should be done. The nurse does not have to make suggestions and must not offer possible solutions. At this point, allow the family unit to explore any number of possible options. Some of the options will not work for a variety of reasons; for example, the option may not be a possible therapeutic outcome. Nonetheless, it is not necessary to point out nonrational ideas. The family unit may still be reacting on the emotional level, without thinking through real solutions. If the family unit has difficulty identifying solutions, ask how many ways there may be to face, change, alter, affect, or resolve the situation. Give the family unit the opportunity to find their own solutions.

Next, write down the suggestions given and then ask, "Which one or ones will you really do?" At this point the intervention may become confrontational because the family unit may feel pushed to come up with a solution. Again, the nurse should have no input into the solution, except to explore the viability of the suggested plan and to determine how it can be implemented. The family unit should think through each of the options and decide which ones are worth acting on.

The home care nurse should then ask, "How can I help?" At this point the nurse becomes involved in the solution. A plan of action is now initiated.

Both parties will provide input and accept responsibility for the solution. However, the family unit must define the what, when, where, how, and who of problem resolution. If the home care nurse knows of factors that may impede the solution, it is important to ask again, "Do you really think that will work?" At this point it is important to have the family unit think and talk things through again and then suggest a different plan.

Finally, it is best to create a written contract about what will be done, which can resemble the format of a care plan. Make the contract measurable in terms of timeframes, with positive steps to be taken toward the anticipated outcomes. The contract should include a follow-up date and time to assess whether the actions have been effective. Follow-up is essential; without it, the trust developed between the home care nurse and the family unit may be lost.[15]

SUMMARY

Health care costs continue to rise, resulting in shorter hospital stays and increased demand for community-based health care. As the "Baby Boom" generation retires, demands on the home care system will rise exponentially. A holistic approach to home care that addresses patient and family health care needs reflects the realities of home care nursing practice. Families can represent an invaluable resource to home care nurses. Mining this largely underused resource can help us provide home care in our new century and in the centuries yet to come.

REFERENCES

1. Altschuler J: Family relationships during serious illness, *Nurs Times* 12(93),48, 1997.
2. Barry P: General systems theory applied to individual and family coping responses. In Barry P, editor: *Psychosocial nursing: care of physically ill patients and their families,* ed 3, Philadelphia, 1996, Lippincott-Raven.
3. Batalden PB, Mohr JJ: Building knowledge of health care as a system, *Quality Manage Health Care* 5(3):1, 1997.
4. Beckman JF and others: A systems model of health care: a proposal, *J Manipulative and Physiolog Therapeutics* 19(3):208, 1996.
5. Chinn PL, Kramer MK: *Theory and nursing integrated knowledge development,* St. Louis, 1999, Mosby.
6. Cohen S, Syme S: Issues in the study and application of social support. In Cohen S, Syme S, editors: *Social support and health,* New York, 1985, Academic Press.
7. Covey SR: *The 7 habits of highly effective people: powerful lessons in personal change,* New York, 1990, Fireside.

8. Dahl RW: Creating the environment necessary to ensure quality patient care in the community setting, *Semin Nurse Manage* 3(3):146, 1995.

9. Dunst C and others: Family support scale: reliability and validity, *J Individual Fam Community Wellness* 1:45, 1984.

10. Duvall EM: *Marriage and family relationships,* ed 5, Philadelphia, 1977, Lippincott.

11. Friedman MM: *Family nursing research, theory and practice,* Stamford, Conn, 1998, Appleton & Lange.

12. Gelmon SB and others: Formulating the mess: lessons from "building knowledge of health care as a system," *Quality Manage Health Care* 5(3):13, 1997.

13. Goodman RM: Principles and tools for evaluating community-based prevention and health promotion programs, *J Pub Health Manage Prac* 4(2):37, 1998.

14. Holkup PA: Our parents, our children, ourselves: a therapy group to facilitate understanding of intergenerational behavior patterns and to promote family healing, *J Psychosoc Nurs* 36(2):20, 1998.

15. Jenkins RL: Effective motivation: empowerment through empathy. In Simendinger EA and others, editors: *The successful nurse executive: a guide for every nurse manager,* Ann Arbor, Mich, 1990, Health Administration Press.

16. Lafaille R: Towards the foundation of a new science of health. In Lafaille R, Fulder S, editors: *Towards a new science of health,* New York, 1993, Routledge.

17. MacPhee M: The family systems approach and pediatric nursing care, *Pediatr Nurs* 21(5):417, 1995.

18. Maugham WS: *The razor's edge,* Great Britain: Coy Wyman, 1944, Reading Penguin Books.

19. McCubbin HI and others: *Family assessment: resiliency, coping and adaptation inventories for research and practice,* Madison, Wisc, 1996, University of Wisconsin.

20. Nelson DB, Edgil AE: Family dynamics in families with very low birth weight and full term infants: a pilot study, *J Pediatr Nurs* 13(2):95, 1998.

21. Nicholas DR, Gobble DC: Worldviews, systems theory and health promotion, *Am J Health Promotion* 6:30, 1991.

22. Oritt E and others: The perceived support network inventory, *Am J Community Psychol* 13(5):565, 1985.

23. Patterson J, McCubbin H: Chronic illness: family stress and coping. In Figley C, McCubbin H, editors: *Stress and the family: vol II, coping with catastrophe,* New York, 1983, Brunner-Mazel.

24. Seigfried RJ: Systems coherence: a method for evolving relationships and measuring system change, *Quality Manage Health Care* 7(1):29, 1998.

25. Smilkstein G: Assessment of family function. In Rosen G and others, editors: *Behavioral science in family practice,* Greenwich, Conn, 1980, Apple-Century Crafts.

26. Speice J and others: In times of transition: an organizational change from a family systems perspective, *Health Care Manage Rev* 24(1):73, 1995.

27. Tsonides A: Family systems medicine: systemic-constructivist perspectives, *Counseling Psychology Q* 8(1):78, 1995.

28. Von Bertalanffy L and others: *General systems theory,* New York, 1971, Brazillier.

29. Weinert C: A social support measure: PRQ85, *Nurs Res* 36:273, 1987.

30. Wright LM, Leahey M: *Nurses and families: a guide to family assessment and intervention,* Philadelphia, 1994, FA Davis.

DEVELOPING THE PLAN OF CARE AND DOCUMENTATION

Robyn Rice

The complexities of managing patient care at home demand a scientific and caring approach. In the hands of knowledgeable and caring nurses, the nursing process provides an organized, step-by-step approach to patient care in the home. Moreover, it is a process that lends integrity and direction to professional home care nursing practice. Finally, precise documentation is a process that co-ordinates and evaluates multidisciplinary care.

The intent of this chapter is to help home care nurses develop a plan of care for their patients based on the nursing process. Steps in the nursing process and guidelines for writing outcomes of care are reviewed. Medicare regulations that influence home care clinical documentation guidelines are also discussed, along with tips for completing paperwork and using laptop computers.

PREPARING FOR THE HOME VISIT

After formal admission of the patient by a home care agency, the referral is sent to the patient service manager in the appropriate service area within the agency. Patient assignments are usually determined by where the patient lives (e.g., zip code) or by the patient's requirements for specialty services (e.g., intravenous therapy). The patient service manager reviews the referral information and then assigns the patient to a home care nurse or therapist.

Before the initial home visit the home care nurse should examine the information on the referral to determine the purpose of the visit. The patient's address and home telephone number, along with any specific orders, should be listed on the referral. It is advisable for the nurse to review the patient's medical record, if available, before the initial visit.

Initial preparation for care will focus on the medical diagnosis as identified by the referral. Once the nurse has assessed the patient and home, subsequent preparation will be directed toward both nursing and medical diagnoses. Nurses should use current research and professional literature, policy and procedure manuals, and resource individuals when preparing the plan of care.

A phone call to the patient is strongly recommended before making the visit. This allows the home care nurse an opportunity to give the patient an approximate time for the visit, to validate or clarify directions to the patient's house (maps should be available from the agency), to request that pets be restrained if necessary, and to inquire about any need for medical supplies. Most important, the phone call allows the home care nurse to begin to assess patient/caregiver needs in developing the plan of care (see Chapter 2). Once these activities have been completed, stocked nursing bags and any other needed supplies or forms should be obtained.

CONDUCTING THE HOME VISIT

Patients in home care are viewed in the context of their household and community. Home care nurses focus not only on patient health care needs but also on familial, sociocultural, economic, and environmental factors that may affect care.

Assessing phase

Data collected during the assessing phase are used to provide the physician with further guidelines for the plan of care and to develop the nursing care plan. At this point it is important to distinguish between the plan of care and the patient care plan. According to the *Health Insurance Manual,* Publication Number 11 (HIM-11), the plan of care (previously called the plan of treatment) is the medical treatment plan that is established by the treating physician.[4,5] In addition, Medicare expects that a discipline-oriented patient care plan be established, when appropriate, by a home care nurse regarding nursing and aide services and by skilled therapists regarding specific therapy treatment. Although under review and revision, Medicare states that these plans of care may be incorporated within the physician's plan of care on Medicare forms 485, 486, and 487 or prepared separately.[4,5] From a quality point of view, it is recommended that the patient care plan be done in the care path format.

A holistic approach in care plan development is recommended. Components of the assessing phase include (1) the initial telephone call, (2) the assessment interview, (3) the assembly of a historical database (including socioenvironmental and family assessment), (4) the nursing health history, (5) the medication assessment, (6) a nutritional assessment, and (7) the physical assessment (including spiritual, mental, and functional status, as well as specific disease or disability issues).

Initial phone call. The assessing phase of the patient begins with telephone contact. During this time the home care nurse receives feedback about the patient's situation and current health status. Most important, the phone call can be utilized to ask patients how they are doing. This information is invaluable when planning visits. It also prevents dramatic surprises when the home care nurse arrives at the patient's home.

Assessment interview. The assessing phase moves next to the initial formal assessment interview. The purpose of this interview is to collect data and obtain other information related to the patient's health.[8] Even though a printed form, checklist, or outline is usually followed, nurses should be receptive to all information offered by patients, families, or caregivers. The assessment interview primarily collects subjective data from the patient's responses to questions, but nonverbal cues should also be noted. The assessment interview is an important step in the establishment of nurse-patient-caregiver therapeutic relationships.

Historical database. An important element of the historical database is the socioenvironmental

assessment, which should present a clear picture of the patient at home in his or her community, including any safety or sanitary issues. In addition to identifying the patient's economic status and living conditions, the home care nurse should focus on factors such as the cooperation of the patient/caregiver regarding self-care issues and the availability of environmental and community resources needed to implement care (see Chapter 2).

In addition, a family assessment is also recommended in recognizing all support systems available to assist with patient care. Learning, communication, and coping styles of patients, families, and caregivers should be identified. Each person's role in the household should be considered when developing the plan of care. This is of particular importance when working with pediatric cases (see Chapter 4).

Nursing health history. The nursing health history deals with patients' responses to and perceptions of their health status. It focuses on patients' feelings regarding their need for health care and their expectations regarding this care. Clues to patients' abilities to deal with current health problems are sought. The nursing health history also helps to identify past patterns of health and illness, the presence of risk factors, and the availability of resources to the individual and family. Caregiver input may be sought to provide a complete picture of patient needs.

If a complete medical health history is not available, additional information should be sought. This additional information should include a description of the patient's present health status, past medical and surgical histories, family medical history, and a review of body systems. The review of body systems consists of the patient's responses to questions concerning each body system. It is not the same as the physical assessment, which seeks objective data.

Medication assessment. Information should be gathered about all prescription and nonprescription medications. Home care nurses should ask to see all of the patient's medicines, including over-the-counter medications. A complete medication assessment provides nurses with the opportunity to verify the name, dosage, and frequency of administration for each medicine. This can provide some invaluable insights as to the patient's learning needs (see Chapter 23). The purpose of the medicine, adverse reactions, allergies, side effects, therapeutic effects, and patient compliance with the medication regimen should be determined.

Medications should be reviewed on each visit to note changes in dose, frequency, or type. These findings should be prescribed by the physician in the patient's record. Consequently, changes in the medication regimen become a basis for new teaching. Always verify, document, and obtain written physician orders for any change in the patient's medication regimen because sometimes the physician's office will notify the patient of such changes but not the nurse.

Nutritional assessment. A nutritional screening can be used to assess patients at high risk for malnutrition.[10] Specifically, the nurse identifies any patient who may be at risk for developing protein-energy malnutrition or specific nutrient deficiencies, malnutrition-related complications, or adverse health reactions related to eating habits. In addition, the nurse assesses the adequacy of any nutritional therapies. A dietary history including eating habits and patient weight are some of the approaches to clinical assessment of the patient's nutritional status (see Appendix V-I).

Physical assessment. The physical assessment is another major source of information. It consists of an evaluation of the patient's health status through the use of the nurse's specially trained senses of sight, hearing, touch, and smell. Patients can be examined in a head-to-toe, systematic manner or according to body systems. Nurses should develop their own approach and should be ready to adapt their assessment skills to the particular patient.

The physical assessment should identify any functional limitations that the patient may experience when ambulating or performing activities of daily living (ADLs). For example, asking the patient to perform a simple activity such as walking or opening a jar may be all that is necessary to determine his or her functional ability.[7] This becomes a basis for a further evaluation by the rehabilitation therapists (see Chapter 17).

Spiritual and mental health assessment. The mental health assessment is typically performed in conjunction with the physical assessment (see Chapter 22). The database may also include a spiritual assessment (Figure 5-1). This will be especially important for hospice nurses because issues of hope and faith play a major role in patient care (see Chapter 24).

Initially, home care nurses should do a complete physical assessment. On later visits it may be necessary to assess only specific problem areas. Any changes noted in later assessments should be reflected in the chart. This serves to keep the database current.

In reporting assessment findings to the physician, home care nurses should primarily report deviations from the patient's baseline status. In home care it is not unusual to find patients with fluctuating vital signs or blood glucose levels. Many physicians, as they continue to adjust medical treatment, may feel it is unnecessary for the nurse to report this information after each visit. When in doubt, home care nurses should obtain written guidelines from the physician regarding when he or she wants to be notified of the patient's status. These guidelines should be placed in the medical record. Home care nurses should **never** hesitate to notify the physician of assessment findings or to send the patient to the emergency room for medical evaluation when their "gut feelings/common sense" tell them to do so.

Diagnosing phase

Once the assessment is completed, the nurse interprets the data and develops nursing diagnoses. A *nursing diagnosis* is a clear, concise statement of the patient's health status.[1] It reflects the patient's healthy and unhealthy response(s) and the supporting factor(s) for each response.

Nursing diagnoses commonly used in home care include knowledge deficit (identify subject), activity intolerance, and self-care deficit.[1] Of note, as documentation systems are moving toward multidisciplinary needs, many home care agencies are utilizing nursing diagnosis to coordinate multidisciplinary care (i.e., nursing diagnosis/identified patient problem).

Planning phase

Plan of care. Trends in health care, such as care paths, are merging nursing care plans with multidisciplinary needs. In addition, with increasing emphasis on patient participation in the plan of care, nursing care plans are now more commonly being referred to as *patient care plans.*

Patient care plan. The patient care plan is established by the home care nurse and the multidisciplinary team, which includes the physician. It reflects the medical treatment plan, interventions, projected outcomes of care, and long-term goals.

Hospice Spiritual Assessment   Client Name: _____

---

1. Client's current and past religious affiliation.

2. Clergy   Name: _____
            Address: _____ Phone: _____

3. What is the religious affiliation of immediate family members, significant other, or caretaker?

4. Which religious/spiritual practices are meaningful to the client (e.g., prayer, sacraments, rosary, Bible readings, hymns, yoga)?

5. Which aesthetic interests enhance the client's life (e.g., art, music, nature)?

6. Which relationships are most important and meaningful to the client?

7. Which holidays, family events, or rituals are significant to the client and family?

8. What are the client's sources of strength in life?

9. How does the client describe his/her life in relation to its meaning, successes, and joys?

10. Is the client at peace? If not, describe.

11. What meaning does pain/disease/terminal illness and death have for the client?

12. What does the client usually do to cope with fear/anger? Stress?

13. Are there relationships where forgiveness/reconciliation is sought?

14. What legacy or message would the client like to leave to others?

Signature: _____   Date: _____

S.M. Hatch/H.L.L.

Figure 5-1 Spiritual assessment. (Courtesy Suzanne Hatch, West Stockbridge, Mass.)

The plan has a specific aim or purpose regarding patient care. It is recorded to maximize quality patient care, to ensure appropriate utilization of resources, to evaluate the delivery of services, and can provide documentation to validate Medicare reimbursement of services.[5,9]

The first step in the planning phase is the establishment of priorities. The nurse, the multidisciplinary team, and patient/caregiver should work together to identify the immediate concerns and patient/caregiver needs. Nursing diagnoses are then derived and outcomes of care are mutually determined. Priorities are constantly changing. As the patient's medical condition changes, the "ranking" of the nursing diagnoses will also change.

Because visit frequency is often limited, home care nurses should plan patient care needs around basic "survival needs." The question to answer is, "What does this patient absolutely need during this visit to manage his or her care at home?" Providing for the patient's basic survival needs often includes teaching the patient when to call the physician, about medication, how to operate home medical equipment, and basic procedural care. Patient input should always be sought when planning and prioritizing patient health care needs and subsequent nursing interventions.

Outcomes of care. The next step in the planning phase is the identification of goals and outcomes of care. Goals and outcomes of patient care should reflect the nursing diagnosis and overall plan of care (POC). They give direction to nursing interventions and pace activities within the patient care plan.[2,6] Both should be written as patient-centered rather than nurse-centered statements. In other words, goals and outcomes of care should contain verbs that reflect responses to be observed in the patient, not activities to be performed by the nurse.

Goals are generalized long-term outcomes of care that should occur by discharge. Statements of long-term goals do not describe the exact process necessary to reach the goal. For example, "the patient's appetite will improve in 4 weeks" is a long-term, patient-centered goal.

Outcomes of care are precise and measurable. They reflect steps leading to the accomplishment of the long-term goal. For example, "the patient will eat 800 calories per day by the end of the week" is a short-term, patient-centered outcome of care. See Box 5-1 on writing outcomes of care. As with pri-

ority setting, patients should be involved in setting their own goals and outcomes of care.

Implementing phase

Once long- and short-term goals have been identified, home care nurses, in partnership with the patient/caregiver and multidisciplinary team, can identify specific interventions, actions, or therapies that will help patients achieve outcomes of care and goal resolution. Although directed by the physician and initiated by home care nurses, intervention within the patient's environment is, by nature, frequently improvisational. What works well for one patient may or may not work well for another. Therefore recommendations for care may be determined by trial and error.

Implementation of the patient care plan by home care nurses functioning in the role of case managers involves exchanging information with patients/caregivers, coordinating referrals, facilitating multidisciplinary conferences, and—as the patient's advocate—seeking resources within the community. Specific home care nursing interventions involve a great variety of procedural skills such as dressing changes, medication administration, intravenous therapy, and foley catheter changes.[4,5,8]

The implementing phase should integrate the plan of care and patient care plan into the patient's environment. Patients/caregivers are then able to take on the responsibilities for self-care management, which will involve learning, assessment, task achievement, evaluation, and personal decision making for best levels of health. They acquire knowledge, judgment, and confidence as home care nurses support and encourage this process. The following principles govern implementation of the patient care plan:

1. Formal guidelines as to what the nurse can and cannot do are determined by the home care agency's scope of services and its policies and procedures.
2. Implementation should be inclusive of the multidisciplinary team and patients/caregivers because all will participate in effecting the plan of care.
3. The relationship between home care nurses, physicians, the multidisciplinary team, and patients/caregivers should be a collaborative and

---

Box 5-1   WRITING OUTCOMES OF CARE TO DOCUMENT PATIENT/CAREGIVER RESPONSE TO THERAPY

Definition

Outcomes of care are objective measurements of the patient's health status to be achieved or worked toward during home care services. They represent a change in the patient's health status from one time frame to another. The main purpose in using outcomes is to guide planning, implementation, and evaluation of the plan of care (POC). Outcomes of care support discharge goals of care. In documenting patient/caregiver response to therapy, outcomes of care should:

1. State the expected behavioral performance.

   Specific performance verbs:

Write	Demonstrate
List	Explain
Cite	Utilize
Verbalize	Achieve
Accomplish	Identify
Perform	Assist

2. State the criteria or measurable level of performance specified. Criteria should include concepts such as amount and accuracy.

   Examples:

   "Patient cites correct medication regimen."

   "Patient identifies complications of disease process (e.g., on list in narrative of visit report, on POC, or on care path) to report to case manager or physician."

   "Patient achieves optimal response to the physical treatment plan as evidenced by wound healing."

   "Patient agrees to the plan of care by explaining treatment principles, use of multidisciplinary services, and estimated length of service(s) without the prompting of the nurse."

3. Reflect the treatment plan and identified primary nursing diagnoses/patient problems.

   Example:

   Medical treatment plan: Decubitus ulcer

   Standard of care: Skin/integumentary

   Primary nursing diagnoses/patient problems:

   Impaired skin integrity

   Impaired physical mobility

   Knowledge deficit: Disease process, risk complications, nutrition, procedural care, infection control, socioeconomic resources

4. Occur within an expected time frame. Set a specific date for outcome achievement.

5. Evaluate the POC using skilled observation, oral questioning, or written measurement. Did the patient's health improve? Were outcomes met? **Was there a positive change in patient behaviors enabling self-care management and promoting best level of function?** If not, why not? Outcomes that are not met should be coded as variances. Identify any variance(s) and determine a corrective plan of action with the physician, the multidisciplinary team, and patient.

Be aware that quality outcome measures are used to evaluate many aspects of service delivery (see Chapter 10).

---

cooperative one, based on a mutually derived plan of care.

4. Improvisation and individualization of interventions and outcomes of care are a fact of life when working in the home milieu.

5. Medicare regulations strongly influence documentation and services rendered and are the basis for reimbursement of Medicare-certified home care agencies.

Evaluating phase

Evaluation is the fifth step in the nursing process. Evaluation measures the effectiveness of medical treatment (nursing actions, as well as multidisciplinary care) and appropriate utilization of resources. It is the act of determining the patient's progress in meeting outcomes of care and achieving long-term goals.[2,9] Finally, it promotes accurate benchmarking for quality improvement (QI) processes (see Chapter 10).

Some patient care plan formats have preplanned outcomes of care based on major patient groups or related patient classification topology; they have been referred to as *care paths, critical pathways,* and *clinical pathways.* Chapter 9 discusses the uses of care paths as evaluation tools for case management. Once goals and outcomes of care are achieved or it has been determined that the patient no longer requires home care or is no longer appropriate for home care services, discharge from the agency occurs.

MEDICARE DOCUMENTATION GUIDELINES FOR REIMBURSEMENT OF HOME CARE SERVICES

Medicare, administered by the Health Care Financing Administration (HCFA), influences the financial operations of Medicare-certified home care agencies. The *Home Insurance Manual,* Publication Number 11 (HIM-11), and Federal Register identify conditions to be met for coverage of home health care services.[4,5] Designated fiscal intermediaries (FIs) throughout the United States are responsible for assuring HCFA that billing and subsequent Medicare payments are in accordance with these requirements.[11,12] Each FI provides a guideline manual explaining Medicare coverage and billing requirements. In addition, each state's Department of Health and Home Health Licensing Bureau regulates the delivery of services. These conditions periodically change pending federal and state review.

HCFA is currently examining ways in which to move home care reimbursement into a prospective payment system. This will influence guidelines and regulations for documenting home care services. The Center for Health Policy Research at the University of Colorado has developed outcome measures for home care.[13,14] The result is the Outcome and Assessment Information Set (OASIS). The purpose of this tool is to provide standardized guidelines for admission and care, as well as a national data base for evaluation, reimbursement, and quality improvement.[6,13,15] To receive reimbursement for services, all Medicare-certified home care

agencies must complete the OASIS instrument as part of the agency's comprehensive patient assessment and will be required to report the OASIS data to the agency's state agency, as well as utilize the information to improve patient outcomes.

Federal regulations for reimbursement of home care services will continue to change. To keep up with such change is beyond the scope of a book. The nurse and home care agency are expected to keep up with federal and state regulations in delivering reimbursement of services. The HCFA (http://www.hcfa.gov) and OASIS (http://www.hcfa.gov/medicare/hsqb/oasis/hhoview.htm) Internet websites may be a valuable resource in this process. At present, use HCFA forms 485, 486, 487 and UB92 for certification and billing of services. At present, to qualify for Medicare-reimbursed home care services the patient must:

1. Be under a physician's plan of care
2. Require the skilled services of a registered nurse, physical therapist, or speech language pathologist
3. Be expected to improve in a reasonable and predictable period of time
4. Be confined to home for medical or psychiatric reasons; before home care services may begin, the patient must understand and sign the following:
    a. Statement identifying and allowing the home care agency to provide services to the patient
    b. Statement identifying the payment source and defining any and all charges for which the patient is responsible
    c. Statement of the patient's rights

At present, the following conditions to be met for the coverage of home care services include but are not limited to:

1. The patient must be under a physician-certified plan of care, which must be periodically reviewed and signed for the duration of services; this is called the *certification period.* (Currently, certification periods are approximately 9 weeks or 62 days). A verbal physician order may precede a signed order. The case manager or patient's primary nurse/therapist must review and sign all oral orders, even though such orders were taken

and signed by other qualified personnel at the home care agency. Oral orders must be countersigned and dated by the physician before the home care agency bills for care.

2. Disciplines and services that are viewed as reasonable and necessary to treat and improve the patient's condition are documented on the HCFA forms 485 and 487.

3. Objective clinical evidence must support the patient's needs for intermittent skilled care. The need for management and evaluation of patient care, as well as procedural care (e.g., tube feedings, ostomy care, venipuncture), patient/caregiver teaching/training activities, and abnormal or fluctuating vital signs, symptoms of drug toxicity, changes in cardiopulmonary or mentation status, or changes in the medication regimen are conditions that validate the necessity for home care visits (see Box 5-2 and Chapter 7). Be aware that the intermediary will not reimburse home care services for the "chronically ill" yet "stable" patient. Documentation should clearly profile exacerbation of chronic disease or demonstrate patient health care needs for skilled home care services as described above (see Table 5-1).

4. Homebound status should be documented each visit. (Boxes 5-3 and 5-4). In addition, most states require that patients notify the home care agency of any homebound status change. Be aware that an individual does not have to be bedridden to be considered homebound. However, the condition of these patients should be such that a normal inability to leave the home exists and, consequently, that leaving the home would require a considerable and taxing effort. If the patient does leave the home, the patient may nevertheless be considered homebound if the absences from the home are infrequent or for periods of relatively short duration or are attributable to the patient's need to receive medical care.

5. All visitor orders on the plan of care (HCFA 485) must state:
   - The service(s)—the assessments, teachings, and/or treatments
   - The discipline—SN, HHA, PT, OT, ST, SW, and/or other services

- The visit frequency for the 9-week period—when daily visits are ordered; an end point must also be stated

The following are examples of visit orders:

a. *Home health aide*—3 wk 4; 2 wk 5 to assist with bath and personal care

b. *Social services*—2 visits q 60 days to help the family identify community resources to pay bills and buy food

c. *Skilled nurse*—3 wk 4; 2 wk 5 to assess patient with infected wound, change wound dressing, instruct patient/caregiver on wound care, and evaluate healing

d. Ranges of 1 to 2 visits may be used in stating the frequency of visits within the certification period. For example, skilled nurse—3-5 wk 2; 1-2 wk 4; 1 wk 2; for home intravenous therapy management and two visits PRN for problems with central venous catheter leakage (Note: A **specific** reason and number of PRN visits must be documented). Review fiscal intermediary guidelines for reimbursement when using ranges to specify visit frequencies. Any changes in the visit frequency or new orders must be authorized and signed by the physician (Box 5-5).

6. The patient's rehabilitation potential, goals of care, and discharge status must be stated on the plan of care. This should reflect the desired outcome and an estimated discharge time. For example, wound to heal by 10/00. Discharge to self-care or physician care. (Note: For anticipated prolonged admissions such as with a severe decubitus ulcer, estimate the discharge by stating the month and year. This period may be reused upon recertification as needed.)

7. If the patient has not achieved stability, identify which discipline will provide which services and the frequency/duration of visits. At this time the physician should receive, review, sign, and return an updated HCFA 485 before the start date of the recent period. If it is not received by this date, an interim or verbal physician order must be obtained to continue services. (Typically, recertification orders are sent out 2 to 4 weeks before the

---

Box 5-2 OUTCOME AND ASSESSMENT INFORMATION SET (OASIS-B1)

This is a dynamic instrument, and home health agencies should use the most recent publication, which may be obtained from the OASIS World Wide Web site: www.hcfa.gov/Medicare/hsqb/oasis/hhsoview.htm

The OASIS items are to be used for all patients 18 years or older who are receiving health services or personal care from a certified home health agency at specific time points. Exceptions include prepartum and postpartum patients and patients who only receive homemaker, chore, or companion services.

Start or Resumption of Care

The OASIS form must be integrated into the agency's initial patient assessment documentation; it may not be used as a separate form. The assessment must be performed within 48 hours of referral or the patient's return home from an inpatient hospital stay, and the form must be completed within 5 days and note the following:
- Start of care—further visits planned
- Start of care—no further visits planned
- Resumption of care (after inpatient stay)

Follow-Up

Follow-up requires a home visit with completion on or between every 57- and 62-day interval from the start of care date and includes the following:
- Recertification (follow-up) assessment
- Other follow-up assessment

Transfer to an Inpatient Facility

The OASIS form must be completed within 48 hours of notification of transfer to inpatient facility and should note the following:
- Transferred to an inpatient facility—patient not discharged from an agency
- Transferred to an inpatient facility—patient discharged from an agency

Discharge From Agency (Not to an Inpatient Facility)

The OASIS form must be completed within 48 hours of death or discharge notification as follows:
- Death at home
- Discharge from agency
- Discharge from agency—no visit completed after start/resumption of care assessment

From Rice R: *Manual of home health nursing procedures,* ed 2, St. Louis, 2000, Mosby.

---

current certification period ends.) An OASIS follow-up assessment is also required on or between the 57th and 62nd day after each start of care or within the 5 days preceding each recertification.

8. A physician or psychiatrist may direct the plan of care for patients who require the services of a psychiatric home care nurse.

9. Complete a visit report each time the patient is seen. Each visit report should stand on its own merit regarding Medicare guidelines for reimbursement (Table 5-1). In addition, documentation on the visit report should directly reflect the medical treatment plan, related nursing diagnosis, interventions, and outcomes of care as identified on the patient care plan (Figure 5-2).

   Subsequent visit reports must document procedures or skilled care that concurrently reflect changes in medical treatment to support continued or increases in services.

10. Obtain physician's orders for multidisciplinary services and follow home care agency policy for consultation services. The orders for multidisciplinary services should identify which discipline is requested, for what purposes, and the frequency/duration of visits needed. Multidisciplinary or team conferences should be held as frequently as needed to coordinate, communicate, and review efficient and quality management of patient care service by all involved disciplines or at least every 60 days. The conference may be face-to-face, by telephone, or by other electronic communication. Document each attendee, the patient's progress with his or her plan of care, any new or remaining patient problems or unmet outcome(s), and the suggested goal(s) or resolution(s). To ensure patient participation in the plan of care, share this information with patients/caregivers to help them identify progress with the plan of care,

---

**Box 5-3   GUIDELINES FOR DOCUMENTING HOMEBOUND STATUS FOR MEDICARE
COVERAGE OF HOME CARE SERVICES**

Medicare requires physician certification of the patient's homebound status. To be certified as homebound the patient must have a physical or medical contraindication for leaving the home. The home health agency and physician work together to assess the continuation or change in the patient's homebound status. Homebound status must be documented frequently and in objective and measurable terms. Include the following in each service visit documentation or at least weekly:

- Why the patient left home
- How long the patient is away
- How often the patient leaves home during a week/month/or other period of time
- The physical effect on the patient (describe the taxing effort)
- Assistive devices and/or personal assistance used

Medicare allows the patient to attend a day care, but this does not waive the homebound status–qualifying criteria or the need to document the preceding criteria, as well as the following additional documentation:

- Medical care provided, if any
- How often the patient attends during a week/month/or other period of time
- Number of hours the patient attends day care per session

Patients with a psychiatric problem and who are otherwise physically able to leave the home may be certified as homebound when their psychiatric problem is manifested in part by a refusal to leave home or when unattended absences are considered unsafe.

As the patient's medical or psychiatric condition improves, the homebound status must be assessed and discussed with the physician for appropriate discharge planning. Remember that homebound status is one of the four qualifying criteria for Medicare reimbursement. When any one of the qualifying criteria are no longer met, the patient must be considered ineligible for Medicare reimbursement and discharged from the home health agency. Medicare allows for a reasonable amount of time for services to be provided before the patient is discharged. Reasonable time is based on national and regional examples of home health agency practices.

From Rice R: *Manual of home health nursing procedures,* ed 2, St. Louis, 2000, Mosby.

---

as well as recognize needed areas of improvement.

11. Obtain physician orders for all medical supplies and home medical equipment (HME). Documentation showing that supplies and equipment are reasonable and necessary for the patient's treatment and recovery is required for Medicare to reimburse the expense. For example, if requesting a bedside commode, document "patient is unable to stand" rather than as "patient has limited mobility." The plan of care (HCFA 485) must reflect any HME already in the home.

12. Establish the patient care plan. Medicare requires that a patient care plan be established by the home care nurse or therapist that reflects all services and disciplines involved in the patient's care.

Document and update patient/caregiver response to the plan of care and any changes in the plan of care weekly. Patient problem areas

or resolution of problems identified on the care plan should be summarized at least every 60 days. Be aware that many home care agencies use the HCFA forms 485/487 at recertification to summarize the patient's progress with the plan of care.

13. Provide the patient with "A Patient's Bill of Rights." Obtain the patient's or caregiver's signature to acknowledge that he or she has received this information. HCFA requires that each patient be made aware of "A Patient's Bill of Rights" on admission to the home care agency (see Chapter 8).

14. Review and document the patient's or legal guardian's wishes regarding HCFA's requirement to document if the patient has or has not advance medical directives. If the patient has advance medical directives, obtain a copy for the patient's medical record. Special issues to consider are the patient's wishes regarding "do not resuscitate" (DNR) orders, organ do-

---

Box 5-4   DOCUMENTING HOMEBOUND STATUS

Be as specific as possible; indications of homebound status include the following:

1. Restricted mobility caused by a disease process, such as unsteady gait, draining wounds, depressed immunity, severe fluctuations in blood glucose level or blood pressure, or pain. When these conditions are present, mobility out of the patient's familiar home environment may further compromise or impair the patient's medical condition.
2. Poor cardiac reserve for stair or distance ambulating as demonstrated by shortness of breath, rapid irregular pulse, abnormal facial color, or other signs of activity intolerance secondary to unstable or exacerbated disease process.
3. Patients who are confined to bed or a wheelchair and who require physical assistance to move any distance.
4. Patients who require caregiver help with assistive devices, such as a cane, a walker, a wheelchair, or other special devices to leave home.
5. Presence of tracheostomy, abdominal drain, Foley catheter, or nasogastric tube that restricts ambulating.
6. Bladder or bowel incontinence that is not controlled by incontinence pads/devices.
7. Home ventilator dependence or the inability to ambulate with portable oxygen.
8. Delusion, hallucinatory or paranoid behavior, confusion, disorientation, anxiety, agitation, or other inappropriate behavior that restricts independent ambulation outside the home.
9. A new colostomy or ileostomy that complicates ambulating.
10. Fluctuating blood pressure or blood glucose level that predisposes patients to syncope or dizziness.
11. Patients who cannot ambulate stairs or uneven surfaces without assistance from a caregiver.
12. One to two days after surgery when the physician has restricted the patient's physical activity.
13. Patients who have sensory deficits such as impaired vision, hearing, or speech and require another's assistance for activities of daily living or self-expression.
14. Any physical or mental inability to independently and safely use a car, taxi, or public transportation.
15. Structural barriers to the patient's environment that do or potentially limit independent mobility, such as using stairs inside the home that lead to toileting, sleeping, eating, or laundry areas or stairs leading to the outside, and/or narrow or obstructed doorways.
16. Geographic barriers, such as dirt roads or islands or natural disasters, that restrict patient activity or make it taxing for the patient to leave.

From Rice R: *Manual of home health nursing procedures,* ed 2, St. Louis, 2000, Mosby.

---

nation, and request or refusal of specific treatments, such as tube feedings and other medical procedures. The chart should reflect these special requests. Follow individual state laws regarding the implementation of advance medical directives and durable power of attorney for health care.

15. When the patient is receiving home health aide service, document a home health aide supervisory visit every 14 days to include the following:
   a. Patient/caregiver satisfaction with the home health aide service
   b. Home health service following the care plan (Figure 5-3)
   c. Continued need for home health aide service
16. Document pertinent conversations regarding the patient's care or caregiver concerns on appropriate home care agency forms, such as the visit report, addendum nursing notes, telephone communique, or multidisciplinary conference forms.
17. When services are no longer required, complete the appropriate patient discharge summary form and the OASIS discharge items within the required time.

Box 5-5   GENERAL DOCUMENTATION GUIDELINES FOR CONTINUED SKILLED CARE

I. Each patient service visit must support the patient's continued need for Medicare services. Pay particular attention to the qualifying skilled discipline's documentation of skilled service. Skilled services refer to the assessment, teaching, and/or treatments ordered by the physician as reasonable and necessary to the patient's condition. Keep in mind the saying, "If it wasn't documented, it wasn't done." The patient's medical record must paint a picture of how the patient qualifies for home health services, why they are required, and the patient's response to the services.

II. Be objective, specific, and brief in all documentation.

III. Describe why the patient has a continued need for home health services. For example:
- "Unable to take medication without use of pillbox and verbal cues."
- "Blood pressure fluctuates between . . . during period of ambulation less than 10 ft."
- "Symptoms poorly controlled with frequent adjustment in treatment and dose monitoring."
- "Symptoms affecting daily functioning, such as . . ."

- "Safety or sanitary hazards impede the patient's ability to obtain/maintain necessary conditions for health to improve."
- "Requires assistance with . . .; patient lives alone with no one identified to assist."

IV. List supplies used during the patient service visit. Be sure that supplies are medically necessary and reasonable for the service (treatment/care) provided.

V. State the specific skilled service provided as supported by the physician's plan of care or subsequent interim order. The service must be reasonable and necessary for the patient's condition and diagnosis. If the service is not recognized treatment for the patient's condition (e.g., snake venom injections for rheumatoid arthritis), the service is not considered reasonable or necessary and therefore not a skilled or reimbursable service.

VI. Services provided by registered nurse; physical, occupational, or speech therapist; or social worker should include any and all assessment, treatments, and teachings to improve, progress, and/or support the patient's health status.

From Rice R: *Manual of home health nursing procedures,* ed 2, St. Louis, 2000, Mosby.

Additional considerations for the medical record

All telephone conversations pertinent to the care of the patient and the performance of the home care nurse should be documented. Documentation should reflect what was discussed, the time and date, who took part in the conversation, and any instructions given to the patient/caregiver.

Always write neatly and legibly. The medical record is a legal document that describes not only patient outcomes of care but also the type of care given. Hence the medical record is a reflection of the expertise of the home care nurse and that of the agency.

Travel charts or patients record should always be handled in a confidential manner so as not to violate patient rights.

Complete patient records in a timely manner consistent with agency policy. It has been said, "If it is not documented, it probably did not happen." This saying may be applied to home care because "if it is not documented correctly, it will not be reimbursed by Medicare." Intermediary denials of payment are processed and documented on the HCFA 488. Home care agencies may contest unpaid claims with their intermediaries.[4,5]

Using laptop/notebook computers to document care

Evidence suggests that home care agencies can successfully use laptop computers to document patient care.[3] The ultimate payoff of such endeavors may well result in increases in nurse productivity, procedural efficiency, and the delivery of quality care. Key issues in selecting appropriate equipment include weight of the laptop, size and brightness of the screen, size and arrangement of the keys, lowest processor speed acceptable to give

Table 5-1 Guidelines for Medicare documentation to validate the need for home care services

Avoid the following words	Use instead
Monitor, supervise. Denotes a stable patient.	**Assess, evaluate.** *Monitor* may be used when managed care is ordered and the skilled nurse is supervising paraprofessionals to ensure safe delivery of the therapeutic regimen.
Healing well. Suggests that visits are unnecessary, and supports patient discharge from home health services.	Objectively describe the wound in terms of size, depth, drainage, color, and odor.
Discussed. Does not require the skills of a professional; anyone can discuss.	**Teach, educate, instruct, demonstrate.**
Prevent/prevention. Not covered. Must be done incidental to a skilled service such as assessment, teaching, and treatment.	Focus on **restorative, rehabilitative,** and/or **palliative** (hospice) interventions.
Stable, independent. Negates medical necessity and supports patient discharge from home health services.	Document response to treatment.
Feeling better. Subjective and supports patient discharge from home health services.	Focus on the patient's physical assessment, functional ability, and problems/needs.
Noncompliant/uncooperative	Document specific problems with coping or refusal to follow the plan of care as source of referral to psychiatric home health nurse or social worker. Document refusal to follow the plan of care as a justification for a learning contract or, per home health agency policy, patient discharge.
Went to the market/going to church, etc. Negates homebound status.	Document equipment, manual assistance, and number of people required for patient to leave home. Verify homebound status each visit. If the patient leaves the home, explain why trips were taken as related to lifestyle or medical necessity.
Patient not at home	**Not available for visit** or **no answer to locked door.** Document on next visit why patient was not available for visit. "At community appointment," for example.
Continue care plan	Describe what your next visit plans are based on, for example, "Assess cardiopulmonary status of CHF patient."
Maintenance. Never use this word because it negates the necessity of visits and supports patient discharge from home health services.	Document response to the plan of care or case management needs.
Confused	Describe disorientation to person, place, or time. Describe ability to follow commands and short- and long-term recall.
Chronic condition. Is indicative of a stable condition.	Describe exacerbation of the chronic condition that requires the services of a skilled nurse.
Reinforce, reinstruct. Repetitive instruction will not be covered unless learning difficulties are documented.	Document comprehension difficulties, attention deficit, or other problems that hamper ability to learn and necessitate repeating instructions. Use words such as **demonstrate, teach, instruct,** or **educate.**
Observed. Anyone can observe.	Use **assess** or **evaluate.** Skilled observation may be used as a component of patient education to document patient/caregiver return demonstration.

From Rice R: *Manual of home health nursing procedures,* ed 2, St. Louis, 2000, Mosby.

SKILLED NURSING CLINICAL VISIT REPORT

❑ Billable
❑ Non-billable

❑ DePaul Home Care   ❑ SSM Home Care   ❑ St. Francis (Maryville)   ❑ St. Mary's Home Health
❑ Good Samaritan   ❑ SSM Hospice   ❑ St. Joseph Home Health (S.C.)   ❑ SSM Home Care of Mid-Missouri
❑ SSM Home Care of Oklahoma   ❑ St. Francis (Blue Island)   ❑ St. Joseph (Kirkwood)

Patient name _____ Record # _____ Time in _____ Time out _____

T _____ AP _____ RP _____ Resp _____ Wt _____ FBS _____ PP _____

BP: (R) lying _____ sitting _____ standing _____ (L) lying _____ sitting _____ standing _____

SYSTEM ASSESSMENT - X boxes that apply. Describe current status.

Emotional/mental
❑ Alert
❑ Oriented: ❑ Time
    ❑ Person   ❑ Place
❑ Disoriented
❑ Confused
❑ Depressed
❑ Forgetful
❑ Anxious
❑ _____

Integument   ❑ NPN
❑ Color_____
❑ Warm/dry
❑ Clammy/diaphoretic
❑ Jaundice
❑ Rash/itching
❑ Bruising
❑ Wound/incision
❑ Oral mucosa lesion(s)
❑ Capillary refill
❑ See body outline

Musculoskeletal   ❑ NPN
❑ Falls
❑ Weakness/paralysis
❑ Assistive devices:
_____
_____
❑ Gait/balance:
   ❑ Steady ❑ Unsteady
❑ Decreased ROM
   Describe: _____
_____

Neurological   ❑ NPN
❑ Dizziness
❑ Headaches
❑ Tremors/seizures
❑ Leg strength: R>=<L
❑ Grasp: R>=<L
❑ Pupil response:
   ❑ Pinpoint ❑ Dilated
   ❑ Fixed ❑ Perrl
   ❑ Other: _____

Cardiopulmonary ❑ NPN
❑ Arrhythmia
❑ Chest pain:
   ❑ Rest ❑ Exertion
❑ Jugular vein distention
❑ SOB:
   ❑ Rest ❑ Exertion
❑ Crepitus
❑ Rales/rhonchi
❑ Wheezing
❑ Diminished R L
❑ Cough
❑ Sputum
❑ O₂ _____ liters/min
❑ Pedal pulse: R _____
          L _____
❑ Sacral edema:
❑ Peripheral edema
   R   L
❑ Dorsum ❑ Dorsum
❑ Ankle ❑ Ankle
❑ Calf ❑ Calf

Gastrointestinal ❑ NPN
Appetite: _____
Fluid intake___glasses/day
❑ Nutritional score _____
❑ Nausea/vomiting
❑ Pain/bleeding
❑ Flatus
❑ Distention
   Abd. girth _____
❑ Ostomy _____
   Stoma _____
   Skin _____
❑ Diarrhea
❑ Constipation
❑ Last BM _____
❑ Bowel sounds _____
❑ Enteral nutrition
   Type NG/GT_____
   Product _____
   Amount _____
   Frequency_____
❑ Pump _____
❑ Gravity
❑ Tube change:
   Type _____
   Size _____
   Date _____

Genitourinary   ❑ NPN
❑ Dysuria/hematuria
❑ Frequency_____
❑ Retention
❑ Incontinent

❑ Cath size ___ /___ cc
   Changed _____
   Urine: Color_____
   Clarity _____ Odor _____
❑ Ostomy
   Skin _____
❑ Penile/vaginal discharge

EENT   ❑ NPN
❑ Dysphagia/aphasia
❑ Hearing loss R L
❑ Drainage
❑ Redness
   Other _____

Pain   ❑ NPN
❑ Location _____
Type _____
   Level (scale 1–10)
   Before med. _____
   After med. _____
❑ Effective relief
❑ Ineffective relief

IV Acess
❑ Type _____
❑ Site _____
❑ Pain/redness/drainage
❑ Occlusion
❑ Infiltration/extravasation
❑ Pump _____
❑ Program - see narrative
❑ Dressing change
❑ Inj. cap change

❑ Rotate site
   ❑ New site _____
   ❑ Device _____
❑ Flush _____ ml NS
_____ml Hep ___ u/ml day
❑ Access/deaccess port
   blood return❑Yes❑No
❑ Change cassette/
   reservoir/tubing
❑ Medication/fluid admin.
   Type ___ Amt. ___
❑ See IV form(s)

Home bound status
❑ Bed bound
❑ Chair bound
❑ CV instability
❑ Visual impairment
❑ Mental status
❑ ↓Strength, endurance
❑ Draining wound
❑ Dyspnea
❑ Severe pain
❑ Impaired mobility
❑ Other: _____

Care pathways

Type:_____
❑ Initiated
❑ Followed
Week/Visit # _____

Skilled care this visit:
❑ Lab spec._____
   Site _____
❑ Wound care as described
❑ Medication instruction:

❑ Instruct pain control
❑ Inst. disease process/tx:

❑ Instruct _____diet
❑ Safety instr._____
❑ Instruct terminal care
❑ D/C planning
❑ Instruction per pathway

Instructions, treatments, additional findings: _____
_____
_____
_____
_____
_____

Communicated with _____ Re: _____
Plan _____
Pt/SO verbalize understanding of instructions given this visit ❑ Yes ❑ No ❑ Partial   Return demonstration ❑Yes ❑No
Next MD appt. _____ Supplied used _____
HHA Supervision: Aide present ❑Yes ❑No   Adheres to care plan ❑Yes ❑No   Personal care needs met ❑Yes ❑No
Positive interaction ❑Yes ❑No   Plan _____
Staff signature _____ Date _____

WHITE COPY - CHART   YELLOW COPY - STAFF

SSMHC-62 (REV. 2/00) **RB&O**

Figure 5-2 Skilled Nursing Clinical Visit Report. (Courtesy SSM Home Care, St. Louis, Mo.)

AIDE VISIT REPORT (INTERMITTENT VISITS)

- ☐ DePaul Home Care
- ☐ Good Samaritan
- ☐ SSM Home Care of Oklahoma
- ☐ SSM Home Care
- ☐ SSM Hospice
- ☐ St. Francis (Blue Island)
- ☐ St. Francis (Maryville)
- ☐ St. Joseph Home Health (S.C.)
- ☐ St. Joseph (Kirkwood)
- ☐ St. Mary's Home Health
- ☐ SSM Home Care of Mid-Missouri

Patient name _____ Record # _____ Certification period _____

✓ Indicates intervention performed.   **X** Indicates intervention declined by patient/already done by S.O.

ASSIGNMENT	Each visit	Range	Sunday	Monday	Tuesday	Wednesday	Thursday	Friday	Saturday
DATE									
TIME IN									
TIME OUT									
BILLABLE									
NON-BILLABLE									
Vital signs									
Weight									
General hygiene									
Complete bath									
Assisted bath									
Shower									
Tub bath									
Skin care/lotion									
Oral hygiene									
Comb/brush hair									
Shampoo/dry hair									
Set hair									
Shave									
Fingernails: clean/file									
Toenails: clean/file									
Assist to dress									
Elimination									
Catheter care									
Last bowel movement									
Nutrition									
Encourage fluids									
Prepare light meal									
Assist at meal									
Feed patient									
Mobility									
Range of motion									
Ambulate with assist									
Other									
Clean work area									
Linen change									
Make bed									
Light laundry									
Aide initials									

SSMHC-4 (REV. 2/00) *RB&O*   **AIDE SIGNATURE / NARRATIVE NOTES ON REVERSE SIDE**

Figure 5-3 Aide Visit Report (Intermittent Visits). (Courtesy SSM Home Care, St. Louis, Mo.)

Continued

NARRATIVE NOTES

SUNDAY
Observations/patient response to care: _____
_____
Problems reported to supervisor/primary RN or therapist: _____
Environment safe ❑ yes ❑ no ❑ final visit
Visit cancelled/reason: _____
Signature _____　Date _____

MONDAY
Observations/patient response to care: _____
_____
Problems reported to supervisor/primary RN or therapist: _____
Environment safe ❑ yes ❑ no ❑ final visit
Visit cancelled/reason: _____
Signature _____　Date _____

TUESDAY
Observations/patient response to care: _____
_____
Problems reported to supervisor/primary RN or therapist: _____
Environment safe ❑ yes ❑ no ❑ final visit
Visit cancelled/reason: _____
Signature _____　Date _____

WEDNESDAY
Observations/patient response to care: _____
_____
Problems reported to supervisor/primary RN or therapist: _____
Environment safe ❑ yes ❑ no ❑ final visit
Visit cancelled/reason: _____
Signature _____　Date _____

THURSDAY
Observations/patient response to care: _____
_____
Problems reported to supervisor/primary RN or therapist: _____
Environment safe ❑ yes ❑ no ❑ final visit
Visit cancelled/reason: _____
Signature _____　Date _____

FRIDAY
Observations/patient response to care: _____
_____
Problems reported to supervisor/primary RN or therapist: _____
Environment safe ❑ yes ❑ no ❑ final visit
Visit cancelled/reason: _____
Signature _____　Date _____

SATURDAY
Observations/patient response to care: _____
_____
Problems reported to supervisor/primary RN or therapist: _____
Environment safe ❑ yes ❑ no ❑ final visit
Visit cancelled/reason: _____
Signature _____　Date _____

ANY CHANGE IN PATIENT'S CONDITION MUST BE DOCUMENTED AND REPORTED TO YOUR SUPERVISOR.

Figure 5-3, cont'd For legend see p. 72.

good software response, smallest hard drive necessary to hold needed information over the useful life of the laptop, and warranty type and services. Key issues in selecting appropriate software include user friendliness of the system and vendor availability to train staff and update the system as needed. An environmental analysis of impact of automation in the workplace, including the nurse's car, should also be conducted before purchasing equipment. If using laptops, home care nurses should ensure that documentation reflects an individualized profile of each patient in the caseload and the skilled care provided on each home visit. Benefits of using laptops to document patient care include[3]:

- *Decreased duplication of paperwork and costs of services.* Automation allows admission information to map from an original entry to other areas requiring the same information, thus preventing recopying of materials.
- *Improved standards of documentation.* Field staff have access to previous visit notes and assessment information while they are in the patient's home.
- *Improved legibility.* Documentation is easier to read and follow when it is generated by a computer.
- *Improved communication and multidisciplinary care.* All levels of patient care personnel have access to current patient information.
- *Reduced mileage and costs of services.* Field staff can download necessary patient data without having to drive to the home care agency to retrieve it.

SUMMARY

Developing the plan of care and precise documentation provides nurses with systematic and scientific methods for delivering patient care. Consequently, the patient care plan becomes a virtual care map, whereby nursing implements and directs cost-effective services and guides patient/caregiver actions in the management of health care needs at home. Careful attention to documentation provides a method for evaluating the quality of care, serves as a basis for reimbursement of services, and creates an enormous database for nursing research.

REFERENCES

1. Ackley BG: *Nursing diagnosis handbook,* ed 4, St. Louis, 1999, Mosby.
2. Antone T, Davis P: Outcomes measurement: fact vs fiction, *HomeCare* 16(10):107, 1994.
3. Briggs S, Pate E: Successful implementation of computerized documentation in home health care, *Home Health Care Manage Prac* 8(3):36, 1996.
4. Health Care Financing Administration: Medicare conditions of participation, *Federal Register* 59(243), December 20, 1994.
5. Health Care Financing Administration: *Home health insurance manual* (Pub No 11), Washington, DC, 1995, U.S. Department of Health and Human Services.
6. Health Care Financing Administration: *Outcome and assessment information set: user's manual,* Washington, DC, 1998, U.S. Department of Health and Human Services.
7. Hieber K: Mobility health assessment, *Orthop Nurs* July/August:35, 1998.
8. Jaffe M, Skidmore-Roth L: *Homehealth nursing: assessment and care planning,* ed 3, St. Louis, 1997, Mosby.
9. Marrelli TM: Handbook of homehealth standards and documentation, ed 3, St. Louis, 1998, Mosby.
10. McLaren S, Green S: Nutritional screening and assessment, *Nutrition* 13(6):s9, 1998.
11. Randall D: The role of the Medicare fiscal intermediary and the regional home health intermediary, part I, *JONA* 22(6):47, 1992.
12. Randall D: The role of the Medicare fiscal intermediary and the regional home health intermediary, part II, *JONA* 22(7/8):24, 1992.
13. Shaughnessy P, Crisler K: *Outcome-based quality improvement: a manual for home care agencies on how to use outcomes,* Washington DC, 1995, National Association for Home Care.
14. Shaughnessy P and others: Outcome-based quality improvement in the information age, *Home Health Care Manage Prac* 10(2):11, 1998.
15. Steinback P, Rebecca Zuber: Preparing for the future: tips for using OASIS now, *Home Healthcare Nurse Manager* 2(5):28, 1999.

Appendix V-I

Medical Nutrition Therapy: Assessment of Patient's Nutrient Requirements*

PURPOSE

- To establish parameters for calories, protein, and fluid level requirements
- To provide instruction on obtaining accurate measurements critical to the nutrition assessment of the patient

GENERAL INFORMATION

Medical nutrition therapy (MNT) is the process of assessing the patient, identifying treatment goals, developing the nutrition care plan, and applying specific interventions through multidisciplinary team approaches. All aspects of MNT must include input from, agreement with, and participation by the patient/caregiver. The nutrition assessment includes but is not limited to the information in Box V-I. In this section, only establishing nutrient requirement parameters is discussed.

EQUIPMENT

Cloth measuring tape
Scales
Calculator
Blood pressure cuff, stethoscope, and thermometer (see Chapter 6)

PROCEDURE

1. Explain the procedure to the patient/caregiver.
2. Obtain the following patient measurements for nutritional care:

a. Vital signs
b. Weight and height; never accept a caregiver's and/or other family member's statement of height or weight of a patient; recent reports from hospital stays or from other institutions may be used as a guide, but accurate height and weight measurements at the time of assessment are preferable; obtain measurements in the following manner:
   - Weight—The frequency of conducting weight measurements depends on the physician's orders but should be done at least monthly; follow correct procedures for the type of scale used; always use the same scale to weigh the patient each time; balance the scale before obtaining the patient's weight; weigh the patient at the same time of the day and have the patient wear the same type clothes, stand without support, and wear no shoes; floor scales should be placed on a solid surface, not carpet; for accurate measurements, obtain an average of two to three weight measurements.
   - Height—Measure without the patient wearing shoes; for accurate measurements, obtain an average of three measurements; measurements may be taken with a cloth measuring tape with the patient standing, lying flat in the bed, or contracted in the bed. For bilateral amputee patients, the measurement of the arm span is roughly equal (within 10%) to original height; as individuals age, height decreases.

---

* Modified from Dantone JJ: Nutritional care in the home. In Rice R: *Manual of home health nursing procedures,* ed 2, St. Louis, 2000, Mosby.

Box V-I   NUTRITION ASSESSMENT

Subjective Data

Interview with the patient to gather information about appetite, food preferences, eating pattern, weight history, reasonable weight for patient

Physical examination to determine condition of skin, feeding and meal preparation ability, dental status, mental status, clinical manifestations of problems related to diagnosis

Objective Data

Anthropometric measurements

Laboratory data

Medical history to include nutrition and medication regimens

Assessment

Interpreting and evaluating the data gathered

Establishing nutrient requirement parameters

Planning

Professional judgment to determine action/nursing intervention needed for each identified problem

Evaluation

Methods to evaluate outcomes of care

---

(1) The following are alternatives to height and weight measurements:
- A midarm circumference (MAC) measurement may be used only to judge changes in the patient's condition (MAC does not determine weight status); use a cloth measuring tape to measure the circumference of the arm at the midpoint—between the elbow and shoulder bone; always measure the same arm; record the measurement in centimeters; measure the MAC monthly at the same time of the month.
- Knee height—Use the guidelines found in Table V-I to estimate height

and weight measurements based on knee height (KH), which is the measure of length in centimeters between the top of the knee to the bottom of the heel when the knee and heel are both positioned at right angles to the tibia.
- Frame size—Measure the wrist circumference just distal to the styloid process at the wrist crease on the prominent arm using a cloth measuring tape; the "quick" method of establishing frame size is found in Table V-II.

c. Desirable (normal or ideal) body weight (DBW)—The National Institutes of Health (NIH) defines desirable weight as the midpoint of the recommended weight range at a specified height for persons of medium build, according to Metropolitan Life Insurance; the following guide may also be used to calculate DBW of medium-frame persons (subtract or add 10% for small or large frame persons, respectively):
- Women—Allow 100 pounds for first 5 feet of height, plus 5 pounds for each additional inch.
- Men—Allow 106 pounds for first 5 feet of height, plus 6 pounds for each additional inch.

d. Body mass index (BMI)—BMI is an index of a person's weight in relation to height; it is determined by dividing the weight in kilograms by the height in meters squared.

Weight status

BMI <20 = Underweight
BMI $20\text{-}25$ = Normal
BMI $26\text{-}30$ = Overweight
BMI >30 = Obese

e. Adjusted body weight (AjBW)—AjBW is recommended for calculating the energy requirements of persons who are 125% or more of their DBW.

AjBW = [(Actual body weight − desirable body weight) × 0.25] + DBW

Table V-I Estimating patient height and weight

Estimating height (cm)		
Males	**Age**	**Formula for calculation**
White	6-18 years	[KH(cm) × 2.22] + 40.54
Black	6-18 years	[KH(cm) × 2.18] + 39.60
White	19-59 years	[KH(cm) × 1.88] + 71.85
Black	19-59 years	[KH(cm) × 1.79] + 73.42
White	60-80 years	[KH(cm) × 2.08] + 59.01
Black	60-80 years	[KH(cm) × 1.37] + 95.79
Females	**Age**	**Formula for calculation**
White	6-18 years	[KH(cm) × 2.15] + 43.21
Black	6-18 years	[KH(cm) × 2.02] + 46.59
White	19-59 years	[KH(cm) × 1.86] − [Age(years) × 0.05] + 70.25
Black	19-59 years	[KH(cm) × 1.86] − [Age(years) × 0.06] + 68.10
White	60-80 years	[KH(cm) × 1.91] − [Age(years) × 0.17] + 75.00
Black	60-80 years	[KH(cm) × 1.96] + 58.72

Use the following formula to convert height from centimeters to inches:

$$\text{Height in inches} = \frac{\text{Height in cm}}{2.54}$$

Estimating weight (kg)		
Males	**Age**	**Formula for calculation**
White	6-18 years	[KH(cm) × 0.68] + [MAC(cm) × 2.64] − 50.08
Black	6-18 years	[KH(cm) × 0.59] + [MAC(cm) × 2.73] − 48.32
White	19-59 years	[KH(cm) × 1.19] + [MAC(cm) × 3.21] − 86.82
Black	19-59 years	[KH(cm) × 1.09] + [MAC(cm) × 3.14] − 83.72
White	60-80 years	[KH(cm) × 1.10] + [MAC(cm) × 3.07] − 75.81
Black	60-80 years	[KH(cm) × 0.44] + [MAC(cm) × 2.86] − 39.21
Females	**Age**	**Formula for calculation**
White	6-18 years	[KH(cm) × 0.77] + [MAC(cm) × 2.47] − 50.16
Black	6-18 years	[KH(cm) × 0.71] + [MAC(cm) × 2.59] − 50.43
White	19-59 years	[KH(cm) × 1.01] + [MAC(cm) × 2.81] − 66.04
Black	19-59 years	[KH(cm) × 1.24] + [MAC(cm) × 2.97] − 82.48
White	60-80 years	[KH(cm) × 1.09] + [MAC(cm) × 2.68] − 65.51
Black	60-80 years	[KH(cm) × 1.50] + [MAC(cm) × 2.58] − 84.22

Use the following formula to convert weight in kilograms to pounds:

$$\text{Weight (lbs)} = [\text{Weight(kg)} × 2.2]$$

Modified from Ross Products Division, Abbott Laboratories, Columbus, Ohio.
KH, Knee height; MAC, Midarm circumference.

Table V-II "Quick" method of establishing frame sizes

Males	Females	Frame size
<6 inches	<6 inches	Small
6-7 inches	6-6½ inches	Medium
≥7 inches	≥6½ inches	Large

Table V-III Quick method

Status	kcal/kg of ideal body weight
Basal energy needs	25-30
Ambulatory with weight maintenance	30-35
Malnutrition with mild stress	40
Severe injuries and sepsis	50-60
Extensive burns	80

The following are methods used to estimate energy (calorie) requirements:

- Harris-Benedict equation (Box V-II)
- Quick method (Table V-III)
  - (1) Determine whether weight loss or gain is desirable; establish a calorie level by adding or subtracting 500 calories from the estimated energy requirements (EER) to produce a 1-pound weight gain or loss per week, respectively; the established calorie level must be discussed with and accepted by the patient for successful diet adherence.
  - (2) Use AjBW to calculate energy requirements of obese individuals who are 125% or more than their DBW.
  - (3) Patients with congestive heart failure (CHF) may have 30% to 50% higher energy requirements than normal.
  - (4) Patients with depleted protein stores (DPS) (e.g., as a result of pressure ulcers, burns, surgery,

---

Box V-II   HARRIS-BENEDICT EQUATION

Estimated Energy Requirement=

Basal energy expenditure (BEE) × Activity factor (AF) × Injury factor (IF)

BEE is calculated using the Harris-Benedict formula below.

English measurements

Males: BEE = 66.5 + 6.3W + 12.7H − 6.8A
Females: BEE = 655.1 + 4.4W + 4.6H − 4.7A
W = Weight in pounds
H = Height in inches
A = Age in years

Metric measurements

Males: BEE = 66.5 + 13.8W + 5.0H − 6.8A
Females: BEE = 655.1 + 9.6W + 1.8H − 4.7A
W = Weight in kilograms
H = Height in centimeters
A = Age in years

Conversions

1 pound = 0.454 kilograms
1 kilogram = 2.2 pounds
1 inch = 2.54 centimeters

Once BEE is determined, energy requirements are calculated by multiplying BEE by the appropriate activity factor and injury factor as listed below.

Activity factor (AF)

Confined to bed	1.2
Ambulatory, low activity	1.3
Average activity	1.5-1.75
High activity	2

Injury factor (IF)

Mild starvation	0.85-1
Minor surgery	1-1.1
Major surgery	1-1.3
Mild infection	1-1.2
Moderate infection	1.2-1.4
Severe infection	1.3-1.8
Skeletal trauma	1.1-1.3
Burns (<20% BSA)	1.2-1.5
Burns (20%-40% BSA)	1.5-1.8
Burns (>40% BSA)	1.8-2

Combined AF + IF

COPD	1.75-2

BSA = Body surface area

Adapted from Harris JA, Benedict FG: *A biometric study of basal metabolism in man,* Washington, DC, 1989, Carnegie Institution of Washington.

cancer, sepsis, and hospitalization) require 150 to 300 calories per gram of nitrogen ratio, depending on the severity of their condition; nitrogen grams are calculated by dividing the required protein grams by 6.25; DPS energy needs are calculated by dividing the required protein grams by 6.25, then multiplying the outcome by 150 to 300 calories.

(5) Patients diagnosed with failure to thrive (FTT) require 30 to 35 calories per kilogram of actual body weight (ABW).

f. Protein requirements—Protein requirements are based on grams of protein per kilogram of ABW or DBW and are condition-specific; the following are formulas used to calculate protein requirements for specific patient statuses:

- Normal healthy adults:

$$ABW (kg) \times 0.8 g$$

- Geriatric patients:

$$ABW (kg) \times 0.8 \text{ to } 1 g$$

- Patients with DPS:

$$ABW (kg) \times 1.25 \text{ to } 1.5 g$$

- Patients diagnosed with FTT:

$$ABW (kg) \times \text{ to } 1.5g$$

- Obese patients: DBW (kg) (used for estimated lean weight) $\times$ 1.5 g

g. Fluid requirements—Fluid requirements are based on milliliters of free water fluid per kilogram of ABW and are condition-specific; a minimum of 1500 ml is recommended unless contraindicated by patient's clinical condition; the following are fluid requirements for specific patient statuses:

- Normal healthy adults:

$$ABW (kg) \times 30 \text{ to } 35 ml$$

- Geriatric patients: ABW (kg) $\times$ 30 ml
- Patients with DPS:

$$ABW (kg) \times 30 \text{ to } 35 ml$$

- Patients diagnosed with FTT:

$$ABW (kg) \times 30 ml$$

- Obese patients: ABW (kg) $\times$ 25 ml
- Patients with CHF:

$$ABW (kg) \times 25 ml$$

3. Use the following to provide nutritional care:
    a. Food diary—Use the food diary form to record a 24-hour recall of the patient's intake.
    b. Feedback questions—Use the following list of questions to determine how well the patient has understood the diet instruction; can patients do the following:
        - Name three foods and portion sizes allowed on their diet?
        - Identify the times of the day they are supposed to eat meals?
        - Identify a 1 cup, 2 cup, 1 tablespoon, and 1 teaspoon measuring utensil from the samples you have shown them or from their own kitchen?
        - Name a snack food they are allowed to eat on their diet?
        - Plan a sample menu for 1 day?
        - Tell you the name of their diet and the reason why it is important to follow the diet?
4. Clean and replace the equipment. Discard disposable items according to Standard Precautions.

NURSING CONSIDERATIONS

This procedure requires the home care nurse to establish nutrient requirements for the patient. This is the cornerstone to teaching the patient/caregiver the appropriate amount of food and fluid that should be consumed. It is important to compare the amount of food and fluid actually consumed by the patient with this *requirement* and make meaningful constructive recommendations for modifying the diet.

DOCUMENTATION GUIDELINES

Document the following on the visit report:

- Vital signs
- Height—Measure at least annually for patients 65 years or older.

- Frame size—Obtain the wrist measurement of the prominent arm whenever height is measured.
- Weight—Obtain per physician's orders or at least monthly.
- Nutrient requirements—State method used and show calculations for listing calories, protein, and fluid requirements; these parameters should be recalculated whenever the patient's condition changes.

- Compare food intake nutrient levels and requirement of nutrients.
- Modifications suggested to patient/caregiver
- Physician notification, if applicable
- Standard precautions
- Other pertinent findings

Update the plan of care.

INFECTION CONTROL IN THE HOME

Robyn Rice and Gail B. Lewis-Rea

The specter of illness moving out of the hospital and into the community has profound implications for home care nursing practice. Increasingly virulent microorganisms coupled with greater numbers of a sicker, as well as an immunocompromised, population in home care pose real concerns regarding the transmission of communicable disease.[1,33,40] In addition, our communities are experiencing multicultural migrations and environmental changes that have the potential to spread communicable disease. As a result infection control policies and procedures, both for patients and staff, are more important to home care nursing practice than ever before.

FROM PAST TO PRESENT: UNDERSTANDING THE NEED FOR INFECTION CONTROL

History is replete with outbreaks of disease such as the bubonic plague, influenza, polio, and now, acquired immunodeficiency syndrome (AIDS). Humans have always been, and most likely will continue to be, exposed to the destructive forces of disease and infection. An example from the 1300s provides insights as to the impact of plague on communities.

In October 1347 Genoese merchant ships landed at Messina, Sicily, with dead and dying men at the oars. The ships had reportedly come from the Crimea. The sick and dying sailors had an infection that manifested itself as black swellings in the armpits and groin that oozed foul smelling blood and pus. Their skin was covered with the boils (buboes) and black blotches caused by internal bleeding.[38] The infection was very painful and the sick died quickly, within a week or less after the symptoms first appeared.[42]

The disease was the bubonic plague, a contagion that reportedly killed approximately 10 million people, one third of the population of the known world in the fourteenth century.[38,42] Caused by the bacillus *Yersinia pestis,* the plague was transmitted by infected rats and fleas. Poor nutritional status and unclean living conditions characteristic of medieval society were believed to contribute to the morbidity and mortality rates. The plague was particularly ferocious in cities where there was close contact between people and usually took from 4 days to a week to kill. Of note, a more lethal and infectious airborne pneumonic variation of the plague developed. The victims of pneumonic plague usually died within 48 hours. Coughing of blood either by itself or as an additional symptom of pneumonic plague was reported by medieval physicians and scholars. It is also believed that a third variant of the bacillus caused septicemia and rapid death within hours after exposure to the infective organism.[38,42]

The black death obliterated entire communities. Physicians, clergy, and sisters of the convents who tried to assist plague victims were literally wiped out; some dying at their patient's bedside.[38] Ignorance of the cause, rapid transmission of the infection, gruesome symptomatology, and high mortality rates served to further terrify the people. Confronted with the horror of the black death, communities in western Europe attempted to isolate themselves from outsiders or strangers who represented the source of the contagion. If this was not possible, contact with the plague-struck victims was discouraged. As the plague approached, those who were able fled from their homes in fear for their lives. In trying to find a "reason" or scapegoat for the plague, the Jews were blamed and accused of poisoning the community drinking water with the plague.[38] As the black death raged across western Europe from 1347 to 1350, so did the massacre of the Jewish communities.[38] From all accounts it was a time when brother turned away from brother and parents abandoned children, when brutality and chaos reigned. Hope seemed all but lost. Chronicling the historical accounts of the plague in medieval times, Philip Ziegler writes:[42]

> "Father abandoned child;" wrote Agnolo di Tura of the plague at Siena, "wife, husband; one brother, another; for this illness seemed to strike through the breath and the sight. And so they died. And no one could be found to bury the dead for money or for friendship . . . And in many places in Siena great pits were dug and piled deep with huge heaps of the dead . . . And I, Agnolo di Tura, called the Fat, buried my five children with my own hands, and so did many others likewise. And there were also many dead throughout the city who were so sparsely covered with earth that the dogs dragged them forth and devoured their bodies."

One may ask, what does the black death have to do with infection control in the home today? Historical accounts of the bubonic plague have meaningful implications for controlling outbreaks of communicable and preventing epidemics. Today nurses working in the community are caring for patients with a variety of infectious diseases including acquired immunodeficiency syndrome (AIDS). Ideally, when faced with a disease such as AIDS, the community response should be an informed one based on scientific principles. In looking at our history, however, fear of the unknown all too often replaces rational thought. This irony still holds true. Although the situation has improved, today many people with the human immunodeficiency virus (HIV) or AIDS infection still find that no one wants to be near them, much less care for them. This avoidance is partly a result of public fear of contracting a disease for which there is no cure, with death as the end result. It is also due to the fact that, like our medieval ancestors, the public still has much to learn about the management of communicable disease. These fears of the unknown and public misconceptions or lack of knowledge regarding the transmission of infectious organisms

can make it difficult for nurses to call on community resources when coordinating care at home for people with communicable disease.

From a historical perspective, some additional points are made. Originally a bloodborne pathogen, the bacillus causing the plague during the 1300s changed into a more lethal respiratory form. Home care nurses should be aware that bacteria and viruses can and do mutate. One has only to follow the historical development of hepatitis A (an oral/fecal pathogen) to hepatitis B and C (bloodborne pathogens) to realize that this is true (Figure 6-1). In addition, when implementing infection control precautions, it is important to recognize that bloodborne pathogens are not the only infectious agents in the community.

Finally, in trying to isolate himself from the plague, medieval man understood that it was something outside of his home that was bringing the contagion to his family. Today we also recognize that patients are not likely to become infected by agents in their own home environment; the real threat arises as the nurse moves from home to home. When caring for populations at risk for communicable disease, home care nurses should be aware that they have the potential to become carriers and therefore are potential sources of infection.

Sound infection control policies and procedures coupled with comprehensive reporting of communicable disease and follow up care, for both patients and staff, will resolve some of these issues. Regulations and recommendations for accreditation and licensure specified by the Centers for Disease Control and Prevention (CDC), the Joint Commission on Accreditation of Healthcare Organizations (JCAHO), and the Occupational Safety and Health Administration (OSHA) are useful resources to direct home care organizational infection control policies and procedures.[2,7-16,26-32]

In addition, community education about communicable disease transmission and basic infection control practices assists the patient, the family, and the public at large to effectively cope with any epidemic. Education *can* change behavior so that fears of the unknown are overcome. As a result the community response to people with communicable disease becomes an informed and humane one. The purpose of this chapter is to describe how and why disease is transmitted and to provide current recommendations for infection control in the home setting.

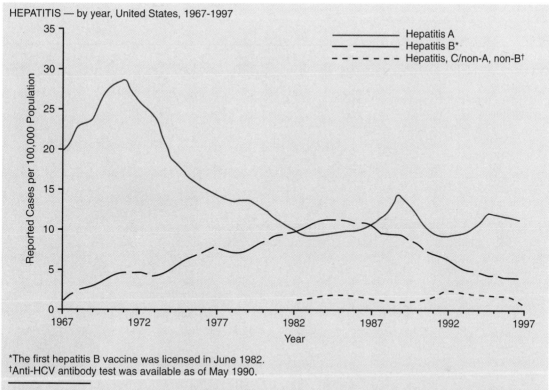

HEPATITIS — by year, United States, 1967-1997

Hepatitis A
Hepatitis B*
Hepatitis, C/non-A, non-B†

*The first hepatitis B vaccine was licensed in June 1982.
†Anti-HCV antibody test was available as of May 1990.

Hepatitis C/non-A, non-B is the most under reported type of viral hepatitis. Nonetheless, the increase observed in this type of hepatitis after 1990 is misleading because, in some states, reported cases have included those among persons identified in routine screening programs who were positive for antibody to hepatitis C virus but who did not have evidence of acute hepatitis.

Figure 6-1 Incidence of hepatitis by year, United States, 1967-1997. (From Centers for Disease Control and Prevention: Summary of notifiable diseases, *MMWR Morb Mortal Wkly Rep* 46(54):56, 1998.)

EPIDEMIOLOGY

Epidemiology is the study and explanation of the interrelationships among the host, the disease agent, and the environment in disease causation.[4] The CDC publishes many reports on the prevalence and mortality rates of communicable disease.[7-16] These reports are useful to track trends or outbreaks of communicable disease that may or may not require some form of governmental intervention and control. See Table 6-1 for the following discussion.

First, almost all communicable diseases are actively being reported in the United States. Of interest, since 1991 there has been a steady increase in the incidence of meningococcal infections reported

each year. The polio vaccine has almost eradicated polio, but isolated cases are still reported. Cases of hepatitis A continue to be reported in significant numbers. However, the incidence of reported hepatitis B has been decreasing since the 1980s. It is speculated that the federal standards for the hepatitis B vaccine and increased public education regarding the transmission of bloodborne pathogens are responsible for this downward trend. Of note, hepatitis C is now the most common bloodborne infection in the United States[15] (see Figure 6-1).

Of interest, the 1992 revision in the CDC surveillance case definition of AIDS, which went into effect in 1993, accounted for the dramatic jump in reported AIDS cases from 1992 to 1993.[15]

Table 6-1 Notifiable diseases—summary of reported cases, United States, 1990-1997

Disease	1990	1991	1992	1993	1994	1995	1996	1997
AIDS*	41,595	43,672	45,472	103,691	78,279	71,547	66,885	58,492+
Amebiasis	3,328	2,989	2,942	2,970	2,983		&	
Anthrax	–	–	1	–	–	–	–	–
Aseptic meningitis	11,852	14,526	12,223	12,848	8,932	——	&	——
Botulism, total (including wound and unsp.)	92	114	91	97	143	97	119	132
Foodborne	23	27	21	27	50	24	25	31
Infant	65	81	66	65	85	54	80	79
Brucellosis	85	104	105	120	119	98	112	98
Chancroid	4,212	3,476	1,886	1,399	773	606	386	243@
Chlamydia**			++			477,638	498,884	526,671@
Cholera	6	26	103	18	39	23	4	6
Cryptosporidiosis				++				2,566
Diphtheria	4	5	4	–	2	–	2	4
Encephalitis, primary	1,341	1,021	774	919	717		&	
Post-infectious	105	82	129	170	143		&	
Escherichia coli 0157:H7	——	——	++	——	1,420	2,139	2,741	2,555
Gonorrhea	690,169	620,478	501,409	439,673	418,068	392,848	325,883	324,907@
Granuloma inguinale	97	29	6	19	3		&	
Haemophilus influenzae, invasive	++	2,764	1,412	1,419	1,174	1,180	1,170	1,162
Hansen disease (leprosy)	198	154	172	187	136	144	112	122
Hepatitis A	31,441	24,378	23,112	24,238	26,796	31,582	31,032	30,021
Hepatitis B	21,102	18,003	16,126	13,361	12,517	10,805	10,637	10,416
Hepatitis, C/non-A, non-B &&	2,553	3,582	6,010	4,786	4,470	4,576	3,716	3,816
Hepatitis, unspecified	1,671	1,260	884	627	444		&	
Legionellosis	1,370	1,317	1,339	1,280	1,615	1,241	1,198	1,163
Leptospirosis	77	58	54	51	38		&	
Lyme disease	++	9,465	9,895	8,257	13,043	11,700	16,455	12,801
Lymphogranuloma venereum	277	471	302	285	235		&	

NOTE: Data in the annual Summary of Notifiable Diseases might not match data in other CDC surveillance reports because of differences in the timing of reports, the source of the data, and the use of different case definitions.
* Acquired immunodeficiency syndrome.
+The total number of AIDS cases includes all cases reported to the Division of HIV/AIDS Prevention—Surveillance and Epidemiology, National Center for HIV, STD, and TB Prevention (NCHSTP) as of December 31, 1997.
& No longer nationally notifiable.
@ Cases were updated through the Division of Sexually Transmitted Diseases Prevention, NCHSTP, as of July 13, 1998.
** Chlamydia refers to genital infections caused by *C. trachomatis.*
++ Not previously nationally notifiable.
&& Anti-HCV antibody test was available as of May 1990.
@@ Numbers might not reflect changes because of retrospective case evaluations or late reports (see MMWR 1986;35:180-2).
*** Cases were updated through the Division of Tuberculosis Elimination, NCHSTP, as of April 15, 1998.
From CDC Summary of notifiable diseases, United States, 1997, *MMWR Morb Mortal Wkly Rep* 46(54):101, 1998.

Table 6-1 Notifiable diseases—summary of reported cases, United States, 1990-1997—cont'd

Disease	1990	1991	1992	1993	1994	1995	1996	1997
Malaria	1,292	1,278	1,087	1,411	1,229	1,419	1,800	2,001
Measles (rubeola)	27,786	9,643	2,237	312	963	309	508	138
Meningococcal disease	2,451	2,130	2,134	2,637	2,886	3,243	3,437	3,308
Mumps	5,292	4,264	2,572	1,692	1,537	906	751	683
Murine typhus fever	50	43	28	25			&	
Pertussis (whooping cough)	4,570	2,719	4,083	6,586	4,617	5,137	7,796	6,564
Plague	2	11	13	10	17	9	5	4
Poliomyelitis, paralytic @@	6	10	6	4	8	6	5	3
Psittacosis	113	94	92	60	38	64	42	33
Rabies, animal	4,826	6,910	8,589	9,377	8,147	7,811	6,982	8,105
Rabies, human	1	3	1	3	6	5	3	2
Rheumatic fever, acute	108	127	75	112	112		&	
Rocky Mountain spotted fever	651	628	502	456	465	590	831	409
Rubella (German measles)	1,125	1,401	160	192	227	128	238	181
Rubella, congenital syndrome	11	47	11	5	7	6	4	5
Salmonellosis, excluding typhoid fever	48,603	48,154	40,912	41,641	43,323	45,970	45,471	41,901
Shigellosis	27,077	23,548	23,931	32,198	29,769	32,080	25,978	23,117
Syphilis, primary and secondary	50,223	42,935	33,973	26,498	20,627	16,500	11,387	8,550@
Total, all stages	134,255	128,569	112,581	101,259	81,696	68,953	52,976	46,540@
Tetanus	64	57	45	48	51	41	36	50
Toxic-shock syndrome	322	280	244	212	192	191	145	157
Trichinosis	129	62	41	16	32	29	11	13
Tuberculosis	25,701	26,283	26,673	25,313	24,361	22,860	21,337	19,851***
Tularemia	152	193	159	132	96		&	
Typhoid fever	552	501	414	440	441	369	396	365
Varicella (chickenpox)	173,099	147,076	158,364	134,722	151,219	120,624	83,511	98,727
Yellow fever			&&&				1	–

Declines in AIDS incidence and deaths, first reported in 1996, have continued (Figure 6-2). This provides evidence of the widespread beneficial effects of new treatment regimens, as well as public education regarding HIV risk-reduction strategies.

In terms of respiratory disease, tuberculosis (TB) reemerged in the United States in the early 1990s. As a result the CDC recommended tuberculosis control laws in 1993 requiring health care agencies to report cases of TB to local or state health departments and direct observational therapy for patients

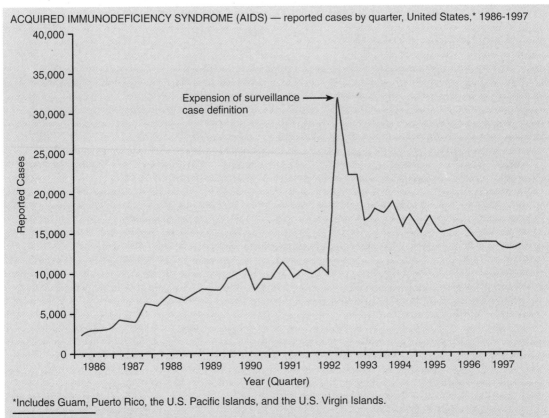

ACQUIRED IMMUNODEFICIENCY SYNDROME (AIDS) — reported cases by quarter, United States,* 1986-1997

*Includes Guam, Puerto Rico, the U.S. Pacific Islands, and the U.S. Virgin Islands.

The expansion of the AIDS surveillance case definition in 1993 resulted in a substantial increase in reported cases during that year. Since 1996, new treatments have slowed the progression from human immunodeficiency virus (HIV) infection to AIDS and from AIDS to death. Consequently, the number of new AIDS cases is declining, and the number of persons living with HIV infection and AIDS is increasing.

Figure 6-2 Incidence of AIDS reported cases by quarter, United States, 1986-1997. (From Centers for Disease Control and Prevention: Summary of notifiable diseases, *MMWR Morb Mortal Wkly Rep* 46(54):38, 1998.)

who were noncompliant with the medication regimen. OSHA now mandates special air purifying masks when caring for patients with TB.[5,30,32] An overall decrease in TB cases since 1992 primarily reflects the substantial decline in cases among U.S. born persons with small increases in cases among foreign-born persons (Figure 6-3). This decline in the overall number of reported TB cases has been specifically attributed to stronger TB control programs that emphasize promptly identifying persons with TB, initiating appropriate therapy, and ensuring completion of therapy.[16]

It is interesting to note that isolated cases of the bubonic plague are still reported in the United

States and worldwide. In 1994 the CDC reported outbreaks of bubonic and pneumonic plague with numerous deaths in India.[10] To the extent that CDC summaries represent an accurate profile of communicable disease in the United States and elsewhere, the following conclusions that affect home care nursing may be drawn[1,7-9,29,39,40]:

- Communicable disease exists in many forms in the community, with the potential for new forms to emerge.
- Although vaccines and increased public awareness of cause and treatment of communicable disease have drastically reduced rates of trans-

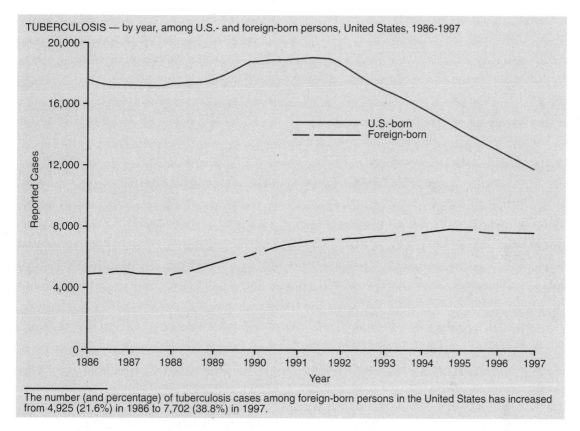

TUBERCULOSIS — by year, among U.S.- and foreign-born persons, United States, 1986-1997

The number (and percentage) of tuberculosis cases among foreign-born persons in the United States has increased from 4,925 (21.6%) in 1986 to 7,702 (38.8%) in 1997.

Figure 6-3 Incidence of tuberculosis by year, among U.S.- and foreign-born persons, United States, 1986-1997. (From Centers for Disease Control and Prevention: Summary of notifiable diseases, *MMWR Morb Mortal Wkly Rep* 46(54):85, 1998.)

mission and incidence, cases continue to be reported.

- AIDS and hepatitis B infection are continuing to be reported, and both are associated with high mortality rates.[15] The incidence of AIDS cases is of particular concern because at present there is no known vaccine or cure. The incidence of hepatitis C, which causes profound liver disease, is increasing.

- The presence of HIV and other infectious disease in home care is being felt. One study shows that 2 of 22 health care workers who acquired HIV were apparently infected in the home care setting.[7] Household transmissions of HIV among family members, although rare, are now being reported.[8] Methicillin-resistant *Staphylococcus aureus* (MRSA) and vancomycin-resistant enterococci are now being reported in home care

and are of additional concern as related to their virulence and impact on the entire household.[1,33,39]

- Common infections treated in the home setting today include pneumonia; scabies; pediculosis; streptococcal pharyngitis; impetigo; urinary tract infections; a variety of skin, fungal, and gastrointestinal infections as a result of HIV infection; gastrointestinal infections resulting from various oral/fecal pathogens; and pseudomonas or staphlococcus in wounds, ostomies, or infected intravenous (IV) sites.[1,18,33,36,40]

- The immediate recognition and identification of infection may be difficult because many communicable diseases are relatively "silent" in initial manifestation of clinical signs and symptoms. It is likely that many such cases go unreported, and the CDC statistics may well represent only the tip of the iceberg (Figure 6-4). The lesson for home care nurses: IF YOU DON'T SEE IT, IT DOESN'T MEAN IT'S NOT THERE.

- A careful, ongoing patient evaluation for infectious disease should be a part of everyday nursing care in the home. In addition, surveillance and tracking of infections and communicable disease should be a part of every home care quality improvement (QI) program (see Chapter 10).

MECHANISM OF INFECTION

Understanding how communicable disease is transmitted is the first step in the implementation and management of infection control. First, an infectious agent must exist. Infective bacteria and viruses, as well as a variety of microbial, plant, and parasitic sources, exist—all with the potential to cause infectious disease. Second, the infectious agent must have a reservoir within which it can live and multiply in such a manner that it can be transmitted to a host. Reservoirs are not usually adversely affected by the infectious agent but rather serve as a medium in which these organisms naturally reside. Any person, animal, plant, or substance capable of sustaining life can serve as a reservoir. Finally, what is needed for infection to occur is a mode of transmission and a susceptible host.[4]

A susceptible host is a person or other living animal that has no specific immunity against the infectious agent. This lack of immunity to the infectious agent is of particular concern for those who work in home care because the majority of their patients are older adults with weakened immune systems as a natural consequence of aging.[2,4]

Mechanisms of transmission vary, the most common types being contact, droplet, airborne, and vector-borne transmission.[2,4,7]

Contact transmission

Contact transmission includes direct and indirect contact.[2,4] Infectious agents may be contracted by direct contact between persons, as by sexual intercourse, touching, and biting (including animal bites). Direct contact may also occur with exposure of susceptible tissue to dust or contaminated soil (fungus/spores).[2,4]

Transmission by indirect contact occurs when an infectious agent is introduced into a susceptible

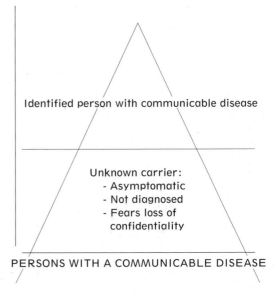

Figure 6-4 Unreported/unknown versus identified cases of communicable disease.

host via food, water, blood products (e.g., blood transfusion), medical equipment, dressings, or anything that serves as an intermediate source.

Droplet transmission

In droplet transmission a droplet containing the infectious agent is emitted by the infected host and infects others who are susceptible to the disease.[2,4] A proximity of 3 to 4 feet is usually required for droplet transmission. A cough is a good example of droplet transmission.

Airborne transmission

Airborne transmission requires the entry of microbial aerosols into the respiratory tract. In this type of transmission the infectious agent could be spread by humidifiers or fans in the ventilation system of the home.[2,4,16]

Vector-borne transmission

Vector-borne transmission occurs when the infectious agent is passed from a nonvertebrate host such as an arthropod (e.g., a mosquito) to a susceptible host (a human).[4] The infection is transmitted when the arthropod bites, regurgitates, or deposits feces or other material containing the infectious agent through the bite wound or an open area of the host's skin.

To summarize, communicable disease and infection occurs as a result of transmission of an infectious agent to a susceptible host. Home care nurses must keep in mind that an infected individual will not necessarily show initial signs or symptoms of the infection but may nonetheless be capable of infecting others. Also, some hosts can become reservoirs (essentially carriers of the disease), and although they exhibit few or no symptoms, they can travel around in the community infecting others.

Understanding mechanisms of transmission of infectious agents provides insights into the management of communicable diseases and infection. The following principles are recommended[2,4,7-16]:

- Clean and sanitary living conditions will reduce the incidence of infection and communicable disease. Although OSHA has stated that it does not hold the home care agency responsible for the living conditions of the patient's home, unclean or unsanitary home conditions should not be tolerated as part of the home care agency's bill of rights[30] (see Chapter 8).
- Good nutrition, personal hygiene, and health will reduce the incidence of infection and communicable disease.
- The routine use of infection control precautions will reduce the incidence of infection and communicable disease.
- The prevalence of the infectious agent is reduced by means of immunizations and antibiotic administration.
- The practice of consistent handwashing with soap and water is to be emphasized.

These principles, incorporated with a philosophy that all patients should be treated as though they have an infectious disease, are elemental to home care nursing practice. In addition, they support the following infection control guidelines recommended by the CDC and others.

HOME CARE APPLICATION
Standard precautions for home care

Standard precautions synthesize the major features from *universal precautions* (originally designed to reduce the risk of transmission of bloodborne pathogens) and *body substance isolation* (designed to reduce the risk of transmission of pathogens

from moist body substances). The following infection control guidelines reflect current recommendations from CDC; OSHA's bloodborne pathogen standard; the Hospital Infection Control Practices Advisory Committee (HICPAC), a CDC-supported committee; and the Association for Professionals in Infection Control and Epidemiology (APIC) and others.[2,7-16,20,24-32]

These guidelines are designed to reduce the transmission of bloodborne and other pathogens and apply to all patients regardless of their diagnosis. These guidelines reinforce the idea that all body substances (e.g., oral and body secretions; breast milk; blood; feces; urine; droplet or airborne spray from a cough; tissue, vomitus, wound, or other drainage) can be a source of infection. *These guidelines also emphasize that the environment is a potential source for infection; they contain recommendations to prevent droplet, direct or indirect contact, and true airborne transmission of infectious disease.* **Good judgment should be used in all circumstances.** In addition, as government regulations change, it is expected that home care agencies will keep current with and adhere to federal and individual state requirements for infection control.

Equipment

1. Personal protective equipment provided to the employee by the home care agency should include the following:
   a. Disposable nonsterile or sterile gloves
   b. Utility gloves
   c. Disinfectants recommended for blood or body substance spills, including:
      (1) Chemical germicides that are approved for use as agency disinfectants and are tuberculocidal when used at recommended dilutions
      (2) Products registered by the Environmental Protection Agency (EPA) with an accepted label that are effective against hepatitis B
      (3) A solution of 5.25% sodium hypochlorite (household bleach) diluted to 1:10 parts with tap water; mix a fresh supply of bleach every day for effective disinfection
   d. Masks; disposable cardiopulmonary resuscitation (CPR) masks; goggles; National Institute of Occupational Safety

and Health (NIOSH)-approved respiratory protection devices; moisture-proof aprons or gowns, shoe covers, and caps; extra uniform stocked in the car

e. Liquid soap (bacteriocidal), soap towelettes, dry hand disinfectants (bleach and alcohol based), hand lotion

f. Paper towels

g. Plastic bags with a seal and marked with a biohazard sign for use when transporting laboratory specimens

h. Leakproof and punctureproof containers marked with a biohazard sign on the outside of the container for use when transporting laboratory specimens

i. Sharps containers

j. Nursing bag that is easily cleaned with soap and water and then disinfected

k. Large plastic container or water-impermeable box to store nursing bag and supplies in trunk of field staff car

l. Impermeable plastic trash bags with twists or closures to secure contents for waste material (e.g., soiled dressings)

m. Sterile bottled water for irrigation (e.g., eyes) in case of accidental exposure to pathogens

Procedures

Handwashing. Hands should be washed before and after patient contact. Wash hands during client care if soiled.[21,22] Wash hands with liquid soap and water immediately after removing gloves. If soap and water are not available, antiseptic hand cleanser or towelettes may be used. Hands should then be washed with soap and water as soon as possible. See a further discussion on handwashing in the section on special home care considerations.

Gloves. Wear gloves if the possibility of contact transmission may occur. Change gloves between each client procedure or when going from dirty to clean (e.g., multiple dressing changes).[41] Wear nonsterile disposable **non-latex** gloves when performing any clinical procedure that may expose you to the patient's blood or other body substances (e.g., with venipuncture and during perineal care).[31] Sterile disposable non-latex gloves are to be worn during certain clinical procedures that require sterile technique (e.g., during certain dress-

ing changes or inserting a urinary catheter). Sterile and nonsterile disposable non-latex gloves are to be discarded after each use in a leak-resistant waste receptacle, such as a plastic trash bag.[31]

Utility gloves are to be used to clean up equipment, the work area, or spills. Utility gloves are to be issued to each household. Utility gloves may be disinfected and reused. Dispose of and replace utility gloves that show signs of cracking, peeling, tearing or puncture, or other signs of deterioration.

Impermeable plastic trash bag. Secure all soiled dressings, disposable gloves, and other waste material in an impermeable plastic trash bag. Place the trash bag in family trash. Follow federal, state, and local ordinances regarding disposal of biohazardous waste in the community.[34]

Additional personal protective equipment. Such equipment is provided to home care nurses by the home care agency for use in appropriate clinical circumstances and includes the following.

Blood spill kit. The blood spill kit travels with the nurse and should be kept in the car supply container. At a minimum, the kit should contain utility gloves, plastic trash bags, and paper towels. The kit should also contain a 1 : 10 bleach solution, bleach wipes, or approved home care agency disinfectant to be used to clean up blood or body substance spills in the patient's home. A new batch of bleach solution should be made daily because chlorine deteriorates and loses efficacy over time.

Blood or body substance spills should be cleaned with soap and water, then a disinfectant should be applied to the contaminated area.[30]

Gowns, aprons, shoe covers, caps. Wear moistureproof disposable gowns or aprons, shoe covers, or caps when there is a reasonable expectation that contact transmission may occur. After use, remove and dispose of personal protective equipment in an impermeable plastic trash bag in the work area.

Masks. Wear disposable face masks whenever there is a reasonable expectation that droplet transmission may occur. Masks should be discarded after they are used.[35]

When respiratory isolation is required, post a homemade "STOP" sign outside the sick child's room. Instruct the family, caregivers, and/or visitors to wear masks when entering the room and/or when caring for the sick child. The "STOP" sign should alert everyone, including children, of the necessity to wear a mask when entering the sick child's room.

- *Disposable CPR masks.* Use disposable CPR masks if you are required to provide artificial mouth-to-mouth or mouth-to-stoma ventilation. Most CPR masks are designed to be used once and then discarded. Follow individual manufacturer's recommendations for usage and care.
- *Respiratory protection devised.* Use a NIOSH-approved respiratory protection device when you are caring for children and families with tuberculosis; fit-testing is required.[29,30] Respirators must be cleaned according to the manufacturer's recommendations and discarded when excessive resistance, physical damage, or any other condition renders them unsuitable for use.
- *Goggles or face shields.* Goggles or face shields are to be worn when there is a reasonable expectation that droplet transmission may occur to the eyes. Clean goggles or shields according to the manufacturer's recommendations and discard them when physical damage or any other condition renders them unsuitable for use.

Sharp objects and needles. Sharp objects and needles should be placed in a punctureproof disposable container that can be sealed with a lid. A needle should not be bent, sheared, replaced in the sheath or guard, or removed from the syringe after use. Do not recap used needles unless using a capping device or one-hand scoop method (nursing staff should be in-serviced on a one-hand method if this technique is approved by the home care agency).

Sharps containers. Sharps containers should be punctureproof, red or opaque (do not use a clear container where needles can be easily identified), labeled or marked with a biohazard sign on the outside, and leakproof.

Never fill sharps containers so that the contents protrude out of the opening. *Do not fill sharps containers over two thirds full.* Store sharps containers in a secure area out of the reach of children and others (e.g., on the top shelf in a bedroom closet). Follow state and local ordinances regarding disposal of sharps containers.

Specimen collection. Wear gloves when handling specimens. Handle all specimens carefully to minimize spillage. Place blood or other body substance specimens in a leakproof plastic bag and secure in a punctureproof/leakproof container during collection, handling, storage, and transport. Label specimens with the patient's name and identifying data. Place the punctureproof/leakproof container in the trunk or on the floor of your car during transport.

In accordance with the home care agency policy, a courier service may be called to pick up laboratory specimens that have been left at the patient's home.

Uniform. Keep an extra, "clean" uniform secured in a water-resistant bag in your car. Store the extra uniform in the supply container located in the trunk of your car. If a uniform becomes soiled during patient care, change into the clean uniform as soon as possible. Place the soiled uniform in a leakproof plastic bag and launder according to individual home care agency policy.[6] (If the home care agency purchases scrubs for nurses to wear or a uniform *specific* for contact with blood and/or body substances, then the agency is responsible for laundering the uniform.[5]) Contact your local OSHA representative with further questions on this subject.

If you choose to launder your uniform or work clothes at home, it is recommended that you wash clothing soiled with blood or body substances separately from household laundry in extremely hot water for about 25 minutes (use a detergent and bleach that won't damage colored clothes). Uniforms or work clothes that are not soiled with blood or body substances may be routinely cleaned in the regular family wash. Store one dry uniform or set of work clothes in a plastic bag in your car for possible future use.

Medical supplies in the home care nurse's car. Maintain medical supplies in a plastic container in the trunk of the car when traveling. Make every effort to ensure that medical supplies including your nursing bag are kept in as clean an area of the car as possible.

Principles of cleaning, disinfecting, and sterilizing in the home. Clean all equipment thoroughly to remove organic material before disinfection or sterilization. Modifications to routine disinfection practices in the home may include the use of the following:

Bleach
Hydrogen peroxide

Boiling water
Hot, soapy water
Phenolic (e.g., Lysol)
Isopropyl alcohol (70%)
Acetic acid (white vinegar)

All items to be disinfected should be cleaned first with a detergent and running water and then cleaned with the disinfectant. The following are cited as disinfectants used in home care: bleach, white vinegar, hydrogen peroxide, boiling water, phenolics, and isopropyl alcohol.[18,21,39] The item to be disinfected will primarily determine the disinfectant to be used. Bleach corrodes metal but is cited as an all-purpose disinfectant in the home for blood and body fluid contamination. White vinegar (acetic acid) may be used to disinfect respiratory therapy equipment, although home medical equipment (HME) vendor guidelines for cleaning respiratory therapy equipment should be reviewed.

Routinely wipe down the bell/diaphragm of the stethoscope with a disinfectant between patients. If you are using a baby scale, wipe the scale down with disinfectant between uses or use a fresh disposable plastic sheath/pad underneath the baby on each visit. For glucose meters, follow specific manufacturer's guidelines for cleaning. If patients do not have their own thermometer, wipe the nursing bag thermometer with an antiseptic wipe before and after use and place a plastic/protective sheath over the thermometer before administering to a patient.

Patient/family laundry. Laundry should be handled as little as possible and with minimum agitation to prevent gross microbial contamination of the air and of the persons handling the linen. Place soiled linens with blood or body fluids in a leak-resistant bag at the location where care was given. See a further discussion in the section on patient education.

Personal practices. Eating, drinking, smoking, applying cosmetics or lip balm, and handling contact lenses are prohibited in patient care areas where there is reasonable likelihood of occupational exposure to blood or body substances. Food and drinks are not to be kept in patient care areas where blood or other potentially infectious materials are present.

Immunizations. It is recommended that all staff involved in direct patient care (touching, working with patients/caregivers) be immunized against hepatitis B. In addition, the Advisory Committee on Immunization Practices (ACIP) strongly recommends that all staff be vaccinated against (or have documented immunity to) influenza, measles, mumps, rubella, and varicella.[12]

Finally, it is mandatory that all staff involved in direct patient care receive an initial two-step tuberculosis skin test (the Mantoux test with 5 tuberculin units of PPD) on employment. Staff must be retested annually. Previous BCG vaccination is not a contraindication for skin testing.[16,32]

Exposure incident. In the event of eye or body contact with the patient's blood or body substances (e.g., deep wound puncture from a needlestick), first irrigate the eye with water or wash the exposed body part with soap and water (use bottled sterile water stocked in the nursing bag or car as necessary), and then contact the home care agency infection control director for follow-up instructions and care. In addition, report suspect exposure to *M. tuberculosis* or any other infectious organism to the infection control director.

OSHA regulations. Infection control standards and policies published by OSHA should be accessible to all home care staff for reference. A copy of these regulations should be placed in the infection control manual or in the appropriate policy/procedure manual located in an easily accessible place at the home care agency. The home care agency is responsible for having an infection control program, including a staff infection control exposure plan that identifies patient risk for infectious organisms on admission to the home care agency and includes guidelines for clinical management.

Miscellaneous. All clinical procedures shall be performed in a manner that minimizes splashing, spraying, splattering, or generating droplets of the patient's blood or body substances. Mouth pipetting/suctioning of blood or other body substances is prohibited.

Consider placing patients with active infectious organisms, such as vancomycin-resistant *S. aureus,* with an "infection control care team" or specific case manager to reduce the risk of staff exposure and transmission of infectious organisms to other patients. Try to visit these patients last or at the end of the day. When possible, use disposable equipment, or keep needed equipment in the home with these patients. Contact the local health department for further surveillance/management guidelines.

Be aware that OSHA is now proposing new rules for staff protection against exposure to TB, including skin retesting every 6 months for all staff who are at risk for exposure to sources of aerosolized TB or who come in contact with patients with suspect or active TB.[29]

Special home care considerations

Bag technique and handwashing. Observe proper technique at all times. The inside of the nursing bag should be regarded as a clean area. Transport the bag in a clean container in the car with a supply of newspapers. Once you are in the patient's home, select the cleanest or most convenient area and spread the newspaper. Place the bag on the newspaper. Prepare a receptacle (trash bag) for disposable items. Open the nursing bag, and remove the items you need to wash your hands (handwashing supplies should be placed at the top of the bag). Close the bag. Go in and out of the nursing bag as few times as possible. Take the items to wash your hands (liquid soap/paper towels) to the sink area. Remember, this is the patient's home. Ask the patient where you should wash your hands.

When at the sink, use one paper towel upon which to place other items. Use a second and third towel for washing and drying your hands before and after care has been given. Remove your watch. Wet your hands and forearms and then lather using vigorous friction, starting at fingertips and working toward the forearms. Hold your hands lower than your elbows while washing your hands. Hold your hands under running water for at least 10 seconds. Rinse and dry your hands from your fingers toward your forearm. Turn the faucet off with a paper towel (return liquid soap to nursing bag after care has been given). Apply lotion as needed. To prevent cross-contamination between patients and staff, wash your hands before and *after* care of the patient. If you are wearing gloves, *wash your hands after you remove the gloves.*[23,26] Avoid using cloth towels or bars of soap; these may become a haven for bacteria. If running water or clean facilities are not available, clean your hands with an antiseptic foam or rinse. If you are providing care for a patient on specific isolation orders, consider use of a antimicrobial scrub.

Return to the bag, open it again, and remove items necessary for the visit. Keep the bag closed during the visit. Leave all plastic containers in the bag. Do not reenter the bag unless your hands are clean. If you wear a plastic apron, do not return it to the nursing bag. Remove the apron by folding the exposed side inward, and discard it in the patient's waste receptacle, along with the newspaper and other used, disposable items. The nursing bag should not be exposed to extreme temperatures or left in the car for long periods. Never place dirty or contaminated items in the nursing bag. Nursing bags should be cleaned, disinfected, and restocked at the home care agency weekly or PRN.

Disposal of soiled dressings. Place contaminated dressings and disposable supplies in a plastic bag for disposal. Disinfection of dressings with a 10% bleach solution before disposal is recommended. Seal the plastic bag and place it in the trash. In most states the patient is responsible for waste disposal in the home setting. The home care nurse is responsible for educating the patient regarding neutralization of infectious waste and safe disposal procedures. Review local ordinances regarding infectious waste disposal in the home.

Patient education issues

As stated previously, patient education is a major focus for home care nurses when providing care (see Appendix VI-I). In a culturally sensitive manner, home care nurses should instruct the patient/caregiver about infectious disease; mechanisms of transmission; signs and symptoms of infection to report to the physician; environmental, health, and personal hygienic habits that reduce the incidence of infection; and specific infection control precautions, such as proper techniques in handwashing, needle disposal, and infectious waste disposal.[37] For example, patients should be instructed to cover their mouths when they cough because this prevents the spread of germs.

Although home care nurses should primarily use an aseptic technique when performing most procedural care, clean technique is usually taught to the patient/caregiver. Information must be imparted so that the patient/caregiver can safely manage infectious disease in the home. With this in mind, the following guidelines are recommended.

Patient laundry. Instruct the family to bag the patient's laundry at the patient's bedside and to wash soiled linens separately in hot, soapy water with a bleach solution. One cup of household bleach in addition to the detergent should be added to each load of laundry. Depending on the amount of drainage on the linens or patient's laundry, the wash cycle may have to be run through twice, and then the laundry should be dried. To clean the washer, the caregiver should run the empty machine through a complete cycle using a commercial disinfectant or 1 cup of full-strength bleach. Rubber gloves should be worn when washing soiled laundry by hand, and then they should be disinfected with a 10% bleach solution.

Bathroom. When others must share a bathroom with a patient whose disease is spread by stool or urine, request that the patient cover the faucet and handles with tissue paper before touching them. The patient should also use his or her own toothbrush and drinking glass. The person cleaning the bathroom should wear rubber gloves. The gloves should be disinfected with a 10% bleach solution after each use, and cracked or torn rubber gloves should be discarded. Damp towels and washcloths should be removed as quickly as possible. Recommend that the family use a liquid soap. If the patient has an outdoor toilet, 3 to 4 cups of lime should be placed in the toilet weekly.[24]

Kitchen. Instruct the family to keep the refrigerator clean and set the temperature at 45° F. Weekly cleaning of the inside of the refrigerator with regular household cleaning agents will help control microbial growth.

There is no need to prepare the patient's food with

Box 6-1   CRITERIA FOR HOME CARE INFECTIONS

Urinary Tract Infection With a Foley: (High risk, high volume)

A positive culture **OR**

☞   Must have two of the following signs and symptoms:
1. Fever ≥38.0° C or chills
2. New flank or suprapubic pain or tenderness
3. Change in character of urine
4. Worsening of mental or functional status

Wound: Cellulitis/Soft Tissue/Wound Infections: (High risk, high volume)

Report only those wound infections that develop while receiving services from home care (not infections that occurred before admission to home care) or report if a patient develops a post-op infection (identify whether ≤30 days or >30 days post-op or up to 1 year for artificial implants).

A positive culture **OR**

☞   One of the following **MUST** be present:
1. Pus at the wound
2. Pus at the skin
3. Pus at the soft tissue

☞   OR, if there is no pus present, four or more of the following signs and symptoms **MUST** be present:
1. Fever ≥38.0° C
2. Worsening of mental or functional status

3. New or increased heat at affected site
4. New or increased redness at affected site
5. New or increased pain/tenderness at affected site
6. New or increased serous drainage at affected site

Primary Bloodstream Infection: (High risk, low volume)

Report only if a line is present.

☞   Two or more positive blood cultures for the same organism; **OR**

☞   A single positive blood culture documented with an organism though not to be a contaminant AND at least one of the following:
1. Fever ≥38.0° C
2. New hypothermia ≤34.5° C
3. A drop in systolic blood pressure of >30mm hg from baseline
4. Worsening of mental or functional status

Case managers need to report ALL post-operative cardiac/thoracic, spinal surgery, and ENT total resection infections. This data will be reported to the hospital infection control specialist. All staff are to report TB cases (suspected or diagnosed). Diagnosed TB cases are to be reported to your infection control specialist and the Department of Health.

separate cooking utensils, but patients should be discouraged from sharing the food on their plates with other members of the household. Likewise, patients with oral/fecal pathogens should be discouraged from food preparation. The patient's utensils and dishes do not necessarily need to be isolated from those used by other household members if they are washed thoroughly with hot, soapy water. However, the use of common or unclean eating utensils should be avoided. Instruct household members to wash the patient's dishes last and then to disinfect the sink with a 10% bleach solution.

Patient's room. Encourage daily cleaning of the room. Items such as toys, books, and games may be cleaned with soap and water or wiped down with alcohol. Trash containers should be washed with soap and water and sprayed with commercial disinfectant. Floors and furniture should be washed with germicidal solution. The room should be aired out, if possible. OSHA has indicated that home care agencies are not responsible for the living conditions in the home.[30] However, as part of admission agreements, unsanitary home conditions should not be tolerated by the home care agency.

Personal hygiene. Patients should be taught to wash their hands in soap and water before and after evacuating bowels or bladder and before handling food. They should cover their mouths when coughing or sneezing and then wash their hands. Paper or tissues used by a patient experiencing a productive cough should be discarded into a plastic trash bag.

Caregivers should wash their hands before and after delivery of patient care. The patient's body should be kept clean with soap and water baths. *Gloves should be worn by caregivers whenever there is a possibility of touching a patient's blood or body substances.*[12]

Pets. Pets sometimes harbor organisms (in excreta or hair) that may pose a threat of serious illness to someone with a compromised immune system. AIDS patients in particular should not be responsible for cleaning the bird cage, cat litter box, or fish tank.[7]

Box 6-2   INFECTION RATE CALCULATION FOR QUALITY IMPROVEMENT

Incidence
The number of new cases during a defined time period.

Incidence Rate

$$\frac{\text{New nosohusial infections for the month}}{\text{Total number of patients receiving services for the month}} \times 1000$$

Device-Associated Infection

$$\frac{\text{The number of new infections related to a specific device for the month}}{\text{Total number of patients receiving services for the month with the same device}} \times 1000$$

Or, if the number of days in which the device was used is available, another method for calculating incidence would be *device days rate*.

Device Days Rate

$$\frac{\text{The number of new infections related to a specific device for the month}}{\text{Total number of days the device was used (in place)}} \times 1000$$

Analyzing and comparing trends of infections allows home care agencies to focus on specific educational and infection control programs. When comparing rates (internal or external comparisons), methods of calculation must be identical (including denominator and the constant). Even when calculation methods are consistent, be aware that infection rates may vary among facilities because of differences in risk factors, disease severity, environment, and definitions used to determine infections.

INFECTION SURVEILLANCE REPORT

Case manager _____ Month _____ Year _____ Agency _____

Report only infections which occur while receiving services from home care, not admitting diagnosis

Patient's name	MR#	Type of infection	Date reported to MD	Positive culture Y/N	Date resolved
		Report only infections which occur while receiving services from home care, not admitting diagnosis. Wound (specify type) ☐ Within 30 days post-op ☐ More than 30 days post-op ☐ Cellulitis ☐ Other wound type ☐ Post-op Cardiac/Thoracic* ☐ Primary bloodstream (IV line only) ☐ Spinal surgery* ☐ TB (suspected or diagnosed) PPD Date _____ Result _____ ☐ UTI with Foley (new occurrence) ☐ Ent total resection*			
		Wound (specify type) ☐ Within 30 days post-op ☐ More than 30 days post-op ☐ Cellulitis ☐ Other wound type ☐ Post-op Cardiac/Thoracic* ☐ Primary bloodstream (IV line only) ☐ Spinal surgery* ☐ TB (suspected or diagnosed) PPD Date _____ Result _____ ☐ UTI with Foley (new occurrence) ☐ Ent total resection*			
		Wound (specify type) ☐ Within 30 days post-op ☐ More than 30 days post-op ☐ Cellulitis ☐ Other wound type ☐ Post-op Cardiac/Thoracic* ☐ Primary bloodstream (IV line only) ☐ Spinal surgery* ☐ TB (suspected or diagnosed) PPD Date _____ Result _____ ☐ UTI with Foley (new occurrence) ☐ Ent total resection*			
		Wound (specify type) ☐ Within 30 days post-op ☐ More than 30 days post-op ☐ Cellulitis ☐ Other wound type ☐ Post-op Cardiac/Thoracic* ☐ Primary bloodstream (IV line only) ☐ Spinal surgery* ☐ TB (suspected or diagnosed) PPD Date _____ Result _____ ☐ UTI with Foley (new occurrence) ☐ Ent total resection*			

* Reported by employees only.

Figure 6-5 Infection surveillance report. (Courtesy BJC Home Care Services, St. Louis, Mo.)

ADMINISTRATIVE CONSIDERATIONS

In developing specific procedures regarding infection control, home care agencies must ensure employee cooperation and safety. The CDC, OSHA, and others suggest that this can be accomplished by doing the following[7,19,29,36]:

- Conduct an initial orientation program for employees that explains epidemiology, modes of transmission, and agency policies regarding infectious disease. The need to recognize that all patients may have a potentially infectious disease should be emphasized, and standard (universal) precautions should be taught. Provide yearly inservice training in infection control to reinforce the initial program.
- Issue medical supplies and clean equipment

and nursing bags to minimize transmission of disease. It is recommended that nursing bags be turned in weekly for cleaning and disinfection.

- Managers should monitor their staff during field visits to evaluate staff technique and compliance. This gives managers an indication of when staff retraining or counseling is needed.
- Clearly define the agency's procedures for internal processing of infectious waste. A local waste hauler may be contracted to remove the agency's infectious waste (e.g., sharps containers) as deemed necessary.
- Instruct employees to report home-acquired infections to the agency for follow-up, surveillance, and evaluation. In addition, infection and

INFECTION SURVEILLANCE

Number of records (N) = _____ Entity = _____ Reported by: _____

Infection Surveillance			
Indicators (Skilled Nursing)	MONTH:		
1. Did infection develop within 30 days of hospital discharge?	YES	NO	N/A
2. Did infection develop within one year of surgery?	YES	NO	N/A
3. Was patient/caregiver instructed regarding care/prevention of infection?	YES	NO	N/A
4. Is assessment of infection complete?	YES	NO	N/A
5. Was treatment initiated in a timely manner and appropriately?	YES	NO	N/A
6 Was patient rehospitalized due to infection?	YES	NO	N/A

NOTE: Please answer in the percentage of *records* not the number of *patients*.

Figure 6-6 Infection surveillance. (Courtesy BJC Home Care Services, St. Louis, Mo.)

communicable disease are to be reported according to individual state law.

• Conduct a quarterly analysis of infection control indicators as part of QI (Boxes 6-1 and 6-2 and Figures 6-5, 6-6, and 6-7).

The home care agency's infection control program should also have written follow-up procedures—including testing, counseling, and appropriate medical intervention—for possible exposure of staff to HIV or HBV. The hepatitis B vaccine, a series of three injections, should be made available to those health care workers who are frequently exposed to blood or blood products on the job.[29]

SUMMARY

The planning and implementation of infection control policies in home care is no easy task because of the scope of services provided. In formulating such policies, it would be well to remember a few simple rules. First, soap and water are still highly recommended because good handwashing is a proven step in basic sanitation. Second, an infection control program should focus on *behaviors* rather than *barrier* precautions. Therefore explain precautions clearly and completely, for unless staff and patients find such recommendations meaningful, compliance is unlikely. Historically, mankind has always experienced the destructive forces of plague and communicable disease. A strong educational focus on staff and public awareness of infection control precautions contributes to the welfare of our communities. In this manner we will all be ready to effectively deal with the plagues of today and the ones that will surely come tomorrow.

Name _____ Month _____ Year _____ Agency _____ Census _____

Summary of Infection Surveillance Reports					
Wound (specify type)	Month	Month	Month	QTR	YTD
≤30 days post-op** (Nosocomial - not included in home care data)					
>30 days post-op					
Cellulitis					
Other wound type					
Primary bloodstream (IV line only)					
TB (suspected or diagnosed)					
UTI with Foley (new occurrence)					
Post-op ENT total resection*					
Post-op cardiac thoracic*					
Post-op spinal surgery*					
Total infections					
Census (# of patients)					
I.C. rate (%) = Total infections ÷ Census					

*Case managers only: Report any post-op cardiac/thoracic, spinal surgery and ENT total resection infections.

**Not to be included in home health infection control rate: surgical wound infections <30 days post-op are nosocomial infections (included in hospital infection control rate, not home health).

Figure 6-7 Summary of infection surveillance reports. (Courtesy BJC Home Care Services, St. Louis, Mo.)

REFERENCES

1. American Health Consultants: VRE, MRSA: hospitals starting to send nasty new bugs to home care. *Homecare Educ Manage* 2(2):16, 1997.
2. Association for Professionals in Infection Control and Epidemiology, Inc: *APIC infection control and applied epidemiology: principles and practice,* St. Louis, 2000, Mosby.
3. Backinger CL: Analysis of needlestick injuries to health care workers providing home care, *Am J Infect Control* 22(5):300, 1994.
4. Benenson AS: *Control of communicable diseases in man,* ed 17, Washington, DC, 1999, American Public Health Association.
5. Bissell W: Conversation with Ms. Bissell, NIOSHA health compliance division, regarding current OSHA recommendations for managing health care worker exposure to bloodborne pathogens, Washington, DC, April, 1998.
6. Callagan I: Bacterial contamination of nurse's uniforms—a study, *Nurs Standard* 139(1):37, 1998.
7. Centers for Disease Control and Prevention: Update: universal precautions for prevention of transmission of human immunodeficiency virus, hepatitis B virus, and other bloodborne pathogens in health care settings, *MMWR Morb Mortal Wkly Rep* 37:377, 1988.
8. Centers for Disease Control and Prevention: Human immunodeficiency virus transmission in household settings—United States, *MMWR Morb Mortal Wkly Rep* 43(19):347, 1994.
9. Centers for Disease Control and Prevention: Guidelines for preventing the transmission of tuberculosis in health care facilities, *Federal Registrar* 59(208):54242, 1994.
10. Centers for Disease Control and Prevention: Recommendations for preventing the spread of vancomycin resistance, *MMWR Morb Mortal Wkly Rep* 44(RR-12):7, 1995.

11. Centers for Disease Control and Prevention: The role of bcg vaccine in the prevention and control of tuberculosis in the United States: a joint statement by the advisory council for the elimination of tuberculosis and the advisory committee on immunization practices (ACIP), *MMWR Morb Mortal Wkly Rep* 45(RR-4):1, 1996.

12. Centers for Disease Control and Prevention: Immunization of health care workers: recommendations of the advisory committee on immunization practices (ACIP) and the hospital infection control practices advisory committee (HICPAC), *MMWR Morb Mortal Wkly Rep* 46(RR-18):1, 1997.

13. Centers for Disease Control and Prevention: Recommended childhood immunization schedule—United States, January-December 1998, *MMWR Morb Mortal Wkly Rep* 47(1):8, 1998.

14. Centers for Disease Control and Prevention: Recommendations for prevention and control of hepatitis C virus (HCV) infection and HCV-related chronic disease, *MMWR Morb Mortal Wkly Rep* 47(RR-19):101, 1998.

15. Centers for Disease Control and Prevention: Summary of notifiable diseases, United States, 1997, *MMWR Morb Mortal Wkly Rep* 46(54):101, 1998.

16. Centers for Disease Control and Prevention: Tuberculosis morbidity—United States, 1997, *MMWR Morb Mortal Wkly Rep* 47(13):253, 1998.

17. Free KW: Infection control and safety: client education in the home, *Home Healthcare Nurse* 14(12):957, 1996.

18. Hanchett M: Implementing standard precautions in home care—getting started, *Home Care Manager*, 2(2):16, 1998.

19. Herrick S, Loos KM: Designing an infection control program, *Home Care Provider* 1(3):153, 1996.

20. Hospital Infection Control Practices Advisory Committee: 1996 guidelines for isolation precautions in hospitals, *Infect Control Hosp Epidemiol* 17(1):53, 1996.

21. Jones RD: Bacterial resistance and topical antimicrobial wash products, *Am J Infect Control* 27(4):351, 1999.

22. Kiernan M: Handwashing in infection control, *Community Nurse* 5(7):19, 1999.

23. Lynch P and others: Implementing and evaluating a system of generic infection precautions: body substance isolation, *Am J Infect Control* 18(1):243, 1990.

24. Magruder C, Hamilton G: Management of tuberculosis in home health care, *Home Health Care Manage Pract* 10(3):9, 1998.

25. Moscati R and others: Comparison of normal saline with tap water for wound irrigation, *Am J Emerg Med* 16(4):379, 1998.

26. Occupational Safety and Health Administration: 29 CFR, part 1910.1030: *Occupational exposure to bloodborne pathogens: final rule, Federal Registrar,* December 1991.

27. Occupational Safety and Health Administration: Guidelines for preventing the transmission of tuberculosis in health-care facilities, *Federal Registrar* 58(195):52810, 1993.

28. Occupational Safety and Health Administration: Occupational exposure to bloodborne pathogens, *OSHA 3127* (revised), Washington DC, 1996, U.S. Department of Labor.

29. Occupational Safety and Health Administration: 29 CFR part 1910: occupational exposure to tuberculosis: proposed rule, *Federal Registrar,* p 54160, October, 1997.

30. Occupational Safety and Health Administration: CPL 2-2.44D: Enforcement procedures for the occupational exposure to bloodborne pathogens—update, November, 1999.

31. Occupational Safety and Health Administration: Latex allergy. OSHA technical links at http://www.osha-slc.gov/SLTC/latexallergy/index.html, December 7, 1999.

32. Occupational Safety and Health Administration: Tuberculosis. OSHA technical links at *http://www.oshaslc.gov/SLTC/tuberculosis/index.html,* January 31, 1999.

33. Qureshi M and others: Concise communications. Controlling varicella in the healthcare setting: barriers to varicella vaccination among healthcare workers, *Infect Control Hosp Epidemiol* 29(7):516, 1999.

34. Ralph IG: Infectious medical waste management: a home care responsibility, *Home Healthcare Nurse* 11(3):25, 1993.

35. Roll D: Shielding eyes against bloodborne pathogens, *Occup Health Saf* 66(3):54, 1998.

36. Rosenheimer L: Establishing a surveillance system for infections acquired in home healthcare, *Home Healthcare Nurse* 13(3):20, 1995.

37. Trask K: The challenges of teaching universal precautions to multicultural, diverse patients and their family members, *J Intravenous Nurs* p S32, 1995.

38. Tuckman B: *A distant mirror-the calamitous 14th century,* New York, 1978, Ballantine Books.

39. Smith PW: Infection prevention in the home health setting, *Asepsis* 16(3):9, 1994.

40. Valenti WM: Infection control, human immunodeficiency virus, and home health care: risk to caregivers, *Am J Infect Control* 23(2):78, 1995.

41. Yangco BC, Yangco NF: What is leaky is also risky, *Infect Control Hosp Epidemiol* 19(12):553, 1989.

42. Ziegler P: The black death, New York, 1971, Harper & Row.

Patient Education Guidelines to Reduce the Risk of Transmitting a Communicable Disease

1. If possible, have your own room.

2. Clean your room daily. Items such as toys, books, and games may be cleaned with soap and water or wiped down with alcohol. Wash trash containers with soap and water; then spray the containers with a commercial disinfectant. Wash the floors and the furniture with a commercial disinfectant. Follow manufacturer's guidelines for cleaning medical equipment. Usually soap and water are fine. When it is possible, open the windows and air out your room.

3. Clean up spills of blood or urine with a 10% bleach solution. Mix 1 part of bleach to 10 parts of water daily. Throw away unused bleach solution at the end of the day.

4. The family should wear disposable gloves if contact with the patient's blood, wound drainage, feces, urine, open areas of the skin, or other bodily fluids is a possibility. The family members should wear utility gloves if they are handling soiled linens, cleaning the patient's living area, or cleaning up spills of blood, urine, or feces.

5. Clean utility gloves with hot soap and water; then disinfect the gloves with a 10% bleach solution. Throw away and replace cracked or torn utility gloves.

6. Bag your trash separately (from that of the family) in a plastic leakproof bag. Double bag as needed to prevent leakage of soiled bandages or disposable items. Keep animals and pets out of your trash. Dispose of home medical waste according to local ordinances; contact your local health department.

7. Place needles, syringes, lancets, and other sharp objects in a hard-plastic or metal container with a screw-on lid or with a lid that fits securely. Don't use a glass container. If you use a coffee can, be sure to reinforce the plastic lid with heavy-duty tape. Keep containers with sharp objects out of children's reach.

8. Family members should maintain personal cleanliness by washing their hands before and after using the bathroom and before handling food. Family members should wash their hands before and after giving patient care. (Keep patient as clean as possible.)

9. Use a liquid soap in the bathroom. Cover the faucet and the handles with tissue paper before touching them. Bathroom surfaces should be washed and disinfected with a nontoxic disinfectant such as 10% bleach solution at least once a day or when soiled. Each family member should use his or her own toothbrush and drinking glass. If you have an outdoor toilet, place 3 to 4 cups of lime in the toilet weekly.

10. Cover your mouth and nose when coughing or sneezing to prevent the spread of germs. Turn your head to avoid droplets from coughs or sneezes.

11. Refrigerate milk and other perishable foods. Drink safe water. The household may use the same cooking pots and utensils; however, commonly used or unclean eating utensils should be avoided. Do not share food from the same plate. Wash your dishes last, or use disposable dishes.

12. Maintain health at a high level by eating a balanced diet and getting adequate amounts of sleep, rest, sunshine, fresh air, and exercise.

13. Obtain and maintain protection against the diseases for which there are no known immunizing agents. Talk to your physician about a family immunization schedule.

14. Call your physician and home health nurse when you have complaints of frequent cough; sudden weight loss; diarrhea; vomiting; in-

creased drainage, increased size, or increased redness of any wounds; elevated temperature; areas of skin breakdown; lethargy; night sweats; aching; rashes; sore throat; headache; burning during urination; painful urination; or stiff neck.

15. Keep in mind the following regarding infection control in the home: (1) good common sense usually provides the best solutions to many situations, and (2) the liberal use of soap and water is still one of the best ways to prevent the spread of infection.

From Rice R: *Manual of home health nursing procedures,* ed 2. St. Louis, 2000, Mosby.

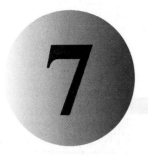

PATIENT EDUCATION IN THE HOME

Robyn Rice, Karen Balakas, Virginia K. Drake,
Patricia E. Freed, and Anne Cahill Schappe

Patient education is a very important component of home care nursing practice. As home care nurses visit patients on an intermittent basis, either the patient or the caregiver must be able to manage health care needs after the nurse has left the home. Therefore a primary focus of patient care in the home is teaching and learning.

Home care nurses also recognize that the patient's "right to know" is intrinsic to quality patient care.[8,49] Patients have the right to know about their illness, treatments, and available resources in the community in order to achieve and maintain their best level of health. This relates to the purpose and goals of patient education in the home.

The goal of patient education in the home is to teach patients how to assume responsibility for their health with an emphasis on patient dynamic self-determination for self-care. Dynamic self-determination for self-care in health (discussed in Chapter 2 and throughout this book) refers to those positive patient activities and health behaviors that keep the patient at home and out of the hospital. On a more fundamental level it reflects the process of the patient choosing what balances him or her. The process is dynamic because it is constantly changing to reflect the fluidity of the patient's awareness, life, and environment. The home care nurse and multidisciplinary team facilitate patient dynamic self-determination for self-care by utilizing teaching strategies that foster personal growth and awareness, active decision making, competence, and judgment in achieving home independence and quality of life.

The purpose of this chapter is to present home care nurses with useful concepts and practical information for providing patient education in the home. A vast amount of literature addresses patient education; to comprehensively discuss all of it is beyond the scope of a single chapter. However, the authors give an overview of information pertinent to clinical needs of field staff. The reader is referred to the rather extensive reference list at the end of the chapter for further information on individual subject matter.

TEACHING AND LEARNING

Teaching is defined as methods of communication that facilitate learning.[1] *Learning* is defined as a primarily purposeful activity that often results in a change in the patient's thinking, behavior, or both.[1]

Learning occurs in three domains: cognitive, affective, and psychomotor. In promoting a change in the patient's thinking or behavior, all are important to consider.[1,34]

Cognitive learning

Cognitive learning refers to intellectual activities such as thought, recall, decision making, drawing inferences, and arriving at conclusions. Applications of cognitive learning involve giving information to patients/caregivers about the disease process, medications, and treatments. Cognitive applications of learning may also include problem solving, empowering patients/caregivers to deal with the health care system, and strategizing lifestyle alterations to maintain household functioning.

Affective learning

Affective learning addresses the patient/caregiver's attitudes, feelings, and beliefs. Feelings, attitudes, and beliefs are often neglected aspects of patient education. Home care nurses may lack confidence in addressing these needs. Patients/caregivers may be reluctant to share this information unless trust and rapport with the nurse have been well established. Miscommunication, cultural misunderstandings, and divergent therapeutic goals between the nurse and patient/caregiver may result when these aspects of learning needs are not fully explored and addressed. Establishing a trusting and caring relationship with patients/caregivers is an essential prerequisite to affective learning. Encouraging and accepting expression of feelings and exploring health-illness beliefs are simple applications of this type of learning.

Psychomotor learning

Psychomotor learning refers to learning physical skills, tasks, or procedures such as a dressing change. Psychomotor learning is the most concrete type of learning; it is therefore frequently the easiest to teach and evaluate. This type of learning is best done in a step-by-step fashion, beginning with the more simple aspects of care and proceeding to the more complex aspects of the procedure.[1] For example, in home intravenous (IV) therapy patients/caregivers are first taught how to hook up IV fluids to the tubing and then move on to the more complicated aspects of IV pump operation.

CONCEPTUAL BASIS

Concepts and theoretical frameworks provide working guidelines for home health nurses in answering the question, "How do we teach?" Concepts and theory are also useful in answering the question, "How do patients learn?"

Behavioral learning theory

Behavioral theorists such as Guthrie, Skinner, and Thorndike proposed a stimulus-response (behavior) reinforcer in associative learning and behavior modification.[18,42,45] In using principles of behavioral modification, home care nurses should plan teaching strategies that elicit the desired behavior. If an undesirable behavior persists, then a more desirable reward must be substituted. Several principles of behavioral modification would be helpful to

consider in designing a teaching-learning plan for patients and their families. These include the following[44]:

- Behavior that is not reinforced will decrease or cease.
- Reinforcement (reward) is a personal issue; a reward for me may not be a reward for you.
- Frequent and consistent reward is required during initial behavior change.
- With demonstrated behavior change, intermittent and variable reward is more sustaining.
- Reinforcement can involve administration of some positively perceived reward or removal of a positive or pleasurable activity.
- Behavioral learning is not aversive (punishment).
- To break the cycle of undesired behavior, the nurse may need to identify the reinforcement the individual is receiving and work toward removing it.

Cognitive-developmental learning theory

Cognitive-developmental learning reflects the work of theorists such as Erickson, Koehler, Koffka, Lewin, and Piaget.[10,17,24,25,27] Cognitive-developmental theories of learning take into account all of the individual's life experiences and perceptions, as well as developmental age. Changes in perception are believed to result in a reorganization of thinking, referred to as the *development of cognitive structures*. Motivation to learn is derived from a need to make sense of the world, solve problems, and develop more cognitive structures in order to process life experiences.

Cognitive-developmental theorists believe that intellectual development is a gradual process that occurs over the life span. As the individual matures, comprehension moves from the concrete to the abstract. As a result individuals are able to develop more extensive and integrated ways of thinking and understanding. Therefore learning is viewed as an ongoing intellectual evolution of insights (or perceptions) and understanding that guides human behavior.

Home care nurses must have extensive knowledge of human growth and development. Applications of developmental theory would include devising a learning plan for a skill involving small incremental steps that build over the course of several scheduled visits, designing age-appropriate activities for a homebound child, and reorganizing the home milieu so that the patient with mild dementia can continue to function as independently as possible.

Humanistic learning theories

Elements of humanistic psychology take a holistic viewpoint in understanding when, how, and under what circumstances individuals learn. Elements such as love, creativity, self-growth, self-esteem, autonomy, and self-direction are emphasized as motivators in the learning process. An active patient role in determining what will be learned is emphasized.[6]

Abraham Maslow's theory of human motivation serves as a framework for a humanistic approach to learning. His theory is based on a hierarchy consisting of physiological, security and safety, love and belonging, self-esteem, and self-actualization needs. As shown in Figure 7-1, these needs are arranged in order of priority for satisfaction. Maslow believed that lower-level needs must first be satisfied before individuals attempt to satisfy higher-level needs. Basic physiological needs (e.g., food, water, oxygen, elimination, rest, and comfort) that are essential for survival were seen as first-level needs that take precedence over other needs. According to Maslow's theory, the patient's basic physiological needs must be met before patient education is attempted. Otherwise, patient anxiety over unmet basic needs is so great that learning is almost impossible. Self-actualization occurs after all other needs are met and is seen as the point at which individuals are capable of truly creative processes.[30]

Home care nurses can apply this information by recognizing that survival needs for home independence are priorities of health teaching for all patients, regardless of ethnic background. For example, when teaching home ventilator-dependent patients, learning how to operate and troubleshoot equipment may well take precedence over understanding the disease process.

Social-cognitive learning theories

According to social-cognitive theorists such as Kohlberg and Rotter, the process of learning occurs as individuals acquire knowledge, values, moral judgments, and standards of behavior by observing others.[26,38] Moral development is believed to occur as individuals proceed through life experiences. Likewise, behavior is thought to be influenced by perceived effects of consequences of actions. In addition, proponents of social-cognitive learning suggest that much behavior is regulated by both internal and external cues for action.

Locus of control. Locus of control relates to patient willingness to take action and readiness to learn. Based on Rotter's social learning theory, locus of control theory depicts people as primarily internally or externally influenced to take health actions.[38] Wallston and others developed this construct further, suggesting that reinforcement for health-related behaviors is primarily internal, a matter of chance, or under the control of powerful others.[48]

"Externals" believe that they are at the mercy of fate, luck, or social environment and have little influence over what happens to them.[5,23,43] In contrast, "internals" believe that they can master their own environment and thus take an active approach toward their own health decisions.[32] Externals are seen as more compulsive and may need more assis-

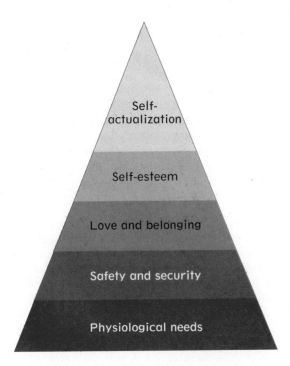

Figure 7-1 Maslow's hierarchy of needs.

tance and guidance for health care, such as a learning contract.[32]

Locus of control in the elderly appears to be influenced by the environment and physical constraints. Research suggests that as the health of the elderly declines, their locus of control orientation becomes more external as dependence on the caregiver is increased.[4,28] Activity is also negatively correlated with an external locus of control, suggesting that health and activity are strong influences on locus of control.[22] Finally, locus of control may also have negative psychological consequences such as depression and learned helplessness; these in turn may lead to detrimental physical changes.[21,33,43]

In general, internals are more likely to desire mutual goal setting and decision making in developing the plan of care, whereas externals may need more structure and guidance in their therapeutic regimen, perhaps relying on the assistance of a caregiver.

MOTIVATIONAL FACTORS FOR LEARNING AND SELF-DETERMINATION FOR SELF-CARE

As discussed in Chapter 2, conceptually patients' self-determination for self-care will be shaped by disease process, socioenvironmental resources, degree of autonomy, interpersonal perceptions, cultural considerations, and many other variables to include the following[37]:

- *Disease process.* Disease process will affect the patient's abilities to care for himself or herself.[21] For example, the learning, as well as physical, needs of a quadraplegic are very different from that of a new onset diabetic. In addition, the nature of the disease or disability will influence just how much a patient is able to care for himself or herself. A severely limiting disease or patient disability may require that the home care nurse also work with a caregiver in the home. In this circumstance teaching strategies may well focus on the learning needs and abilities of the caregiver.
- *Socioenvironmental resources.* Socioenvironmental resources that influence patient self-determination for self-care are numerous and must be considered within the context of each patient's health care needs. Such resources may include things such as proper housing; the presence of heat or air-conditioning; working utilities in the home, including running water and connected telephone; the availability of a caregiver or family member to assist the patient with self-care; available community resources such as Meals-On-Wheels; the patient's ability to purchase medications or medical products necessary for care; and the geographic location of the patient's home and/or patient access to transportation and medical care.[6,28]

- *Degree of autonomy over individual health practices—locus of control.* See the previous discussion.
- *Interpersonal perceptions of health beliefs, self-efficacy, and worldview.* Interpersonal perceptions of wellness and illness, although certainly influenced by a person's cultural background, can also be very individualistic. Such perceptions as related to self-determination for self-care involve patient thinking regarding the following:

Is this treatment or procedure really necessary for me?

How will this treatment or procedure help me?

How will this treatment or procedure affect me? Will it hurt?

What will be required of me in order to do this treatment or procedure in my home?

What will I have to do? What will I have to learn?

Do I have the abilities and/or resources to do this treatment or procedure in my home?

Can I do it? Can I learn it?

Can I afford this treatment or procedure (what will be the cost to me)?

Do I want this treatment or procedure? Am I going to do it? Am I going to try to learn it?

Home care nurses can promote patient self-determination for self-care by providing information to clarify any possible patient misunderstandings regarding the nature of the care. It is very important to make it clear to the patient how he or she will benefit (what will be the gain or outcome) from any health care recommendation. A discussion of any potential cost to the patient, particularly when implementing procedural care, must be included as part of the teaching. Last, in promoting a change in the patient's behavior through patient education, it is important to encourage the patient to believe that he or she can learn new skills and ways of doing things.

- *Cultural considerations.* Self-determination for self-care can best be understood within a cultural context. In examining different ethnic groups, research indicates that participation with the plan of care is not solely achieved by health teaching. Those who work in home care know that a successful plan of care is one that is mutually determined by the patient and nurse. This implies a partnership (e.g., patient as partner rather than dependent object of care) as fundamental to the working relationship between the patient and home care nurse. Such a partnership must accommodate the patient's value and belief system (Table 7-1). When identifying areas for health teaching, consider asking the following questions to assess patient knowledge and beliefs from a cultural perspective[11,15,19,46]:

   What is your concern or what do you think your problem is?

   What do you think caused the problem?

   Why do you think it started when it did?

   What do you think the sickness does? How does it work?

   How severe or bad is the sickness? How long do you think it will last?

   What kinds of treatment do you think you should receive? What are the most important results you hope to receive from the treatment?

   What are the chief problems that have resulted from the sickness?

   What do you fear most about the sickness?

   Certain beliefs and health practices are unique to ethnic group and class. For example, many patients have a strong belief in religion as a means of healing. Evil or a broken cultural taboo may be seen as the cause of the illness. Likewise, as so poignantly written in Fadiman's book, *A Spirit Catches You and You Fall Down,* certain diseases such as epilepsy or seizure can be seen by some cultures as divine blessings.[11] Certain patients and their families may consider prayer and religious worship to be paramount to recovery. In addition, some patients may wish to utilize folk medicine or complementary therapies, as discussed in Chapter 27. These practices may include things such as herbal therapies; meditation; traditional dietary practices, such as eating kosher foods or special soups; poultices; amulets; crystal therapy; aromatic therapy or incense; and religious practices and rituals.

To the greatest extent possible, home care nurses should respect ethnic and religious beliefs. For example, when encouraging dietary changes, nurses should be careful not to recommend foods that are restricted by the patient's religion.[15] It is important to notify the physician of patient use of any over-the-counter medications or home remedies, but unless they are viewed as harmful to the patient's health, they should be tolerated and accepted as part of the home milieu. Understanding cultural diversity within the home milieu permits home care nurses to provide a realistic and achievable plan of care.

PRINCIPLES OF ADULT LEARNING

Adult learners have their own characteristics that must be considered when teaching. These include more varied life experiences, stressful economic and family responsibilities, specific goals and desires for learning, a slower pace in learning style, a preference for self-directed problem-solving approaches to studies, and increased physical limitations (e.g., declining vision and hearing or poor circulation).

Adults learn best when the problems they study are important to their own interests. In working with adults, it is important to address what they believe to be their immediate problem. Therefore the home care nurse should provide adult patients with material or information that has personal relevance for the patient. Home care nurses should acknowledge the adult learner's experiences and draw from them when using examples to illustrate a point during teaching. Ignoring or devaluing adult learners' experiences or questions may be perceived as a rejection of their personhood or life's work. This phenomenon may be one reason why adults express deep resentment when they return to school or learning situations; they may feel they are not treated like professionals or "grown-ups."[1]

Home care nurses can use the conceptual applications of learning discussed so far to (1) develop a plan of care that is realistic for the patient's abilities, desires, and resources; (2) promote participation with the plan of care by evaluating the patient's perceptions of the value of the treatment or therapy and determination for best level of health; and (3) understand complex human behavior in finding better ways to teach.

Table 7-1 Communicating with people from different cultures

Group	Spoken language	Nonverbal communication	Literacy skills	Greetings
American Indians	Most people speak English; 150 indigenous languages continue to be spoken	Avoid eye contact to show respect	At least 56% of the people are high school graduates	Light touch handshake
Arab Americans	Arabic; different dialects	Expressive, warm, other-oriented; traditional women may avoid eye contact	Inquire if able to read and understand written English	Greet using title; shake hands; smile warmly; eye contact may be helpful
Black/African Americans	English; some dialects Ebonics or Black English	Silence may indicate a lack of trust of caregiver	Inquire as to schooling completed	Address as Mr., Mrs., or professional title; handshake appropriate
Cambodians Khmer	Khmer	Inappropriate to touch heads without permission; silence; eye contact not made	Older adults may not read Khmer or English; young may read English	*Sompeah*—both palms brought together and pointed up
Central Americans	Spanish and dialects	Nonverbal gestures used	Many people do not read	Friendly and outgoing
Chinese Americans	Cantonese, Mandarin, and dialects	Eye contact avoided with strangers	Ability to read English varies	Address people as Mr./Mrs.; use of first names is disrespectful
Cubans	Castilian Spanish	Outgoing; eye contact expected	High degree of literacy in Spanish and English	Only formal with initial meeting; handshake common
Ethiopians	Amharic, Tigrigna, and Oromigna	Polite; reserved; little eye contact	Many people are able to read some English	Hugging, touching, kissing among family and friends; handshake and often bowing
Haitians	French and Creole	Avoid eye contact	Many people do not read or write	Polite and respectful greeting is a handshake
Japanese Americans	Japanese and English	Quiet and polite	Read both Japanese and English	Formal handshake and/or small bow

Continued

Table 7-1 Communicating with people from different cultures—cont'd

Group	Spoken language	Nonverbal communication	Literacy skills	Greetings
Koreans	Korean	Touching considered disrespectful; direct eye contact infrequent	Elders may not read English	Use Mr. or Mrs.; bow is common
Mexican Americans	Spanish or English; many people are bilingual	*Respeto* (respect); direct eye contact avoided	Diversity in reading skills; many people read Spanish but not English	Handshake used
Puerto Ricans	Spanish and English	Respect and affectionate; eye contact avoided	Depends on years of education	Handshake; hugs among friends
Russians	Russian and other languages	Eye contact used	Many immigrants read English	Use Mr., Mrs., or professional title
Vietnamese	Vietnamese, French, and Chinese	Gentle touch; avoid eye contact to show respect	Many people do not read English	Use Mr./Mrs. with last name mentioned first; older people may smile and bow

Modified from Lipson J and others: *Culture and nursing care,* San Francisco, 1996, University of San Francisco Press.

PATIENT EDUCATION AND THE NURSING PROCESS

Although the majority of home care patients are elderly, home care nurses are likely to encounter patients and caregivers of all ages with diverse ethnic backgrounds and educational needs. Age, developmental stage, cognitive level, and focus of care (rehabilitation versus terminal care) will all influence educational content and teaching strategies. The nursing process of assessment, diagnosis, planning, implementation, and evaluation provides a general framework for patient education. Consider the following guidelines[1,34]:

- *Assessment.* Collect data. Identify who will receive teaching; include caregivers or family members who will assist patients with care and thus also require teaching. Determine readiness to learn (recognize motivational, developmental, and sociocultural background). Mutually assess learning needs with the patient/caregiver; identify appropriate learning strategies and tools.

Next identify availability of resources, supplies, or equipment needed for undertaking the therapeu-

tic regimen at home. Initiate referrals and/or consultations as needed. Determine whether the patient's environment is conducive to learning or appropriate for the recommended therapeutic regimen; make adjustments as needed.

- *Diagnosis.* Identify nursing diagnoses/patient problems. Nursing diagnoses commonly used in home care include those of knowledge deficit, self-care deficit, and activity intolerance. (See Chapter 5 for further information on nursing diagnoses.)
- *Planning.* Assign priorities to learning needs. Mutually plan learning goals and outcomes of care with the multidisciplinary team and the patient. Give priority in health teaching to the patient's immediate self-perceived survival needs in the home (e.g., medication or equipment issues).
- *Implementation.* Initiate and implement activities designed to meet learning outcomes; activities should focus on cognitive, affective, and psychomotor learning. (See Chapter 5 for infor-

mation regarding writing behavioral outcomes of care.)

- *Evaluation.* Determine whether outcomes and goals of care were met. See Chapters 9 and 10 for outcome evaluation. In recommending discharge from home care services, evaluate the patient's participation in self-care and the patient's ability to make appropriate decisions regarding health care needs. Is there a change in the patient's behavior toward positive health actions? How is this measured? Determine if the patient has knowledge of the therapeutic regimen (e.g., treatments, procedures, and medications) and disease process. Determine if the patient is satisfied with the teaching plan and home care services; provide this feedback to the QA/QI committee.

Encouraging patient/caregiver active participation in the plan of care

Self-determination for self-care requires the patient's *active participation* with the plan of care. Patients are taught to recognize problems with equipment and detrimental changes in health status that should be reported to the nurse and physician.[31] For example, patients with chronic obstructive pulmonary disease are taught the importance of reporting the first signs of a cold, because the immediate use of antibiotics can prevent respiratory infections and hospitalization. Likewise, treatments specific to the health care needs at home (e.g., medication regimen and wound care), use of equipment and supplies (e.g., IV pump, walker, home whirlpool, and dressings), and personal care (e.g., diet, elimination, mobility, bathing, and dressing) all become part of active patient/caregiver tasks through the process of patient education.

If the patient is not able to learn, the home care nurse must identify a caregiver, family member, or friend who will receive health teaching. It may be necessary for patients with extensive health care needs and no available caregiver to consider alternate health care strategies such as homemaker services or long-term care placement.

Medicare documentation guidelines for patient education

As stated in Chapter 5, Medicare considers teaching to be skilled care and reimbursable. Box 7-1 provides guidelines for teaching and training activities considered reimbursable by Medicare. Since reimbursement is based on documentation, the documentation of patient education should be very specific. Describe what was taught and to whom, state goals of teaching activities that were met, give an evaluation of the patient/caregiver's ability to learn, and present plans for future teaching sessions.[20]

TEACHING STRATEGIES AND TOOLS

Teaching strategies in the home primarily include discussion, storytelling, and demonstrations. Ample time should be allowed for comments and patient/caregiver questions. As discussed in Chapter 9, in leadership roles home care nurses may find that they are occasionally requested to lecture to groups of people or for organizations (Box 7-2).

Teaching tools provide visual and audio guides for learning. Examples of teaching tools useful for patient education include videos, models, audio-cassette tapes, flip charts, pamphlets, posters, photographs, checklists, and cartoons. See Table 7-2 for features of various teaching materials and Figure 7-2, which demonstrates using symbols as teaching tools.

Preprinted patient education guides regarding disease process, procedures, and treatments, as well as computer-assisted programs, are a useful learning resource and an upcoming trend in home care (Figure 7-3). In addition, they free the home health nurse from the burden of documenting in the narrative of the visit report what was taught. Keep a copy of the education guide in the patient's folder at the home and a copy in the medical record (see Box 14-4, p. 246, which provides an example of a wound care patient education guide). As discussed in Chapter 9, consider developing patient education guides for each care path. In evaluating the usefulness of teaching tools, ask yourself the following questions[49]:

Is the teaching tool accurate?

Can the teaching tool help the learner meet behavioral outcomes of care?

Is the material relevant to the learning needs of the patient?

Do the materials reflect the developmental and functional needs of the patient?

Is the teaching tool written at a level the patient can understand?

Box 7-1   TEACHING AS A SKILLED SERVICE: MEDICARE REGULATIONS

Teaching and training activities are covered by Medicare because of the skill required to teach, even though the task may be nonskilled. For example, a nonskilled activity such as using a blood glucose monitor may be taught because nursing skills are needed to explain how and why to test blood glucose. The following questions may be used to determine whether the teaching and training criteria are met:

- Is the teaching necessary to manage the patient's plan of care?
- Is the skill being taught reasonable and necessary to the patient's condition?

There is no requirement that the patient, family member, or other caregiver be taught to provide the services if he or she cannot or chooses not to provide the care.

Teaching may not continue forever. If the patient/caregiver cannot learn, then document that no further teaching or training would be helpful. Document what methods were tried and what behaviors were demonstrated.

Repeat teaching is usually not covered by Medicare unless there is a **change** in treatment, the patient's condition, or the person who will perform the treatment or when the patient/caregiver is not doing the treatment properly.

Teaching activities specific to Medicare include the following:

- Injectable medication or a complex range of medication administration
- Diabetes management for newly diagnosed patients
- Oxygen administration
- Wound care, when the complexity to the overall condition requires teaching
- Recent or reinforcement of ostomy care
- Care and maintenance of central or peripheral infusion devices or medication administration
- Bowel or bladder training
- ADL training when special techniques and/or adaptive devices are required (may be physical therapy [PT] or occupational therapy [OT] services)
- Transfer techniques and adaptive devices (may be PT or OT services)
- Proper body alignment, positioning and turning for bedbound patients
- Special dressings or skin treatments
- Oral medication administration including purpose, how and when to take, potential side effects, and special precautions
- Preparation and maintenance of a therapeutic diet

Modified from Rice R: *Manual of home health nursing procedures,* ed 2, St. Louis, 2000, Mosby.

TEACHING STRATEGIES FOR SPECIAL PATIENT GROUPS IN HOME CARE
The older adult patient

It has been shown that with normal aging there is little change in intelligence.[2] However, with chronic disease there does appear to be a slight decrease in intelligence. Likewise, older adult patients often require more time to learn. Psychomotor skills in particular may take longer to master.[4,5] However, the old adage, "you can't teach an old dog new tricks," is false; adults maintain the ability to learn throughout life.

The normal changes associated with aging, which are described in Chapter 23, will certainly affect teaching strategies (Table 7-3). This will require an adjustment of teaching techniques to accommodate specific age-related physical and psychosocial changes.[49] It is important that home care nurses be aware of these normal aging changes when they develop an educational plan.[8]

Because many standard teaching tools are devised for younger patients, it is important that home care nurses be creative in their approaches to health education for the older adult. Figure 7-4 summarizes effective teaching techniques for the older adult patient. Be aware that older adults don't like to be patronized any more than younger adults do so don't tell them information they already know.

The noncompliant patient

Noncompliance by patients with their prescribed health care regimen remains one of the most challenging and frustrating behaviors with which home health nurses contend. Frequently, noncompliant behavior is interpreted by the home care nurse as personal rejection by the patient. Internally the nurse is thinking, "Don't you realize I am trying my best to help you, and you (the patient) won't even cooperate with me." Home care nurses may feel

---

Box 7-2   GROUP TEACHING STRATEGIES

1. Relax! They want to hear what you have to say.
2. Dress the part and look professional.
3. Mentally rehearse the sequence of your presentation. Make sure you have practiced your session beforehand!
4. Arrive at least one half hour early so you can settle in and troubleshoot the room setup or equipment.
5. Use your prepared session notes but do not read from them.
6. Check your session notes and transparencies/slides for correct sequencing before you start your presentation.
7. Establish credibility at the beginning of your presentation. Tell the audience a little about yourself. A joke or humorous story will capture their attention early on.
8. Tell your audience when they can expect their break or lunch before you begin your presentation. Also, tell them where the bathrooms and phones are located.
9. Give your audience an outline of events and topics. Go over handouts as needed.
10. Move around. Do not stand in one spot.
11. Keep eye contact with your audience.
12. Use all the principles of adult learning. Ask questions. Be comfortable answering questions. Use brainteasers. Be enthusiastic. Use relevant storytelling to capture and recapture your audience's attention. *Work your audience.*
13. Plan for a morning and afternoon interactive learning experience if you are giving an all-day program. For example, have the audience get into groups and do some group work that is relevant to the presentation topic.
14. Understand the psychology of the group and use it to your advantage. Find out in advance who your participants will be. The group will have individuals from varying backgrounds. Some individuals in the group will have very little knowledge of your subject matter, whereas other individuals will feel that they are experts on all subject matter. Serve the majority. Recognize that you cannot meet everyone's needs.
15. Do not let one person take over your program. Some individuals are needy for attention. Make time for them during breaks or at lunch. Give them a leadership role during the interactive experience, but limit it to that. Be aware that security can remove disruptive individuals.
16. Get feedback from your audience.
17. The key to a successful presentation is to entertain and educate. Share your knowledge and creative talents with your group so that when they leave you, they are energized and empowered by your subject matter.

---

angry, discouraged, frustrated, hopeless, and helpless that their offerings of care are being rebuffed by the patient. These feelings may lead the nurse to interpret the patient's uncooperative behavior as a rejection of the nurse's competency, professional acumen, and personhood. This sets the stage for an adversarial relationship with the patient rather than one of advocacy. Home care nurses may unconsciously retaliate against the presumed ungrateful or uncooperative patient by ignoring, rejecting, or prematurely discharging the patient from services.

Remember, all behavior is purposeful and all behavior has meaning.[14] Consider that noncompliant patients/caregivers cannot be helped unless the reasons for their behavior are understood. In trying to alter maladaptive or unhealthy behaviors, consider the term *nonparticipation.* Why is the patient not participating with the plan of care? What behaviors underlie nonparticipation?

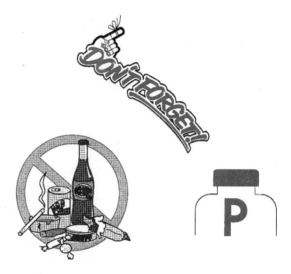

Figure 7-2 Using pictures and symbols as teaching tools.

Table 7-2 Using teaching tools in home care

Type	Advantages	Disadvantages	Helpful hints
Video recordings	Best possible substitute for actual experience Easily obtainable Easy to remake and update Can be stopped and rerun Familiar to many	Patient/caregiver may not have a VCR/TV Technical skill with film-making helpful Expensive initial investment	Must be compatible with the VCR Can take three times longer than expected to make a tape
Objects and models	Depict the real thing as closely as possible Can be handled and studied at the patient's pace Replicas—static Analogues—dynamic Appeal to kinesthetic learners	Can be bulky and heavy Inconvenient to transport Time consuming Expensive Analogues—demand conceptual sophistication	Require advance planning if borrowed
Audiocassette tapes	Can be used with individuals or groups Good for developing listening skills Accessible Cheap Can be tailor made, erased, or remade Good for enhancing stress management skills	Patient/caregiver may not have a cassette player Can be dull if used by themselves Can be damaged easily	Must be protected from temperature and moisture extremes Should be of high quality Must be long enough
Pamphlets and posters	Portable, attractive, and attracting Can be used before, during, and after a presentation Can be studied at patient's pace Readily available Often free Posters can be used to clarify the patient's medication regimen or aspects of procedural care	Time consuming to make Need a prop Bulky to carry and store Pamphlets—too many may overwhelm patient	Pamphlets—must be checked for currency and must be passed out at the most propitious time Should contain few words and lots of space Posters—figures and drawings can be placed on the poster
Photographs and cartoons	Easily personalized Can elicit emotions Can portray many more thoughts than words alone Allow the patient to control the pace	Inappropriate for large groups Can be distracting if passed during talk Will yellow with age Cartoons—can inadvertently offend or confuse	Should be tried out on people of similar ages and backgrounds as your patients Look more lively if in color May require explanations

Table 7-2 Using teaching tools in home care—cont'd

Type	Advantages	Disadvantages	Helpful hints
Computer-assisted instruction (CAI) programs	Allow the patient to control the pace Reinforce correct responses immediately Good for sequential thought processes Allow the patient to repeat the lesson if necessary	Patient/caregiver may not have necessary equipment for home CAI programs Time consuming to monitor and do Are of a limited value if the teacher is not available Require patients who are visual learners and computer literate Can be boring	Allow the teacher to select the more user-friendly software available Work best if the teacher spends enough time with the patient to ensure that he or she is comfortable with the program
Flip charts	Versatile, portable, used like a chalkboard May be prepared before or spontaneously during the presentation	Require artistic talent and good handwriting	Teacher should have a good supply of black and colored pens and should use masking tape or soft, gummy adhesive to affix flip charts to the wall
Patient education guides	Versatile, portable Easy to leave in the patient's home health agency folder	Require patients who are visual learners and who are literate	Develop patient education guides to correspond to the clinical pathway

Modified from Babcock D, Miller M: *Client education: theory and practice,* St. Louis, 1994, Mosby.

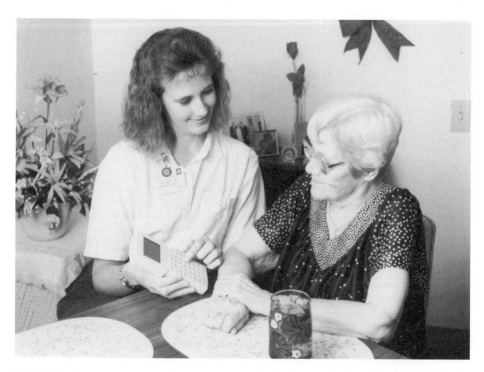

Figure 7-3 Using a handheld computer to teach patient care to the older adult. (Courtesy St. Anthony's Health Center, Alton, Ill.)

Table 7-3 Age-related changes and alterations affecting teaching techniques

Age-related changes	Teaching techniques
Reaction time	
Lengthens	Slow pace of presentations.
	Do not rush patient response.
	Provide liberal practice time.
	Give small amounts of information at each session.
	Repeat information frequently.
	Use analogies.
	Reinforce teaching with videos; practice.
Vision	
Lens yellows and thickens	Avoid blue and green paper.
	Use white paper.
	Use nonglossy paper.
	Make sure eyeglasses are worn.
	Use 12- to 16-point type.
	Use bold type.
	Use black or red ink.
	Use simple sentence structure.
Decreased lens accommodation	Use magnifying mirror.
	Make sure eyeglasses are worn.
	Use large graphic illustrations.
Hearing	
Ability to discriminate sounds decreases	Speak slowly.
	Use short sentences.
	Do not shout.
	Face patient when speaking; make sure lighting allows your face to be seen clearly.
	Use slightly louder tone.
	Eliminate background noise.
	Have patient wear hearing aid.
	Use amplifier.
	Determine whether patient hears better with one ear.
	Allow time for patient to repeat information.
Memory	
Decreased short-term memory	Teach one concept at a time.
	Use oral and written demonstration techniques.

Modified from McCaffrey B, Boyle D: The elderly patient with cancer: teaching/learning considerations for ostomy, wound, and continence management, *Progressions* 6(1):11, 1994; and Weinrich S, Boyd M: Education in the elderly, *J Gerontol Nurs* 18(1):17, 1992.

It is "crucial" to be nonjudgmental; accept the patient's behavior and work to change it. Likewise, do not view nonparticipation and noncompliance as de facto negative, uncooperative behavior on the part of the patient but rather as the patient's way of trying to communicate that there is something unacceptable, uncomfortable, or unsatisfactory about the plan of care. It is important to assess what the patient is trying to convey by the noncompliant behavior.

By working together, the home care nurse and patient can identify a mutually satisfactory plan of care with which the patient will be "willing" and "able" to comply. Once this task is achieved, both the home care nurse and patient will feel less dis-

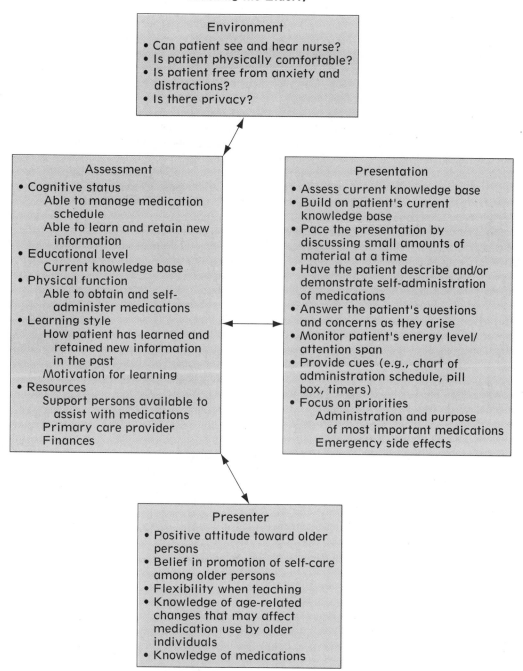

Teaching the Elderly

Environment
- Can patient see and hear nurse?
- Is patient physically comfortable?
- Is patient free from anxiety and distractions?
- Is there privacy?

Assessment
- Cognitive status
    Able to manage medication schedule
    Able to learn and retain new information
- Educational level
    Current knowledge base
- Physical function
    Able to obtain and self-administer medications
- Learning style
    How patient has learned and retained new information in the past
    Motivation for learning
- Resources
    Support persons available to assist with medications
    Primary care provider
    Finances

Presentation
- Assess current knowledge base
- Build on patient's current knowledge base
- Pace the presentation by discussing small amounts of material at a time
- Have the patient describe and/or demonstrate self-administration of medications
- Answer the patient's questions and concerns as they arise
- Monitor patient's energy level/attention span
- Provide cues (e.g., chart of administration schedule, pill box, timers)
- Focus on priorities
    Administration and purpose of most important medications
    Emergency side effects

Presenter
- Positive attitude toward older persons
- Belief in promotion of self-care among older persons
- Flexibility when teaching
- Knowledge of age-related changes that may affect medication use by older individuals
- Knowledge of medications

Figure 7-4 Teaching the elderly. (Modified from Dellasega C and others: Nursing process: teaching elderly clients, *J Gerontol Nurs* 20(1):31, 1994.)

tressed and will be better able to partner together in future health care situations.

When working with noncompliant patients, begin with a comprehensive assessment, focusing first on the positive behaviors of the patient and then moving to the noncompliant behavior. To establish rapport it is important to acknowledge those behaviors with which the patient has complied.

It may be surprising to learn that the patient is unaware of any intentional noncompliance. This information indicates a knowledge deficit that can be corrected by additional patient education. Perhaps the patient did not understand the directions, the importance of following the directions, or some other part of the process. The patient may have misplaced the directions and not known whom to contact for help. The point is that home care nurses *must not* assume that the patient is being noncompliant just to be rebellious or uncooperative.

Noncompliance may also be influenced by the family or friends. Others may genuinely believe they are contributing to the patient's best interests and be unaware that their "helping" efforts are undermining the patient's well-being. Unfortunately there are situations when others interfere as a result of their own agendas, which are *not* in the best interest of the patient. If such a situation exists, the involved persons must be confronted about their detrimental effects on the patient's welfare.

There are many varied reasons for noncompliance. These include knowledge deficits related to the plan of care, lack of financial resources to comply, lack of support systems to assist the patient with compliance, lack of trust in the multidisciplinary team and physician, negative side effects of treatment, insecurities with self-care management, ethnic barriers, value differences, disease process, or cognitive aberrations (e.g., dementia, depression, or psychosis) that impair the patient's ability to comply.

Home care nurses have the responsibility to supportively inquire about all issues that have bearing on noncompliance including sensitive, personal issues such as sexuality, family problems, or financial concerns. The home care nurse might say, "As your nurse I am concerned that you have not been following your plan of care. I am willing to help you find a way to do whatever is best for your health. What can you tell me about the things that are preventing you from complying with the recommendations for your plan of care?" By asking the patient

for specific information, the home care nurse increases the chances of obtaining useful data.

Proceed by asking the patient to share his or her understanding of what behaviors are necessary to achieve compliance with the plan of care. Encourage the patient to weigh and discuss the advantages and disadvantages of the requested change.[35]

Inquire about possible side effects of medication, fear and anxiety about managing illness at home, lack of resources or other forms of support, or other factors interfering with compliance. At this point the home care nurse may state, "It has been my experience with some other patients having difficulty following the treatment regimen, that they experienced (state side effect of medication or problem). I'm wondering if perhaps the same thing is happening to you?" This gives the patient the knowledge that the nurse understands some of the problems and will be comfortable hearing them and discussing them with the patient. This approach encourages the patient to identify reasons for noncompliance. Until all the reasons are understood, minimal (if any) progress will be made toward compliance.

If patients are unable to change with information alone, consider behavioral strategies. Consider the following recommendations[35,36]:

- Identify the behavior to be changed.
- Analyze the behavior. (Consider the meaning of the behavior to the patient and socioenvironmental factors or events that influence the behavior.)
- Identify environmental factors or events that would facilitate the desired behavior.
- Gradually add behaviors that enhance the accomplishment of the new behavior.
- Assist the patient to find new ways to meet needs that old behaviors previously met.
- Help the patient identify means within his or her own environment to build continuous reinforcement.

Participating with the therapeutic regimen can be difficult. Step-by-step planning that focuses on incremental changes may be more successful than planning that focuses on immediate and drastic changes in behavior (e.g., diet modifications).[36] It is very important to encourage patients for the positive things they have done since the last visit. In giving praise, focus on achievements; stress the difficulty of the level of accomplishment.

As a matter of routine home care agency policy, it should be made clear to the patient during the admission process that participation or compliance with the plan of care is expected. It should also be made clear that failure to work with the nurse and multidisciplinary team could result in termination of home care services. If the patient demonstrates continued unacceptable health behaviors, a learning contract is recommended (Box 7-3.) If the patient fails to adhere to the learning contract, consult with supervisory staff and follow home care agency policy; these situations will have legal, as well as ethical, implications (see Chapter 8).

Unless a patient is consciously or unconsciously self-destructive, it is rare to find a person who totally refuses to participate with the plan of care once the significance is understood and the obstacles are removed. When working in the home milieu, nurses focus on those patient behaviors they can change and accept that there may be certain behaviors that the patient will not change. In delivering services, a middle ground of patient adherence with the plan of care is usually acceptable (*how* acceptable will ultimately be up to the professional judgment of the nurse).

The illiterate patient

Low literacy indicates a lack of reading skills but also limits the patient's ability to organize perceptions and thoughts about the therapeutic regimen. Patients with low literacy skills may react to a complicated, fast-paced learning situation by withdrawing from or avoiding the experience because their process of interpretation is slow.[1,34] If questioned about understanding, the patient may well smile and nod that the information was understood while mentally wishing the home care nurse to be gone. Such a response may be due to low self-esteem and a lack of vocabulary, comprehension, or problem-solving ability to verbalize what was not understood. Teaching strategies for the illiterate patient include[1,34]:

- Simplified therapeutic regimens, medication schedules
- Techniques such as cuing (combining timing with the situation that reminds the patient to perform the task [e.g., teaching a patient with diabetes to examine the feet during morning care]) and tailoring (allowing the patient to decide on a schedule that is acceptable to the

---

> **Box 7-3   ELEMENTS OF THE LEARNING CONTRACT**
>
> 1. Date
> 2. People in attendance (it is recommended that the social worker or supervisor attend this session with the nurse and patient/caregiver)
> 3. Identified problematic behavior
> 4. Identified interventions for problem resolution:
>   a. Nursing actions/therapies
>   b. Patient/caregiver actions
> 5. Method of evaluation of care
> 6. Time frame for problematic behavior to resolve (in most cases give the patient/caregiver one visit to turn things around)
> 7. Home care agency course of action should the problematic behavior continue or resurface during the course of the patient's care (consult with your legal team, consider discharging the patient to the physician's care if problems continue)
> 8. Signatures and dates

patient and is within the realm of the physician's orders [e.g., the patient may wish to schedule medications around mealtimes])
- Simplified teaching tools, use of pictures or stick figures
- A slow-paced teaching style, lots of reinforcement, information repeated as needed
- A warm, nonjudgmental approach (e.g., fostering patient self-esteem by acknowledging that academic degrees and advanced levels of education are not always equated with good common sense and they are not a requirement for learning or for having a desire to better one's life)

The mental health patient

Today, many individuals with mental illness are being cared for in their home. Often such individuals have dual diagnosis (i.e., a physical and mental illness). Therefore it is not unusual for home care nurses to visit these patients and their families. When doing so, it is essential that nurses be able to provide information about the disease, medication, and treatment; information to help patients cope with the illness in their daily lives; and information to help them live with the stigma of mental illness.[16,39] In addition, patients may experience emotional needs that take priority over physical needs. Anxiety, fear, distrust, and misperception are not uncommon behaviors in patients/caregivers experiencing health alterations. Therefore home care nurses must also use relational and therapeutic communication skills to decrease anxiety, provide security, and promote trust.

In some instances patients in the home experience profound alterations in thought, feeling, and behavior that are associated with mental illness. Medicare reimbursement now allows for provision of services to homebound individuals with a psychiatric diagnosis who have impairments in cognition or judgement that restrict their ability to function in the community.[12] These patients should routinely be seen by the psychiatric home care nurse or by an advanced practitioner in mental health (see Chapter 22).

Educational approaches to patients with mental illness should aim at empowerment and active decision making within an egalitarian patient-nurse relationship.[39] Patients and their caregivers need to learn to recognize when the patient's behavior warrants immediate medical attention or hospitalization. In addition, home care nurses should educate the patient and family about the importance of forming alliances within the community as a part of discharge planning. Several general guidelines may be helpful for home health care nurses to consider when planning teaching-learning activities in the home for patients with mental illness. These include the following[13]:

Make assessments, not assumptions.

Avoid challenge and confrontation; build trust and acceptance.

Demonstrate a positive attitude that improvement/change can occur and support this attitude in the patient/caregiver.

Emphasize strengths and contributions to family tasks to build self-esteem.

Foster self-esteem, share goals, and teach about self-esteem.[16]

Use relevant, brief, clear, and nonmoralistic teaching strategies.

Avoid overload and overstimulation.

Set a slow pace to decrease stress and promote concentration.

Provide verbal and written information (remember that psychotropic medications can affect vision).

Balance teaching about compliance with teaching about self-care practices.

Find additional resources in the community for the patient and family.

Patient and family education is a major component in the home care of individuals with mental illnesses. The home care nurse must provide educational interventions related to the illness and its treatment and general health promotion information, including sexuality, safe-sex practices and the importance of avoiding or limiting the use or recreational drugs, tobacco, and alcohol. The nurse must also provide practical information that helps the patient and family live and cope with the illness. In a qualitative study, Vellenga and Christenson found that stigmatization, loss, pervasive distress, and need for acceptance characterized mentally ill persons' perceptions of their illnesses.[47] Keeping these themes in mind can help the home care nurse remain sensitive to important concerns and issues and direct teaching interventions to effectively meet the needs of mentally ill patients and their families.

The pediatric patient

As individuals become more responsible for their own health care, the role of the home care nurse in home pediatric care becomes even more important. If given information that is accurate and delivered at their level of understanding, children can learn to make appropriate decisions regarding their own health and participate in their own care. Whether the nurse is making a well-baby visit and discussing immunizations, caring for an acutely or chronically ill child or family member, or preparing the family for death, children must be included in the health teaching. Children listen attentively and observe behaviors. They piece together bits of information and use their imagination to draw erroneous conclusions if their teaching needs are not met. Education should be directed in a very specific manner to ensure the child's understanding of the information.

A child's thinking and reasoning abilities mature over time. At most stages of development, children are capable of some participation in their own care. Home care nurses need to be able to assess the child's level of understanding and motivation to learn. The child's developing memory and fine motor skills should also be assessed.

Home care nurses will need to draw on their knowledge of growth and development, as well as theories related to personality and cognitive development, when planning teaching strategies for children. A child's current ability to cope with illness will affect his or her level of comprehension. For example, during periods of stress and illness, many children will regress to earlier, more familiar patterns of behavior.

Caring for children involves working closely with the family. Since the home health nurse will need to design a teaching plan that will provide for at least two people—the child and the caregiver—it is helpful to ask the children or parents how they best learn. The following descriptions of personality and cognitive stages of development will give home care nurses a general framework that will be helpful in planning individualized teaching.

Infants (birth to 2 years). According to Piaget, an infant in the *sensorimotor* period develops behaviors and responses to stimuli in the environment that will be the base for perceptive and intellectual development.[17] Children in this age group learn through their senses: seeing, hearing, smelling, tasting, and touching. Infants are acutely aware of the parental response to any situation. For this reason it is important that home care nurses initiate health teaching with the parent before any procedure that involves children.

Toddlers and preschoolers (2 to 6 years). The preschool period is characterized by *preoperational* thought. Children of this age have beginning memory and begin rudimentary problem solving, relying more on their own perceptions than on logical reason.[50] Preschoolers have a very active imagination and little understanding about how the body works. Health teaching has to be delivered in language they can understand. Simple explanations regarding how something will feel, look, smell, taste, or sound can be understood by the child. For example, the nurse might tell a child that the blood pressure cuff is going to "hug your arm." Teaching for these children should occur just before or during the nursing intervention.

When teaching young children, home care nurses should be very careful with the words that are used. These children take words literally. When someone speaks of a "CAT" scan, children may imagine a huge cat looking them over; a voice box may be perceived as a boom box in the neck.

During these years, children have many fears concerning the intactness of their bodies. Bandages can help heal real or imagined injuries. If a parent or someone in the household is sick, children may wonder if they too will become ill. Children should be reassured about who will care for them when they or someone in their home is sick.

An effective strategy for teaching preschoolers may be to use dolls or stuffed animals for "practice" (Figure 7-5). Letting children handle equipment before using it will often decrease their fears. Videos may also help explain things to children in a language they comprehend. Published animal stories can be used to help children cope with illness. Make-believe play and fantasy storytelling work well with small children. Home care nurses may wish to use puppets, models, stuffed toys, or coloring books as teaching tools.

In make-believe play (Box 7-4) the child assumes the characteristics and desired behaviors of a caregiver and a doll/puppet represents the child. Anticipated stressors or problems are identified in the process as a means of teaching the child positive coping strategies with illness or disability.

Box 7-4   MAKE-BELIEVE PLAY

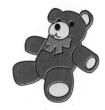

Suggested Equipment
Doll, puppet, stuffed animal
Bandages
Syringes
Splints
IV tubing and bags
Any other medical equipment
   used for the child

Procedure
1. Invite the child to pretend a puppet/doll/stuffed animal is "sick."
2. Invite the child to be the caregiver (e.g., nurse, doctor, therapist).
3. Ask the child what is wrong with "Teddy" (generally it will be the same thing that is wrong with the child).
4. Ask appropriate questions. For example, "How did Teddy get sick"? "What are you going to do to make Teddy feel better?" "How does Teddy feel when he has to get _____ (e.g., an IV, his dressing) changed?" "What is important for the caregiver (e.g., nurse, doctor, therapist) to tell Teddy?"
5. Use the information that the child gives you to clarify misperceptions over the course of the next few visits. (Keep in mind that children's ability to understand reasons for treatment is limited by their cognitive development.)

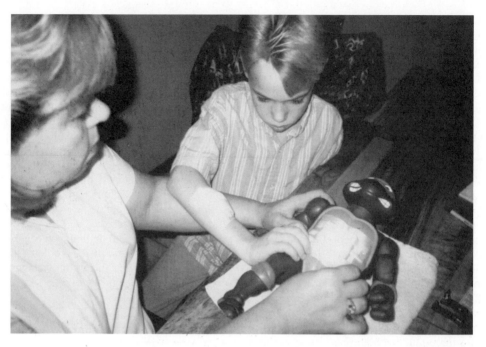

Figure 7-5 Using a model to teach a child about dressing changes. (Photograph courtesy Robyn Rice.)

Storytelling with children is different than with adults. For adults, real-life situations may be used to make a point or share an experience. With children, the nurse begins a fantasy story and lets them finish the story. This identifies insecurities and provides a means to establish positive coping for the child.

School-agers (6 to 12 years). During the school-age years, children are in the stage of cognitive development Piaget termed *concrete operations.* "Operations" are mental actions that allow the child to do mentally what previously had to be done physically.[40] Children are able to use their thought processes to experience events and actions. Their developing cognitive abilities now allow them to understand and accept another's viewpoint.[50] However, this understanding is still limited to immediate reality. These children cannot conceptualize abstract or hypothetical reality.

Since the child is still unable to understand concepts such as infection or the function of the neuroendocrine system, health teaching should be delivered using concrete examples. A newly diagnosed diabetic child may be able to use the analogy of gasoline in an automobile to understand the need for insulin. Pictures, models, books, videos, and Internet games are very helpful for these children.[29] School-agers learn best when they are able to see and handle equipment as they are being taught how to use it.

School-agers enjoy being productive and will usually participate in care when given the opportunity. They also may use medical terminology in conversation without understanding the meaning of the terms. Misconceptions and inaccuracies are common, and home care nurses will need to clarify the child's understanding of the information. Providing children with knowledge will help them gain a feeling of mastery and control over their health.

Adolescents (12 to 18 years). Around the time of adolescence, individuals develop a more sophisticated type of thinking. Piaget termed this stage *formal operations* and identified it as involving a transformation of thought and the assumption of adult roles.[17] Part of this transformation includes being able to imagine possibilities. Through their study of science and biology, adolescents have an understanding of the physiology of the internal body. They understand cause and effect, so a concept such as bacteria causing a disease can be processed.

Illness is contrary to everything that is important to an adolescent: the future, independence, and physical prowess. Although an adolescent can intellectually understand illness better than a younger child, coping on an emotional level becomes more difficult. An adolescent faced with a serious acute or chronic illness may have difficulty imagining his or her future adult role.

Individuals in this age-group should be increasingly more involved in decisions concerning their health. They need truthful information. Occasionally adolescents will test reality concerning their health. For example, adolescents may stop taking medication or stop following a certain diet to see if these treatments really do affect their health. Information on substance abuse and sexuality is very important to this age-group.

The caregiver

There is scant literature on educating caregivers in the home setting. It is estimated that 50% of adults in the United States will at some point be caregivers for an ill or disabled friend or loved one.[3] As caregivers these adults will need new skills and knowledge required to provide a variety of physical and emotional interventions.

Research indicates that caregivers' expressed needs for assistance from professionals are markedly similar across studies.[7] They want (1) information and skill training for managing the requisite tasks and activities of caregiving, (2) affordable and accessible community resources, and (3) recognition and reassurance that the care they provide is important.

Davis (1992) presents a model of professional interventions with caregivers, which include the following: (1) caregiver education: content-defined teaching programs designed to increase caregiver knowledge about the patient's problems, symptoms, prognosis, and available resources; (2) caregiver support: problem-focused counseling and supportive actions that encourage or enable the caregiver to express feelings and concerns; (3) caregiver skill training: structured activities designed to enable a caregiver to master new skills; and (4) caregiver substitution: the provision of day care or respite services. All of these may be used by home care nurses to maintain an effective caregiving unit in the home.

Specific techniques for teaching caregivers have been described in relation to hospital-based units that simulate a home environment and allow the caregiver to practice care activities with the support of nursing staff.[41] Consider the following suggestions:

- *Assess caregiver knowledge and abilities before beginning any teaching.* Caregivers may be unable to perform part or all of certain tasks because of diminished vision, arthritic deformity of hands, poor upper body strength, or cognitive deficits. Home care nurses need to break down new tasks into their component parts and assess the caregiver's ability to perform each part; other caregivers or adaptive equipment may be able to compensate for specific steps in a sequence that the primary caregiver is unable to perform.
- *Provide written instructions for teaching caregivers, with each step clearly and concisely stated.* (The caregiver receives a copy for reference, and another copy becomes a part of the patient's medical record.) Document outcomes of teaching.
- Home care nurses must be aware that failure to carry out the activities taught may not always be a case of "diagnosis: knowledge deficit." Work with caregivers to mutually achieve reasonable goals and to keep expectations to a manageable level.[9]
- *Observe for signs of caregiving unit breakdown, burnout, and a need for respite,* which include: (1) feelings of exhaustion and resentment; (2) feelings of inadequacy; (3) loss of loving and caring feelings; (4) lack of pride in care activities; (5) destructive coping methods; (6) refusal to think of self; (7) shutting out others who offer help; (8) breakdown in family relationships because of caregiving pressures; (9) continuing in a no-win situation to avoid being a failure, even if the situation is detrimental to the patient; and (10) feelings of being alone.[9] If the patient's needs overwhelm the abilities of the caregiver, consult with social services; alternate assistance including long-term care placement may have to be considered.

The intermittent visits of the home care nurse to teach and support caregivers often cannot meet all of their educational and support needs, 24 hours a

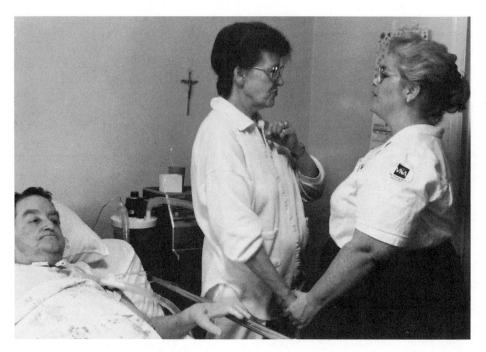

Figure 7-6 Caring for the caregiver. (Photograph courtesy Robyn Rice.)

day, over the course of a chronic progressive illness. An innovative strategy that may become widely accessible to caregivers in the future is described by Brennan and others.[3] In a randomized field experiment, caregivers of patients with Alzheimer's disease were assigned to a telephone support group, or a ComputerLink group. The 22 caregivers in the ComputerLink group received a computer, modem, and training. The computer system provided three kinds of resources: (1) an electronic encyclopedia with 200 factual entries about Alzheimer's disease; (2) a decision support system that helped caregivers select among alternative actions; and (3) a communications pathway, with access to a caregiver-to-caregiver discussion group and access to a nurse expert.

This innovative approach to caregiver education and support utilizes the principles of adult learning, making information available whenever the learner needs and wants it and at a pace the learner selects.

As caregiver needs for education increase and nursing time becomes a scarce commodity, home care nurses need to use all available and appropriate teaching methods described in this chapter. It is also important to recognize that when fostering learning about patient care, caregivers will also need nurturing and lots of hugs in the process (Figure 7-6).

SUMMARY

The unique role of home care nurses is to help patients/caregivers learn new behaviors that have a positive impact on their health and their lives. Much of this is accomplished through patient education. As we enter the patient's world, we work with the patient in mutually deciding what to teach, when to teach, and how to teach. Disease process, age, family, sociocultural background, and other elements of the home milieu will influence the process.

Success in patient education is primarily achieved when patients accept responsibility for their own quality of life, actively participate in the plan of care, and are self-determined to manage their health care needs at home. The true measure of the value of patient education lies in the patient's ability to sustain positive health behaviors after discharge from the home care agency and to avoid unnecessary hospitalizations. When these goals are achieved, we close our nursing bags and move on.

REFERENCES

1. Babcock D, Miller M: *Client education: theory and practice,* St. Louis, 1994, Mosby.
2. Botwinick J: *Aging and behavior,* ed 2, New York, 1978, Springer.
3. Brennan PF and others: ComputerLink: electronic support for the home caregiver, *Adv Nurs Sci* 13(4):14, 1991.
4. Brothen T, Detzner D: Perceived health and locus of control in the aged, *Percept Mot Skills* 56:946, 1983.
5. Burgess C: Application of the rotter scales of internal-external locus of control to determine differences between smokers, non-smokers and ex-smokers in their general locus of control, *J Adv Nurs* 19:699, 1994.
6. Davis C and others: An interactive perspective on the health beliefs and practices of rural elders, *J Gerontol Nurs* 17(5):11, 1991.
7. Davis LL: Building a science of caring for caregivers, *Fam Community Health* 15(2):1, 1992.
8. Dellasega C and others: Nursing process: teaching elderly clients, *J Gerontol Nurs* 20(1):31, 1994.
9. DeMeneses M, Perry G: The plight of caregivers, *Home Health Care Nurs* 11(4):10, 1993.
10. Erickson E: *Childhood and society,* New York, 1963, WW Norton.
11. Fadiman A: *A spirit catches you and you fall down,* New York, 1997, Farrar, Strauss, & Giroux.
12. Ford J, Rigby P: Focus on mental health nursing. Aftercare undersupervision: implications for cmnn's, *Br J Nurs* 5(21):1312, 1996.
13. Freed P, Rice R: Managing mental illness at home, *J Geriatr Nurs* 18(13):134, 1997.
14. Freud A: *The ego and mechanisms of defense,* New York, 1958, International Universities Press.
15. Germain C: Cultural care: a bridge between sickness, illness, and disease, *Holistic Nurs Practice* 6(3):1, 1992.
16. Greenburg JS and others: Contributions of persons with serious mental illness to their families, *Hosp Community Psychiatry,* 45(5):475, 1994.
17. Gruber H, Voneche J, editors: *The essential Piaget,* New York, 1977, Basic Books.
18. Guthrie E: *The psychology of learning,* New York, 1935, Harper & Row.
19. Hahn JA: Transcultural nursing in home health care: learning to be culturally sensitive, *Home Health Care Manage Prac* 10(1):66, 1997.
20. Health Care Financing Administration: *Health insurance manual* (Pub No. 11), Washington, DC, 1995, U.S. Department of Health and Human Services.
21. Horgan P: Health status perceptions affect health-related behaviors, *J Gerontol Nurs* 13(12):30, 1987.
22. Hunter K and others: Discriminators of internal and external locus of control orientation in the elderly, *Res Aging* 2(1):49, 1980.
23. Kist-Kline G, Lipnicky S: Health locus of control: implications for the health professional, *Health Values* 13(5):38, 1989.
24. Koehler W: Gestalt psychology, *Am Psychol* 14:727, 1958.
25. Koffka K: *Principles of gestalt psychology,* New York, 1935, Harcourt, Brace & World.
26. Kohlberg L: Moral development. In *International encyclopedia of science,* New York, 1968, McMillan.
27. Lewin K: *Field theory in social sciences,* New York, 1957, Harper & Row.
28. Lumpkin J: Health versus activity in elderly person locus of control, *Percept Mot Skills* 60:228, 1985.
29. Manworren RC, Woodring B: Evaluating children's literature as a source for patient education, *Pediatr Nurs* 24(6):548, 1998.
30. Maslow A: *Motivation and personality,* New York, 1970, Harper & Row.
31. McCaffrey B, Boyle D: The elderly patient with cancer: teaching/learning considerations for ostomy, wound, and continence management, *Progressions* 6(1):11, 1994.
32. Nemcek M: Health beliefs and preventative behavior, *AAOHN* 38(3):127, 1990.
33. Pollock S and others: Responses to chronic illness: analysis of psychological and physiological adaptation, *Nurs Res* 39(5):300, 1990.
34. Redman B: Patient education at 25 years: where we have been and where we are going, *J Adv Nurs* 18:725, 1993.
35. Reed A: Simple strategies that improve compliance, *RN* 60(9):35, 1997.
36. Reutter L, Ford JS: Enhancing diet compliance: melding professional and client knowledge in public health nursing practice, *Pub Health Nurs* 14(3):143, 1997.
37. Rice R: Key concepts of self-care, *J Geriatr Nurs* 19(1):52, 1998.
38. Rotter JB: Generalized expectancies for internal versus external control of reinforcement. In Rotter J and others, editors: *Applications of a social learning theory of personality,* New York, 1972, Holt, Rinehart, & Winston.
39. Ryglewicz H: Psychoeducation for clients and families: a way in, out, and through in working with people with dual disorders, *Psychosoc Rehabil J* 15(2):80, 1991.
40. Santrock JW: *Life-span development,* Boston, Mass, McGraw-Hill.
41. Shivley S and others: Lessons in caring: a care by caregiver program, *Geriatr Nurs* 14(6):304, 1993.
42. Skinner B: *Beyond freedom and dignity,* New York, 1972, Random House.
43. Smith R: Who is in control—an investigation of nurse and patient beliefs relating to control of their health, *J Adv Nurs* 19:884, 1994.
44. Swenson L, Skinner B: Reinforcement or operant conditioning. In *Theories of learning: traditional perspectives/contemporary developments,* Belmont, Calif, 1980, Wadsworth.
45. Thorndike E: *Animal intelligence,* New York, 1911, Macmillan.
46. Tripp-Reimor T, Anna L: Cross-cultural perspectives on patient teaching, *Nurs Clin North Am* 24(3):613, 1989.
47. Vellenga BA, Christenson J: Persistent and severely mentally ill clients' perceptions of their mental illness, *Issues Ment Health Nurs* 15(4):359, 1994.
48. Wallston K and others: Development of the multidimensional health locus of control (MHLC) scales, *Health Educ Monogr* 6:161, 1978.
49. Weinrich S, Boyd M: Education in the elderly, *J Gerontol Nurs* 18(1):15, 1992.
50. Wong D: *The essentials of pediatric nursing,* ed 5, St. Louis, 1997, Mosby.

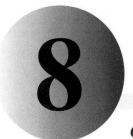

LEGAL AND ETHICAL ISSUES IN HOME CARE

Gayle H. Sullivan, Joanne P. Sheehan, and Robyn Rice

- An elderly home care patient who has clearly stated his wish to not be resuscitated arrests at his home while the home care nurse is present, but there is no DNR order in his medical record.
- A home care nurse who has been threatened by a patient's family member refuses to provide care in the home, and the patient later dies from lack of care.
- The spouse of a patient falls, suffering possible injury while the home care nurse is in the home, but refuses any assistance.
- A patient's condition is deteriorating, but attempts to reach her physician fail.
- A home care nurse is requested to perform a procedure that he or she does not feel qualified to do.

Home care nurses are likely to encounter at least one of these dilemmas in the course of their work. Although home care has been confronted with ethical and legal issues since the early 1900s,[9] the practice of home care nursing has become increasingly complex and the corresponding ethical and legal accountability has increased as well. Consequently a heightened awareness of the legal requirements and ethical guidelines that direct nursing practice within the home milieu is critical.

UNDERSTANDING OUR LEGAL SYSTEM

Home care nurses should be aware of three types of actions in our legal system: criminal actions, administrative law actions, and civil actions. All three are important to consider.

Criminal actions

Criminal actions are brought by states against defendants accused of crimes as defined by the state. Although health care providers are not typically involved as defendants in criminal actions, they have been prosecuted for crimes such as negligent homicide, insurance fraud, falsification of a business record, and theft of narcotics. The consequences of being found guilty generally involve some restriction on conduct, such as a jail sentence or probation, and sometimes a fine payable to the state.[15] The victim is not compensated in a criminal proceeding.

Administrative law actions

Administrative law actions are brought by state agencies empowered by the legislature to investigate complaints and take specified actions. The State Board of Nursing in each state and the Department of Health may investigate complaints against nurses. Complaints may be filed by patients or their families. Many health care organizations, and in some cases individual practitioners, have obligations under state law to report instances of misconduct, revocation or suspension (including voluntary suspension) of privileges, disciplinary action, or termination. Pursuant to any investigation, a hearing may be held. As part of this process, the State Board of Nursing is empowered to take actions including revoking, suspending, or restricting the nurse's license; requiring the nurse to undergo treatment; requiring the nurse to pursue continuing education in certain areas; and publicly censuring the nurse.

A nurse's license is a property right and cannot be taken without due process of law. Therefore nurses have constitutional rights in the administrative law process. To ensure that their rights are adequately protected, home care nurses should retain experienced counsel if they suspect that their conduct is being investigated.[1,2,15]

Home care nurses should also be aware that not all malpractice insurance policies provide coverage for disciplinary defense; however, some policies do. When applying for malpractice insurance, check your policy carefully for disciplinary defense coverage. Disciplinary defense coverage may also be purchased separately from some carriers. Most disciplinary defense policies cover attorney's fees up to a specified dollar amount. Keep in mind that any action taken against your license can result in the revocation of your license. Therefore retaining the services of an attorney is a small price to pay.[6]

Case example: Administrative law action. A complaint was filed against a health care nurse alleging failure to initiate CPR in a timely fashion. After an investigation and a hearing, the actions taken by the state board included requiring the nurse to successfully complete an adult CPR training course and placing the nurse on probation for 1 year. This action limits the nurse's ability to change employment because he or she may not do so without written permission of the state board.

Civil actions

Civil actions are designed to resolve disputes between individuals. Home care nurses, by virtue of their familiarity with patients and their families, may become entangled in many types of civil actions, including personal injury suits, workers' compensation claims, and divorce and custody proceedings. One of the most common types of civil actions in which home care nurses and their agencies can be involved is a malpractice or professional negligence suit. Malpractice (discussed later in this chapter) is a specific type of negligence. Anyone can be negligent, but only a professional can commit malpractice.

The purpose of civil action is to compensate with money for injuries caused, not to punish the person who committed the harm. Therefore the consequence of being found liable in a negligence or malpractice claim typically involves the payment of money for damages to the injured party.

Case example: Civil law action. A home care nurse administered an injection of Demerol and Vistaril IM to the right deltoid of an elderly patient with poor muscle mass. The patient developed erythema, which developed into a third degree burn and was accompanied by severe pain. According to the home care agency's policies, the deltoid was not a site approved for this type of IM injection. A civil suit alleging negligent administration of medication was brought against the nurse and agency. A $200,000 settlement was demanded.

UNDERSTANDING MORE ABOUT MALPRACTICE

Malpractice is defined by four distinct elements, all of which must be proven by the plaintiff. Elements of malpractice include the following:

1. Duty: established by a professional relationship
2. Breach of duty: an act or omission in violation of the standard of care
3. Injury: hurt, damage, or loss sustained
4. Causation: nurse's breach of duty caused the patient's injury

A duty is created by a professional relationship. With that in mind, consider the following example.

Case example: Establishing a duty. A home care nurse stops at a grocery store on his or her way home from work. The nurse sees that an elderly gentleman is lying on the sidewalk just in front of the store and that a small crowd has gathered. The spouse of a former patient recognizes the nurse and calls out for the nurse to help. The home care nurse does not want to become involved, and even though he or she can initiate lifesaving action, the nurse shouts back, "I'm not a nurse anymore," and then enters the store to shop. The elderly man dies.

Will the family of the deceased be successful in an action against the home care nurse if they claim that the nurse had an obligation to stop and help and that failure to do so caused their family member's death? Conflicting answers to this question illustrate the difference between what the law and ethical codes require. In this situation ethical codes dictate that nurses should assist;[3] however, the law does not require it. A malpractice claim against home care nurses under these circumstances will surely fail because the first element, duty (a professional relationship), is lacking.

Suppose that in this case, a home care nurse does attempt to help. However, after determining that the patient has no pulse, the nurse announces that there is nothing more he or she can do and leaves the scene. How does this change the analysis of liability? This represents a Good Samaritan situation, generally referred to as an emergency located away from the provider's place of employment. Each state has a Good Samaritan statute, and although these laws generally do not require nurses to assist at the scene of an emergency, immunity for negligence is provided if they do. Gross negligence is not protected, however, and abandoning a patient under these circumstances would most likely rise to that level, eliminating the Good Samaritan shield. Consider the following Good Samaritan guidelines:

- If you choose to stop at the scene of an emergency, stay until the ambulance arrives or someone of equal or greater skill takes over for you.
- Do not accept payment for services rendered.

The establishment of a professional relationship in the home care setting is created by the home care agency's contract to provide care to the patient. The duty is to meet the standard of care or, put another way, to act like a reasonably prudent nurse under the same or similar circumstances. The standard of care is determined by evaluating a variety of sources including the home care agency's policies and procedures, the individual state nurse practice acts, other state statutes and regulations, clinical guidelines promulgated by professional organizations, job descriptions, pertinent literature, and expert witness opinions.

It is particularly important for home care nurses to be aware of the significance of the home care agency's policies and procedures. The plaintiff's attorney will review the medical record, request copies of applicable policies and procedures, and then compare what the policy says should have been done with what is documented. Discrepancies provide an opportunity to argue that nonadherence with policies and procedures is evidence of malpractice.[8] A lay jury will find this compelling.[12] Consider implementing the following guidelines for policies and procedures:

- All employers should have written policies and procedures.

- Policies and procedures should be accessible to all staff members.
- Beware of mandatory language (e.g., "the nurse shall . . ." and "in every case . . .").
- Encourage discretionary language (e.g., "when appropriate . . ." and "in the nurse's professional judgment . . .").
- In-services should be provided on changes or additions to policies and procedures.
- Policies and procedures should be reviewed annually for accuracy.
- Annual reviews should be documented.

In addition to establishing the duty, the plaintiff must show that a breach of duty or violation of the standard of care occurred. Failing to use correct procedural technique when indicated, delegating specialized functions to untrained assistants, failing to notify a physician about significant changes in the patient's condition, and failing to teach the patient/caregiver how to operate home medical equipment, can all constitute a breach of duty.

A successful malpractice claim also requires that the plaintiff suffer an injury. Generally, this must be a physical injury such as paralysis, brain damage, fracture, or scarring. Emotional damages may be claimed in connection with the physical injury. In malpractice actions, damages based on purely emotional injuries are prohibited in most jurisdictions.

Causation, the last element of malpractice, can be the most problematic. There must be evidence that the nurse's breach of duty caused the patient's injury.

Case example: Elements of malpractice. A 40-year-old male patient was visited by a home care nurse at 10:00 AM, 1 day after discharge from the hospital and 5 days post gallbladder surgery. The nurse noted signs of infection at the incision site and an elevated temperature. The home care nurse left a message with the attending physician's answering service requesting the physician to return the call but did not document this. The physician never called back and the nurse forgot to follow up. At 4:00 PM that day, the patient suffered a massive cardiac arrest and died. The autopsy report indicated myocardial infarction as the cause of death.

This case example can best be analyzed by considering each of the four elements of malpractice:

- *Duty.* A professional relationship existed by virtue of the home care agency agreement to provide services to the patient.

- *Breach of duty.* The home care nurse should have followed up with the physician and documented these efforts. A failure to do so is arguably a breach of duty. If there was a question regarding medical coverage, the patient service manager should have been contacted.
- *Injury.* Cardiac arrest and death are physical injuries.
- *Causation.* It would be difficult to argue that the home care nurse's omission was the cause of the patient's injury in this case. However, note that if the patient had become septic and died, the outcome would likely be different.

WHAT ALL HOME CARE NURSES SHOULD KNOW BEFORE ACCEPTING EMPLOYMENT

Before accepting employment with any home care agency, home care nurses should ascertain the following information regarding future employment: (1) Will the home care nurse be an employee of the home care agency or an independent contractor? (2) Is the home care nurse familiar with the type of care and treatment patients require and the type of equipment that will be used? (3) Has the home care nurse been properly oriented and familiarized with his or her responsibilities to the patient and the home care agency? (4) Will the home care nurse be provided with a safe environment in which to work? (5) Is the home care nurse familiar with requirements to report to state agencies?

Home care agency employee versus independent contractor

Whether home care nurses function as independent contractors or as employees may determine whether the home care agency will provide malpractice insurance, unemployment compensation benefits, and workers' compensation benefits; make social security payments (FICA); withhold income tax; and whether the Fair Labor Standards Act would apply. The ultimate question is whether the employer has the right of general control over the means and method of work of the employee. The employer of an independent contractor is ordinarily not liable for the negligence of the contractor; however, the employer can be liable when the employer has selected an incompetent independent contractor.[7]

If the patient reasonably believes that the home care nurse, even though an independent contractor, was acting on behalf of the home health agency, the home care agency faces potential liability for the conduct of the nurse.

Nursing malpractice coverage. Home care nurses should be aware of the dollar amount of the professional liability coverage provided by their employer. The home care agency's policy should provide coverage for its employees within the scope of employment. It would not, then, apply to situations arising outside of work (e.g., assisting at the scene of an emergency or administering an injection to a neighbor). Therefore home care nurses should consider purchasing an individual policy to ensure coverage for any situation that may arise. Home care nurses should also determine the type of policy that is in effect.

A professional liability policy can be either a claims made or an occurrence policy. The claims made policy will cover home care nurses for incidences that occur *and* result in a claim during the policy period. If the policy includes a retroactive date, incidents that have occurred before purchase of the policy may also be covered.

An occurrence policy will provide coverage if a negligent act occurs during the time period that the policy is in effect, and if that negligent act gives rise to a claim for malpractice at any time in the future, even after the policy has expired. Home care nurses who change employers and liability coverage may experience a period of time in which they are uninsured. It is important to avoid this. Only by knowing the type of policy in force, its expiration date, and limits of liability can nurses be prepared to protect themselves from gaps in coverage.

Workers' compensation

As an employee you will also be entitled to workers' compensation if you are injured on the job. Workers' compensation insurance is paid for by the employer and provides benefits regardless of the employee's negligence. It may not provide benefits if the injuries are caused by willful or serious misconduct or intoxication. If the home care nurse is injured during the course of employment, he or she must file a written notice of claim with his or her employer or workers' compensation commissioner within the time specified by the workers' compensation act in the appropriate state. The notice filed should specify the date and place of the incident, the nature of the injury, and the name and address of the employee and employer. Keep in mind that any incident that may cause injury in the future should be recorded in the same manner. For example, a needle stick injury that may cause hepatitis C in the future should be documented.

Other insurance

Before accepting employment, home care nurses must also determine whether their employer will provide automobile liability insurance for the motor vehicle that will be used during the course of employment to get to patients' homes. Typically it is the nurse who provides this insurance.

Familiarity with type of care, treatment, and equipment required by patient

Before accepting employment, home care nurses should inquire as to the orientation provided by the home care agency for new hires. They should inquire whether a supervisor or a preceptor will be assigned to them for any period of time. If so, during the period of supervision, home care nurses should especially request experiences for work that is unfamiliar to them.

A standard checklist should be completed before and after orientation to document exposure to different situations and devices that are used in the home. A thorough review of the job description and the state's nurse practice act should be part of any orientation. The home care agency's policies and procedures should also be reviewed.[19] In addition, the home care agency should provide staff with inservices and educational offerings designed to build clinical skills and foster competence with work expectations.

Home care agency responsibilities to patient

After the home care agency admits the patient, no matter how complex the care, the agency is obligated to provide reasonable and competent care to that patient. If the patient's care needs progress beyond the ability of the home care agency, the agency is obligated to assist the patient to identify an acceptable alternative health care provider.

Appropriate supervision must be available during all service hours. In addition, home care agencies should provide access to qualified consultants when supervisors have neither appropriate clinical training nor experience for clinical practice needs.[10]

Provision of safe work environment

Home care nurses must know how to protect their patients and themselves from harm. (See Chapter 3, which discusses safety in the community.) As an employer, the home care agency should provide staff with a safe working environment. Any form of sexual or physical harassment or abuse of staff should be reported to the nurse's supervisor and director of nursing. Such problems may also be a matter for review by the professional consultation or ethics committee.

Home care nurses should adhere to their agencies' policies and procedures in documenting and reporting such incidents. In the event of assault, the nurse should consider filing a complaint with the local police department.

Familiarity with requirements to report to state agencies

Home care nurses must be familiar with the state requirements for reporting suspected abuse or neglect of patients. Every state has a law that specifies a state agency to which suspected cases of child abuse/neglect and elder abuse/neglect must be reported. Neglect can be defined as not providing for necessary physical, emotional, medical, or surgical needs, thereby endangering the person's health. Abuse is a form of cruelty to an individual's physical, moral, or mental well-being. In most states it is mandated that an RN or LPN who has reasonable cause to suspect or believe that an elderly person has been abused, neglected, exploited, or abandoned or is in the need of protective services, shall report such information to the Commission on Aging. It is also mandated in most states that an RN or LPN who has reasonable cause to suspect or believe that any child under the age of 18 has been subjected to physical injury, maltreatment, sexual abuse or exploitation, deprivation of necessities, or emotional maltreatment or neglect, must report the same to the applicable state agency and the local police department. Failure of home health nurses to file such reports will subject them to an imposition of a fine and to disciplinary action within some states. Any and all observations of suspected abuse or neglect should be documented in the patient's medical record.

Appropriate home care agency forms should be completed. If the person suspected of being abused or neglected is not a patient, the home care agency should have specific policies and procedures to follow and forms to document clinical concerns and actions taken. In most states if the reporting of abuse and/or neglect is done in good faith, the reporter will be immune from civil and criminal liability. However, any individual who willingly makes a false abuse and/or neglect report may be liable for civil and criminal penalties as provided in the state's statutes.[4]

If home care nurses observe and/or suspect a co-worker or supervisor of abuse or neglect, the same reporting procedures should be followed. In addition, home care nurses and/or home care agencies should report the professional misconduct to the State Department of Public Health and/or the State Board of Nursing.

Reporting communicable diseases. Home care nurses must also report communicable diseases to the appropriate state and community agencies. If a home care nurse is exposed to a communicable disease, the agency's appropriate policies and procedures should be followed. In addition, the home care nurse should consider filing a workers' compensation claim, which will put the employer and local workers' compensation commissioner on notice of the potential injury. (See Chapter 6 for information on infection control in the home.)

DOCUMENTATION ISSUES

The medical record has become an increasingly public document that is open to review by state surveyors, insurance carriers, attorneys, and jurors as circumstances warrant. The home care nurse's documentation constitutes the bulk of the record and serves as a crucial piece of evidence in ethical dilemmas and legal proceedings.

The medical record can prevent malpractice suits from being brought. If the record is complete and legible and documents that the standard of care was met, the case will be of less interest to the plaintiff's attorney.

The medical record can also protect home care nurses in the event that suit is brought. Years may pass between the time of an incident and the time the defendants become aware of the potential for liability. However, the medical record should be written at the time the events take place, while the events are clear and fresh in the writer's mind. It is sometimes referred to as *"the witness that never dies."*

Record keeping in home care

Complete, accurate, and truthful documentation is the cornerstone of the defense of any malpractice claim. The following are some important guidelines for recording assessments and documenting treatments and other actions taken in the home care setting:

- Document all assessments objectively. Objective documentation states the nurse's assessment based on facts, observations, patient's statements, and other measurable criteria. Subjective documentation states the nurse's conclusions without supporting facts and should be avoided (Table 8-1).

- Provide the date and time of each visit report at the time it is written, even if it is well after the visit has taken place. Also indicate the date and time of the visit. The visit report is often used to determine the chronology of events. Therefore accurate dating and timing of visit reports are critical.

- Sign all entries. The visit report should be signed with the home health nurse's first name or initial, last name, and title. Certain documentation may be initialed, such as an IV flow sheet or medication administration record. This is legally acceptable provided there is a space for each writer to initial and sign the document.

Table 8-1 Subjective vs objective documentation

Subjective documentation	Objective documentation
Skin good	Client's right hand and fingers are pink and warm to touch. There are no complaints of pain or tingling. Nail beds blanch well.
Appears depressed	Client is tearful. States, "I have never been this depressed in my life."
Teaching client to give own insulin	Client is able to give own insulin, demonstrates correct technique, and has no additional questions.

- Be certain that the patient's name appears on each page of the medical record.
- Accurately document all patient/caregiver teaching. In malpractice litigation, health care providers often face claims that they provided insufficient information to patients regarding use of equipment, techniques for procedures, recognizing signs and symptoms, side effects of medications, and so forth. Without supporting documentation, it's the patient's word against the home care nurse's word. To fully protect yourself, document all patient and family teaching, including what was said and who was present. In addition, document any return demonstrations given and by whom and that an opportunity to ask questions and instructions to follow in the event of a problem were provided.
- Maintain professionalism in documentation, particularly with regard to patients and their families. Remember, patients have a right to the information contained in their record. Documentation that subjectively characterizes a patient as "uncooperative," "obnoxious," "rude," or "snotty" (all examples from real charts), may be so offensive to the patient and family that they seek legal counsel. In a malpractice action this type of documentation will allow the plaintiff's attorney to argue that the nursing staff did not like the patient and that substandard care was delivered as a result. Therefore if a patient is truly uncooperative, be certain to document the objective reasons for this conclusion. For example, "Patient is noncompliant with medication regimen or diet," "Patient refuses to perform range of motion exercises," or "Patient does not follow instructions for dressing change."
- Use approved home care agency abbreviations.
- Properly correct mistakes on the visit report and other parts of the record. A failure to do so could constitute an alteration of the record, rendering a case indefensible. Every agency should have a written policy on how to correct a mistake, add information, and make late entries. Although the law does not require that nurses document perfectly, it does require corrections to be made pursuant to policy (Box 8-1).
- Do not rewrite notes, even to obtain reimbursement for the patient or agency. This is an unethical practice that can create significant legal exposure for both the home care nurse and the

home care agency. Insurance fraud allegations, loss of credibility in a malpractice action, and investigation by the State Board of Nursing are but a few of the problems a nurse who participates in this practice could face.

Physician orders and nursing implications

Although home care nurses have a duty to follow physician orders, there are five major exceptions to this general rule: (1) the order is illegible, (2) the order is illegal, (3) following the order could cause harm to the patient, (4) the order is against the policy of the home care agency, and (5) the home care nurse is not trained to carry out the order. In any of these situations the home care nurse's ethical and legal obligation to protect the patient rises above the duty to follow the physician's orders.

If there is a question regarding the appropriateness of a physician's order, home care nurses should first confer with the physician who wrote the order and then document this in the record. For example, "Discussed lasix dose with Dr. Smith; no changes ordered." If the home care nurse is still not comfortable with the order, he or she should not hesitate to invoke the home care agency's chain of

---

Box 8-1   CORRECTIONS, ADDITIONS, AND LATE ENTRIES

To correct a mistaken entry:
Draw a single line through the entry, date and initial it, and continue your documentation.

To enter an addendum to an existing note:
Write the date and time of the new entry on the next available space in the record (even if several days have passed) and state, "Addendum to note of [*date and time of prior note*]."

To make a late entry:
Late entries can be made in situations where no note was written at all; for example, the nurse forgot to document a home visit.
Write the date and time of the new note on the next available space in the record or on a visit report and state, "Late entry for visit of [*date and time of visit*]."

command and document this as well. The documentation could read, "Supervisor Jones notified of above conversation with Dr. Smith. Medication not given." Bear in mind that collaborative decision making to resolve complex ethical and legal issues can protect home care nurses from making erroneous choices.[16]

It is important to remember that the nurse always has the right to refuse to carry out an order. Although disciplinary action may be threatened, the nurse should prevail if the chain of command is followed and documented.

Incident reports

A patient falls out of bed while the home care nurse is in the home. Assessing him and initiating treatment for any injury are obvious priorities, but eventually an incident report must be completed. Situations requiring completion of an incident report will vary from agency to agency, but the usefulness of these forms in detecting and preventing recurring problems is universal.

Although incident reports are intended exclusively for home care agency use, they can be important in legal proceedings as well. The plaintiff's attorneys can sometimes gain access to incident reports, which often contain valuable information such as names, phone numbers, and addresses of witnesses; the cause of the incident; and corrective actions taken. It is important therefore to report information factually. Avoid making statements that affix blame, express opinions, or draw conclusions. The facts should be documented as follows:

- Date, time, and location of incident
- Family member notified (name, time, and by phone or in person)
- Name of physician notified and time
- Facts of the occurrence (e.g., in the case of medication that was not ordered for the client, "10 mg Inderal given PO," not "10 mg Inderal given PO by mistake because I picked up the wrong med.")
- Direct quotes from third parties (e.g., the patient)
- Assessment of the patient, using objective documentation
- Action taken

Incidents involving staff members, such as needlestick injuries, may also require completion of an incident report and should be documented in the same fashion. Every home care agency should have written procedures for completing incident reports and seeking medical treatment for on-the-job injuries.

Patient incidents should be documented on the visit report as well. Because an attorney would look at the record to determine whether the standard of care was met, include the details of any follow-up care and the patient's response to treatment. Do not document that an incident report was completed, however. At a minimum, this is a red flag to the plaintiff's attorney who could argue that reports mentioned in the record are part of the record and must be disclosed.[18]

Keeping incident reports confidential can be facilitated by implementing a few basic security procedures. First, stamp all incident reports "confidential." Be certain that incident reports are completed and routed to the appropriate persons within 24 hours. Limit distribution to those involved in reviewing the incident, and store reports in a locked file cabinet. Do not make copies of incident reports for patients or their family members, because this would surely destroy any hope of preserving confidentiality. Home care nurses should not make copies of incident reports for personal use. This would not only constitute a breach of confidentiality but also would likely be a violation of home care agency policy.

Patient rights and responsibilities

Home care nurses must be familiar with the patient's rights and the patient's responsibilities and review both with the patient (Box 8-2 and Box 8-3).

It should be documented in the medical record that the patient's bill of rights and the patient's responsibilities have been given to and reviewed by the patient, and the patient has acknowledged an understanding of each. Signed copies are to be maintained in the patient's medical record.

With this information in the record, the home care agency may be better positioned to discharge abusive and noncompliant patients from care without exposing the home care nurse and home care agency to allegations of abandonment. Home care agencies do have the right to discharge patients from home care. To terminate this relationship effectively, a certified letter should be sent to the patient (return receipt requested), and a copy

Box 8-2   PATIENT RIGHTS

Statement of Rights

A person who receives home care services has these rights:

1. The right to receive written information about rights in advance of receiving care or during the initial evaluation visit before the initiation of treatment, including what to do if rights are violated.
2. The right to receive care and services according to a suitable and up-to-date plan and subject to accepted medical or nursing standards and to take an active part in creating and changing the plan and evaluating care and services. *The provider must advise the recipient in advance of the right to participate in planning the care or treatment.*
3. The right to be told in advance of receiving care about the services that will be provided, the disciplines that will furnish care, the frequency of visits proposed to be furnished, other choices that are available, and the consequences of these choices, including the consequences of refusing these services.
4. The right to be told in advance of any change in the plan of care and to take an active part in any change *and the planning before any change is made.*
5. The right to refuse services or treatment.
6. The right to know, in advance, any limits to the services available from a provider and the provider's grounds for a termination of services.
7. The right to know, *and to be advised both orally and in writing,* in advance of receiving care whether the services are covered by health insurance, medical assistance, or other health programs, the charges for services that will not be covered by Medicare, and the charges that the individual may have to pay. *The provider must advise the recipient of home care services, both orally and in writing, of any changes in such coverage and the recipient's liability for charges as soon as possible but no later than 30 calendar days after the provider becomes aware of a change.*
8. The right to know what the charges are for services, no matter who will be paying the bill.
9. The right to know that there may be other services available in the community, including other home care services and providers, and to know where to go for information about these services.
10. The right to choose freely among available providers and to change providers after services have begun, within the limits of health insurance, medical assistance, or other health programs.
11. The right to have personal, financial, and medical information kept private and to be advised of the provider's policies and procedures regarding disclosure of such information.
12. The right to be allowed access to records and written information from records in accordance with section 144.335.
13. The right to be served by people who are properly trained and competent to perform their duties.
14. The right to be treated with courtesy and respect and to have one's property treated with respect.
15. The right to be free from physical and verbal abuse.
16. The right to a reasonable, advance notice of changes in services or charges.
17. The right to a coordinated transfer when there will be a change in the provider of services.
18. The right to voice grievances regarding treatment or care that is, or fails to be, furnished or regarding the lack of courtesy or respect to the patient or the patient's property.
19. The right to know how to contact an individual associated with the provider who is responsible for handling problems and to have the provider investigate and attempt to resolve the grievance or complaint. *The provider shall document in writing all complaints, as well as document, in writing, any resolution of the complaint against anyone furnishing services on behalf of the provider.*
20. The right to know the name and address of the state or county agency to contact for additional information or assistance.
21. The right to assert these rights personally, or have them asserted by the patient's family or guardian when the patient has been judged incompetent, without retaliation.

I have reviewed and understand my responsibilities as described above.

Signature of patient: _____   Date: _____

Relationship if not
signed by patient: _____   Date: _____

Case manager: _____   Date: _____

Source: Carla Scheffert, RN, Minneapolis, Minn.

Box 8-3   PATIENT RESPONSIBILITIES

Statement of responsibility

A person who receives home care has the following responsibilities:

1.   Every patient shall provide accurate and thorough information regarding his/her health history, mental health history, hospitalizations, present status, allergies, medications, and any other information pertinent to his/her well-being.
2.   Every patient shall report any significant or unexpected change in his/her status.
3.   Every patient shall participate and adhere to the development and update of the Home Care Plan of Care with the health team or collaboration with the attending physician.
4.   Every patient shall have the right to refuse treatment, programming, and/or instructions, as well as the responsibility for his/her actions and consequences.
5.   Every patient, to the best of his/her ability, shall make it clear that he/she comprehends requests and expectations. The patient will request further information concerning anything he or she does not understand.
6.   Every patient shall adhere to the stipulations of the Home Care Admissions Agreement.
7.   Every patient will inform the home care services when unable to keep a home care visit.
8.   Every patient will assist in developing and maintaining a safe environment.
9.   Patients are responsible for fulfilling the financial obligations of their health care as promptly as they are able.

I have reviewed and understand my responsibilities as described above.

Signature of patient: _____   Date: _____
Relationship if not
signed by patient: _____   Date: _____
Case manager: _____   Date: _____

Source: Carla Scheffert, RN, Minneapolis, Minn.

---

should be placed in the record. It is always advisable to consult legal counsel before discharging patients with conditions requiring regular medical attention. A sample letter for discharging a noncompliant patient is shown in Box 8-4.

ADVANCE DIRECTIVES

The advance directive allows a competent patient to advise others of his or her choices and treatment in the event of future incapacity.

The Patient's Self-Determination Act, which is part of the Omnibus Budget Reconciliation Act (OBRA), became effective December 1, 1991. To continue to be eligible for Medicare and Medicaid funds, health care facilities (including home care agencies) must determine at the time of admission whether the patient has an advance directive. If not, the patient must be provided with education concerning the applicable state laws on advance directives and the home care agency's policies on advance directives. If the patient has an advance directive, it should become part of the medical record.

Living will

The living will is one type of advance directive. It is a written statement of a patient's wishes regarding the use of medical treatment when the patient is in a terminal state or determined to be permanently unconscious. Although state laws vary, a terminal condition can generally be defined as one that is incurable or irreversible and, without the administration of life support systems, will result in death. The living will may list life support systems the patient does not want, such as artificial respiration, cardiopulmonary resuscitation, and artificial means of providing nutrition and hydration.

Health care agent or proxy

In addition to the living will, some state statutes provide for the appointment of a health care agent. If the patient's physician determines that the patient is unable to understand and appreciate the nature and consequences of health care decisions and to reach and communicate an informed decision regarding the treatment, the health care agent may be authorized to state the patient's wishes con-

---

Box 8-4 SAMPLE LETTER FOR DISCHARGING A NONCOMPLIANT PATIENT

Dear Client:

The agency finds it necessary to inform you that as of (date), it will no longer provide home care services as a result of (reason). Since your condition requires continued attention from a home care provider, it is suggested that you place yourself under the care of another agency without delay. The above termination date should give you ample time to select an agency of your choice from the home care providers in this city. If you are not acquainted with another agency, you should consult with your attending physician or contact the (town agency or professional association and phone number). Should a medical emergency arise before the termination date indicated above, you should contact your attending physician; you may contact us as well. The agency will make your medical records available to the agency you designate below. Since your records are confidential, your written authorization is required. Please complete the enclosed form and return it to (agency) (enclose an authorization to transfer records).

Very truly yours,
AAA Agency

cc: (Patient's attending physician)

---

cerning medical care. Depending on the jurisdiction, this may include the withholding or removal of life support systems. The agent may also take whatever actions are necessary to ensure that the patient's wishes are given effect. It is imperative that the home care agency and the home care nurse know who the patient's appointed health care agents are and how to reach them in case of an emergency. This should be documented in the patient's medical record.

A patient may revoke the living will or appointment of a health care agent at any time in any manner. If the patient does so, it should be well documented in the patient's medical record, and the physician should be notified so that the physician's record may also be documented.

Case example: Advance directives. The patient has executed a valid living will. The living will indicates that the patient does not wish CPR, artificial respiration, and artificial means of hydration and nutrition. The patient has appointed her son as her health care agent. Copies of the living will and appointment of health care agent are contained in the patient's medical record. The home care nurse assumes care of the patient, at which time the patient lapses into a coma and dies. Based on the patient's living will no CPR or artificial means of respiration are given by the home care nurse. The next day the home health agency that employs the nurse is notified by the patient's son that his mother had changed her mind and wanted to live as long as possible. However, this information was not given to the patient's health care providers. Is the home care nurse liable for malpractice and professional misconduct for not taking aggressive measures?

In the absence of knowledge of the revocation of either a living will or appointment of health care agent, a health care professional is not subject to civil or criminal liability or discipline for unprofessional conduct for carrying out the living will. If the health care provider or agent is unwilling to comply with the wishes of the patient, care of the patient should be transferred as promptly as possible to a health care provider who is willing to comply with the wishes of the patient within the confines of the applicable state law.

Do not resuscitate orders

"Do not resuscitate" orders may differ from state to state. The order must be written by the patient's physician. In addition, "do not treat" or "do not hospitalize" orders should also be written by the physician and kept in the patient's medical record.

INFORMED CONSENT

Before initiating any medical intervention, valid consent of the patient and/or the legally authorized substitute decision maker must be obtained. Lack of informed consent that proximately causes an injury to a patient may give rise to a claim of professional negligence and/or malpractice.

Historically it has been up to the clinician, typically physicians who perform the procedure, to discuss treatment with the patient and obtain required consent. Thus far no duty to obtain informed consent has been established for home care nurses, and no home care agency has been successfully sued for a failure to obtain informed consent. However, it is the home care nurse's obligation to speak up when the patient appears not to understand, seems to be incompetent, or may have been coerced into agreeing to a procedure. Although not required in most instances, written informed consent is preferable to a conversation that is not documented.[5] The consent must be given voluntarily from an informed competent person. In providing informed consent, the elements of disclosure should include (1) the nature of the procedure, (2) the risks and hazards of the procedure, (3) the alternative to the procedure, and (4) the anticipated benefits of the procedure.[13]

According to the patient's bill of rights the patient also has the right to refuse treatment and/or care. If patients refuse treatment or care, they should not be forced to cooperate. The nurse should document such refusal and communicate the same to the treating physician.

RIGHT TO CONFIDENTIALITY
IN MEDICAL RECORDS

As with all patients, home care patients have the right to confidentiality of medical records. The patient's medical records may not be released to a third party without the written consent of the patient. Authorizations should be scrutinized carefully to determine the scope of the allowed disclosure. Limitations that may be included in the authorization include time frames of treatment, reference to a particular injury and/or disease entity, and to whom the records may be released. The authorizations should not be more than 1 year old. If the authorization does not provide for the disclosure of psychiatric treatment, then the same should not be released. In some states a health care provider may not release records that make mention of the HIV virus and/or its related symptoms without the express consent of the patient.

Confidentiality and security of the field or travel chart should be addressed by home care agency policy. The practicalities of delivering quality patient care dictate that certain patient information must be available to caregivers in the home. The confidentiality and security of this information should be discussed with the patient and/or family pursuant to home care agency policy.

TELECARE

Telecare is the use of communications technology to transmit health information from one location to another. The proliferation of telecare projects has prompted uncertainty about legal responsibilities and potential liability. Although many vexing legal issues must still be resolved, solutions to most common problems do exist. Home care nurses should be aware of the telecare regulations in their state. Few courts have addressed the subject and there is no consensus on practice standards; however, malpractice for telecare is likely to present the same basic question as in any malpractice case: Did the nurse breach his or her duty to the patient, thereby causing an injury? See Chapter 27 for further discussion and practice guidelines.

COMMON AREAS OF LIABILITY
AND HOW TO AVOID THEM
Inadequate staff training for assigned tasks

Case example. An inexperienced home care nurse was assigned a patient on a portable ventilator. The home care nurse was worried about her lack of training and experience with ventilator-dependent patients, but as a new graduate, she felt pressured to take the assignment and talked herself out of these concerns. She thought it best not to question her superior's judgment and accepted the case.

Guidelines to avoid liability

- Before you accept or refuse a patient you think you are untrained to competently handle, determine precisely what type of care will be required and whether you will receive any supervision.
- Be thoroughly familiar with the care your patient requires. You must know how to operate any equipment in use, provide associated care, make relevant clinical assessments, and detect potential problems.
- Be certain that you are not being asked to perform a function that violates your home care agency's policies and procedures.
- Refuse to perform any treatment not permitted by your state's nurse practice act. If you do not know whether a particular procedure is beyond the scope of nursing practice in your state, contact the state board to find out.
- Insist on proper training and information before you accept an assignment of a patient with whose care you are unfamiliar. Request an inservice as necessary before implementing care.

- Refuse to accept an assignment if you are not familiar with the care the patient requires. Put the reasons for your refusal in writing in a memo to your supervisor. State your objections factually. For example, "I have never irrigated a patient's colon using traditional equipment without supervision and my training was over 10 years ago," as opposed to "I'm not comfortable using traditional equipment to irrigate a patient's colon."
- Express a willingness to take a comparable assignment in the future provided you receive appropriate training and supervision. If you are the supervisor, you are responsible to ensure that employees to whom you delegate have the proper training and authority to perform assigned tasks. If you knew or should have known that the employee was not sufficiently trained, you could be liable for negligent delegation.
- Familiarize yourself with the skills and abilities of anyone you supervise, including nurses and nursing assistants. The supervisor or primary care nurse should discuss the proper care for each patient with the nursing assistant who will be involved in the care. Clarify circumstances under which the case manager is to be notified. If you are forced to make an assignment you think may be unsafe or you are unable to properly supervise another, put someone in your chain of command on notice before you take this action.
- Implement an annual criteria-based performance evaluation that documents clinical abilities and skills of all nursing staff members.

Patient falls

Case example. The patient is an 88-year-old male with poor eyesight. He ambulates with a walker. While the home care nurse leaves the room to get something for the patient, he gets out of his chair and attempts to ambulate to the bathroom. Unfortunately, his walker is nowhere near his chair and he walks unaided. The patient falls and fractures his hip.

Guidelines to avoid liability

- Evaluate the patients who are at risk for falling at home because of impaired senses, decreased physical capabilities, side effects of medications, or their environment. Initiate a referral to rehabilitation services as necessary.

- Document your assessment and the fall prevention plan, including all patient and family teaching.
- Keep all ambulating devices and corrective lenses within reach of the patient.
- Routinely educate and remind the patient how to avoid falls and document this completely.
- Evaluate the patient's environment for potential risks, such as loose carpeting, poor lighting, and steep stairs.

When environmental hazards exist or a patient is noncompliant with the fall prevention plan, consider having the patient and/or family sign a statement indicating their understanding that a fall resulting in serious injury is possible in these circumstances. Keep a copy in the patient's medical record.

Medication errors

Case example. A home care nurse is assigned to a cardiac patient. The home care nurse notes that the patient's blood pressure is lower than usual and that the patient is complaining of being tired all of the time. The home care nurse reviews the patient's medication record and sees that the patient is taking two antihypertensive medications. The nurse phones the patient's physician and reviews the medication orders. The order for the first antihypertensive medication had expired when the second medication was ordered. However, the first medication was never discontinued; therefore the home care nurse continued to give the medication.

Guidelines to avoid liability

- Before administering medication, check and double-check the patient's name, route of administration, the correct dosage, the correct medication, and the time(s) of administration.
- Be familiar with the medication administered, its side effects, and its compatibility with other medication the patient may be taking.
- Observe the patient for potential side effects of the medication; document and report the same to the patient's physician.
- Adhere to the home care agency's policies for medication renewal by the physician.
- Immediately report medication errors to the patient's physician and your supervisor. Complete an incident report form as required.
- Validate patient self-reported changes in medications with the physician's office.

- Report instances of patient self-medication error or dangerous home remedies to the physician, and follow home care agency policy regarding this matter.

Faulty equipment

Case example. Your patient is a 69-year-old male with chronic obstructive pulmonary disease, and he is on a portable ventilator. You routinely check the flow rate during your visits and document this. The patient complains that for the past 3 days, he has awakened with a headache. You wonder whether the ventilator is properly calibrated and whether the patient is receiving too much oxygen.

Guidelines to avoid liability
- Be thoroughly familiar with any equipment used in the care of your patient. You must know how to operate the equipment, monitor it, provide associated care, and detect potential problems.
- Insist on proper training and information before you accept an assignment of a patient whose care involves the use of equipment you are not familiar with.
- Refuse to accept an assignment if you are not familiar with all applicable medical devices and their operation.
- Be certain that nursing assistants providing care to your patients are thoroughly familiar with any equipment in use.
- Provide the patient and the patient's caregivers with complete instructions on the use of all equipment.
- Carefully document in the record all teaching you have done with the patient and caregivers on the equipment in use.
- Request and observe patient/caregiver return demonstrations with procedural care and equipment and document this in the record.
- Ensure that the manufacturer's instruction manual is attached to the equipment in the home.
- Contact the company "Write it Right"* for assistance in evaluating and preparing medical device user instructions.[11]

---

*Small Manufacturers Assistance Office and Health and Industry Program Center for Devices and Radiological Health, Food and Drug Administration, HF2220, 1350 Piccard Drive, Rockville, MD 20850.

- If equipment failure could be life threatening, determine the availability of a backup generator and/or backup equipment in the home. Provide specific instructions to follow in the event of equipment failure, and keep a copy in the record.
- If you suspect that a device is malfunctioning, call for immediate service, notify your supervisor and the patient's attending physician, and document in the record the steps you have taken.
- Complete an incident report detailing any equipment malfunction or failure.
- If you plan to use any of your own equipment on the job, have it inspected by the home care agency and get the home care agency's written approval for its use. This may protect you from liability if a problem occurs.

The Safe Medical Devices Act of 1990 requires the reporting of any equipment malfunction resulting in serious injury, illness, or death. The suspected malfunction and details of the occurrence should be reported by the home care agency within 10 weekdays to the FDA and the equipment manufacturer.[21]

Communication and safety problems

Case example. You have accepted assignment of a new patient, an 86-year-old female stroke victim who lives with her daughter and 27-year-old grandson, a chronic schizophrenic with a history of violence. At 7:30 PM on the day after your first home visit, you receive a call from the daughter, who thinks her mother has had another cerebral vascular attack. You arrive at the home and are met by the grandson, who threatens to harm you if you enter.

Guidelines to avoid liability
- If you feel your safety is threatened, immediately leave the home and notify your patient service manager of the problem.
- All home care agencies should have an administrator or patient service manager on call 7 days a week, 24 hours a day to assist with clinical decision making. This person should carry a beeper and be available immediately by telephone to consult with and advise you.
- Before you accept your first patient assignment, know your chain of command, including names and phone numbers of your supervisor, Director

of Nursing, Agency Administrator, and Medical Director. If you cannot reach your immediate supervisor, call the Director of Nursing and so on. If your immediate supervisor is not responsive to your clinical needs, continue to follow the chain of command for assistance in appropriate decision making.

- Nonclinical emergencies should be covered in the home care agency's policy, but even if they aren't, invoke the chain of command when you need assistance. Be assertive enough to initiate the chain of command. Remember, it is your legal duty, and a failure to do so could result in patient injury and professional liability.
- Carry the name and telephone number of the patient's attending physician with you on all home visits. Do not hesitate to involve the patient's physician.
- Factually document in the record your efforts to communicate with others. Specify who was called and the time.
- If you are the supervisor, know who is available to you before you start your shift, including names and phone numbers. If you contact the Agency Administrator or Medical Director in response to a problem, document this in a memo and keep one copy for your files.
- Remember, whether you are a manager or primary care nurse, putting someone in authority on notice of the problem is critical.

If you are unable to reach anyone in your organization, use your best judgment in response to the situation, bearing in mind that in most instances it is better to be overcautious. Documenting all efforts to obtain assistance and acting in good faith should serve to protect you in the event of litigation.

Inadequate medical response

Case example. An 83-year-old patient suffers an apparent transient ischemic attack while you are in the home. You do not want to leave without speaking to the patient's physician, who you suspect will want to see the patient and probably adjust the medication orders. By the time you are ready to leave, the physician has not returned your call. This physician is known to ignore nurses' calls and then complain to administration that he has not been kept informed.

Guidelines to avoid liability

- Note in the record every attempt to reach the patient's physician, including the time, content of messages left, facts conveyed in each conversation, and efforts you have made to go up the chain of command.
- If the patient's condition is rapidly deteriorating, do not hesitate to get medical treatment for the patient. Invoke your chain of command; in an emergency, call emergency medical services (EMS).
- When a particular physician routinely ignores nurses' calls or provides otherwise inadequate care, bring it to the attention of your supervisor in a memo. Document factually, noting, for example, instances in which you attempted to reach the physician but did not receive a timely response. Keep one copy of the memo for your files.
- If a physician's response rises to the level of incompetence, report it to your supervisor in a memo.
- Contact the patient's physician whenever you detect more than a minor exacerbation of the patient's condition or whenever the physician has asked to be notified.
- Always alert a physician whose patient is en route to the hospital.

Trust your instincts when the patient's condition seems serious. You have a duty to be an assertive advocate when the physician does not respond appropriately to your patient's needs.

Admitting inappropriate patients into home care

Case example. The home care nurse is assigned to a patient with a history of mental health, as well as physical, problems. The patient is continually changing residences to various shelters. Often the home care nurse cannot locate the patient, or the patient is not home at the time of the scheduled visit.

Guidelines to avoid liability

- Carefully screen patients, including their home environment for equipment needs before accepting them.
- Consider whether home care services can reasonably be expected to meet the needs of the patient. Review government regulations for re-

imbursement; Medicare will not reimburse home visits in which the patient is noncompliant or no longer homebound (see Chapter 5).

Document all of the patient's noncompliance in the medical record. Be specific by using actual examples of noncompliance and report the same to the physician. Let the physician know that the patient is in jeopardy of discharge.

Request a multidisciplinary conference to evaluate the patient's needs and whether a referral to a different agency may be appropriate.

Provide the patient with a written letter indicating that he or she is discharged from the agency (see Box 8-4). If possible, have the patient sign the letter and return it to the agency. If you cannot locate the patient, send a letter (return receipt requested) to the last known address. Be sure to inform the patient's physician before the patient's discharge, then send the physician a copy of the discharge letter.

Maintain a copy of any correspondence with the patient in the patient's medical record.

SUMMARY

Home care is growing and will continue to become increasingly complex in service delivery. For home care nurses this means caring for more acutely ill patients and using the associated technology within the sometimes unpredictable environment of the home milieu. In these circumstances careful attention to legal and ethical ramifications of patient care is a must.

REFERENCES

1. Aiken T, Catalano J: *Legal, ethical and political issues in nursing,* Philadelphia, 1994, FA Davis.
2. The American Association of Nurse Attorneys, 420 Light Street, Baltimore, MD 21230-3816, (410-752-3318).
3. American Nurses Association: *Code for nurses with interpretive statements,* Kansas City, 1985, The Association.
4. Brendt N: The home health care nurse and suspected child abuse and/or neglect, *Home Health Care Nurs* 12(4):10, 1994.
5. Cat M, Bigot A: *Geriatrics and the law: patient's rights and professional responsibilities,* New York, 1985, Springer.
6. Catalano J: *Ethical and legal aspects of nursing,* Springhouse, Pa, 1991, Springhouse.
7. *Darling v. Burrone Brothers, Inc,* 162 Conn 187, 1972.
8. De Marzo D: Policies and procedures: protection or peril? *RN* 56(7):61, 1993.
9. Haddad A, Kapp M: *Ethical and legal issues in home health care,* Norwalk, Conn, 1991, Appleton & Lange.
10. Joint Commission on Accreditation of Healthcare Organizations: *Home health standards,* 1989, Chicago, The Commission.
11. Kingsley P and others: Medical device user instructions: the patient's need, the nurse's role, *Home Health Care Nurs* 13(1):27, 1993.
12. Laska L, editor: Medical malpractice verdicts, settlements & experts, 11(2):19, 1995. Case reported: *Ballon v. St. Joseph Hospital and Janet Reyes, RN,* Passaic County (NJ) Superior Court, Case No. PAS-L-3271-90.
13. Meisel, Kabnick: Informed consent to medical treatment: an analysis of recent legislation, *Upitt Law Rev* 41:407, 1980.
14. Northrop CE, Kelly ME: *Legal issues in nursing,* St. Louis, 1987, Mosby.
15. *People v. Coe,* 131 Misc 2d 807, 1986.
16. Rubsamen DS, editor: A fatal case of aspiration pneumonitis, *Professional Liability Newsletter* 24:10, 1994.
17. Sullivan G: Home care: more autonomy, more legal risks, *RN* 57(5):63, 1994.
18. Sullivan G: The right way to fill out an incident report, *RN* 57(12):53, 1988.
19. Sullivan G: When assignments don't match skills, *RN* 58(4):57, 1995.
20. Sweeney M: Your role in informed consent, *RN* 54(8):55, 1991.
21. Tammelleo A: Who's to blame for faulty equipment? *RN* 53(10):67, 1990.

CASE MANAGEMENT AND LEADERSHIP STRATEGIES FOR HOME CARE NURSES

Robyn Rice

The cost of health care in the United States has skyrocketed out of control. The rise in home care expenditures demonstrates this increase in costs. From 1989 to 1996, spending in home care increased by more than 800%, whereas the percentage of Medicare beneficiaries using the home care benefit only doubled.[4] Within this economic climate of spiraling expenditures, the public and congress are demanding cost-effective, quality patient care.

In 1997 the Balanced Budget Act was primarily passed by the U.S. Congress in order to maintain the solvency of the Medicare program. Numerous payment revisions were introduced in this act in order to control Medicare spending. The home care Medicare benefit was targeted in these revisions because of its soaring costs and industrywide complaints of abuse, fraud, and waste. As discussed in Chapter 1, Medicare is now moving toward prospective payment and the establishment of a national database through the Outcome and Assessment Information Set (OASIS), which will be used to define costs and quality of care.[4,25,28] These reforms, along with the growing influence of managed care, are challenging home care nurses to essentially plan and implement outcome-based patient care with a specific amount of monies or visits. As a result, professional accountability for efficient and effective employment of home care services will be more important than ever before.[1,2,6]

How is accountability for efficient and effective patient care to be addressed by a caring profession such as nursing? In dealing with the regulatory and economic restructuring of health care in this country, home care nurses must provide innovative approaches to patient care that maximize efficiency and utility of service. They must also maintain professional standards of practice. Hence, in balancing economics with a professional commitment to serve the public, home care nurses must not only implement patient care but also have a *say* in how quality patient care and clinical policies are determined, implemented, and evaluated.

Refer to Chapters 1 through 10 and the clinical chapters in this book that build on principles of case management. The purpose of this chapter is to provide an overview of case management and leadership strategies that empower home care nurses to address issues of fiscal accountability for services, to deliver quality patient care in the home setting, and to maintain professional standards of practice.

MANAGEMENT AND LEADERSHIP STRATEGIES

More patients, sicker patients, regulatory issues influencing the availability of resources, and increasing professional responsibilities for patients are realities for home care nurses. Yet the milieu of home care is rewarding to those nurses who enjoy the tremendous amount of freedom and autonomy of nursing practice that home care offers. For these nurses, their experience is not "Nurse do this," but rather "Nurse, what do we do?" In other words, in addition to providing hands on patient care, home care nurses often consult with physicians and patients to make recommendations for service coordination and treatment. In order to rise to this expectation and maintain the public's trust that quality patient care will be given, home care nurses must be expert clinicians. As a result, familiarity with disease processes, medical treatments, wound-care products, community resources for referral, and a sensitivity to the home milieu are required. In maintaining professional standards of practice, home care nurses must also have a strong voice in governing clinical policies. They must be managers and leaders.

Management versus leadership

Bennis and Goldsmith differentiate management and leadership in the following manner, "A good manager does things right. A good leader does the right things." In the management role, home care nurses are concerned with the implementation, organization, structuring, and evaluation of systems, procedures, and policies. In the leadership role, nurses are not only concerned about providing quality patient care but also have definite ideas and opinions about how patient care and home care agency policy should be determined. The implication is that a leadership role is more likely to involve visionary, innovative, and inquiry-based approaches. Management is about implementing and evaluating policy. Leadership creates such policy.[3] In the following sections, clinical applications of how home care nurses can be effective managers and leaders are presented.

TRENDS IN MANAGEMENT: CASE MANAGEMENT
Historical perspectives

Home care and community-based nurses have traditionally utilized principles of case management when providing and coordinating services for their patients. However, models of case management continue to be shaped by the government and the private sector of the health care market. Historically, case management models have been around since the turn of the century when Visiting Nurse Associations emphasized service coordination of patient care. The term *case management* first appeared in social welfare literature in the 1970s.

Case management broadly refers to the process of delivering patient care according to patient "case type" or individual needs. *Case type* refers to groups of patients who share a common medical or nursing diagnosis. As discussed in Chapter 10, case management focuses on the achievement of patient outcomes of care within an effective and appropriate time frame (length of stay). As a cost-containment initiative, case management largely operates under the umbrella of managed care.

Managed care became a popular term in the 1980s. *Managed care* refers to the systems that provide the structure, regulations, and guidelines for implementing cost-effective patient care. These systems link the provider with the public in managing cost, access to resources, and quality patient care.[8,9] Examples of public managed care systems include Medicare and Medicaid. Examples of privately managed care systems include health maintenance organizations (HMOs) and preferred provider organizations (PPOs). These organizations are increasingly seeking providers (home care agencies) who can show an improvement in the patient's health status while exhibiting appropriate resource utilization.

Reimbursement of health care services is intricately tied to the principles of case management and managed care. As described above, Medicare's reimbursement of home care services is moving toward prospective payment or capitation of fees for an episode of care. Using utility screens, HMOs and PPOs are already limiting the number of home visits nurses can make. As prospective payment becomes the future of home care, there will be increased emphasis on more efficient utilization of services through the process of case management, as well as care path development. In order to secure managed care contracts and meet future Medicare guidelines for reimbursement of services, home care agencies are now focusing their attention on case management models in which care is structured by patient care plans that are based on a working knowledge of case type or disease process, anticipated outcomes, and appropriate resource utilization.[7,11,15] In addition, trends in documentation systems are moving toward multidisciplinary notation. The goals of the model are as follows:

- To demonstrate positive health outcomes
- To use resources more effectively
- To maximize patient, physician, nurse, and payer satisfaction
- To enrich clinical practice

Home care definitions of a case manager and case management

The case manager is an expert clinician who is responsible for maintaining standards of care, coordinating multidisciplinary services, utilizing community resources, and ensuring that patient/caregiver outcomes of care are met within a reasonable time frame. The Commission on Insurance Rehabilitation Specialists provides certification for case managers, and the National Association of Case Managers serves as a support and accreditation organization for case managers.[10] The registered nurse (RN) usually serves as the case manager in home care. The only exception to this would be if the patient is receiving only rehabilitation services. In this case the physical therapist may serve as case manager.

There are many models of case management. This chapter will present a home care agency point-of-service case management model. In this model, case management is broadly defined as a process of multidisciplinary care in which nursing coordinates its services with those of other disciplines[1,2,18,19,23] (Figure 9-1).

In this model, home care nurses work with many different physicians and care for patients with a variety of diseases and functional disabilities. Therapeutic interventions are based on a patient classification system or case type such as a specific medical diagnosis or disease.[26] Documentation systems with predetermined patient goals, outcomes of care, and anticipated learning needs for patient case types are emphasized. The result is a standardized, high-quality, cost-effective plan of care.[29] Elements of case management in a home care-based case management model include the following[9,20,22]:

- Autonomy in practice; encouraged decision making of case managers and support services; an emphasis on decentralized decision making

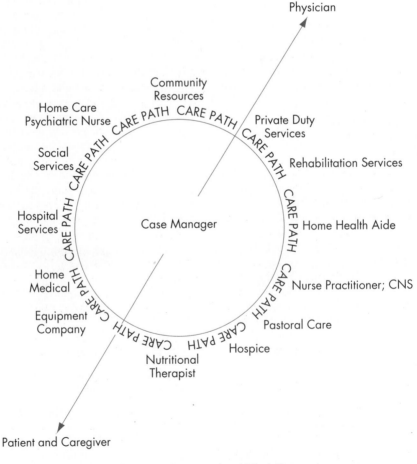

Figure 9-1 The case manager and multidisciplinary resources.

- Accountability for practice as case managers are vested with the authority and responsibility for clinical and financial outcomes for their caseload; an emphasis on risk management strategies that decrease the probability of incurring adverse outcomes
- Decreased fragmentation of services; the patient is followed by an individual or group of individuals who are responsible for assisting the patient/caregiver through the system; an emphasis on coordination of care
- Outcome evaluation; expected outcomes are determined during the admission process and compared with actual outcomes in identifying opportunities for benchmarking improvement of services
- Satisfaction of customers and consumers (including the managed care organization, patient/caregiver, physician, and home care staff); improved patient outcomes and coordination of services, decreased rework, recognition of service and accountability for role, consistency in policy implementation, and increased satisfaction for all
- Use of the primary nurse (RN) as case manager; an emphasis on full-time salaried field staff as case managers
- Efficient and effective resource utilization; an emphasis on multidisciplinary referrals for service
- Collaborative practice between case manager, physician, and the multidisciplinary team; the case manager merges each discipline's plan of care into one collaborative plan with mutually agreed on goals; an emphasis on increased communication systems via the plan of care
- Comprehensive patient/caregiver assessment and reassessment
- Emphasis on patient/caregiver education
- Emphasis on active patient/caregiver participation with the plan of care
- Appropriate discontinuation of care
- Caseload organization

CLINICAL APPLICATIONS OF CASE MANAGEMENT IN THE HOME

As discussed in Chapter 5, outcomes of care are derived from the intake referral and admission assessment. In the role of case manager, it will be important for home care nurses to meet with the patient/caregiver and mutually develop the plan of care. For example, when identifying outcomes of care, the patient/caregiver's perceptions of learning needs should be assessed. This information would then be incorporated into the plan of care (Figure 9-2).

Typical questions regarding the implementation of home care services and caseload organization often involve the number of patients to be seen and the time that the home care nurse should spend in each patient's home. The information in Box 9-1 may provide insights for answering these questions.

The caseload will require basic organization so that all of the patients are seen and services rendered as ordered by the physician and authorized (reimbursed) by Medicare or the managed care organization. Home visits are primarily made from 8 AM to 4 PM during the workweek. However, additional staff coverage is provided for after hour and weekend visits.

Many nurses carry a travel chart for each patient. Information in the travel chart includes the physician's up-to-date orders for treatments and medications, a copy of the plan of care, and a calendar to indicate patient/caregiver visit frequency and dates for specimen collection, specific procedural requirements, physician office visits, or when recertification orders should be sent in. As discussed later, if laptop computers are used, all information can be easily stored in the computer. In addition, a folder including basic service information about the home care agency, a copy of the plan of care or care path, and related information is usually kept in the patient's home.

A calendar outlining visit frequency services of all disciplines is advised (Figure 9-3). As case managers, home care nurses should use calendar planning to ensure that multidisciplinary visits are spread across the workweek. This way everyone does not show up at the patient's home on the same day, which does little to maximize quality care and can be exhausting for the patient/caregiver. Share the calendar with patients as a means to involve them in their own care.

As technological advances increase, trends in organizing the caseload include the use of mobile cellular phones and dictaphones to maximize the efficiency of communications and the use of laptop computers with a modem to record and transmit patient data from the car (Box 9-2).

Questions to Use in Assessing Dynamic Self-Determination
for Discharge Planning to Home Care Services

Patient's Name _____

	Yes	No	Comments

1. Patient is under the care of a physician.   ____ ____

2. A reasonable expectation exists that the patient's
   medical, nursing, rehabilitation, and social needs
   can be adequately met by the home care staff in
   the patient's home.   ____ ____

3. The home care agency has adequately trained staff to
   provide services to the patient.   ____ ____

4. The home environment is safe for visiting staff.   ____ ____

5. The home environment supports required technology for
   home care services.   ____ ____

6. The patient is willing to work with the home care agency
   staff in learning self-care management at home.   ____ ____

7. The patient is trainable.   ____ ____

8. If the patient is unable to assist home care agency staff
   with self-care management, a caregiver or family
   member is available to do this.   ____ ____

9. The patient/caregiver participates with the plan of care.   ____ ____

10. The patient/caregiver understands his or her rights and
    responsibilites for home care services.   ____ ____

11. Primary nursing diagnosis/patient problems:

12. Patient/caregiver educational needs (include patient/caregiver self-perceived needs):

13. Patient/caregiver advocacy needs (procedural care required?):

14. Patient/caregiver case management needs (Multidisciplinary referrals for care?
    Community resources? Recommended care path, standard, or plan of care?):

15. Patient/caregiver spiritual needs:

Professional's signature: _____ . Date: _____

Figure 9-2 Admission assessment questions. (Theoretical framework: The Rice Model of Dynamic
Self-Determination.)

Teamwork is very important in home care because patients are often visited by many disciplines. A collaborative relationship is fundamental to teamwork so that everyone understands their role and gives their best effort toward achieving patient/caregiver outcomes of care.[21,22] This includes the patient/caregiver.

Medicare and most managed care organizations will deny payment for duplication of home care services.[17] Home care nurses should work with the multidisciplinary team so that this does not happen. For example, if the patient requires instruction on energy conservation techniques, this should be done either by the occupational therapist or the

---

Box 9-1　RESEARCH IN HOME CARE: A NATIONAL SURVEY[26]

During 1994 while giving a national lecture series for home care nurses, the author surveyed seminar attendees regarding average caseload and visit frequency.[27] The results of the survey may have useful applications in planning the caseload. Neither laptop computer utilization nor the impact of OASIS on documentation time was assessed.

An average caseload for home care nurses ranged from 15 to 46 patients. It was noted that some of the patients in the nurse's reported caseload were seen only monthly (e.g., patients receiving services for a monthly indwelling foley catheter change).

Patient acuity levels and service area (or expected miles driven) influenced the size of the caseload. For example, nurses who reported a smaller caseload stated that they "drove great distances" or cared for patients who received high-tech services such as intravenous (IV) therapy. Also, nurses in Florida and Texas reported increases in caseload during the winter months when older adults migrated to areas with milder climates.

Patient acuity levels, mileage, extra time required with patient admissions, work with student nurses, and planned office time were also cited as factors that influenced the number of patients that the nurses were able to see in 1 day. Typical daily visits fell in the range of 3 to 9 patients with a mean of 5.6 patients, again depending on patient needs and other work-related expectations that the home care nurse may have had. For example, nurses providing high-tech services such as home IV therapy reported daily visits in the range of 2 to 5 patients with a mean of 3.4 patients. It was interesting to note that home care nurses in New York City reported an average daily visit schedule higher than nurses in most other parts of the country. This could possibly be related to the fact that the New York City nurses who were surveyed reported that they typically walked to work and that most of their patients were located in one apartment building or on a city block.

In terms of length of visits, nurses surveyed reported a mean of 45 minutes for a Medicare repeat visit* with a mean of 2 hours required for Medicare openings or patient admissions.* High-tech services such as an initial TPN visit or an initial visit for a ventilator-dependent patient took longer. Reported estimates varied with a mean from 3.8 hours.*

Average driving time or average miles driven in the course of a day by home care nurses was not assessed in the survey.

*This included time allotted for paperwork.

Box 9-2　TIPS FOR ORGANIZING THE CASELOAD

Plan patient visits to maximize efficient mileage.
　Look at the patient's address and find the location of the residence on the street map; avoid unnecessary driving.
Plan to visit patients requiring lab work in the morning because test results are usually requested by the afternoon.
Use the travel chart, calendar, or laptop computer database as a reminder of when certain procedures, lab work, or recertification orders are due.
If possible, visit patients with a communicable disease last or at the end of the day.

nurse but *not* by both disciplines. Multidisciplinary conferences are one way for case managers to bring the team together.[31,32]

A multidisciplinary conference for each patient is recommended once a month in order to review patient/caregiver progress toward meeting identified outcomes of care. Conferences should make use of present day electronic communication systems (e.g., telephone conferences, e-mail communications via the Internet, and electronically recorded care plans) to increase efficiency in service. During the conference the role of each team member should be reviewed relative to achieving patient/caregiver outcomes of care. Progress toward goals of care, as well as variances or identified problems, should be reviewed. An action plan would be implemented for problem resolution (Box 9-3). Variances would then be tracked in the quality improvement (QI) program (see

Patient's name _____
Current certification period _____
Recertification orders required by _____

Sunday	Monday	Tuesday	Wednesday	Thursday	Friday	Saturday
	SN (AM FBS) hha	PT	SN hha	PT MSW	SN hha	
	SN hha	PT	SN hha *hha supervisory visit	PT	SN hha	
	hha	SN PT	hha	SN MSW	hha PT	
	hha	SN PT	hha *hha supervisory visit	SN (AM FBS)	hha PT	
	hha	SN PT	hha	SN (no SN visit as patient has MD office appointment)	hha PT	

SN=RN   PT=Physical therapy services
hha=Home health aide   MSW=Social worker

Figure 9-3 Using a calendar to plan Medicare-certified home visits.

Box 9-3   OUTCOME FAILURE ANALYSIS

1. Identify the outcome(s) that was not met.
2. Identify all possible causes.
3. Evaluate the likelihood of each.
4. Select the most probable cause(s) of outcome failure.
5. Identify all possible corrective actions.
6. Select the optimal corrective action(s).
7. Evaluate the efficacy of the action plan.

Chapter 10). If the patient's physician is unable to attend the conference, the case manager should send the physician a copy of the conference summary and seek feedback as appropriate. It is also important to share the conference summary with the patient/caregiver in order to identify those outcomes of care that have been accomplished and those that require further work.

Adjusting the visit frequency during services and planning for patient discharge are also part of case management for home care nurses. Typically the patient will require more visits at the beginning

---

Box 9-4   WORKING WITH MANAGED CARE ORGANIZATIONS TO SECURE EXTRA HOME VISITS

Questions to Consider

Whom do you have a contract with?

What are the terms of the contract regarding referral and payment?

Who is the gatekeeper (utilization review person) at the managed care organization?

Does the managed care organization request that you work with a certain supply company or service that they contract with? If so, who are these people and how will business be handled?

What are the charges (e.g., for visits, skilled care, and supplies)? Find out if there is a deductible or patient co-payment and make the patient aware of this before making the visit.

How is prior approval for home visits (e.g., for phototherapy) handled?

What documentation will the managed care organization require from you?

Tips to Secure Extra Visits

Contact the gatekeeper or managed care organization case manager and negotiate for extra visits on a weekly, not monthly, basis.

Focus on patient physiological instability as a medical necessity for extra visits (e.g., fever, draining wounds predisposing the patient to sepsis, lung con-

gestion predisposing the patient to hypoxia, or any condition that places the patient at risk for [more expensive] hospital readmission).

To promote the good will of the managed care organization and position yourself to ask for extra visits in the future, turn back those visits that you believe are unnecessary or that you do not use. The managed care organization will see you as an efficient and caring provider—good politics for future contracts.

To speed things up, send a preprinted letter of request for the physician to sign.

When All Else Fails

Take your concerns up the chain of command to the managed care utilization review committee or president (leaders do want to see the right thing done, so give them a chance).

Take your concerns to your legal or ethics committee for advice.

Consider filing a complaint with your state's insurance organization (be aware that this action will likely cost you some business).

Consider the implications of the patient's rights and choices.

---

of services. After the initial needs are met and the patient is stabilized, the visit frequency should decline as the patient/caregiver becomes more comfortable with self-care management of health care needs at home. To obtain provider reimbursement for services, fluctuations in visit frequency, the need for increased visits during services, and the need for continued home care services must be supported by clinical documentation that indicates outcomes of care that were not met or the instability of the patient/caregiver's health status[13,17] (Box 9-4). When goals of care are met and the patient is stabilized at home, discharge occurs (Box 9-5).

An operational model for service delivery

Many home care agencies are moving toward an evaluation system whereby nurses have a set number of efficiency points to earn each week rather than "numbers of patients seen." In this

---

Box 9-5   PATIENT DISCHARGE CRITERIA

Goals of care met
Outcomes of care achieved
Stabilization of disease process
Maximal potential with rehabilitation program achieved
Moved outside of service area
No longer homebound
Does not participate with the plan of care
At the patient's or physician's request
Rehospitalization
Death
Other

model, field staff are evaluated not only on clinical expertise but also on service to the agency. As described later in this chapter, service could take on the form of committee work. In this model, part-time and LPN staff would typically cover Thursday afternoon visits while the case managers went to the agency to attend to paperwork; participate in committee work, conferences, or in-services; and set up the next week's visits.

These quotas or point systems, mutually determined by staff and administration, are based on the miles that the home care nurse must drive each day, patient acuity levels, the mentoring of student nurses, and the amount of committee work or service that the nurse has agreed to take on. Overtime pay typically is discouraged. Operational models, like the one described, tend to promote efficient operation of clinical services as expectations of job performance are clearly defined and talents of staff are fully utilized.

How can case managers implement and track multidisciplinary care? Described as "the road map to home care" and as "the critical tool of case management," care paths are becoming an increasingly popular means of bringing managed care to home care.[11,16,24]

A tool for case managers: care paths

A care path is a standardized multidisciplinary plan of care that enables home care nurses to plan, implement, coordinate, and evaluate the care for certain groups of patients based on a shared medical or nursing diagnosis or some form of patient classification system based on a standard of care.[2,16,19] Originally described as a critical pathway, its purpose is to evaluate whether quality patient care is being delivered in a cost-effective and timely manner.[30,31] The term *care path* is recommended for home care agencies instead of *clinical pathway* or *critical pathway* because patients at home provide self-care management that is neither clinical nor critical.[19] Care paths in home care are used as follows:

- Patient care plans
- Standards of care
- Orientation tools for staff in learning home care
- Educational tools for student nurses in learning home care

- Multidisciplinary conference guides
- Documentation and tracking tools for the QI program and Medicare or managed care organization
- A patient database for purposes of research in future decision making to improve quality of care and utilizations of services

Care paths in home care involve standardized patient outcomes based on patient groupings that should allow for individualization of content, which is determined by the multidisciplinary team and the patient/caregiver during the admission process. It is important to share the content of the care path with the patient/caregiver so that the delivery of services, as well as patient/caregiver expectations with the plan of care, are clearly understood by all. Patient/caregivers should be able to articulate who they are being seen by, the purpose of each discipline, what *they are supposed to accomplish* during home care services, and an expected date of discharge.[14] Care paths can be very specific in format and outline day-to-day care, or they can be more general in describing the overall course of service. A care path outlining care on a per visit or weekly basis is recommended for patients at home.

The care path model in Appendix IX-I is designed to replace the patient care plan and multidisciplinary conference guide. For ease and simplicity of use, the care path is designed to fit front to back on an 8½ by 11 inch piece of paper. It could also be modified into a computer software program. Specific dates for achieving the outcomes of care designated on the care path would be selected by the case manager, the patient/caregiver, and the multidisciplinary team (including the physician) after initial patient assessment. In this particular form, outcomes also serve as critical events or actions that the nurse would take in order to facilitate patient home independence and discharge. Daily visits would be documented on the visit report (see Chapter 5). The case manager would be responsible for updating the care path each week with documented input from the multidisciplinary team at least once a month. If the case manager is working for a Medicare-certified agency, a new form would be used each recertification period that would carry over outcomes yet to be achieved.

Note that the care path presented in Appendix IX-I has predeveloped patient education guides that would be issued with the form (see Box 14-4 to examine the education guide). A patient edition of the care path can be found in Appendix IX-II. Patients would be provided with a stamped self-addressed envelope and encouraged to complete their care path survey and mail it back to the agency after discharge. This should be used as data for quality improvement processes.

TRENDS IN LEADERSHIP: EMPOWERMENT

In striving toward innovation in health care, philosophies of leadership and management are changing. Trends in leadership suggest a flattened hierarchy within organizational systems in which a shared governance is represented by councils, committee work, and internal restructuring for creative and inquiry-based change.[3] Innovative leadership builds an environment in which staff feel free to voice recommendations or dissent. Innovative leadership utilizes the creative talents of staff to create a work environment that fosters trust, integrity, competence, and a vision of shared objectives or outcomes. Innovative leaders lead creative people. Creativity is a basis for empowerment.

Empowerment, within the context of this chapter, refers to those partnerships within the home care agency that emphasize innovative and creative approaches to the business of home care. It also promotes individual expression for quality patient care. For example, empowered home care nurses believe that they are at the center of things and that what they do makes a difference to the success of their home care agency. Empowerment obligates nurses to focus their attention not only to the patient's bedside but also to the organization and operation of the home care agency. It obliterates a "pay per visit" mind-set in which the nurse's only concern is to make the home visit and get paid. It discourages home care agencies from increasing daily visit frequencies to the point where it becomes impossible for staff to provide quality patient care. Likewise, empowerment puts aside autocratic managers who do not listen or care to listen to what their staff have to say. Through service such as committee work, home care nurses become more than bedside clinicians. They are given opportunities to apply their talents toward discovering the solutions to the complex problems facing health care today.[3] This is the essence of empowerment and the spirit of good business.

To effectively work within these changing organizational systems and govern clinical practice, home care nurses need to know how to be leaders, as well as case managers.

CLINICAL APPLICATIONS OF LEADERSHIP: COMMITTEE WORK

Group work does not come easily to people in the United States, which is truly a country that values individualism. Yet active, organized committees with shared objectives can be one of the most politically effective means to determine and drive policy at the home care agency. Most important, committee work allows home care nurses a platform from which to speak. The following questions are frequently asked by home care nurses: What types of committees should home care nurses be involved in? How do home care nurses get the administration to support committee work? How does one chair a committee and run a meeting?

Committees a home care agency can't afford to be without

Clinical practice needs, economic constraints, regulatory issues, and the specter of legal or ethical issues in the milieu of home care drive the need for committee work (Box 9-6).

Consider using a professional consultation committee to assist staff in coping with some of the very difficult legal and ethical issues they face in home care. For example, abusive or noncompliant patients, inadequate medical treatment, and safety concerns may be very real problems for home care nurses. In these matters, the professional consultation committee would become an advisory board for an appropriate course of action. Because government and regulatory agencies seem to continuously redefine operational policy for home care agencies, consider the advantages of addressing changes in standards through the professional practice committee. Who better able to determine clinical policies and procedures than the nurses and other home care staff who practice them?

Consider this question: Does the home care agency have the best alcohol prep pad at the best cost? The professional research committee could ensure this by evaluating different vendor brands of alcohol prep pads for cost efficiency. Committee

---

Box 9-6 RECOMMENDED COMMITTEES FOR HOME CARE AGENCIES

Professional Standards Committee
QA/QI
Staff preparation for state and regulatory review
  (mock survey)
Care path development and implementation

Professional Consultation Committee
Legal/ethical issues
Staff safety
Employee grievance

Professional Research Committee
Product evaluation
Research projects

Professional Practice Committee
Policies and procedures
Forms
Technology
Infection control

Professional Service Committee
Educational in-services
Fund raising
Town hall
Christmas party and summer picnic

---

members would squeeze each brand of prep pad and determine how many drops of alcohol were obtained. In this manner, the committee would be able to recommend that the home care agency purchase the lowest cost brand of alcohol prep pads that have the most drops of alcohol. In reality, the cost effectiveness of alcohol prep pads is a *little thing*. However, it is the little things that bespeak a mutual concern for quality when doing the *big things* such as patient care. The professional research committee should meet with suppliers, evaluate products, and pass information along to field staff so that what is stocked in the medical supply room is relevant to clinical practice needs.

How do you get administrative support for committee work? In approaching administration regarding the need for committees, it is important to present the benefits of committee work to the home care agency. What are the economic advantages? How can the home care agency strengthen services from committee work? Improved patient care, improved outcomes, improved employee satisfaction, improved working relationships, improved communications among the multidisciplinary services, and reduced liability are only a few of the benefits derived from committee work.

How to chair a committee and run a meeting

There are several ground rules that are important to understand when chairing a committee. First, the chair should be prepared to accept responsibility for the committee. Chairing a committee is definitely a leadership role and it will be necessary for home care nurses to handle the politics of leadership. It is important to understand one's role as the chair, whether appointed or elected. Although committee member input is to be highly valued and expected, a primary role as chair is to keep the committee on track so that goals are met. It is the chair's responsibility to ensure that the committee's designated assignments are achieved.

Second, the chair should consult with the administrator or director. As chair, it is important to find out the administrator's expectations of what the committee should be accomplishing. When meeting with the administrator, the chair should take notes as a matter for future reference. The chair should periodically review the committee's goals and progress with administration. There are some issues that may require the administrator's political clout or authority in order to get the committee work accomplished. For example, the chair may require administrative assistance in handling an uncooperative intraagency department or unresponsive committee member. Therefore the chair should keep administration informed and involved. When initially assuming the position of chair, the individual should make sure lines of authority are clearly understood. If the home care agency has made committee work mandatory as part of staff's job descriptions, the chair should find out up front from the administrator who is responsible for ensuring that staff attend the meetings.[12] A chair should **never** accept the responsibility for ensuring member attendance or performance without some kind of authority to back up this responsibility. Such a situation will make a chair ineffectual and frustrated.

Third, the chair should meet with the committee. At this time, administrative ideas regarding the purpose and goals of the committee should be shared with the committee members. The administrative charge to the committee must be very clear and priorities must be set. It is important to mutually incorporate administrative assignments with goals that the committee members wish to achieve. A written action plan outlining committee goals and member responsibilities in meeting assignments with time lines for completion should be given to each committee member and the chair's administrator. At the end of the year (or whenever committee work is completed) the chair should report a summary of the committee's work and accomplishments to administration or to the home care agency's governing body. DeVries's book, *How to Run a Meeting,* based on Robert's Rules of Order, provides some basic guidelines for running a meeting[12] (Box 9-7).

Chairs should get to know the committee members and utilize their talents to the committee's advantage. For example, a particular committee member who enjoys research could perhaps be assigned to work that involves statistical analysis. As chair, it will be important to delegate committee assignments to the committee members. Issues will have to be thoroughly researched and analyzed before the committee makes recommendations to the home care agency. The chair should periodically touch base with committee members to make sure that assignments are being completed within the designated time frame.

Wess's book, *Victory Secrets of Attila the Hun,* provides some interesting perspectives in leading groups and cultivating followers.[30] Trust, integrity, enthusiasm, competence, consistency, and caring are qualities of leaders that followers appreciate and are drawn to.

As chair, it is important to recognize that being a leader is no easy job. Leaders are often risk takers. The Japanese have a saying that, "The nail that sticks out is the one that gets hit." Job promotion, recognition, and professional achievements can, at times, make for jealous and hostile colleagues. If intraagency politics get rough, home care nurses should document any concerns they may have regarding their job and look to their *true colleagues,* as well as family, for support and guidance. In advocating that the right things are done, it is impor-

---

Box 9-7	TIPS FOR CHAIRING A COMMITTEE AND CONDUCTING COMMITTEE WORK

- Arrange to reserve a room or place for all committee meetings.
- Consult with committee members in arranging times and dates to hold meetings; choose the most convenient meeting time for the group.
- Send out an announcement of the next committee meeting to all members at least 1 week before the meeting is scheduled; include an agenda on the announcement.
- Arrange to keep a record of the minutes of the committee meetings. Send out copies of the minutes to committee members and administration no later than 1 week after the meeting.
- Review the past minutes at the start of a new meeting to clear up old business.
- Consider providing refreshments; the sharing of food often relaxes the atmosphere and may enhance teamwork.
- Stick to time frames and schedules.

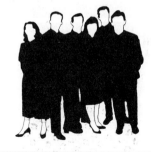

---

tant for nurses, as leaders, to understand that change can be an exhausting yet very rewarding process. It is also important to recognize that *hard work and dedication to improvement are the keys to success.*[5]

SUMMARY

As managers and leaders, home care nurses appreciate that learning and competence are elemental to accountability for professional practice. In working with the public, such a philosophy is also essential for good business.

Where there is management, there is leadership. Where there is leadership, there is a team. As described in this chapter, through the process of teamwork, as well as individual expression for innovative approaches to service delivery, home care nurses can provide cost-effective, quality patient care *in caring ways.*

REFERENCES

1. American Nurse Association: *Nursing case management,* Kansas City, Mo, 1988, The Association.
2. Becker-Weilitz P, Potter P: A managed care system: financial and clinical evaluation, *JONA* 23(11):51, 1993.
3. Bennis W, Goldsmith J: *Learning to lead,* Reading, Mass, 1994, Addison-Wesley.
4. Briggs E, Nelson K: The changing home health care environment, *Phys Ther* 7(4):12, 1999.
5. Brown H: *On success,* Nashville, 1994, Rutledge Hill Press.
6. Bulger S, Feldmeier C: Developing standards and quality measurements for case management practice, *J Case Manage* 7(3):99, 1999.
7. Cesta T: Case management: its value for staff nurses, *Am J Nurs* 99(5):48, 1999.
8. Cesta T and others: The case manager's survival guide: winning strategies for clinical practice, St. Louis, 1998, Mosby.
9. Chan F and others: Foundational knowledge and major practice domains of case management, *J Case Manage* 5(1):10, 1999.
10. Cline K: Preparing for the first CM examination, *Case Manage* 4:19, 1993.
11. Crummer M, Carter V: Critical pathways-the pivotal tool, *J Cardiovasc Nurs* 7(4):30, 1993.
12. DeVries M: *How to run a meeting,* New York, 1994, Penguin Books.
13. Eposito L: Home health case management: rural caregiving, *Home Healthcare Nurse* 12(3):38, 1994.
14. Feldman C and others: Decision making in case management of home health care clients, *JONA* 23(1):33, 1993.
15. Hamm T, Callahan H: Functional model for centralized intake and care management within a home health integrated delivery system: a case study, *Home Health Care Manage Prac* 11(3):58, 1999.
16. Hawkins J, Goldberg P: Planning, implementing and evaluating a chemotherapy critical pathway, *Oncology Med,* p. 24, March/April 1994.
17. Health Care Financing Administration: *Health insurance manual* (Pub No. 11), Washington, DC, 1995, U.S. Department of Health and Human Services.
18. Huggins C, Phillips C: Using case management with clinical plans to improve patient outcomes, *Home Healthcare Nurse* 16(1):15, 1998.
19. Leininger S, Laux L: The continuum of health care: highlights of orthopaedic and general medical pathways, *Home Health Care Manage Prac* 10(4):1, 1998.
20. Lyon J: Models of nursing care delivery and case management: clarification of terms, *Nurs Econ* 11(3):163, 1993.
21. Maturen V, Van Dyck L: Using outcome-based critical pathways to improve documentation, *Home Health Care Manage Prac* 8(2):48, 1996.
22. Migchelbrink D and others: Population-based managed care: one hospital's experience, *NAQ* 17(3):45, 1993.
23. Molloy K: Defining case management, *Home Healthcare Nurse* 12(3):51, 1994.
24. Nyberg D, Marschke P: Critical pathways: tools for continuous quality improvement, *NAQ* 17(3):62, 1993.
25. Packard N: The price of choice: managed care in America, *NAQ* 17(3):8, 1993.
26. Reeder L: Anatomy of a disease management program, *Nurs Manage,* p. 41, April, 1999.
27. Rice R: *Reported findings of average caseload and visit frequency.* Unpublished national survey of home health nurses conducted during 1994. Funded by American Nursing Development, Maryville, Ill, 1994.
28. Shaughnessy PW, Crisler K: Outcome-based quality improvement, Denver, 1995, National Association for Home Care.
29. Trinidad E: Case management: a model of CNS practice, *Clin Nurs Special* 7(4):221, 1994.
30. Wess R: *Victory secrets of Attila the Hun,* New York, 1993, Dell.
31. Zander K: Managed care within acute settings: design and implementation via nursing case management, *Health Care Supervisor* 6(2):24, 1990.
32. Zander K: Physicians, care maps & collaboration, *New Definition* 7(1):1, 1992.

Care Path (CP) Standard:
Skin/Integumentary System

Physician _____   Primary diagnosis_____

Case manager_____   Secondary diagnosis _____

ADM date _____   _____

DC date _____   Surgical procedure(s) and dates_____

Certification period from _____ to _____   _____

Admission assessment and initial visit forms completed □

Identified nursing diagnosis/patient or caregiver health care needs [check as appropriate]

_____ 1. Impaired skin integrity

_____ 2. Impaired physical mobility

_____ 3. Knowledge deficit re: disease process, risk complications, health management, infection control, socioeconomic resources

_____ 4. Pain

_____ 5. Other [list] _____
_____

CP standard utilized: #1; [list if adjunct CP utilized]: _____

Multidisciplinary services utilized (check as appropriate)

RN	□	PT/PTA	□	MSW	□	Other: [list] (volunteer, chaplain,
LPN/LVN	□	OT/COTA	□	RD/NT	□	other agencies, vendors,
HHA/HMK	□	ST	□	Specialty nursing	□	suppliers, etc.)

SN total visits _____   Rehabilitation services total visits _____

Personal care total visits _____   Other disciplines/services total visits _____

Patient education guides utilized: [check as appropriate]

_____ 1. Patient/caregiver home CP

_____ 2. Wound care

_____ 3. Infection control

_____ 4. Medications

_____ 5. Home safety

_____ 6. Other [list]:   (skin care)_____
_____
_____

**Pressure relief/reduction devices or home medical
equipment utilized: [list]** _____
_____
_____

CP treatment codes:

T1. Wet to dry NS   T3. Topical moisturizer   T5. Calcium aginate   T6. See medication record

T2. Dry dressing   T4. Hydrocolloid   Other: [list] (skin care) _____

Courtesy American Nursing Development, Maryville, Ill.

Week 1   Progress toward meeting patient/
caregiver outcomes

Outcomes: [list code]   Variance(s):   [list code-
Treatment: [list code]   OV; TV]

[Brief narrative of patient/caregiver progress with CP
including patient/caregiver learning, changes in
physician orders/treatments, or identified problems.
Utilize the variance tracking guide for problem
resolution or plan of action.]

Case manager's
signature:_____ Date:_____

Week 5   Progress toward meeting patient/
caregiver outcomes

Outcomes: _____Variance(s): _____
Treatment: _____

Case manager's
signature: _____ Date: _____

Week 2   Progress toward meeting patient/
caregiver outcomes

Outcomes:_____ Variance(s):_____
Treatment: _____

Case manager's
signature:_____ Date:_____

Week 6   Progress toward meeting patient/
caregiver outcomes

Outcomes:_____ Variance(s): _____
Treatment: _____

Case manager's
signature:_____ Date: _____

Week 3   Progress toward meeting patient/
caregiver outcomes

Outcomes: _____ Variance(s):_____
Treatment: _____

Case manager's
signature: _____Date: _____

Week 7   Progress toward meeting patient/
caregiver outcomes

Outcomes:_____Variance(s):_____
Treatment: _____

Case manager's
signature: _____Date: _____

Week 4   Progress toward meeting patient/
caregiver outcomes

Outcomes:_____ Variance(s):_____
Treatment: _____

Case manager's
signature: _____ Date: _____

Week 8   Progress toward meeting patient/
caregiver outcomes

Outcomes:_____Variance(s):_____
Treatment: _____

Case manager's
signature: _____ Date: _____

Week 9   Progress toward meeting patient/caregiver outcomes and discharge goals of care
Outcomes: _____Variance(s): _____
Treatment: _____
[*Brief narrative including medical reasons for patient discharge or need for recertification.*
Were goals achieved? Were objectives or patient outcomes of care met?
Utilize the variance tracking guide for problem resolution or plan of action.]   ☐Continue services

Identify outcomes with
related variances not met [list]_____
_____

Goals met?☐Yes ☐No_____
_____

☐Discharge
# of patient/caregiver outcomes_____
# of patient/caregiver outcomes met_____
% of patient/caregiver outcomes met _____
Goals met?☐Yes ☐No
Discharge summary completed ☐

Case manager's
signature: _____   Date: _____

EVALUATION CRITERIA

Patient/caregiver discharge goal codes. The patient/caregiver:
G1. Will demonstrate knowledge of disease process and self-care management; skilled __ personal care __other __
G2. Will stay outside of the hospital for three months
G3. Provide self-management for continued wound care; wound healed or no evidence of infection
G4. Will be satisfied with the CP and delivery of home health agency services
G5. Other [list] _____

Patient/caregiver outcomes of care codes. The patient/caregiver:	Date/Week	Met	Not met	N/A
[Summarize at end of cert. period.]				
O1. Demonstrates correct medication regimen	—	—	—	—
O2. Demonstrates correct diet regimen	—	—	—	—
O3. Demonstrates correct wound and skin care regimen	—	—	—	—
O4. Identifies complication of disease process to report to case manager; physician	—	—	—	—
O5. Identifies community resources to buy food and pay bills; LTC placement				
O6. Verbalizes when to call 911 for help	—	—	—	—
O7. Demonstrates correct use of equipment and home safety precautions				
O8. Agrees to CP by explaining treatment principles, purpose/use of multidisciplinary services, and length of service(s) without prompting of nurse	—	—	—	—
O9. Achieves maximal rehabilitation potential: ADLs __Ambulation __ Other__	—	—	—	—
O10. Achieves optimal response to treatment plan (physician) evidenced by wound healing	—	—	—	—

O11. Other [list]_____
_____
_____

Variance codes:
V1. Learning difficulties/comprehension deficits
V2. Noncompliance; nonparticipation; self-neglect
V3. Exacerberation of disease process
V4. Lack of adequate response to medical treatment plan
V5. Lack of caregiver or family to assist with care
V6. Lack of socioeconomic resources to support home health care needs
V7. Infection
V8. Rehospitalization [state reason] _____
V9. Other [explain]_____
_____
_____
_____

Variance Tracking Guide

CP standard# _____

Date	OV-TV	Problem resolution	Initials
	[list codes]	[brief description of action plan]	

Patient/Caregiver Care Path: Home Guide

Hello and **welcome** to_____ home health agency. The home health agency has been asked to visit you for _____ and related medical care so that you can reach your best level of health.

Our services will be approximately [*state visit frequency or projected length of service*]. During this time we will be following your physician's orders for your medical treatment. We will also be sharing information with you about how to get better and make the best decisions for your health!

During our services we will be following a plan of care designed specifically for your medical diagnosis. We call this plan of care a care path because it outlines all the important information, services, and medical treatment you will need to improve your health. We will periodically review your specific care path with you. This way you will always be updated and informed about your medical treatments, the delivery of the home health agency's services, and your progress with your care path.

A copy of your care path will be kept in a folder in your home to review at your convenience.

Your care path has specific tasks which we call outcomes of care for you and your nurse or therapist to accomplish in order to improve your health. These outcomes involve assisting you to manage your health care needs at home. For example, we will be teaching you how and when to take your medicines. Most important you will have an opportunity to add to your care path for your specific learning needs. Our philosophy is that **YOU HAVE A SAY IN YOUR HEALTH CARE!**

The care path is directed by your physician and carried out by your primary nurse or therapist. We call your primary nurse or therapist a case manager because they will coordinate all of your care including any additional services provided to you by the home health agency and your community. Your case manager's name is _____. Your case manager can be reached at _____.

Your case manager will go over your care path with you and update it each week. When you are ready for discharge, we will ask you to fill out a brief survey to let us know what you thought of your care while receiving our services. We appreciate your ideas and suggestions! Always call and speak with your case manager or physician if you have any questions or concerns regarding your health or the delivery of your health care services.

Thank you for choosing _____. We value you as an important customer and wish you great success with your care path!

Patient name:_____
Admission date:_____
Certification period: To: _____From:_____
Primary diagnosis or reasons for home visits: _____
_____
CP standard #:_____
Case manager's signature:_____ Date:_____

Courtesy American Nursing Development, Maryville, Ill.

Based on our assessment of your primary diagnosis and your individual needs, the following is a list of tasks which we call outcomes that we would like you to achieve during our services. We believe that achieving these outcomes improves your chances of getting better and being ready for discharge. The outcomes of care that we would like to help you accomplish during [*state visit frequency or projected length of service*] are: (list CP outcomes; consider revising them to the patient's level of understanding)

Patient/caregiver outcomes   **Date/week met**

You may also benefit from other home health agency services such as the home health aide, physical therapist, or social worker. Talk to your case manager to see if these services are right for you. Services utilized: [list]

[*state discipline and visit frequency*]

Do you agree to work with us on your care path?   ❏ Yes   ❏No

Is there anything else you would like to learn or do in order to get better? If so, list them below and we'll try to help you with this.

Patient/caregiver signature:_____ Date:_____
Case manager's signature:_____ Date:_____

Patient/Caregiver Guide: CP Standard#_____

Date	Vital signs, treatments, progress meeting patient/caregiver outcomes	Initials

Patient/Caregiver Discharge Survey: CP Standard#_____

We would appreciate it if you would take a few minutes to complete the following survey. Check the boxes below as appropriate. Please mail the survey to us in the enclosed, preaddressed envelope at your earliest convenience.

Yes	No	
☐	☐	1. Did you feel that your care path helped you understand your medical treatment and the purpose of your home health services?
☐	☐	2. Did you feel that your care path allowed you to be involved in your own health care decisions?
☐	☐	3. Were you satisfied with your physician's care?
☐	☐	4. Were you satisfied with your patient care? Nursing __ Therapy __ Aide __ Other __
☐	☐	5. Were you satisfied with the medical supplies and equipment services you received?
☐	☐	6. Were your educational guides and the instructions given to you by your case manager helpful in assisting you to learn about your health?
☐	☐	7. Did you feel your case manager adequately answered your questions and addressed your health concerns?

If you answered "no" to any of the questions above, could you briefly tell us why? This is your opportunity to let us know what you liked or disliked about our services and let us know if there is anything we can do to improve our services.

Comments

We thank you for selecting_____as your home health agency. If we can serve you or your family in the future, please do not hesitate to let us know!

10

QUALITY PATIENT CARE

Saundra J. Triplett and Robyn Rice

The early writings and thinking of W. Edward Deming and Joseph Juran and recent work by Dr. Paul Ellwood serve as a basis for quality improvement (QI) models seen in home care today. Deming and Juran stated that "lapses in quality were rarely rooted in workforce ineptitude but almost invariably stemmed from poor job design." In 1988 Dr. Ellwood introduced the word "outcomes" as a public accounting system for health care with bottom lines of health, functioning, and well-being. In 1989 Donald Berwick, MD, encouraged colleagues to adopt these same principles in health care in a landmark article in the *New England Journal of Medicine.*[5,22,25] This chapter builds on these principles of QI to include prioritizing interventions, measuring results, analyzing findings, defining or redefining best practices or processes, demonstrating improvement, and benchmarking results. It should be emphasized that true QI is a continuous and ongoing process that dynamically reflects positive change in the health care environment.

Home care nurses and Medicare's Outcome and ASsessment Information Set (OASIS) are critical links in QI, from assuring the presence of quality patient care (quality assurance, or QA) to continually improving quality patient care (quality improvement, or QI).[13] Why is the home care nurse a critical link? The nurse has the knowledge, experience, and commitment needed to best define, measure, analyze, and implement improved outcomes of care. Moreover, home care nurses provide grassroots clinical expertise that fosters realistic and achievable goals of patient care. Hence they are an integral part of the QI process.

Why is OASIS a critical link? It is critical because the OASIS data items were developed by Medicare for purposes of outcome-based QI and mandated as part of the conditions of participation for federal reimbursement of home care services. Data items in OASIS measure home care patient outcomes. It is not a comprehensive assessment instrument and therefore must be integrated into the agency's clinical assessment tool.

OASIS provides patient demographic and medical history information, living arrangements and supportive assistance, clinical status and functional ability assessments, emergent care and discharge information.[1,18,20,26] Comparison of certain OASIS data items at admission and discharge measures the patient's response to care. The OASIS database provides a universal data set for ease in benchmarking results with other home care agencies locally, regionally, or nationally. The OASIS database can be found on the website http://www.hcfa.gov/medicare/hsqb/oasis/hhoview .htm.

The purpose of this chapter is to demonstrate the importance of quality improvement tools and measures and to introduce the home care nurse to philosophies of QI. This chapter builds on the groundwork laid in Chapters 5, 8, and 9, which discuss care plan development and documentation issues, legal and ethical issues, and case management strategies in home care. Furthermore, this chapter empowers the home care nurse to work collaboratively with the home care agency to define patient outcomes of care based on evidence-based practice (EBP) models that reflect both practice and process outcomes.[2,16,22]

PHILOSOPHY OF QUALITY IMPROVEMENT

A QI program selects key indicators that will signal actual or potential patient care practice or process problems that alter expected patient care outcomes.[1,8,19,21] The traditional QA program of quantifying and qualifying structure, process, and outcome standards remains basic to this approach. A newer addition to QI is the movement toward EBP, which is care guided by research findings, expert consensus, or a combination of the two. Evidence-based practice strengthens the link between standards of practice and outcomes of patient care.[2,16]

Most home care programs have a QI program focused on nursing or home care services to ensure compliance with Medicare's home health agency conditions of participation (COPs) and, where required, annual state licensure. Traditional QA programs reported the adherence to structure and process standards through deficiency (negative) ratings to defined minimum-rating goals of structure, process, or outcome standards. (See discussion on structure, process, and outcome standards.) Outcome standards have recently gained significance over structure or process standards by replacing deficiency ratings with compliance ratings and minimum standards with expected compliance percentage.*

The home care agency leaders' support is key for a successful QI program. The leaders must support strategies that provide the vision and spirit for the new effort. The leaders must demonstrate a belief that quality patient care is everyone's responsibility. And the leaders must create an environment that encourages inquiry and the creative effort needed to achieve ever-increasing quality patient care goals.[8,22,25] Finally, a QI program must be allowed to grow by both successes and failures, empowered to address its own patient care practices and processes, and encouraged, through teamwork, to improve practices and processes that affect patient care.[19,22]

QUALITY IMPROVEMENT TEAM

The composition of the QI committee (typically referred to as the team) should recognize all levels of agency and nonagency staff for their contribution

to the delivery of quality patient care. An effective QI team should consist of no more than five to eight members. Larger groups will slow the group process and make decision making and consensus more difficult.[25] Members represent those directly involved in the home care agency's patient care practices and processes. This structure keeps the program reality based and focused on collaboration or teamwork.[11,25] Depending on the type of care or service provided, members of the QI team may include the following[24,28,31]:

- Caregiver staff providing the hands-on direct patient care, for example, home care nurse, home care aide, physical therapist, occupational therapist, speech language pathologist, medical social worker, and specialty staff (e.g., nutritionist, infusion nurse, pediatric nurse, maternal-child nurse, or enterostomal therapist)
- Representatives from agency management for support and assistance with possible program and/or policy improvements
- Patients, or information from patients, who are receiving or have received the home care services (Use survey, focus group, or individual comment information gathered by patient satisfaction surveys, patient compliment/complaint records, patient focus groups, conversations during patient visits by home care nurses or other patient care staff or patient calls to the office.)
- Nonagency suppliers who provide home medical equipment, medical supplies, infusion therapy products, or other services
- Agency medical director for support and understanding of possible program and/or policy improvements
- Physicians, or information from physicians, who refer or may refer to the agency (Use survey, focus group, or individual comment information gathered by physician surveys, focus groups, and conversations during phone calls or office visits by home care nurses and/or other agency staff, etc.)
- Data processing representatives or a person who is knowledgeable about computers if the agency records or accounts are computerized

The QI team will select the key indicators for review, analysis, comparison with other agencies,

---

*References 8, 10, 15, 18, 27, 30, 32.

and identification as needing improvement. This method of continuously comparing and measuring the work processes of other agencies for information that will help improve agency performance is called benchmarking.[2,22,32]

The QI team will also use data from agency reports (Box 10-1) for analysis and outcome reporting.[2,32] Before using these data, the team needs to determine their usefulness by considering their source, how they are compiled, what is being re-ported, and if the data make sense based on the team's knowledge of the practice or process being evaluated. It is not unusual for a QI team to find that such information needs to be updated, eliminated, or replaced with better material before it can be used as a data source.[7,22,30] This is an example of the critical role that the home care nurse has on the QI team. In other words, because the home care nurse is both patient care provider and patient care manager and has a vital role in many of the clinical practice and

---

Box 10-1   EXAMPLES OF QUALITY IMPROVEMENT TEAM DATA

Clinical Practice
Infection rates—new and continuing (patient and staff)
Medical record audits, peer reviews, or other reports
Supervisory home visit reports
Variance reports from care plans, clinical decision/practice algorithms, process flowcharts, etc.
Team conference reports

Clinical Practice Outcomes
Change in ambulation/locomotion ability
Change in ability to self-administer medications
Change in pain management in relation to activity
Change in any of the OASIS functional areas
Health status at discharge

Patient/Physician/Employee Satisfaction
Customer compliment and/or complaint reports and/or notes
Patient satisfaction surveys
Physician satisfaction surveys
Staff satisfaction/opinion surveys

Agency Process Monitors
Physician order list by date obtained, returned by staff, and mailed to physician
Recertification list by
• Last date of service on present certification
• Date staff requested to complete
• Date returned by staff
• Date mailed to physician
Number of physician orders past signature return/filing date
OASIS and/or ORYX completion date reports
OASIS and/or ORYX submission data reports

Service Utilization
Number of patients by diagnosis
Number of patients by types of services (registered nurse, home health aide, physical therapist, occupational therapist, speech therapist, medical social worker, other)
Number of patients by type of supply or any supply
Average length of stay by diagnosis, payer, or other
Number of patients by discharge codes
Disposition at discharge (e.g., discharge to home, acute facility, skilled nursing home, other agency, death)

Service Cost
Cost by diagnosis
Cost by specialty service (e.g., newborn mother-baby, infusion service, mental health or psychiatric nursing)
Cost by disease management program or ICD9 groupings (e.g., congestive heart failure, chronic skin ulcers, asthma, newly diagnosed diabetes, community-acquired pneumonia)
Cost by payer type

Risks—Real or Potential
Readmissions within 48 hours of admission
Deaths within 48 hours of admission
Acquired patient or staff infections
Incident reports—patient and staff
Service complications identified in medical record review but not recorded elsewhere (e.g., hematoma after blood draws, urinary tract infection after catheterization, increasing wound size)

Triggers for QI Review
Deaths within 48 hours of admission
Acquired patient or staff infections

process measures, the nurse can best determine a report's usefulness or applicability.[11,19,20,30]

THEORETICAL FRAMEWORK

Several movements are shaping the nature of QI and are identified in the following discussion.

Quality improvement model

Theorists such as Deming and Juran have written extensively on the topic of quality improvement. Their emphasis is on a leadership open to change based on the ideas and work of those involved in the change.[10,12,25] When this happens, customer-mindedness permeates the organization. Many agencies are using such theories to shape a QI model that keeps moving to improve patient care practice or processes.[3,8] This is a key point in this chapter.

A QI model recognizes the system in which we work (not the people we work with) as the primary barrier to quality improvements. The model identifies areas for improvement at all levels to create better overall understanding, communication, and improvements. Changes made by one level working alone would not achieve the same improvements. Moreover, improvements made by those not involved in the process are not sustained. It puts the power for change (improvements) into the hands of those involved in the process (empowerment).[8,12,19,20]

Steps in the QI model to improve care include the following:

1. Identify real or potential problem(s) by measuring patient care outcomes (Figure 10-1, *Identify Opportunity*).
2. Define the care practices or processes being followed (Figure 10-1, *Current Situation*).
3. Identify ways to improve care practices or processes to improve results or outcomes using best-practice models or clinical practice standards (Figure 10-1, *Analysis*).
4. Try new care practices or processes (Figure 10-1, *Proposed Solutions*).
5. Use visual, not just written, descriptions to improve analysis and understanding (e.g., flowcharts, graphs, surveys, case studies, Pareto charts, fish-bone diagrams). Program evaluation then becomes both quantitative and qualitative in nature (see Figure 10-2).

6. Compare the improved process results with previous results to identify the degree of improvement or variance (Figure 10-1, *Results*).
7. Reach for and achieve increasing levels of performance, including those with other businesses (benchmarking).
8. Continue the process to continually maintain and/or improve outcomes.

Key elements in a successful QI model include the following:

- Acceptance and support by the home care agency administration, the leaders
- Knowledge and belief of all others in the leaders' support of QI.
- Collaborative input and decision making of others supported and promoted by the home care agency leaders
- Active involvement and teamwork among home care agency clinical and support staff and nonagency workers involved in the services the agency provides (e.g., community resources, patients, equipment suppliers, infusion companies, or contract workers)
- Commitment from the top down to make customer satisfaction the agency's number one goal, recognizing that customers include patients, families, physicians, employees and ancillary staff, and related services/suppliers
- Continuous drive to meet and improve all agency functions
- A focus on improving industry quality goals

Care standards: the Marker model

Carolyn Smith-Marker developed the Marker model to facilitate the development and implementation of standards that are useful in a QI program.[17] The Marker model reflects Donabedian's framework of structure, process, and outcome standards of care.[9]

Structure standards define how a system operates. They encompass all aspects of the home care system except the process of giving care and the desired outcomes. They define optimal conditions that support staff function, agency operation, and patient care. Expressed as policy, structure standards have legal, regulatory, and professional implications. Because of this, Medicare regulations and state licensure requirements form the basis for

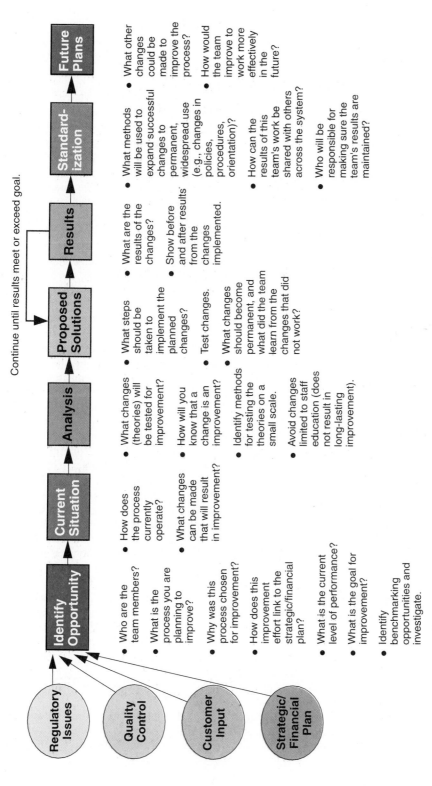

Figure 10-1 CQI model. Process improvement approach. (Courtesy SSM Health Care, St. Louis, Mo.)

each home care agency's operational policies and procedures or structural standards.

Process standards define the actions, knowledge, and skills needed to provide quality patient care. These standards make up the bulk of any agency's set of standards because they cover such a wide range of nursing activities and patient care. They can be directed toward the home care nurse, another discipline, or the patient. Process standards may assume many different forms: job descriptions, performance standards, procedures, protocols, guidelines, and patient care standards.

Outcome standards specify the end to be achieved. These standards define the benefit from the service or care received.[2,26] The home care nurse and other disciplines use outcome standards as short-term and long-term goals in the patient care plan. (See Chapter 5 for information about developing outcomes of care.)

In the Marker model, "structure" defines home care agency organization, including staff qualifications; "processes" defines policies or procedures for appropriate service delivery; and "outcomes" identifies the expected patient service results.[17]

Evidence-based practice model

Evidence-based practice is gaining importance in health care and especially in home care nursing practice. The EBP model asks for scientific evidence or expert consensus or both to support a specific intervention or clinical practice. There are two standards for EBP: the Agency for Healthcare Research and Quality Clinical Practice Guidelines (see website http://www//.ahrq.gov) and the Cochrane Collaboration (see website http://hiru/mcmaster.ca/cochrane/cochrane), which originated in the United Kingdom.[6,17] In both, expert practitioners of many disciplines are convened to review available research-based evidence and to provide clinical practice guidelines and standards of care. Using the EBP model, the QI team would make sure that agency standards of care and clinical practice are researched based.

To determine the best patient care practice using the EBP model, the home care nurse should ask these questions: What is the best or right patient care practice for defined patient care situations? Are such practices supported by research or shared clinical experiences? Is the research of adequate quality, and is it generalizable to home care popula-

tions? How do such practices affect the patient's quality of life and outcomes of care?[8,33] The OASIS data set is a tool that may also be used to assess and answer these questions.

Outcome quality improvement model using OASIS

An outcome reflects the measurable changes in a patient's condition between two or more points. The change can be attributed to performance (including patient behavioral changes with self-care) or process of care.[2,22] The outcome measurement must include both a beginning and ending point (two points of measure) to determine the effect (outcome).[2,32] Key to this measurement is the controlling of influences on the outcome. For example, if the care delivery system changes, such as when the patient is hospitalized, the measurement needs to compare the admission to the agency and the admission to the hospital. In this case the care practice result may show the patient's health status worsening, but the care process result may show a quicker identification of patient symptoms and physician reporting for a shorter hospital stay. Finally, when evaluating outcomes, it is important to remember to keep reporting periods free of other (non–home care) patient care delivery systems.

In 1999 HCFA required the use of OASIS as part of the home health agency conditions of participation (COPs)[1,19,20] (see website http://www.hcfa.gov/medicare/hsqb/oasis/hhregcop.htm). Significantly, OASIS gives home care nurses and home care agencies a common language and method for comparison of patient care practices. In addition, in order for certification, the Joint Commission on Accreditation of Healthcare Organizations (JCAHO) accreditation program now requires home care agencies to collect and quarterly submit select QI indicators to JCAHO for review. This requirement is called ORYX: The Next Evolution in Accreditation[11,12] (see website wwwb.jcaho.org/perfmeas/oryx/oryx__qa.html). The indicators used and approved in the ORYX requirement are typically data obtainable from the OASIS database.

QUALITY IMPROVEMENT PROGRAM COMPONENTS

The QI team should identify the improvement opportunities that can be acted on and set priorities. The criteria established by JCAHO for setting pri-

Table 10-1 Ranking opportunities for improvement

Improvement area	Expected impact	High volume	High risk	Problem prone	Resources available	Ranking
Increase physician satisfaction score	High	Yes	Potential	Potential	Yes	3
Decrease patient-acquired infection rate	High	No	Yes	Yes	Yes	1
Decrease employee needle sticks	High	No	Yes	No	Yes	2
Decrease patient complaints	High	No	No	Yes	Yes	4

orities include three considerations: (1) the expected impact on performance, selecting high-risk, high-volume, or problem-prone processes, (2) the relationship of potential improvement to the dimensions of performance and functions, and (3) the home care agency's resources.[12]

Key patient services and regulatory issues help determine and prioritize the improvement opportunities. For example, patient and/or physician satisfaction may be something an agency always wants to improve. In a customer-driven business such as home care, patient and physician satisfaction with the delivery of home care services is always an expected outcome. A key element in obtaining JCAHO accreditation is to provide evidence of patient satisfaction with all provided services, skilled (registered nurse, physical therapist, occupational therapist, speech therapist, medical social worker) and nonskilled (aide, homemaker).[12]

To get started the QI team should select two or three operational or service areas in which the data show improvements are needed. The team should rank the opportunities for improvement according to the expected impact on performance (classification as a high-volume, high-risk, or intrinsically problem-prone area) and the agency's available resources.[12] The team should next discuss options and a plan of action (Table 10-1). By following these guidelines the QI team begins the task of quality improvement.

MEASURING QUALITY
Measures

Measures serve as signals of potential or actual problems or barriers to the delivery of quality patient care. They do this by quantifying and qualifying patient care events identified as important aspects of care. "Quantifying" means counting the number of events compared to all events. This is best presented in a ratio[7,14]:

$$\frac{\text{Number of patients for whom a specified event occurs}}{\text{Number of patients experiencing condition or procedure that indicator is measuring}}$$

For example:

$$\frac{\text{Number of patients with hematomas following venipuncture}}{\text{Number of patients receiving venipuncture}}$$

"Qualifying" refers to the quality and appropriateness of the event. Quality measures may measure efficacy, appropriateness, availability, timeliness, effectiveness, continuity, safety, efficiency, respect, and caring. For example:

$$\frac{\text{Number of patients involved in their own care decisions}}{\text{Number of active patients}}$$

Measures are categorized by the type and seriousness of the event they measure.[12,14,26,32]

Structure measures measure whether or not agency policies are followed. For example, if the important aspect of care is timeliness and the agency policy states all patients are evaluated for admission within 24 hours of referral, the structure indicator may read as follows:

$$\frac{\text{Number of patients evaluated within 24 hrs}}{\text{Number of patients admitted}}$$

This would be further categorized as a rate-based, desirable indicator.

Process measures measure specific processes or steps critical to quality patient care. For example, the agency may define wound care management techniques or treatment in a standard of care based on the wound description. A rate-based, desirable process indicator may read as follows:

$$\frac{\text{Number of wound} - \text{care}}{\text{patients with management techniques}}$$
$$\frac{}{\text{Number of wound} - \text{care patients}}$$

Outcome measures measure what happens or does not happen after something is or is not done. For example, the agency may evaluate goal achievement based on the patient care plan. With effectiveness as the important aspect of care, the rate-based, desired outcome indicator may read as follows:

$$\frac{\text{Number of patients reaching stated goals}}{\text{Number of active patients}}$$

Desirable outcome measures are expected to improve or be maintained. Unexpected or undesirable outcomes may include worsening of a condition, a new complication, rehospitalization, and unexpected death.

To keep the QI program manageable, the selection of quality measures should be based on the home care agency's services that have the greatest impact on care. When selecting the events or measures, consider the following:[11,22,23,27]

1. Include large numbers of patients (e.g., wound-care patients).
2. Include measures that entail a high degree of risk for patients or produce problems for patients or staff (for example, acquired infections).
3. Involve low-volume but complex services (for example, infusion therapy).

Patient satisfaction is a desired outcome in all home care services. As such it should be included in these three activities and defined separately to gauge overall home care agency performance.[22,23,27]

It is important to recognize that, when asked what is important regarding their health care needs, patients' perceptions may differ greatly from those of the home care nurse or home care agency.[22,23,27] Therefore involving patients is very helpful when the QI team is defining and measuring patient satisfaction.[5,15,22,23] To summarize, patient care stan-

dards define quality whereas quality measures measure and monitor quality.

Threshold parameters or ranges

Outcomes may be measured against threshold parameters (ranges) or finite numbers. Ranges allow for natural variances in the performance of the patient care standard. The range is determined by calculating a standard deviation for the sample used and determining an acceptable and safe deviation from the standard. The range may also be set by the team members based on their knowledge, experience, and discussion of acceptable and unacceptable thresholds. Finite numbers give specific thresholds for the study group to achieve. When the number is less than 100% or more than 0% (depending on how the indicator is stated), variances are allowed as a rare occurrence.

Finite numbers, such as 98%, are preferred because they are less ambiguous and keep the expectation simple and clear to the patient, the nurse, and the agency. For example, when monitoring staff availability as an important aspect of patient care, the indicator threshold may read 98% or higher of physical therapy (PT) cases opened within 2 days:

$$\frac{\text{Number of patients opened by PT within 2 days}}{\text{Number of patients with orders for PT services}}$$

Sentinel or undesirable events are measured against finite thresholds because of the seriousness of their outcome. For example, when monitoring safety as an important aspect of care, the outcome indicator threshold for patient falls may be 0%:

$$\frac{\text{Number of patient falls during a patient visit}}{\text{Number of patient visits}}$$

Safety of patient discharge should also be evaluated. This is especially important to do when the patient goals are not met and the patient is not being discharged to another health care delivery system. In addition, issues of patient safety are a prime consideration when working with a case management payment program and limited patient visits.

QUALITY IMPROVEMENT TOOLS

The following discussion lists some scientific QI tools available to help the team visualize a process, pinpoint problems, discover causes, and identify solutions[12,25] (Figure 10-2):

Flowcharts or diagrams are excellent tools to use when reviewing the steps in a process. Self-stick

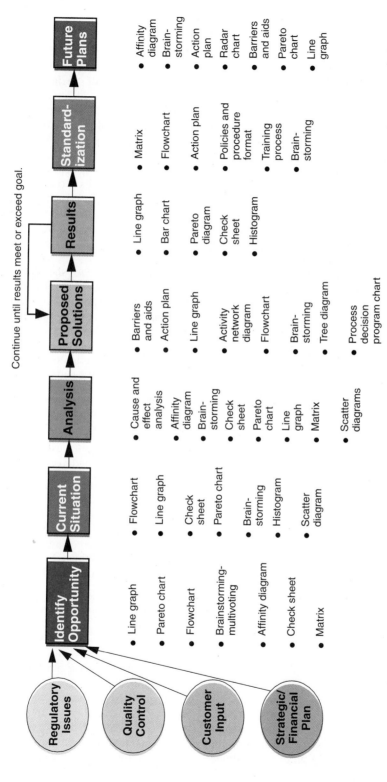

Figure 10-2 CQI model. Process improvement approach: possible tools. (Courtesy SSM Health Care, St. Louis, Mo.)

notes are useful in developing and revising a flow-chart because they can be moved quickly and the process steps are easily seen.

Time plots and control charts are simple tools to plot points along a time line. Threshold parameters or numbers can be added to the chart to see if the values are above, below, within, or at the threshold parameter.

Cause-and-effect or fish-bone diagrams are used to identify all the possible causes of a stated effect or result. This type of tool can be used to classify possible causes under five headings: people, measurements, materials, method, and machines.

Pareto charts are bar charts organizing the significance of data by quantity and significance percentage. It assumes 80% of the problems result from 20% of the causes. Because the data is shown in descending bar graph order, major and minor factor(s) may be discussed for significance to the improvement and the ability to effect process improvement.

Scatter diagrams compare two variables such as time and frequency. The clustering of points shows the time the monitored event has the highest frequency.

Solution models include assigning values to a proposed method's effectiveness multiplied by ($\times$) the feasibility to obtain an overall score for determining if action is appropriate.

Charts help quantify and visualize data to improve understanding and decision making among team members.

The creation of charts has been made easier by computer spreadsheet and database software that allow data manipulation, make data display suggestions, compute complex formulas (e.g., standard deviations), and create charts with ease.

Analysis and evaluation

Once evaluation methods are identified, data is collected; then analysis and evaluation follow. Effective groups for analysis and evaluation are typically made up of five members plus a group leader.[25]

Variation and trending

Variation and trend reporting are two ways to analyze measures not meeting threshold(s). Variation reporting is the variance from threshold for individual measures on separate monitoring periods. Trend reporting is the threshold ratings from several monitoring periods plotted on a time graph.

These types of reports reveal the direction of trend lines as being stable, increasing, or decreasing. Trend lines are of special interest in evaluating care practices and identifying future program needs. For example, if pressure ulcers developed on patients during the course of services and the incidence was associated with bedbound or severely functionally limited patients, patient and nursing skin care practices may need to be altered to reduce the risk of pressure ulcer formation. As assessed by the home care nurse, such practices could be applied to all future patients who are assessed to be at risk for pressure ulcer formation.

Analysis

The QI team reviews the data; identifies the system, staff, or patient problem along with trends and variances; develops a corrective plan; and evaluates the indicator for improvement.[14,19]

Evaluation

To be effective, program evaluation must answer the following structure and process questions:

- Was the care delivered according to agency policies and procedures? (structure)
- Was the care delivered as ordered? (process)

Program evaluation must also answer the following outcome-related questions:

- Was the delivered care appropriate to the patient need?
- Was the delivered care effective based on expected patient response and outcome?
- Was the delivered care efficient according to parameters defined by the agency, clinical path, or national statistics?

JCAHO offers clear definitions of QI terms that may be included in your agency's QI program.[12]

COST VERSUS BENEFIT IS THE FUTURE

Today health care consumers and payers want the best quality of care for the lowest cost. This has created dramatic changes in the health care delivery system. Now cost-accounting methods must not only give overall costs by expense categories but also by specific patient service or condition type. This emphasis on costing out services is being led by federal, state, and managed care

```
┌─────────────────────────────────────────────┐
│              Box 10-2   QI PRINCIPLES         │
├─────────────────────────────────────────────┤
│                                               │
│ Patients and other customers are our first priority. │
│ Quality is achieved through people.           │
│ All work is part of a process.                │
│ Decision making by facts.                     │
│ Quality requires continuous improvement.      │
│                                               │
└─────────────────────────────────────────────┘
```

Courtesy SSM Health Care, St. Louis, Mo. Posted in meeting rooms.

providers who are gatekeeping home care and other health care services.[1,11,32] Home care agencies must be able to look at the mix and cost of services they provide and, based on the achieved patient outcomes, maintain or improve their competitive place in the home care market.

Never before have two opposing groups needed each other more: administration and staff. Each has much to offer the other in improving agency systems and practices in order to achieve better patient outcomes. In the past, administration may have focused on costs, whereas staff focused on quality. The QI team now serves as a melting pot for both focuses to be addressed[8,19,20] (Box 10-2).

Paying more or less for a product does not always mean the product is better or worse. The same may be said of a service such as home care. By defining and measuring important aspects of patient care, the QI team and agency staff become aware of the cost of quality care. When alternatives or revisions are needed, the cost benefits of the change must be analyzed for more informed decision making. Acknowledging the importance of the budget, tempered by a concern for quality patient care, is the heart of an effective QI program.

SUMMARY

However quality is defined and measured, every home care patient wants it and every agency wants to deliver it.[5,29] The direction of home care quality and performance improvement programs is clear: every home care agency activity should be directed toward achieving the best possible care for each patient.[4,19]

The changes in home care reimbursement and documentation are giving the home care nurse the opportunity to focus emphasis on using evidenced-based practice models, measuring patient out-

comes, and ultimately improving quality patient care. Pay by visit is being replaced by pay by disease or patient classification. The OASIS data set gives home care agencies a core tool for evaluating and improving their practices and processes and gives the federal government a tool to determine payment to agencies.

In the final analysis, the quality of patient care is only as good as the involvement and commitment of the home care agency to achieve that quality. The extent to which agency operations provide quality patient care will depend on the support of the agency leaders and active involvement of the agency staff with the commitment of home care nurses in defining the QI process. Home care nurses are needed to keep quality patient care the focus of all agency operations and to promote professional standards of practice.

Self-directed home care nurses ultimately have the power to effect improvements in the delivery of services and to participate in other QI functions. This promotes nurses' autonomy and responsibility for meeting the health care needs of the public today and tomorrow. For it is recognized that "no one owns healing" and those who evaluate the performance of a profession *control it.*

REFERENCES

1. Adams CE, DeFrates DS, Wilson M: Data-driven quality improvement for HMO patients, *JONA* 28(10):20, 1998.
2. American Nurses Association: *Scope and standards of home health nursing practice,* St. Louis, 1999, The Association.
3. Apter J: Compare an apple to an apple, *Success in Home Care,* p 19, November/December, 1999.
4. Berhang-Doggett J, Lowenstein A: Quality assurance: achieving compliance with home care regulations, *Caring* 10:37, 1991.
5. Brook R and others: Assessing quality of care: three different approaches, *Bus Health,* p 27, August 1990.
6. Davis PL, Madigan EA: Evidence-based practice and the home care nurse's bag, *Home Healthcare Nurse* 17(5):295, 1999.
7. DePalma J: Measuring outcomes related to nursing, *Home Health Care Manage Prac* 11(4):67, 1999.
8. Dienemann J: *CQI: continuous quality improvement in nursing,* Washington, DC, 1992, American Nurses Publishing.
9. Donabedian A: *Explorations in quality assessment and monitoring, vol 2, The definition of quality and approaches to its assessment,* Ann Arbor, Mich, 1980, Health Administration Press.
10. Hawk AB, Miyamuara JB: Quality improvement: how does it differ from quality assurance? *Hawaii Med J* 52(2):34, 1993.

11. Huston CJ: Outcomes measurement in healthcare: new imperatives for professional nursing practice, *Nurs Case Manage,* p 188, July/August 1999.

12. Joint Commission on Accreditation of Healthcare Organizations: *1999-2000 Accreditation manual for home care,* Oakbrook Terrace, Ill, 1999, The Joint Commission.

13. Joint Commission on Accreditation of Healthcare Organizations: *Quality improvement in home care,* Oakbrook Terrace, Ill, 1993, The Commission.

14. Katz J, Green E: *Managing quality: a guide to monitoring and evaluating nursing services,* St. Louis, 1992, Mosby.

15. Largen CW: Bringing quality to the customer: a new paradigm for quality managers, *J Nurs Care Qual* 8(2):81, 1994.

16. Madigan EA: Evidence-based practice in home healthcare: a springboard for discussion, *Home Healthcare Nurse* 16(6):411, 1998.

17. Marker C: *Nursing standards* (audiocassette), Baltimore, 1985, Resource Applications.

18. Munchus G and others: The US home health care industry: past, present, and future, *Home Health Care Manage Prac* 11(4):21, 1999.

19. Ondeck DA: Emerging best practices through performance improvement, *Home Health Care Manage Prac* 10(5):58, 1998.

20. Pace KB: The information challenge in home health care, *Home Health Care Manage Prac* 10(4):39, 1998.

21. Rhinehart E: The synergy of quality management and risk management in home care, *Caring* p. 32, 1996.

22. Rieve JA: Benchmarking and using outcomes data, *Case Manager,* 8(4):55, 1997.

23. Riley PA and others: Developing consumer-centered quality assurance strategies for home care, *J Case Manag* 1(2):39, 1992.

24. Saba VK: Diagnoses and interventions, *Caring* 3:50, 1992.

25. Scholtes PR: *The team handbook: how to use teams to improve quality,* Madison, Wis, 1988, Joiner Associates.

26. Shaughnessy PW and others: *Measuring outcomes of home health care,* Denver, 1994, Center for Health Policy Research, University of Colorado Health Sciences Center.

27. Smit J, Spoelstra S: Do patients and nurses agree? *Caring* 10:34, 1991.

28. Souza J: Benchmarking basics: how to select a performance measurement system, *Success in Home Care,* p 65, Spring, 1998.

29. Souza JA: A measure of quality outcomes for home medical services, *Case Manager* 8(4):42, 1997.

30. Wagner DM: QA in home care: the staff nurse's challenge, *JHQ* 14(2):30, 1992.

31. Wagner DM: Quality indicators: an approach to quality improvement in home healthcare, *JHQ* 14(3):8, 1992.

32. Wilson AA: Policy trends in outcomes and OASIS, *Home Health Care Manage Prac* 10(6):38, 1998.

33. Zlotnick C, Decker R: Home visiting outcomes and quality of life measures, *J Community Health Nurs* 8(4):207, 1991.

INTERNET RESOURCES

Agency for Healthcare Research and Quality
  http://www.ahrq.gov/clinic
American Nurses Association
  http://www.ana.org
Cochrane Collaboration
  http://hiru.mcmaster.ca/cochrane/cochrane
HCFA's OASIS information
  http://www.hcfa.gov/medicare/hsgb/oasis
Joint Commission on Accreditation of Healthcare Organizations
  http://www.jcaho.org
National Committee for Quality Assurance Guidelines
  http://www.ncqa.org/
National Guideline Clearinghouse
  http://wwwguideline.gov

PART II

CLINICAL APPLICATION

THE PATIENT WITH CHRONIC OBSTRUCTIVE PULMONARY DISEASE

Robyn Rice

Breathing, like the beating of our hearts, is largely taken for granted. Consider for a moment what life would be like if the simple act of breathing became an everyday struggle to survive. Picture the changes in our lives if we could not even walk from the kitchen table into the bathroom without becoming short of breath. These scenarios are real experiences and concerns of patients with chronic obstructive pulmonary disease (COPD).

DESCRIPTION

Chronic obstructive pulmonary disease describes a group of diseases that often overlap each other in presentation and are manifested by obstruction of the small airways within the lungs. Such diseases include chronic bronchitis, asthmatic bronchitis, and pulmonary emphysema.

Chronic bronchitis is a clinical disorder caused by inflamed and edematous bronchial mucosa. Excessive mucus production results, producing a chronic, productive cough (minimal duration of 3 months per year for at least 2 successive years).[14,30]

Asthma is caused by bronchospasm and subsequent hypersecretion of mucus into the airways. Patients with asthma experience severe attacks of wheezing and coughing. Allergies, exertion, changes in temperature or environment, and emotional factors can trigger an asthmatic attack. Childhood asthma is usually attributed to allergies and may dissipate as the child grows older. Adult asthma, however, is associated with COPD. In adults with asthma, scarred and hypertrophied lung tissue resulting from repeated allergy attacks gives rise to asthmatic bronchitis.[30]

Emphysema is a pathological disorder characterized by destruction of lung tissue and overinflation of the small airways. Patients with emphysema develop structural defects in the lungs that hamper exhalation. Collapse of airways and subsequent air trapping prevent these patients from exhaling the "old" air and inhaling fresh, oxygenated air.

Chronic obstructive pulmonary disease is a progressive, debilitating disease for which, at present, there is no cure. Initial diagnosis is usually made between 30 and 50 years of age, and the course of the disease progresses for 25 to 30 years from origination to death. At the time of initial diagnosis, usually some degree of irreversible damage to the lungs is already present.[30]

Symptoms of COPD usually begin with a chronic, productive cough, repeated "chest" colds, and dyspnea or shortness of breath upon exertion. The underlying problem of all COPD patients is a decrease of airflow in and out of the lungs. Hypoventilation, shunting, diffusion impairment, and—most commonly—ventilation-perfusion abnormalities contribute to hypoxemia and the severe dyspnea experienced by these patients.

Advanced stages of COPD are characterized by a decline in mental and physical functioning, decreased activity levels, heart failure, and recurrent pulmonary infections. Such infections can precipitate acute respiratory failure and are a frequent cause of repeated hospitalizations. Dyspnea, fatigue, and limited physical endurance are common problems experienced by patients with COPD, and they become a focus of home care intervention.

The purpose of this chapter is to review what is known about COPD in order to assist home care nurses in developing a plan of care for these patients. Patient education emphasizing home pulmonary rehabilitation and ongoing biopsychological interventions recommended in this chapter can be used to prevent exacerbations of COPD, to promote self-care management for patients and their families, and to offer patients with COPD respite from the enormous financial and emotional stressors associated with repeated hospitalizations. It is likely that home care nurses will visit many patients with COPD because of the large number of reported cases in the United States.

EPIDEMIOLOGY

In 1995 an estimated 16.4 million Americans suffered from COPD, representing an increase of 60% since 1982.[19] The reported incidence of COPD is higher in urban areas and within lower socioeconomic classes.[19] It is more prevalent in men than in women and in smokers than in nonsmokers. Chronic obstructive pulmonary disease is one of the primary chronic conditions afflicting the US population and is now the fourth leading cause of death.[19] The most common causes of COPD-related deaths are respiratory insufficiency, pneumonia, and cor pulmonale.[20]

In addition, COPD takes a heavy toll on the US economy. According to estimates made by the National Heart, Lung, and Blood Institute, in 1998 the annual cost to the nation for COPD was $26 billion dollars.[19] This included $13.6 billion in direct health care expenditures, $6.4 billion in indirect morbidity costs, and $6 billion in indirect mortality costs.

ETIOLOGY AND PATHOPHYSIOLOGY

Understanding the basics of alveolar gas exchange in relation to the structure of the lungs provides a framework for understanding the causes and effects of COPD (Box 11-1).

Causes of COPD that determine specific disease manifestations are interrelated. They commonly include smoking, environmental factors, and familial or hereditary factors.[23]

Smoking

Cigarette smoking is primarily responsible for nearly all COPD deaths. Smoking destroys cilia

lining the airways and represses the formation of alpha$_1$-antitrypsin (AAT) (see the section on familial factors). Excessive mucus production results when particles and irritants, previously cleared by the cilia, collect in the airways and cause inflammation and edema. A chronic cough develops. This further stimulates hypertrophy and hypersecretion of mucosal glands, which are characteristic of chronic bronchitis.

Ideally a sterile area, the lungs accumulate mucus and debris from continued smoking and become a breeding ground for infection. In addition, smoking encourages further migration of inflammatory cells into the lungs, which intensifies tissue irritation and edema. These repeated infections cause more damage, eventually destroying the smaller air passages and narrowing the larger ones.

Environmental factors

Occupation, air pollution, and allergens can influence the development of COPD. Exposure to cold air or substances such as molds, fungi, nitrogen or sulfur gases, asbestos, animal hair, hairsprays, and household pollutants may trigger bronchoconstriction. During acute attacks, spastic contractions of the airways make breathing very difficult and create an overwhelming feeling of suffocation. An increase in mucosal goblet cells, thickening and hypertrophy of airways, and copious, thick mucous secretions are typical of chronic asthmatic bronchitis.

Familial factors

Many diseases, including those of the respiratory system, tend to run in families. Genetic predisposition and household habits passed from one generation to the next can affect disease manifestation. For this reason, taking a health history is important.

Although emphysema is primarily associated with smoking, it may also result from an inherited deficiency of AAT. Alpha$_1$-antitrypsin is a nonspecific, antiproteolytic enzyme. It normally represses the release of proteases, which are enzymes that can disintegrate and lyse lung tissue.[23,30] Proteases are released by blood leukocytes, alveolar macrophage, and bacteria as part of the inflammatory response. If unchecked, proteases destroy the structural elastin of lung tissue, and functional elastic recoil of the smaller airways is lost. Enlargement of air passages distal to the terminal bronchioles develops. Upon loss of elastic recoil, airways tend to

Box 11-1   THE PHYSIOLOGICAL RELATIONSHIP BETWEEN THE LUNGS AND COPD

As air is inhaled, it moves through the upper airways, where it is warmed, cleaned, and moisturized. Air then descends through the large and smaller airways and onward into the alveoli.

Cilia covered by a thin mucous layer (secreted by bronchial glands and goblet cells) line the epithelial airways. Cilia beat in a rhythmic, upward movement that impels the mucous layer toward the mouth and clears the lungs of debris left unfiltered by the upper airways. If mucus becomes too thick or if the amount is excessive, the cleaning action of the cilia is retarded. A cough is elicited in response to irritants or when the capability of the mucociliary system is overwhelmed. A chronic cough, however, is not a "normal" lung defense mechanism and suggests destruction of the mucociliary system.

Inflated with air, the alveoli become the final pathway for diffusion of oxygen and carbon dioxide. A fine capillary network from the pulmonary vessels brings blood to the membranes of the alveoli. Across these membrane surfaces, oxygen attaches and is transported in combination with hemoglobin (a component of red blood cells) to tissue capillaries, where it is absorbed by tissues. Concurrently, as a by-product of metabolism, carbon dioxide moves out of the cells and eventually diffuses across pulmonary capillary membranes into the alveoli for exhalation.

During exhalation, elastic recoil and structural support of the airways force air out of the alveoli in preparation for inspiration. Elastic recoil is the tendency of the lung to return to its resting volume. A hallmark of COPD is the destruction of the mucociliary clearance system and the structural support and elastic recoil of the lungs. Consequently, arterial oxygen falls (hypoxemia) while arterial carbon dioxide increases (hypercapnia), giving rise to further sequelae of COPD.

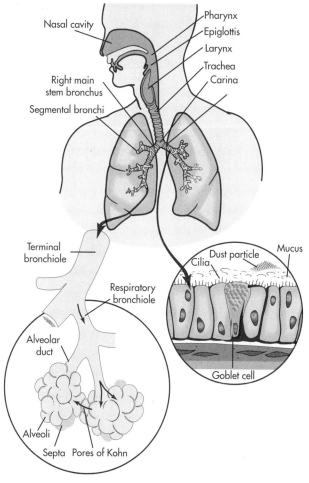

(Illustration from Lewis SM and others: *Medical-surgical nursing: assessment and management of clinical problems,* ed 5, St. Louis, 2000, Mosby.)

collapse with exhalation. Overinflation and air trapping may cause the already distended alveolar walls to rupture. Large pockets filled with stagnant air called bullae may form. As the functional number of alveoli declines, dyspnea increases. Therapy by replacement of AAT is now available.[4] In addition, patients with AAT may be candidates for lung resection or transplantation.

Problems with airflow and hypersecretion of mucus create additional complications for patients with COPD. For example, when oxygen (O_2) does not reach the capillary network within the alveoli, the amount of O_2 in the blood decreases. In response, pulmonary vessels constrict. As a result, some areas of the lung will be well ventilated but have almost no blood flow while other areas may have good blood flow but no ventilation. This phenomenon, referred to as ventilation-perfusion imbalance, is common in COPD and is related to obstruction of airways, poor ventilation of alveoli, and constriction of pulmonary vessels. The net effect is low arterial O_2 content (hypoxemia) and increased concentrations of arterial carbon dioxide (CO_2), or hypercapnia. As a consequence of vessel constriction, pulmonary hypertension develops. The heart must work harder to circulate blood through these narrowed vessels. In response to a magnified cardiac workload, the right ventricle thickens and enlarges. Right-sided failure, or cor pulmonale, can develop, and left-sided failure may follow.[23,30]

An increase in the production of red blood cells, or polycythemia, related to hypoxemia may also occur as a consequence of COPD. Initially the increase in the number of oxygen-carrying red blood cells is helpful in compensating for hypoxemia. However, when the hematocrit exceeds 50%, blood viscosity increases so much that the blood actually clogs the vessels, which can lead to emboli, heart failure, and stroke.

Additional effects of hypoxemia result in a decreased blood flow to the kidneys. The glomerular filtration rate declines, and conservation of sodium occurs. This promotes fluid retention and exacerbates heart failure. In summary, patients with COPD frequently have elements of chronic bronchitis, emphysema, and asthma in the pathogenesis of their disease. The predominant manifestation becomes dyspnea and fatigue, which is a primary focus of nursing care.

HOME OXYGEN THERAPY

Oxygen is used to treat hypoxemia that is associated with COPD. It is a colorless, odorless, tasteless gas that constitutes approximately 21% of the atmosphere. The purpose of O_2 administration is to enhance the O_2-carrying ability of the blood. The method selected depends on factors such as fraction of inspired oxygen (FiO_2), humidification needed, and patient-specific issues, including costs, comfort, and environmental factors.

Oxygen delivery systems are classified as low- or high-flow systems based on whether the system provides the entire inspired atmosphere to a patient in a fixed O_2 concentration.[22] Common methods of O_2 administration are low-flow devices, such as a nasal cannula, that deliver O_2 concentrations that vary with a person's respiratory pattern.[24] In contrast, Venturi masks are high-flow devices that deliver fixed concentrations of O_2 independent of the patient's respiratory pattern or effort. Mechanical ventilators described in Chapter 13 are another example of a high-flow O_2 delivery system seen in home care. See further discussion in the section on ancillary oxygen equipment.

Many studies have documented the benefits of low-flow continuous or as-needed (PRN) O_2 therapy for patients with COPD.[13,15,21] A general improvement of primary organ function, along with increased mobility and cognitive processes such as abstraction and memory, is associated with low-flow O_2 administration to COPD patients. In addition, reduced mortality rates are noted in these study groups. Cardiac output, hemoglobin concentration, and the partial pressure of arterial O_2 saturation (PaO_2) primarily determine O_2 transport, tissue perfusion, and the need for O_2 therapy. Generally speaking a patient whose PaO_2 is less than 55 mm Hg on room air will require supplemental oxygen.[22]

Home oxygen therapy is expensive, but Medicare reimbursement can be obtained for eligible patients. Medicare guidelines specified on the Health Care Financing Administration's (HCFA's) form 484 (certificate of medical necessity, or CMN) outlining the appropriateness of O_2 therapy include the following:

1. A PaO_2 of 56 to 59 mm Hg (or O_2 saturation to 89% on room air by ear oximetry); and
2. Evidence for end organ damage to include a diagnosis of COPD, cor pulmonale suggested

by congestive heart failure, electrocardiographic evidence of heart disease, persistent erythrocytosis (a hematocrit of 57% or more), impairment of cognitive function, and dependent edema.

A written order for home O_2 therapy by the patient's physician is necessary for Medicare reimbursement. The prescription should provide a specific patient diagnosis indicative of end organ damage and specific laboratory evidence of hypoxemia and should include flow rate and O_2 concentration, frequency of use, and duration of need.

The goal of O_2 therapy is to maintain an O_2 saturation of 90% to 93%.[22,23] This can easily be measured by home care nurses by using pulse oximetry. Pulse oximetry does not measure carbon dioxide (CO_2). An arterial blood gas (ABG) measurement is recommended if the patient is suspected of retaining carbon dioxide. In addition, a low blood pressure or inadequate blood flow can result in an erroneous pulse oximetric reading.[24]

Complications of oxygen therapy in the home

Oxygen is a very combustible gas. There should be no smoking or open flames in the area in which oxygen is being used.

Carbon dioxide narcosis may result with an inappropriate O_2 flow rate. Normally CO_2 accumulation is a major stimulus of the respiratory center. When CO_2 levels remain chronically high, as with COPD, the body relies on low O_2 levels, or the hypoxic drive, as a stimulus for breathing.[20,30] Although not all COPD patients are CO_2 retainers, the administration of O_2 at levels greater than 3 L/min may suppress the hypoxic drive in these patients and lead to respiratory arrest. Signs and symptoms of CO_2 narcosis include confusion, lethargy, and a patient who cannot be aroused.[22] Home care nurses should stop O_2 administration if inappropriately high O_2 levels are noted and should alert the physician as soon as possible. If tampering with the flow rate is suspected, the home medical equipment (HME) vendor can be asked to put a lock on the flow meter.

Oxygen toxicity and atelectasis may also result from prolonged exposure to high concentrations of O_2.[22,30] Symptoms are varied and include nausea, vomiting, changes in mucus production, and malaise. Respiratory arrest can occur with both.

Therefore it is critical that the amount of O_2 administered should just be enough to maintain the patient's Pa_{O_2} within a normal or acceptable level. Once the patient is at home, ABGs should be monitored monthly or PRN to evaluate the effects of therapy.

Infection is another problem associated with O_2 administration. Heated nebulizers and humidification systems can support bacterial growth that may cause harmful respiratory infections.[32] Cleaning of equipment is important; see a further discussion in the section on infection control issues.

Oxygen equipment in the home

There are several basic types of O_2 delivery systems used in home care. The type the patient uses is often determined by the insurance company or Medicare; however, the ordered liter flow, Fi_{O_2}, and geographic location of the home must also be taken into consideration[24] (Figure 11-1).

Oxygen tanks. Tanks of O_2 (H or K cylinders), 4 to 5 feet tall and weighing about 150 pounds, serve as the stationary O_2 supply in the home. A smaller tank (E or D cylinder) is available as a portable system for travel. The oxygen concentration delivered from a compressed gas system is 100% pure O_2. The liter flow available from a compressed gas O_2 system ranges from 0.03 L/min to 15 L/min. The manufacture, storage, and shipment of compressed gas cylinders is regulated by the Department of Transportation (DOT). The Department of Transportation requires that all oxygen cylinders be painted green for ease of identification and that all cylinders must be supported in a stand so they do not fall over. Other safety issues regarding compressed gas cylinders include the following: when transporting portable tanks in a car, the tanks should be secured on the seat and not stored in the trunk; portable tanks should not be stored in a car; care should be taken when changing regulators to avoid having O_2 leak from the tank; and tanks should be turned off at the valve stem when they are not in use in order to avoid leakage. The HME vendor schedules the pickup of empty tanks and the delivery of full tanks based on the patient's O_2 use (the higher the liter flow ordered, the more frequent the delivery of tanks).

Liquid oxygen. Liquid O_2 base stations are round tanks about 3 to 4 feet tall made of stainless steel that work like a thermos. The liquid O_2 con-

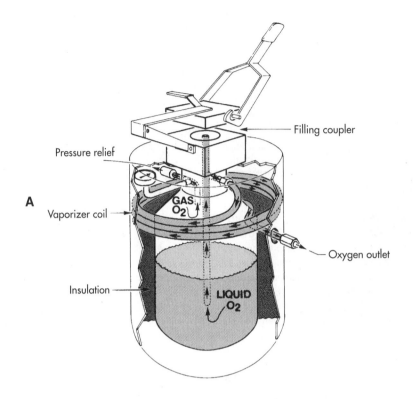

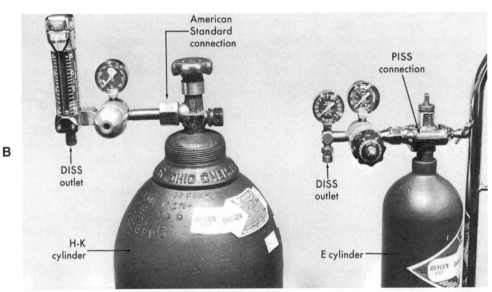

Figure 11-1 Oxygen systems. **A,** Liquid oxygen system. **B,** Tank oxygen system. **C,** Molecular sieve concentrator (Nellcore Puritan Bennett Companion 492). **D,** Oxygen-conserving device. (**A** from Brashear RE, Rhodes M: *Chronic obstructive lung disease,* St Louis, 1978, Mosby; **B** from Scanlan CL and others: *Egan's fundamentals of respiratory care,* ed 7, St Louis, 1999, Mosby; **C** and **D,** courtesy Nellcore Puritan Bennett, Lenexa, Kan.)

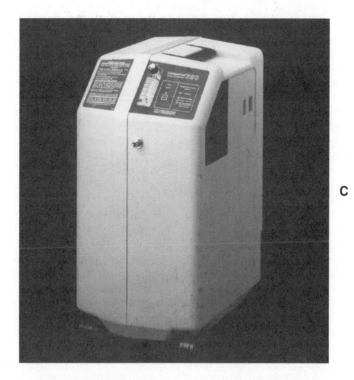

C

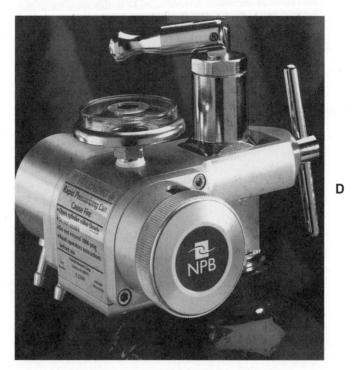

D

Figure 11-1, cont'd. For legend see opposite page.

verts to gaseous O_2 by evaporation. A small portable liquid O_2 system is used for travel. The portable tank is filled from the liquid O_2 base station when the family/caregiver wishes to take the patient out of the home (review manufacturer or HME instructions for filling portable tanks at home). The O_2 concentration delivered from a liquid system is 100% pure O_2. The liter flow available from a single liquid O_2 base station ranges from 0.25 L/min to 6 L/min. The main safety consideration with a liquid O_2 system is the potential for frostbite if the skin comes into contact with the liquid O_2. The liquid O_2 base station is refillable in the patient's home. Home medical equipment vendors schedule the refill based on the patient's O_2 use.

Oxygen concentrators. Oxygen concentrators make a clinically useful concentration of O_2 by drawing in room air and concentrating it to about 95% pure O_2. They run on electricity and do not require refilling. A patient who uses an O_2 concentrator is always supplied with a compressed gas O_2 system to act as a backup O_2 source in the event of a power failure. The liter flow available from an O_2 concentrator ranges from 0.25 L/min to 6 L/min depending on the manufacturer; however, because of the way these devices work, a higher liter flow will supply a lower O_2 concentration. If the patient cannot be adequately oxygenated on 4 L/min or less, then an O_2 concentrator may not be the best choice.

Oxygen-conserving devices. These devices are a special type of O_2 regulator. They conserve gas by providing the patient with O_2 on inspiration only. No gas flows from the regulator when the patient is exhaling. There are several brands of O_2-conserving regulators, and depending on the brand, the portable tank can last from 2 to 8 times as long as with a standard regulator. The HME respiratory therapist will perform an O_2 desaturation walk study with a pulse oximeter when the O_2-conserving device is set up to ensure that the patient is adequately oxygenated on the new device. The portable tank provided with the conserving device is small and lightweight (about 7 pounds), and it comes with a carrying bag for the patient's convenience. An O_2-conserving regulator should only be used with a nasal cannula.

The operation, maintenance, and cleaning of O_2 systems and related equipment should be a routine part of patient education. This training is usually initiated by the HME vendor's respiratory therapist as part of discharge planning and is reinforced by the home care nurse.

Ancillary oxygen equipment

The nasal cannula, Venturi mask, and more recently, transtracheal therapy are prominent methods of O_2 administration in the home.

Nasal cannula. The nasal cannula, by far the most popular, provides flows of 1 to 6 L/min with an O_2 concentration of 24% to 45%. This equipment is easily tolerated by most patients. It is simpler than a mask but provides less humidification. The patient can use extension tubing to promote mobility (up to 50 feet) without adversely affecting the O_2 flow delivery.

To reduce the amount of O_2 that is wasted with use of the nasal cannula, reservoir nasal cannulas are becoming more popular in home care. A reservoir nasal cannula stores oxygen in a 20-cc collapsing chamber during exhalation (Figure 11-2). This allows the patient to use lower flow rates than would otherwise be needed. Reservoir cannulas at a flow rate of 0.5 L/min provide saturation equivalent to that of continuous flow at 2 L/min.[22]

Many patients wearing nasal cannulas complain about irritation from plastic prongs in the nose or soreness where the tubing rests on the ears. Alternate styles for the nasal cannula can be recommended by the HME vendor to promote patient comfort. Cotton balls placed over the ears or a number of home improvisational techniques can alleviate pressure and soreness. If sores should develop in the nose from tubing irritation, instruct patients to rub vitamin E and *not* a petroleum product (such as Vaseline) over the area.

Venturi masks. Venturi masks provide more controlled O_2 concentrations from 35% to 45% with flows of 4 to 6 L/min (Figure 11-3). This mask comes with a set of interchangeable or adjustable adapters. Each adapter is calibrated by the manufacturer to provide a precise FiO_2. Refer to individual package inserts regarding flow-rate setting and resulting FiO_2 level. A Venturi mask can provide a patient with COPD a precise FiO_2 level that does not change with ventilatory pattern. These masks are especially efficacious for patients who are chronically hypercapnic and rely on the hypoxic drive to breathe. Bubble humidifiers are *not* recommended for use with Venturi masks.

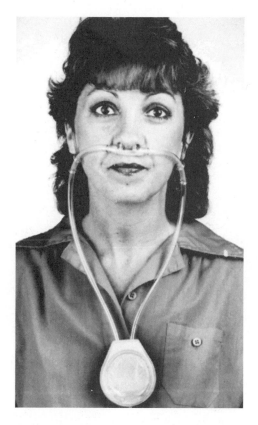

Figure 11-2 Nasal oxygen-conserving device. (From Lewis SM and others: *Medical-surgical nursing: assessment and management of clinical problems,* ed 5, St Louis, 2000, Mosby.)

Transtracheal oxygen therapy. Transtracheal O_2 therapy (TTOT) is accomplished by administration of O_2 directly into the trachea via a SCOOP catheter held in place by a bead chain necklace (Figure 11-4). Advantages of TTOT include a cost savings of 50% to 60% for the same flow provided by nasal cannulas, improved appearance, and increased patient mobility. [26]

Disadvantages include catheter dislodgment, tenderness, and a potential for subcutaneous emphysema around the catheter site. In addition, a mucous plug may form at the opening of the catheter, causing a potentially fatal obstruction. To prevent this complication, the patient should be well hydrated; mucolytic agents may be used. Patients with TTOT should be taught to recognize the

signs of mucus deposition—unexplained dyspnea, back pressure resulting in pop-off of the humidifier, persistent cough, etc.—and to irrigate the catheter or cough the mucus out if they notice these signs. [26]

SCOOP catheters should be cleaned at least daily to prevent infection and should be replaced every 3 months. Cleaning requirements should be reviewed with the supplier. If the catheter accidentally comes out and the patient is unable to reinsert it, the patient should be instructed to loosely cover the insertion site with a lint-free gauze pad, put on the nasal cannula, and notify the physician.

HUMIDIFICATION AND AEROSOL THERAPY
Humidification

Dry O_2 irritates delicate mucous membranes and dries secretions. The bubble-through humidifier is commonly used in home care today to prevent such complications. It is a small, plastic jar filled with distilled water that is attached to the O_2 source. Oxygen passes through the jar, bubbles through the water, and then goes through the tubing to the patient's cannula, mask, or catheter. See section on infection control issues.

Aerosol therapy

Aerosol therapy is used to clear mucus and improve breathing. Although aerosol therapy is ordered by the physician, home care nurses should monitor patients' abilities to administer medication, as well as the therapeutic effects of medications. Aerosolized medication orders must include the medication, dose, diluent, and whether it is to be nebulized with O_2 or compressed air. Microscopic droplets of medication can be inhaled by intermittent positive pressure breathing (IPPB), by compressor nebulizer, or by a cartridge inhaler. Sterile normal saline is frequently used with aerosol therapy and can be made in the home (Box 11-2).

Intermittent positive pressure breathing therapy. Prescribed IPPB treatments should be given before meals. When ready to begin treatments, patients should be instructed to sit upright in a comfortable position. After the machine is turned on, a mist forms at the mouthpiece. Patients then close their lips around the mouthpiece and breathe slowly, letting the machine fill their lungs. To conserve the medicine, the machine should be turned off if any interruption (coughing) occurs and

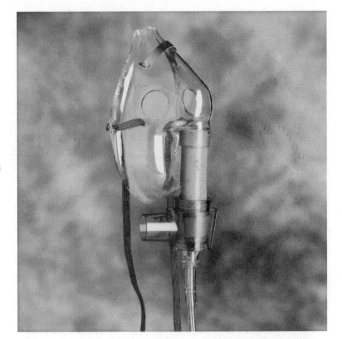

Figure 11-3 Venturi mask. (Courtesy Hudson Respiratory Care, Inc, Temecula, Calif.)

Figure 11-4 Transtracheal catheter for oxygen administration. (From Lewis SM and others: *Medical-surgical nursing: assessment and management of clinical problems,* ed 5, St. Louis, 2000, Mosby.)

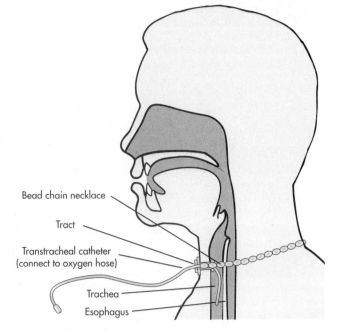

Bead chain necklace

Tract

Transtracheal catheter
(connect to oxygen hose)

Trachea

Esophagus

Box 11-2　HOMEMADE STERILE NORMAL SALINE

1. Add 1 teaspoon of noniodized table salt to 1 cup of tap water in a small clean glass jar with a screw-on lid.
2. Loosely place the lid on the jar.
3. Place the jar in a saucepan of water (water level in the saucepan should be three-fourths the height of the jar).
4. Cover the top of the saucepan.
5. Put the saucepan on the stove and boil the water for about 25 minutes.
6. Remove the saucepan from the stove and cool the solution. Remove the jar and tighten the lid.
7. If rapid cooling is desired, place the hot saucepan in another pan that contains water and ice cubes. Take care that the ice water does not flood over the rim of the saucepan and thereby contaminate the sterile saline. Do not place the hot glass jar directly in ice water as the glass may crack.
8. Store saline solution in the refrigerator. Important: Make fresh solution every week. Discard any solution that has become discolored or cloudy.

Box 11-3　INHALER ADMINISTRATION

Open-Mouth Technique
1. Shake the inhaler canister 15 to 20 times.
2. Remove the protective cap.
3. Inhale a deep, slow breath and then exhale completely.
4. Open your mouth wide.
5. Hold the inhaler canister 1 to 2 inches from your lips.
6. Gently compress the inhaler canister. Take a deep breath.
7. Hold your breath for as long as is comfortable.
8. Exhale slowly through pursed lips.
9. As prescribed by your physician, wait 1 minute between puffs and then repeat steps 1 through 7.

Inspirease Technique
1. Take a slow breath in and exhale completely.
2. Insert the inhaler canister in the mouthpiece.
3. Make sure the bag is connected to the mouthpiece.
4. Shake the inhaler canister 15 to 20 times.
5. Insert the mouthpiece between teeth, and close lips.
6. Gently compress the inhaler canister.
7. Take three to four deep and slow breaths from the bag. Do not make the inspirease whistle. Hold your breath as long as is comfortable between breaths to allow the medicine to deposit in the lungs.

---

should be used until all the medicine is gone (10 to 20 minutes).[24]

Routine administration of IPPB therapy is generally becoming less popular in home care today. It is usually used as a last resort for patients who cannot inhale deeply. It may induce pneumothorax in patients with emphysema.[7,22] Generated pressures may also reduce cardiac output because increased intrathoracic pressures diminish venous return to the heart. Hyperventilation and infection from contaminated equipment are additional complications associated with IPPB.

Compression nebulizers. Compression nebulizers require that the patient be able to take a deep, slow breath and cough effectively. They are similar in operation to IPPB. Two basic types of nebulizers are currently available, a continuous mode and one operated by a finger valve. Use large-size tubing to connect the nebulizer to a face mask or T bar in order to prevent any condensation from occluding the flow of oxygen.

Cartridge inhalers. Very popular in home care, cartridge inhalers are handheld canisters that are pocket sized and metered dosed. Each canister contains approximately 200 puffs. If the patient is taking a total of 8 puffs a day, the canister should be good for about 25 days. Spacers used in the inspirease technique are helpful for the elderly or those patients who lack coordination for the open-mouth technique of administration (Box 11-3).

INFECTION CONTROL ISSUES

All home respiratory equipment should be routinely cleaned to prevent potential infection. Soap and water are effective for cleaning equipment such as nasal cannulas, masks, tubing, the cap and mouthpiece of cartridge inhalers, and humidifiers.

Home respiratory equipment is then usually soaked in a white vinegar/water (1:3 cups) solution for 20 minutes, thoroughly rinsed with warm running water, and allowed to air dry.

Surfaces of all equipment should routinely be wiped with a disinfectant. For most equipment, cleaning should be done daily or at least 2 to 3 times per week. Cleaning of equipment is also recommended after each IPPB or aerosol treatment.[22] After being cleaned, humidifiers should be refilled with fresh distilled water to prevent bacterial growth. All equipment should be dry when stored. Cleaning recommendations from the HME vendor and product manufacturer should be reviewed. For a more detailed discussion of infection control guidelines, see Chapter 6.

SCREENING FOR CHRONIC OBSTRUCTIVE PULMONARY DISEASE

Home care agencies, including home pulmonary rehabilitation programs, should screen all smokers for signs of COPD, including symptoms of dyspnea, cough, increased sputum, and slowed expiration.[7,14] In addition, pulmonary function tests may be used to diagnose, classify, and monitor COPD progression or efficacy of interventions. For example, a forced expiratory volume in 1 second (FEV_1) measurement is a pulmonary function test that can easily be done in the home. This test may also be used as an assessment tool because FEV_1 correlates with several clinical findings, such as the degree of physical impairment and ABG abnormalities.[7,30] Patients with an FEV_1 of 1500 cc usually experience mild forms of shortness of breath. An FEV_1 of 1000 cc usually manifests as shortness of breath with activity. Patients with an FEV_1 of 500 cc or less usually experience shortness of breath at rest and are at high risk for respiratory arrest.

HOME CARE APPLICATION

Providing home care for patients with COPD is not an easy task. These patients and their families are frequently overwhelmed by the physical and psychological complexities of a progressively debilitating disease.[12]

Developing the plan of care

The plan of care and visit frequency will largely depend on the home care nurse's assessment of

Box 11-4   PRIMARY NURSING DIAGNOSIS/PATIENT PROBLEMS

- Ineffective breathing pattern
- Ineffective airway clearance
- Knowledge deficit: disease process and risk complications, medications including home oxygen therapy, operation of home medical equipment, procedural care, diet, pulmonary rehabilitation, infection control, socioeconomic resources, available community services, etc.
- Altered nutrition: less than body requirements
- Activity intolerance: ___ Ambulation, ___ Activities of daily living (ADLs), ___ Other (Specify)
- Self-care deficit: ___ ADLs, ___ Feeding, ___ Toileting, ___ Other (Specify)
- Risk for pulmonary infection
- Ineffective individual coping
- Hopelessness
- Altered sexuality patterns

patient/caregiver needs for care (Box 11-4). Patient care should be directed toward the following goals:

- Relief of physical symptoms, including dyspnea
- Relief of psychosocial symptoms, including anxiety and depression
- Patient education regarding self-care management of COPD and disease process; financial considerations, including billing and reimbursement issues; and home "survival needs"
- Increased independence and activity tolerance; general physical reconditioning
- Prevention of exacerbations of COPD

A multidisciplinary approach is a must for patients with COPD. The home care program will involve nursing (includes use of the home care aide and/or homemaker services), rehabilitation services, respiratory therapists, nutritional therapists, and possibly the services of the social worker in assisting the patient to achieve his or her best level of health. The home care team should coordinate activities to assist the patient in building strength and endurance, clearing excess mucous secretions, and overcoming fears of breathlessness.

Physical assessment

Clinical manifestation of COPD is similar to that of congestive heart failure (CHF). In addition, many ventilator-dependent patients have a diagnosis of COPD (see Chapters 12 and 13).

General. Patients with chronic bronchitis are stocky, typically cyanotic, and bloated due to heart failure. Patients with emphysema often have barrel-shaped chests and ruddy complexions resulting from constant lung inflation and secondary polycythemia. In addition, patients with emphysema tend to be thin and underweight as a result of oxygenation problems and hypermetabolic processes that are still poorly understood.

Observe patients' outward appearance in terms of dress and personal hygiene. Patients with COPD may not dress or bathe because the effort required to do so increases shortness of breath. Be aware that complaints of extreme fatigue, shortness of breath, sudden disorientation, or belligerency may be signs of hypoxemia and impending respiratory failure.

Assess the patient's activity tolerance. Does shortness of breath occur at rest? Does it occur after 5 minutes of conversation or with 10 to 30 feet of ambulation? Use a rating scale to have patients identify how they describe their shortness of breath on a scale of 0 to 10. This is especially useful in caring for patients with changes in the treatment regimen as a means to evaluate the effectiveness of oxygen, bronchodilators, and corticosteroid therapy.

Obtain a health history to identify factors that may contribute to COPD such as smoking, occupation, and environmental or familial considerations. Does the patient look well nourished, overweight, or underweight? Does the patient look rested? Many patients with COPD are afraid to sleep for fear they will stop breathing. Some patients may do a lot of pointing and speak in short, abrupt phrases because they are short of breath.

Cardiopulmonary. Inspect the chest, noting size and shape. A barrel-shaped chest with an increased anteroposterior diameter $(1:1)$ results from chronic hyperinflation of the lungs. An irregular heart rate, clubbing of the fingers, jugular venous distension, dependent edema, and oliguria are some of the clinical manifestations of hypoxemia and pulmonary hypertension. Limited bilateral excursion of the diaphragm and a decreased area of cardiac dullness, along with faint heart sounds, may be detected as a result of hyperinflation of the lungs.

Auscultate the lungs for abnormal or adventitious lung sounds. Specific abnormal lung sounds include the following:

- Wheezes (continuous whistling noises resulting from narrowed airways)
- Crackles (discontinuous popping sounds associated with the movement of fluid in the airways; crackles may be described as fine, medium, or coarse)
- Rubs (coarse scraping or grating noises resulting from the rubbing of inflamed pleura)

A productive cough and dyspnea on exertion are common with bronchitis. Patients with emphysema tend to have minimal coughing with little or no sputum. If patients cough, ask them how often they cough and at what times of the day. Ask if the cough is productive or nonproductive of mucus. If productive, ask about the consistency, color, and amount of mucus. If possible, inspect the mucus when it is coughed up. A green or yellowish color is characteristic of a pulmonary infection and should be immediately treated with antibiotics.

Gastrointestinal. Peptic ulcers are associated with COPD.[30] Ask the patient if he or she is having stomach pains or heartburn. Assess appetite and ability to eat. Perform guaiac testing of stools for blood as indicated.

The physician should be notified of any changes in the patient's baseline status. An awareness of complications from COPD or coexisting health problems—including diabetes, poor nutrition, depression, heart failure, and hypertension—should be a routine component of patient assessment.

Medications

Patients with COPD are frequently on multiple medications. Primary medications used to treat COPD are oxygen, bronchodilators, corticosteroids, and antibiotics.[7,23,30]

Oxygen. Oxygen is usually administered at 1 to 3 L/min by nasal cannula. (See discussions of oxygen therapy, including patient education issues.)

Bronchodilators. Bronchodilators (beta-adrenergic agonists, anticholinergics, and methylxanthine derivatives) relax smooth muscle around the bronchial tubes. They are usually inhaled, or they may be administered orally. Inhalation is preferred to oral administration because a lower dose is needed and systemic side effects are reduced.

Beta-adrenergic agonist inhalers include iso-etharine (Bronkosol), metaproterenol (Alupent), and albuterol (Proventil).[7] They are usually administered via a metered-dose inhaler. Recommended dosage is 1 to 2 puffs 4 times a day. They are indicated for short-term relief of bronchoconstriction and are the treatment of choice for exacerbation of COPD.

Although beta-adrenergic agonists are used "as needed" for intermittent symptoms, ipratroprium bromide (Altrovent) is the anticholinergic agent of choice for patients with persistant symptoms.[7]

Cromolyn sodium (Intal) is a mast cell stabilizer and acts prophylactically like a bronchodilator to prevent anaphylactic reactions. It is used with asthmatics and should be administered before possible contact with an asthmatic agent. Cromolyn sodium may be administered at 2 to 4 puffs 4 times daily by metered-dose inhaler (MDI).[30]

Methylxanthines and theophylline derivatives are not as effective as inhalers but do improve diaphragmatic contractility and act as a mild diuretic.[3] Optimal benefits occur with plasma levels of theophylline between 10 and 20 mg/ml.[3]

Excessive use of bronchodilators may increase tolerance. Side effects include increased heart rate, muscle tremors, and palpitations. Be aware that signs of theophylline toxicity also include anorexia, nausea, headache, tremors, and cardiac dysrhythmia.[29]

Corticosteroids. Corticosteroids decrease inflammation and mucous secretion.[1,16] They may be inhaled or given orally. Their onset of action is delayed compared with that of bronchodilators. They usually must be inhaled for 4 to 5 days before a therapeutic effect can be seen.

Oral doses of 40 mg of prednisone daily for 14 days are recommended when other therapies do not improve the patient's ability to breathe.[1] If the patient responds, the drug should be administered at the lowest effective dose. When being discontinued, steroids should be tapered off slowly.[1]

Oropharyngeal candidiasis, hoarseness, and dry cough may be caused by inhalation of corticosteroids. These problems may be reduced by having the patient use a spacer with the MDI and

by gargling with water after each use. Other side effects of corticosteroids include weight gain, cataracts, glucose intolerance, edema, hypokalemia, brittle bones, and a "moon face." In addition, poor wound healing and depressed immunity may occur.[1]

If using both, the bronchodilator should be administered before the corticosteroid. Numbering the inhalers in order of use may be helpful to patients. Also, if prolonged steroid therapy is considered, a preliminary tuberculin test is recommended.

Antibiotics. Antibiotics should be administered when sputum becomes purulent.[32] *Haemophilus influenzae* and *Streptococcus pneumoniae* are the organisms most commonly isolated from the sputum of COPD patients.[34] Treatment for 7 to 10 days with tetracycline, penicillin, ampicillin, or trimethoprim-sulfamethoxazole is typically used.[34] Be aware that many antibiotics have drug and food interactions that require the patient to take the drug 1 hour before or 3 hours after eating or taking an antacid. Emphasize the importance of completing antibiotic therapy for effectiveness even if the patient feels better.

Other. The major side effect of a number of antianxiety medications is respiratory depression. Antidepressants, narcotics, analgesics, and sedatives should be used sparingly for the same reasons.[12]

Antacids (e.g., Titralac or Amphojel) and histamine H_2-receptor antagonists (for example, Tagament or Pepcid) are commonly used to treat peptic ulcers. These medicines should be used with caution in older adults and patients with renal disease as related to acid/base balance.

Activities of daily living

In planning care, it will be important to determine what activities of daily living (ADLs) the patient can perform. Self-care activities include cooking, cleaning, laundry, shopping, etc. Can the patient move around in the home? Consider a referral to rehabilitation services for problems identified in this area. A request for home care aide services to assist the patient with ADL care may be needed.

Nutrition

Nutritional support will be an important part of nursing care because many patients with COPD are malnourished.[31] Be aware that malnutrition is associated with decreased ventilatory muscle strength, endurance, and force of contraction.[9,31]

A high-fat, low-cholesterol diet to maintain an adequate weight is recommended.[9] Carbohydrate metabolism creates increased blood levels of CO_2 as a by-product. Because CO_2 is excreted primarily by the lungs, calories from fat and protein sources rather than carbohydrates are preferred for CO_2 retainers. Note that total parenteral nutrition (TPN) products and many nutritional supplements have a high carbohydrate content and therefore may produce shortness of breath in patients with COPD.[31]

Gas-forming foods such as beans, brussels sprouts, and cabbage should be avoided. Patients may wish to refrain from drinking milk because it tends to thicken mucus. Alcohol depresses respiration and should be discouraged. Because caffeine is a stimulant, coffee, tea, and sodas should be avoided by patients in danger of heart failure.

Unless contraindicated, encourage the patient to drink 6 to 8 glasses of water a day to thin mucous secretions and promote hydration.

If the patient is using steroids, a monitored regimen of oral calcium and vitamin D may be recommended to prevent osteoporosis.[7] Frequent oral hygiene improves the sense of taste. To conserve energy, if possible, encourage patients to use their oxygen when they eat. See Chapter 5 for nutritional assessment guidelines; also see Appendix XI-I.

Home air quality

Instruct patients to avoid respiratory irritants such as smoke-filled rooms, animal hair, feather pillows, sudden changes in room temperature, pollen, and aerosol sprays. Air-conditioning should be used in hot weather. Recommend that a humidifier be used, if possible, to keep airways from drying out, particularly in dry climates or during the winter, when heated air is dry. Tell patients to stay indoors on days when pollen counts are high or air quality is poor. Recommend that scarves or masks be worn over the face during cold weather to prevent bronchospasm. See Chapter 25 for further environmental precautions.

Psychosocial considerations

Patients with COPD are often depressed, lonely, and socially isolated.[12] The role losses associated with COPD are greater than those of other illnesses

and contribute to the depression. Shortness of breath and easy fatigability are primary factors. It may be necessary to alter the home environment to prevent patient isolation. Encourage patients to have their bedroom on the main floor with easy access to the bathroom and kitchen.

Because the spouse assumes the family roles that the patient with COPD is no longer able to perform, the spouse is also placed under severe stress. Caregiver or family conflicts may arise as a result of role changes and redefinition of lifestyles, or they may be caused by financial strain arising from the impact of a chronic disease. Likewise the spouse or caregiver may absorb some of the patient's overwhelming sense of deprivation and loss.

Dyspnea causes many patients with COPD to withdraw from day-to-day activities and hobbies. In addition, patients with COPD have been shown to have higher levels of anxiety during times of high dyspnea compared with periods of low dyspnea.[17] Research indicates that effective treatment strategies include pharmacological therapy, including tricyclic antidepressants, exercise, individual and caregiver or family therapy, and caregiver or family interventions.[4,6,10,17] It is important to facilitate positive coping by encouraging patient/caregiver communication and by being attentive to behaviors that stress household relationships.

The frustrations and anxiety of air hunger should be reviewed with caregivers or families to promote their understanding of patients' labile emotional states and sudden outbursts of anger. However, manipulative behaviors by patients are not acceptable. When coping with patient discomfort or distress, caregivers or families should be instructed to remain calm and encourage patients to control their breathing, use their inhaler, put on their O_2, and sit still until breath is regained.[17,18,27] Also, it may be necessary to remind caregivers "not to do everything for the patient" in balancing household support with the patient's best interest, which is to promote activity.

Refer patients to social services for assistance with financial planning. Instruct patients in stress reduction and relaxation techniques such as visual imagery. Support groups such as the Better Breathers Club can help patients and their caregivers explore activities that can be done together such as walking, reading, or driving. See Chapter 4 for further information regarding family care.

Sexual counseling

Sex is an important aspect of life for all people, including those with COPD. Sexual dysfunction often parallels the course of lung disease.[8] Loss of touch or fear of intimacy may increase feelings of anger and isolation. The fear of dyspnea and fatigue may limit participation in sexual activities. The subject may be broached with a simple question such as, "Are problems with your breathing affecting your sex life?" If the patient and/or spouse wishes to discuss the subject, the home care nurse can suggest the following measures to improve breathing[8,11]:

- Have sex in a familiar environment with a room temperature controlled at 68° to 72° F and 40% humidity to promote comfort.
- Use the inhaler before sex or keep the metered-dose inhaler by the bedside for quick relief if shortness of breath occurs.
- Use O_2 via a nasal cannula during sex.
- Try positions that do not require the patient to support all the body weight. Lying side by side, lying with the non-COPD partner on top, or using an armless chair with the non-COPD partner on top may alleviate patient dyspnea.
- Encourage patients and their spouses to take rest periods during sex as needed. Sometimes simply hugging can provide the greatest intimacy of all.

PATIENT EDUCATION

Home management of COPD is complex. There is much patients and their families can learn to better their lives (Box 11-5). Patient education regarding home "survival needs" should be a priority of health teaching. Survival needs include information about procedural care, medications, operation of equipment including home oxygen safety precautions, what to do in emergencies, when to call the physician, etc. Never forget to ask patients what they perceive their immediate learning needs for care are.[18,25] Emphasize that smoking cessation is a must because it is the only intervention that produces an improvement in FEV_1 and slows the decline in FEV_1 to levels of normal, nonsmoking individuals.[7] In addition, adherence to nebulizer therapy and other medicines is necessary in order

---

Box 11-5   PRIMARY THEMES OF PATIENT EDUCATION

- COPD: signs and symptoms of disease process to report to the case manager and physician
- When to call 911
- Pulmonary infection: recognition and treatment
- Breathing techniques to conserve energy
- Postural drainage to clear mucous secretion
- Home oxygen therapy: operation and maintenance of equipment
- Medications: purpose, action, dosage, side effects, and methods of administration
- Diet
- Energy conservation
- Positive coping strategies to use when living with a chronic disease
- Adaptations to promote positive sexual relationship with significant other
- Socioeconomic resources
- Community services available for people with COPD
- General self-care strategies

---

to improve breathing and prevent complications of the disease. This means that the patient has to believe in the importance of the treatment in order to fully participate in the plan of care.[25,28]

An exacerbation management plan should be developed and reviewed periodically with the patient. This would include a discussion regarding the early signs of respiratory infection (e.g., fever, increased sputum, color changes in sputum, extreme shortness of breath, or lung congestion) and emphasis on starting antibiotic therapy promptly.[32] In addition, patients should know that a sudden weight gain (greater than 2 pounds in 1 day) should be reported to the physician as a possible sign of heart failure. Caregivers or family members should be taught that patient behavioral or mental status changes (e.g., the patient may suddenly become combative) may indicate hypoxemia and should be immediately reported.

Patients should be taught that although O_2 is not addictive, it is a prescribed drug and should be respected as such. It is important to explain to COPD patients that O_2 should be used when needed but only at the prescribed amount because with certain patients high flow rates can lead to respiratory arrest. Patients receiving home O_2 therapy should be instructed that although O_2 does not burn, it is combustible. Contact with a spark or flame is to be avoided because this can cause an explosion. Hence O_2 should be kept at least 10 feet away from any potential explosive hazard such as people smoking, gas burners, or electrical appliances.[24] Patients should notify the local fire department that they have O_2 equipment in the home.

Patients with COPD often complain of lack of sleep related to shortness of breath. Teach them that pillows or a foam wedge obtained from the HME vendor can ease the effort of breathing and may encourage rest. Instruct them to keep medicines, clothes, tissues, personal articles, and the telephone by the bedside for convenience and ease of use.

Morning is typically a very difficult time for patients with COPD because mucus has accumulated in the lungs throughout the night. The day is begun by coughing and expectoration of mucus, which can be exhausting. Instruct patients to use their inhaler in the morning to ease breathing and to use their O_2 when needed.

Encourage patients to use their O_2 with extension tubing when bathing. They should shower with warm water because extremes of temperature increase energy consumption. Bath blankets and robes help prevent chilling when drying. Shoes of the slip-on variety and shirts, dresses, and trousers with Velcro fasteners ease dressing.

As discussed in the remainder of the chapter, techniques to increase strength, clear excess mucous secretions, and conserve energy are a focus of patient education.

PULMONARY REHABILITATION

Pulmonary rehabilitation involves breathing retraining and chest physiotherapy. The goal of such therapy is to improve the patient's breathing, oxygenation, and endurance. This is accomplished by strengthening muscles, learning proper breathing patterns, and using effective mucus expectoration and clearance methods.[33]

The physical therapist will develop a home exercise program helpful in building the patient's strength and endurance. In developing the plan of care, physical therapy will focus on functional loss. For example, if the patient is unable to walk, ambulation will be a priority of training.[10]

An occupational therapist may be utilized to teach COPD patients to perform ADLs in a way that conserves their energy. Patients should learn to plan their day so that activities are coordinated with rest periods in order to prevent shortness of breath. Expending energy wisely reduces the effort of breathing. Box 11-6 provides energy conservation tips.

Specific techniques

Breathing techniques. There are a number of breathing techniques useful for COPD patients. Pursed-lip and diaphragmatic breathing are commonly taught (Box 11-7). Consider hooking the patient up to a pulse oximeter during breathing exercises as a means of biofeedback.

Pursed-lip breathing helps keep the airways open, thus improving oxygenation. In diaphragmatic breathing, patients use their diaphragms for respiration instead of accessory muscles of the chest and neck. This promotes a more normal breathing pattern and reduces the work of breathing. Patients learn to exhale as they work because exhalation requires less effort than inhaling.

Chest physiotherapy. Chest physiotherapy consists of procedures that cause postural drainage and clear the lungs of mucus. Flutter mucus clearance devices may be used by patients in order to vibrate their airways and loosen mucus from airway walls. In addition, patients are taught to clear secretions from the lungs with effective breathing techniques such as the huff cough and the cascade cough. Appendix XI-II describes chest physiotherapy frequently used in the home.

SUMMARY

Breathing affects every aspect of life. A simple and largely automatic process, breathing may become a daily struggle for people with COPD. Anger, depression, and withdrawal are the understandable consequences of a lifestyle restricted by the effort of breathing.

A multidisciplinary approach to treating COPD is especially important for these patients because of their special diet, exercise, educational, and psychosocial needs. As case managers, home care nurses are in an excellent position to refer patients to various agency and community services. Networking with other disciplines strengthens the plan of care. COPD is a chronic, but not hopeless, disorder. With successful home management, men and women with COPD can resume optimal participation in life activities.

Box 11-6   TIPS FOR ENERGY CONSERVATION FOR THE PATIENT IN THE HOME SETTING

If you have COPD, save your energy for daily activities. Avoid rushing. A slow, steady rate of work with frequent rest periods is best. Never work so long or hard that you feel very weak, tired, or short of breath. High-energy tasks never should be done back-to-back. Use pursed-lip or diaphragmatic breathing as you do your work so your energy will not be wasted. Take your inhaler or use your oxygen as prescribed and needed. Remember, one of the best ways to conserve your energy is to assign priorities and preplan your day.

Ways to Conserve Energy

1. Plan rest periods of at least 5 to 15 minutes between activities.
2. Ensure adequate room ventilation and a comfortable temperature. Excessive heat, cold, or humidity may cause shortness of breath. Avoid places with dirty air such as dusty or smoke-filled rooms. Avoid animal hair, scented soaps, colognes, powders, cleaners, aerosol sprays, glues, or paints if they cause problems with your breathing.
3. When possible, sit while performing activities such as bathing, brushing teeth, or washing dishes. Avoid unnecessary walking or standing. Try to push or slide objects rather than lifting them (use a portable cart).
4. Ask family or friends to help with heavy work as needed. Delegate particularly strenuous chores such as mowing the lawn or vacuuming the carpet to other family members as needed.
5. Let dishes air dry instead of toweling them dry.
6. Space personal activities such as shaving, bathing, and washing hair over several hours or days.
7. Take a quick shower if the moisture in the air makes it difficult to breathe. Turn on tepid water and wet yourself. Turn off the water and soap yourself all over. Turn the water back on to rinse. Immediately towel dry to prevent shivering.
8. Wear loose-fitting clothes with elastic waistbands or Velcro fasteners and front closures. Wear shoes that are easy to slip on, such as loafers or thongs.
9. To stand, first take several slow, deep breaths. Then, while breathing out through pursed lips, stand up.
10. To climb stairs, first breathe in deeply through your nose while standing. Next, exhale through pursed lips as you climb a couple of stairs. Stop, rest, and breathe deeply and slowly. Continue climbing two or three steps *while you exhale.* Stand still when inhaling. Hold onto the stair rails whenever possible for extra support.
11. Always remember to exhale when lifting or pushing heavy objects or when performing the action part of any activity.

Box 11-7   BREATHING TECHNIQUES

Controlled breathing exercises help get the maximum amount of air in and out of the lungs with the least amount of effort and should be practiced every day so that they become a natural way of breathing.

Pursed-Lip Breathing

Relax. Breathe in slowly. Purse lips into a whistling position and exhale slowly and evenly. Exhalation should be 2 to 3 times longer than inhalation. Count 1-2-3 for inhalation and 5-6-7-8-9 for exhalation.

Diaphragmatic Breathing

Sit down. Relax your abdominal muscles with inhalation. This moves the diaphragm down. Tense the abdomen with exhalation. This helps push the diaphragm up. Place your hand over the abdomen just below your breastbone. With correct diaphragmatic breathing, your hand will move out as you inhale and move in as you exhale.

REFERENCES

1. Alberts W, Corrigan K: Corticosteroid therapy for chronic obstructive pulmonary disease, *Postgrad Med* 81(5):33, 1987.
2. American Thoracic Society: Standards for the diagnosis and care of patients with chronic obstructive pulmonary disease, *Am J Respir Crit Care Med* 152:S78, 1995.
3. Aubier MA, Roussos C: Effect of theophylline on respiratory muscle function, *Chest* 86(2):91, 1985.
4. Barker AF and others: Replacement therapy for hereditary alpha$_1$-antitrypsin deficiency: a program for long-term administration, *Chest* 105:1046, 1994.
5. Brundage D and others: Self-care instruction for patients with COPD, *Rehabil Nurs* 18(5):321, 1993.
6. Bush AL, McClements JD: Effects of a supervised home exercise program on patients with severe chronic obstructive pulmonary diseases, *Phys Ther* 68:469, 1998.
7. Carr-Lopez S and others: Medication use in home care patients with COPD, *Home Care Provider* 3(3):144, 1998.
8. Curgian L, Gronkiewicz M: Enhancing sexual performance in COPD, *Nurs Pract* 13(2):24, 1988.
9. Dantone JJ: Medical nutrition therapy: the patient with COPD. In Rice R, editor: *Manual of home health nursing procedures,* ed 2, St. Louis, 2000, Mosby.
10. Gift A, Austin D: The effects of a program of systematic movement on COPD patients, *Rehabil Nurs* 17(1):8, 1992.
11. Gift A and others: Relaxation to reduce dyspnea and anxiety in COPD patients, *Nurs Res* 41(4):242, 1992.
12. Gift G, McCrone S: Depression in patients with COPD, *Heart Lung* 22(4):289, 1994.
13. Goldstein R: Effect of supplemental nocturnal oxygen on gas exchange in patients with severe obstructive lung disease, *N Engl J Med* 310(7):9, 1984.
14. Gravil JH and others: Home treatment of exacerbations of chronic obstructive disease by an acute respiratory assessment service, *Lancet* 351:1853, 1998.
15. Heaton R and others: Psychologic effects of continuous and nocturnal oxygen therapy in hypoxemic chronic obstructive pulmonary disease, *Arch Intern Med* 143:1941, 1983.
16. Keatings VM and others: Effects of inhaled and oral glucocorticoids on inflammatory indices in asthma and COPD, *Am J Respir Crit Care Med* 155:542, 1997.
17. Kohlman-Carrieri V, Janson-Bjerklie S: Strategies patients use to manage the sensation of dyspnea, *West J Nurs Res* 8(3):44, 1986.
18. McBride S: Patients with chronic obstructive pulmonary disease: their beliefs about measures that increase activity tolerance, *Rehabil Nurs* 19(1):37, 1994.
19. National Center for Health Statistics: *Trends in chronic bronchitis and emphysema: morbidity and mortality,* Washington, DC, November 1999 The Center.
20. Niederman MS: Introduction: mechanism and management of COPD, *Chest* 113:23S, 1998.
21. Nocturnal Oxygen Therapy Trial Group: Continuous or nocturnal oxygen therapy in hypoxemic chronic obstructive lung disease, *Ann Intern Med* 93(391):42, 1980.
22. O'Donahue WJ: Home oxygen therapy, *Med Clin North Am* 80:611, 1996.
23. Rennard SI: COPD: overview of definitions, epidemiology, and factors influencing its development, *Chest* 113:235S, 1998.
24. Rice R: Cardiopulmonary care. In Rice R, editor: *Manual of home health nursing procedures,* ed 2, St. Louis, 2000, Mosby.
25. Scherer YK, Schmieder LE: The effect of a pulmonary rehabilitation program on self-efficacy, perception of dyspnea, and physical endurance, *Heart Lung* 26:15, 1997.
26. Spofford B and others: Transtracheal oxygen therapy: a guide for the respiratory therapist, *Respir Care* 32:345, 1987.
27. Stempel J, Meek P: Managing breathlessness, *Home Health Focus* 2(2):14, 1999.
28. Turner J and others: Predictors of patient adherence to long-term nebulizer therapy for COPD, *Chest* 108(2):394, 1998.
29. Weinberger M, Handels L: Theophylline therapy in asthma, *N Engl J Med* 334:1380, 1996.
30. West J: *Pulmonary pathophysiology,* ed 5, Baltimore, 1997, Williams & Wilkins.
31. Wilson DO and others: Nutritional aspects of chronic obstructive disease, *Clin Chest Med* 7(4):643, 1986.
32. Wilson W: The role of infection in COPD, *Chest* 113:242S, 1998.
33. Yeaw E: The effect of body positioning upon maximal oxygenation of patients with unilateral lung pathology, *J Adv Nurs* 23:55, 1996.
34. Yoshikawa TT: Antibiotic treatment of lung infections, *Respir Ther* 6:26, 1996.

Medical Nutrition Therapy: Chronic Obstructive Pulmonary Disease

PURPOSE

- To instruct the patient/caregiver to maintain adequate intake of calories and protein
- To instruct the patient to maintain a stable, reasonable body weight
- To maintain immunocompetence
- To promote self-care in the home

GENERAL INFORMATION

Chronic obstructive pulmonary disease (COPD) is defined as a variety of respiratory diseases characterized by chronic airflow obstruction, namely, chronic bronchitis, asthmatic bronchitis, and emphysema. Signs and symptoms include chronic cough and productive sputum daily for 3 or more months during at least 2 consecutive years, dyspnea, and general difficulty in breathing. COPD is also characterized by shortness of breath, in part as a result of taking in decreased amounts of oxygen and expelling inadequate amounts of carbon dioxide.

The type of foods eaten affects the amount of oxygen and carbon dioxide in the blood. Oxygen is used to change food into fuel, and during this process carbon dioxide is formed as a waste product. Patients with COPD have a lack of oxygen and an increase of carbon dioxide in the blood. This situation leads to lactic acidosis, which makes the patient feel weak.

Malnutrition is a risk factor of respiratory failure. The progression of COPD can be slowed by providing nutrients in correct proportions that place the least amount of stress on respiratory function. Nutritional status is determined by the following:

From Dantone JJ: Nutritional care in the home. In Rice R: *Manual of home health nursing procedures,* ed 2, St. Louis, 2000, Mosby.

- Body weight
- Lean body mass
- Biochemical markers
- Skinfold measurements

The following are the most common symptoms of COPD that affect the patient's nutritional status:

- Early satiety
- Bloating
- Anorexia
- Dyspnea
- Fatigue
- Constipation
- Dental problems

The following are recommended calorie distributions for patients with COPD and normal healthy adults:

COPD	Normal
55% fat	30% fat
15% protein	20% protein
30% carbohydrate	50% carbohydrate

A high-fat diet places low stress on respiratory function. Protein intake should be monitored to prevent overfeeding. The use of long-term steroids can cause protein catabolism. Low-protein intake coupled with high-carbohydrate intake decreases theophylline elimination. Some studies indicate that diets high in vitamins C and E and omega-three fatty acids provide some protection for smokers against developing COPD.

Low body weight is a common problem for patients with COPD because these patients experience the following:

1. Increased calorie expenditure from infection and increased work from breathing, which

can be 10 times greater than what a healthy person requires

2. Decreased calorie intake from the following:
   - High doses of theophylline, causing nausea and/or vomiting
   - Chronic sputum, causing poor appetite
   - Full stomach, causing the diaphragm to be restricted after a large meal and resulting in difficulty in breathing
   - Shortness of breath and weakness, causing difficulty in preparing meals
   - Depression
   - Bronchodilators, which are gastric irritants
   - Peptic ulcers or gastrointestinal distress (experienced by up to 25% of patients with COPD)

EQUIPMENT

1. Cloth measuring tape
2. Scales or recent weight history of patient
3. Calculator
4. Food labels
5. Blood pressure cuff, stethoscope, and thermometer

PROCEDURE

1. Explain the procedure to the patient/caregiver.
2. Consider implementing the following:
   a. Assessing vital signs on each visit; weigh the patient at least once weekly; report abnormal findings to the physician
   b. Setting nutritional requirements for the patient; see nutritional assessment in Chapter 5.
   c. Recording a 24-hour recall of the patient's nutritional intake on the food diary form; analyze the calories, fat, carbohydrate, and protein content of the diet intake
   d. Instructing the patient/caregiver on the COPD diet instruction sheet and menu (Box XI-I and Table XI-I); use food labels to demonstrate calorie, fat, carbohydrate, and protein content in various foods
   e. Comparing the patient's 24-hour diet recall to his or her prescribed diet order as instructed; make appropriate recommendations to the patient/caregiver for modifying any nutrient intake that is found

to be inappropriate on the food intake record
   f. Making suggestions to improve calorie intake, keeping in mind the need to increase fat, monitor protein, and limit carbohydrate intake; use the following feeding strategies:
      - Eat high-calorie foods first, especially those high in fat
      - Use low-cholesterol fatty food sources instead of high-carbohydrate foods for snacks (e.g., eat peanut butter on whole wheat bread rather than a candy bar)
      - Eat small multiple meals
      - Drink liquid 1 hour before meals
      - Do not drink a lot of fluids with meals
      - Rest before meals
      - Take breathing treatments before meals
      - Take oxygen during the meal
      - Have the patient take advantage of the times he or she feels good by eating more
      - Treat food like a medication—take it seriously, sufficiently, and on time
      - Avoid gas-forming foods
      - Eat in a relaxed atmosphere and preferably with a companion

3. Clean and replace equipment. Discard disposable items according to standard precautions.

NURSING CONSIDERATIONS

Beneficial interventions for COPD include smoking cessation; avoiding irritants such as dust, fumes, and air pollutants; and avoiding extreme temperature changes. It is important that the patient with COPD receive influenza and pneumonia vaccines to avoid complications with infection and protect against further digression.

Medications and other therapies such as corticosteroids, antibiotics, bronchodilators, pulmonary rehabilitation, oxygen therapy, exercise, and reconditioning can help maintain functional independence, but no therapy can reverse lung damage. As previously mentioned, many of these therapies have poor nutritional side effects associated with them.

Since COPD is commonly associated with weight loss, low body weight, and calorie-protein malnutrition, prognosis is particularly poor—especially for patients who require mechanical ventilation. Because of high rates of infections and poor lung function, COPD is a common

---

Box XI-I   DIET FOR PATIENTS WITH COPD (High Fat, Low Carbohydrate, Moderate Protein)

Reason for the Diet

By increasing the fat and decreasing the carbohydrates (sugars and starchy foods) in the diet, the lungs are able to lower the amount of carbon dioxide in the blood, so you can breathe much better and easier.

How Much and/or What to Eat

Breakfast	Lunch and dinner (same)
1 serving unsweetened juice	2 ounces meat with fat
1 serving cereal with fat	1 serving starch with fat
1 serving egg with fat	1 serving vegetables with fat
1 serving bacon, ham, or sausage	1 serving bread
1 serving bread	2 servings fat
2 servings fat	1 serving unsweetened fruit
Diet jelly or syrup	1 serving whole milk
1 serving whole milk	Tea or coffee
Coffee	

10 AM	2 PM	Bedtime snack
1 serving meat or substitute	1 serving bread	1 serving whole milk
1 serving bread	1 serving whole milk	1 serving bread or sandwich
1 serving fruit or juice		

Do Not Eat These Foods

Regular sugar	Pies
Syrup	Cakes
Jam	Cookies
Jelly	Doughnuts
Candy	Dried fruits
Regular soft drinks	Anything with a lot of sugar in it

Do not take medicines with sugar in them, such as cough syrups.

Special Instructions

- The COPD diet listed here is approximately 2200 calories, distributed as 55% fat, 30% carbohydrate, and 15% protein.
- Eat small frequent meals, six meals a day if possible. This will keep you from feeling too full at one time. See Table AXI-I for sample menus.
- If you feel too full, it will seem harder to breathe. If you can't breathe you won't eat as well as you should and then you'll lose weight.
- Following the six-meal plan above will help prevent weight loss.

Modified from Dantone JJ: *Bridging the gap diet manual,* Grenada, Miss, 1997, Nutrition Education Resources.

---

source of morbidity and mortality in older adults.

Because of the aforementioned nursing considerations, it is imperative that the following be done:

- Weigh the patient each visit

- Report to the physician a weight change of 2 pounds in 1 day or 5 or more pounds between visits
- Observe the patient for increased difficulty in breathing or shortness of breath
- Fill out a food intake record once a week and compare it to nutrient requirements

Table XI-I   Menu for COPD diet (High fat, low carbohydrate, moderate protein)

	Sunday	Monday	Tuesday
Breakfast	Juice of choice	Juice of choice	Juice of choice
	Oatmeal with margarine	Grits with margarine	Cream of wheat with margarine
	Fried eggs	Fried eggs	Fried eggs
	Sausage	Bacon	Ham
	Biscuit or toast	Biscuits or toast	Biscuit or toast
	2 tsp margarine	2 tsp margarine	2 tsp margarine
	Diet jelly	Diet jelly	Diet jelly
	Whole milk	Whole milk	Whole milk
	Coffee	Coffee	Coffee
Lunch	Fried chicken	Cheeseburger with:	Roast turkey
	Dried beans or peas	Bun	Giblet gravy
	Seasoned greens of choice	Lettuce/pickle/onion	Cornbread dressing
	Buttered cornbread	Mayonnaise/mustard	English peas
	Banana	Chips of choice	Buttered roll
	Unsweetened tea	Diet apple cobbler	Diet jelly
	Whole milk	Unsweetened tea	Angel food cake
		Whole milk	Unsweetened tea
			Whole milk
Dinner	Ham	Beef tips	Potato salad
	Potato salad	Gravy	Tuna salad sandwich
	Seasoned green beans	Rice	Sliced tomatoes
	Buttered roll	Buttered broccoli	Crackers
	Diet pineapple tidbits	Buttered biscuit	Mayonnaise/mustard
	Whole milk	Prunes	Fresh orange
		Whole milk	Whole milk

From Dantone JJ: *Bridging the gap diet manual,* Grenada, Miss, 1997, Nutrition Education Resources.

DOCUMENTATION GUIDELINES
Document the following on the visit report:

- The procedure and patient toleration
- Vital signs
- Weight
- Food intake/appetite
- Patient/caregiver instructions and response to teaching, including understanding of the diet and adherence to nutritional recommendations
- Physician notification, if applicable
- Standard precautions
- Other pertinent findings

Update the plan of care.

Chest Physiotherapy at Home

Maneuvers used to assist in the removal of secretions:

Percussion is performed by clapping the cupped hand on the chest wall over the area of lung to be drained. Rhythmic clapping increases vibrations that stimulate the movement of secretions and helps clear secretions sticking to the bronchial walls. The hand is cupped to create a cushion of air against the chest wall (Figure XI-I). Raise hands 3 to 4 inches above the chest wall and alternately clap lungs to vibrate secretions. Clapping should be vigorous but not painful.

Vibration is used to stimulate the flow of secretions into the larger airways where they can be removed by coughing. To accomplish this technique, the home health nurse's hand should be pressed firmly over the area of the chest wall to be vibrated. The muscles of the home health nurse's upper arm and shoulder are tensed (isometric contractions) to produce fine tremors on the chest wall as the patient exhales. Vibration is done with the flattened, not the cupped, hand.

Deep breathing by the patient assists in the movement of secretions and may stimulate coughing. A deep rapid inhalation followed by a slow, prolonged expiration may move secretions into larger airways for removal by coughing. Encourage deep breathing during chest physiotherapy.

Productive coughing is enhanced by placing the patient in a sitting position, leaning forward. Encourage coughing after chest physiotherapy.

a. Cascade cough: Have the patient take a deep slow inhalation, then cough 2 to 3 times in a row at the end of the breath to move secretions to larger airways.
b. Huff cough: Have the patient take a deep breath and make a "huff" sound when exhaling instead of the usual cough.

Postural drainage uses specific positions to let the force of gravity assist in removing lung secretions. A physician's order must be obtained before the home health nurse can carry out this procedure. There are six basic drainage positions commonly used in home care. Each is specific for major areas of the bronchopulmonary segments. Drainage positions should be maintained for 10 to 15 minutes each. During this time, alternate 2 to 3 minutes of percussion with 10 to 12 vibrations. These exercises should be performed before breakfast and at bedtime or PRN. **Administer the inhaler before postural drainage.**

Primary drainage positions commonly used at home: Use a sturdy ironing board and a couch or other sturdy object of appropriate height to achieve the tilt of the Trendelenburg position. Place the narrow end of the board on the couch. Adjust the angle of the board to about 30 degrees. Brace the end of the board to prevent slipping. Pillows placed under the patient's hips/torso can also be used to achieve correct positioning (hips/torso should be elevated 12 to 20 inches to facilitate proper drainage). Exercises should be done to drain the lower bases of the lung first and proceed to the upper bases (Figure XI-II).

1. To drain base of left lung (left lower lobe): Have patient well turned into right side-lying position. Percuss and vibrate over lower rib area.
2. To drain base of right lung (right lower lobe): Have patient well turned into left side-lying position. Percuss and vibrate over lower rib area.
3. To drain right middle lobe: Have patient in left side-lying position with right side of body supported. Percuss and vibrate over midchest/nipple area.

4. To drain left middle lobe: Position patient as in step 3, but in right side-lying position. Percuss and vibrate over midchest/nipple area.

5. To drain anterior upper lobes: Have patient sit up and lean back. Percuss and vibrate over collarbone/shoulder area.
6. To drain posterior upper lobes: Have patient sit up and then lean forward over a pillow. Percuss and vibrate over shoulder area.

When performing chest physiotherapy, have a cup or basin and paper tissue available for draining mucus. Offer mouthwash and assist with oral care as needed following postural drainage. Encourage patients to rest after the procedure. Note: Observe for potential contraindications of the Trendelenburg position, such as abdominal distension or irregular heart rate. If any of these conditions exist, check with the physician before positioning the patient.

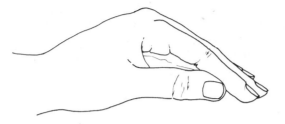

Figure XI-I Cupped hand. (From Wade JF: *Comprehensive respiratory care: physiology and technique,* ed 3, St. Louis, 1982, Mosby.)

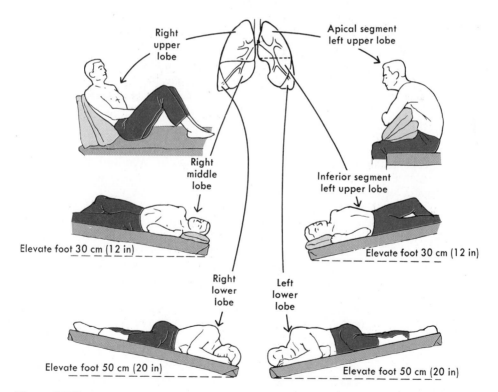

Figure XI-II Postural drainage positions frequently used in home care. (From Phipps WJ and others: *Medical-surgical nursing: concepts and clinical practice,* ed 6, St. Louis, 1999, Mosby.)

12

THE PATIENT WITH CONGESTIVE HEART FAILURE

Robyn Rice and S. Troy McMullin

Congestive heart failure (CHF) occurs when the heart is no longer able to pump and circulate blood effectively. The resulting circulatory overload or congestion is accompanied by clinical symptoms related to fluid pooling in body tissue. Long-term pharmacological therapy, functional disability, and frequent rehospitalizations associated with this syndrome pose severe financial and emotional stress for patients and their families.[4,7,13,20]

SIGNIFICANCE AND PREVALENCE

An estimated 4.8 million Americans have CHF, and many are treated in their homes. Increases in CHF death rates from 1980 to 2000 are attributed to a growing elderly population and longer survival of persons with hypertension or cardiac disease who subsequently develop CHF at an older age.[3,24]

Congestive heart failure may be acute or chronic and is associated with a poor prognosis.[3,25] According to the American Heart Association, half of the patients diagnosed with CHF will be dead within 5 years. It is the most common diagnosis in hospital patients age 65 years and older, and more than 65,000 persons with CHF receive home care each year.[3]

Incidence data indicate that CHF is twice as common in persons with hypertension than in normotensive persons and 5 times greater in persons who have had a heart attack compared with persons who have not.[3] Prevalence is at least 25% greater among the black population than among the white population.

Patient assessment and education regarding precipitating factors of CHF with recommendations for lifestyle changes to control hypertension and reduce the incidence of myocardial infarction are primary focuses of this chapter.

PATHOPHYSIOLOGY

An understanding of the pathophysiology of CHF provides a framework for intervention and treatment and is based on two key concepts[10,16]

1. The relationship among stroke volume, heart rate, and cardiac output
2. The heart as a two-system pump

The relationship among stroke volume, heart rate, and cardiac output must be considered when describing mechanical and physical factors that determine cardiac workload and the circulation of blood.

Stroke volume

Stroke volume represents the amount of blood pumped into the circulatory system by each myocardial contraction (normally 60 to 130 ml of blood are ejected with each contraction). The following forces determine stroke volume:

Preload. This refers to filling pressures, or the amount of blood in the left ventricle at the end of diastole, just before systole (ejection). It is also referred to as left ventricular end-diastolic pressure (LVEDP). In a normally functioning heart, an increase in preload is matched by an increase in the amount of blood pumped out of the ventricles and into the circulatory system. This phenomenon is referred to as "Starling's law," which says that up to a point, increases in ventricular blood volume parallel the strength and force of contractions as the ventricle is stimulated to eject additional volume.

However, in patients with CHF, sustained increases in preload lead to signs of clinical deterioration because overstretching and overworking of the myocardial muscle cause the heart to be unable to pump even moderate amounts of blood. Preload is the major determinant of myocardial oxygen consumption.[16]

Afterload. This refers to pressures in the aorta and peripheral vascular system that the heart must pump against to eject blood out of the ventricle. It is a function of both arterial pressure and left ventricular size. It is a direct reflection of blood pressure. Any increases in vascular pressure or resistance will increase ventricular contractility as the heart attempts to maintain stroke volume and heart rate. Hypertension is one of the major factors that increase afterload.

Contractility. This refers to the strength and force of the mechanical pumping action of the heart. Increases in contractility are associated with a reduction in afterload.

Heart rate

Heart rate determines the timing and pattern of myocardial contractions and is controlled by specialized conduction cells of the heart and the autonomic nervous system. Normally increases or decreases in heart rate serve as compensatory mechanisms for variations in physical activity, emotional state, blood composition, and fluid balance. However, an irregular or abnormally slow heart rate impairs blood circulation and tissue oxygenation just as an extremely rapid heart rate shortens ventricular filling time and produces a smaller circulating blood volume. Therefore inappropriate extremes of heart rate (lower than 60 beats/min or higher than 120 beats/min) may produce clinical signs and symptoms associated with oxygen deprivation and hypoxemia.

Cardiac output

Cardiac output describes the amount of blood pumped by the left ventricle per minute. A normal cardiac output is about 4 to 8 L/min. The relationship among cardiac output, stroke volume, and heart rate is expressed by the following equation:

cardiac output = stroke volume × heart rate

When stroke volume or heart rate declines, cardiac output also decreases. As cardiac output

falls, so does blood pressure. If left untreated, the patient may progress to a state of cardiogenic shock. In addition, limited increases in stroke volume and heart rate cause increases in cardiac output. However, overloading the ventricle with too much fluid in patients with CHF may only serve to aggravate failure because the pumping ability of the heart cannot manage sustained increases in workload.

In maintaining fluid balance, the heart essentially functions as two pumps that are regulated by the left and right ventricles. Any damage to the heart can result in reduced pumping ability of either or both ventricles.

Left ventricular (LV) failure refers to backward failure, in which blood is not pumped into the arterial system and instead backs up into the pulmonary vessels and lungs. Of note, pulmonary vascular congestion and edema are the dominant clinical features of LV failure. The most common form of initial heart failure is LV failure. Left ventricular failure will usually lead to and be the cause of right-sided failure. Heart failure rarely remains one-sided.

Right-sided failure results from a diseased right ventricle (RV) and is often caused by LV failure. It occurs when venous blood is unable to be pumped into the pulmonary circuit where carbon dioxide is exchanged for oxygen. Venous blood subsequently backs up into the systemic circulation, enhancing cardiac anoxia and failure. Systemic edema and circulatory congestion are the dominant clinical features of RV failure. Cor pulmonale (right ventricular dilation and hypertrophy caused by pulmonary pathologic condition) can also cause right-sided failure. Causes of cor pulmonale include chronic obstructive pulmonary disease and pulmonary emboli (see Chapter 11).

Left- and right-sided CHF are interrelated, and both result in an insufficient cardiac output[23] (Box 12-1). Compensatory mechanisms of the body functioning to offset a low cardiac output and restore volume may only aggravate fluid overload and pump failure. For example, as the anterior pituitary gland reflexively senses a decrease in blood pressure, the adrenal cortex is stimulated to secrete mineral corticoids, causing sodium and chloride retention. This electrolyte retention can increase fluid volume and place additional stress on the heart. Also, in response to a decrease in blood pressure, the posterior pituitary releases antidiuretic hormone (ADH), which causes the kidneys to conserve fluid and intensifies circulatory congestion.

In summary, the causes of CHF are related to an inadequate tissue perfusion and are primarily associated with the following clinical disorders[7,9,16]:

1. An increase in afterload (hypertension)
2. An increase in preload (circulatory overload)
3. A decrease in preload (hypovolemia, sepsis)
4. Impaired heart rate and contractility (electrolyte imbalance, myocardial infarction, pacemaker failure, coronary artery disease, congenital heart disease, cor pulmonale, valvular heart disease, cardiomyopathy)

All four may result in decreased cardiac output. The home setting presents another variable that impacts CHF. External and environmental factors will certainly influence the physiological response and clinical manifestations of a weakened heart and must be considered when developing a plan of care.

CLASSIFICATION OF CONGESTIVE HEART FAILURE

The New York Heart Association has developed guidelines for classifying people with CHF. This classification system is based on the person's tolerance to physical activity (Box 12-2).

HOME CARE APPLICATION

Patients typically seen in home care are those with unstable CHF; acute exacerbations will require hospitalization. Observation and assessment of the patient's condition regarding abnormal or fluctuating vital signs, weight changes, edema, respiratory changes, medication compliance, and dietary habits are the basis for home visits. Outcomes of care include an achievement of optimal health. For the heart failure patient, this may include a blood pressure that is less than 140/90 mm Hg or greater than 80/50 mm Hg; absence of orthostatic hypotension; a pulse that is greater than 50 and less than 100 beats per minute; weight that is equal to or less

---

Box 12-1 CLINICAL MANIFESTATIONS OF HEART FAILURE COMMONLY SEEN IN THE HOME

Right-Sided Ventricular Failure
Signs
Murmurs, peripheral edema, weight gain, dependent edema (sacrum, lower extremities, and feet), ascites, anasarca (generalized body edema), jugular venous distention (greater than 2 cm), hepatomegaly (liver enlargement)

Symptoms
Fatigue; dependent edema; anorexia and gastrointestinal bloating; nausea; weak or absent pedal pulses; dry, flaky skin

Left-Sided Ventricular Failure
Signs
Pulsus alternans; point of maximal impulse (PMI) displaced inferiorly and posteriorly, pulmonary edema, S_3 and S_4 heart sounds

Symptoms
Fatigue; dyspnea; orthopnea; dry, hacking cough; pulmonary edema; clubbing of the fingers; nocturia; paroxysmal noctural dyspnea; capillary refill greater than 2 seconds

---

Box 12-2 NEW YORK HEART ASSOCIATION FUNCTIONAL CLASSIFICATION OF PERSONS WITH CONGESTIVE HEART FAILURE

Class 1
No limitation on physical activity; ordinary physical activity not resulting in symptoms

Class 2
Slight limitation on physical activity; no symptoms at rest, but symptoms possible with ordinary physical activity

Class 3
More severe limitation; patient usually comfortable at rest; clinical manifestations with usual physical exercise

Class 4
Inability to carry on any physical activity without producing symptoms; symptoms possible at rest

than that at admission, absence of adventitous lung sounds; decreased fluid retention to the abdomen or lower extremities; and demonstrations of patient self-care strategies for best level of health.[6,17,19]

Planning visits

Home care nurses usually see patients with CHF 2 to 4 times per week depending on patient acuity level, the patient's support systems, and teaching needs. Daily visits may be necessary if the patient has a new medication regimen, new diet, or changes in oxygen therapy. Visit frequency and the plan of care are based on the nurse's ongoing physical assessment and identification of patient health care needs. However, studies indicate that increased age and fewer available caregivers may increase the need for professional home care services.[13, 14, 25] In addition, deficits in performing activities of daily living and functional limitations reported by CHF patients may reflect a continued need for care after discharge from traditional Medicare-based services.[18,21]

Physical assessment

When evaluating decompensation (failure of the heart to maintain adequate circulation), compare any variations in the physical assessment with the patient's baseline status and vital signs. Be aware that fatigue will be a major problem for these patients. In addition, always assess mentation and affect because confusion, combativeness, or unusual expressions of anger may be a sign of oxygen deprivation and hypoxemia. Ask patients if they are experiencing fatigue, weakness, shortness of breath, or dizziness; these may be signs of pump failure.

Cardiac. Auscultate heart sounds for rate, rhythm, and intensity. Extra heart sounds, such as an S_3 caused by turbulent blood flow within a weakened and damaged ventricle, are characteristic of left ventricular failure in adults. Assess for tachycardias or dysrhythmias when recording the apical-radial pulse and check blood pressure. A rapid or irregular heart rate in CHF is often caused by atrial fibrillation and may manifest as a low blood pressure.

Palpate the point of maximal impulse (PMI). Normally the PMI is palpated at the fifth left intercostal space (fifth LICS) at the midclavicular line. The PMI represents the contraction of the ventricle as it pushes upward against the chest wall.[5] With left ventricular failure (LVF), the PMI is displaced to the left. With right ventricular failure (RVF), the PMI shifts to the right of the fifth LICS.

Patients with CHF may exhibit pulsus alternans, which is an alternation of strong and weak pulse amplitudes, frequently accompanied by alternating loud and soft heart sounds.[5] Pulsus alternans is common with left-sided failure and is best palpated in the radial or femoral arteries. Evaluate all peripheral pulses, noting rate, amplitude, and quality. Patients with CHF may have diminished or faint pulses because of edema and poor circulation.

Inspect patients for signs of jugular venous distension (JVD), which is characteristic of right-sided failure. To evaluate for the presence of JVD, have patients sit in the bed with the head elevated at a 30-degree angle. Neck veins are considered abnormally distended when distension of the jugular veins can be measured at a horizontal line more than 2 cm above the sternal angle.[5] Jugular venous distension is a sign of elevated central venous pressure and fluid retention.

Determine whether patients have a positive hepatojugular reflex, which is symptomatic of hepatic congestion and elevated central venous pressure. Have patients lie down, and exert firm pressure over the right upper quadrant of the abdomen while observing the neck veins. Patients are positive for a hepatojugular reflex if an increase of more than 1 cm is visible in neck veins as pressure is applied over the liver.[5] A positive hepatojugular reflex is characteristic of right-sided CHF.

Pulmonary. In LVF, blood backs up into the pulmonary circuit, causing fluid to diffuse into the alveoli and creating adventitious lung sounds. If left untreated, pulmonary congestion may progress to pulmonary edema, which presents with cyanosis, noisy respirations, and frothy pink sputum. Assess oxygenation status with arterial blood gas or by pulse oximetry. Be aware that the patients with CHF are at risk for hypoxemia and hypercapnia.[11]

Evaluate for a cough. Is the cough dry or productive of sputum (phlegm)? Ask the patient, "How much do you think you cough up within 24 hours? A teaspoon, a tablespoon, a cup, or what?" Of note, purulent sputum has a green or yellowish color. Be aware that a cough is an important symptom of LVF.[16]

Auscultate the lungs for crackles and wheezes. These occur when air moves into the fluid-filled alveoli and are characteristic of LVF. Patients also may have coarse gurgles that clear with coughing. Note the use of accessory muscles (such as the diaphragm and sternomastoids) and the respiratory rate in assessing the degree of failure. Normal resting respiratory rates in adults are about 12 to 20 breaths per minute.[5] Assess for breathing patterns associated with LVF such as the following[10]:

- Dyspnea with activity: shortness of breath that occurs with an increase in physical activity (exertional dyspnea). Ask patients to identify activities that cause shortness of breath, and ask them what they do to alleviate shortness of breath. Ask patients to ambulate to determine if shortness of breath occurs with activity.
- Orthopnea: shortness of breath that occurs when patients lie down, causing excess fluid within the vessels to move into the alveoli. To assess orthopnea, have the patient lie down. Next, raise the patient's legs and observe for orthopnea. In evaluating the severity of orthopnea, ask if the patient uses extra pillows at night to make breathing easier and, if so, how many.
- Paroxysmal nocturnal dyspnea: shortness of breath that occurs suddenly, waking patients up. Associated with sudden fluid shifts, paroxysmal nocturnal dyspnea may be accompanied by nightmares that cause patients to complain of feeling anxious and frightened.

Skin. The skin and hair can show signs of cardiac failure. The color of the skin and paleness of mucous membranes may indicate poor circulation. Of note, patients with CHF often have skin that is dusky, cool, and dry or scaly. Hair may be coarse and brittle with partial loss present.

Nail beds may show signs of poor capillary refill. Capillary refill can be evaluated by depressing the nail bed of a finger until the skin blanches. Release pressure and observe the length of time it takes for the patient's normal color to return. Return of color to the nail bed that takes longer than 2 seconds is considered abnormal and may be a sign of poor circulation.[5]

Clubbing of nail beds, indicative of poor peripheral circulation, may also be present. The angle between the normal fingernail and nail base is normally 160 degrees. The nail base feels firm to palpation. In late stages of clubbing (associated with hypoxia), the base of the nail is visibly swollen and the angle between nail and nail base is greater than 180 degrees.[5]

Fluid/electrolyte and blood chemistry levels. On each visit measure the circumference of the ankle, dorsum, and calf of both legs to objectively evaluate dependent and peripheral edema, which are characteristic of right-sided failure; be consistent in measurement. Pitting edema may or may not be present; it is evidenced by a depression left in the swollen extremity when compression is removed.

Observe for weight gain by weighing patients on the same scale and at the same time on each visit. A weight gain of 3 to 4 pounds in 1 week or 2 pounds in 1 day is an indicator of decompensation or problems in lifestyle habits.

Laboratory work should be obtained to assess fluid and electrolyte imbalance, which can cause problems with heart rate and contractility. Blood chemistry values should be checked every other week, particularly if the patient is on intravenous furosemide (Lasix). Verify the frequency of laboratory work with the physician. See the appendix at the end of this book, which indicates normal ranges of blood chemistry values. Observe for signs and symptoms of hypokalemia, hyperkalemia, hyponatremia, and hypochloremia, which may result from medication and fluid retention (Table 12-1).

Gastrointestinal. Note patient complaints of nausea, vomiting, or diarrhea. These symptoms are related to congestion of the gastrointestinal tract and typify right-sided heart failure. Abdominal distension or ascites can be evaluated by measuring abdominal girth; be consistent in measurement.

Assess for ascites by having the patient lie down. Place the palm of one hand against the side of the patient's abdomen, and tap the opposite side of the abdomen with the other hand. A wave of fluid shifting across the abdomen indicates ascites.[5]

In RVF, fluid backs up into the hepatic system, causing liver failure. This is associated with a rise in blood urea nitrogen (BUN) and creatinine levels and jaundice. Palpate for an enlarged liver. Normally the liver should not be felt below the ribs after expiration.[5]

Renal. CHF affects all body organs, including the kidneys. A decline in cardiac output is accompanied by a decrease in the glomerular filtration rate. The kidneys respond by conserving fluid, and reduced urine output results. The minimal 24-hr urine output for adults is about 750 ml, or about 30 ml per hour.[5] The urine of CHF patients is often dark amber in color with a high specific gravity (greater than 1.030).[5] Assess for proteinuria and

Table 12-1   Signs and symptoms of primary fluid and electrolyte imbalances associated with congestive heart failure

Imbalance	Signs and symptoms
Electrolyte	
Hypokalemia	Generalized weakness and fatigue, irregular heart rate, hypotension, nausea, vomiting, apathy, coma
Hyperkalemia	Muscle twitching, musculoskeletal weakness, oliguria, nausea, diarrhea, abdominal distension
Hyponatremia	Thirst, decreased skin turgor, anorexia, nausea, vomiting, headaches, restlessness, apprehension
Hypochloremia	Hyperexcitability of nervous system and muscles, shallow breathing, hypotension, tetany
Fluid	
Hypovolemia	Weight loss, hypotension, oliguria, poor skin turgor, skin that is cool and dry, thirst
Hypervolemia	Puffy eyelids, peripheral and dependent edema, ascites, pulmonary edema, wheezes in lungs, sudden weight gain

glucosuria as BUN and creatinine rise with a decreased glomerular filtration rate. Be aware that the patient is at risk for metabolic acidosis or alkalosis with a decline in cardiac output.

Evidence of cardiac decompensation can be identified by a meticulous physical assessment. Any variation from the patient's baseline status should immediately be reported to the physician. Signs and symptoms of pulmonary edema and changes in level of consciousness warrant prompt medical attention. Under such circumstances home care nurses should place the patient in a high Fowler's position, administer oxygen, and stay with the patient, fostering a calm environment, until emergency medical services arrive.

Developing the plan of care

Box 12-3 lists primary nursing diagnoses for patients with CHF. Medical treatment and home care nursing interventions for patients with CHF should be directed toward the following[4,10,18,21]:

- Controlling symptoms
- Stabilization of CHF at home through patient education regarding precipitating factors of cardiac failure: for example, knowledge of medications, diet, activity regimen
- Increasing functional abilities
- Preventing unnecessary hospital readmissions
- Fostering self-care in the home
- Improving quality of life

Box 12-3   PRIMARY NURSING DIAGNOSIS/PATIENT PROBLEMS

- Fatigue
- Decreased cardiac output
- Fluid volume excess
- Knowledge deficit: for example, disease process and risk complications, medications, operation of home medical equipment, procedural care, diet, activity, socioeconomic resources, available community services
- Activity intolerance: __ Ambulation, __ ADLs, __ Other (*Specify*)
- Self-care deficit: __ ADLs, __ Feeding, __ Toileting, __ Other (*Specify*)
- Ineffective individual coping
- Potential for nonparticipation with the therapeutic regimen

Medications.   A variety of medications are prescribed for patients with CHF. Review Box 12-4 for pharmacological guidelines for patients with CHF and Table 12-2, which lists oral medications commonly used to treat CHF in the home.[1,2,15,22] These medications are basically used to reduce afterload and/or preload and to increase contractility in an effort to improve cardiac output and restore fluid balance (Figure 12-1).

Box 12-4   HOME HEALTHCARE NURSE ASSOCIATION CONSENSUS PANEL: OVERVIEW OF THE RECOMMENDED CLINICAL MANAGEMENT FOR HEART FAILURE

- All patients with confirmed reduced left ventricular failure receive angiotensin converting enzyme inhibitors (ACEI) or isosorbide dinitrate–hydralazine combination therapy.
- Angiotension II receptor blockers are initiated as indicated.
- Patients presenting with fluid overload receive diuretic therapy.
- Patients not responding to ACEI and diuretic therapy receive digoxin.
- Patients receiving diuretic therapy are evaluated for hypokalemia and may require potassium supplementation.
- Patients with atrial fibrillation are placed on anticoagulation therapy, unless contraindicated.
- Beta-blockade therapy is initiated as indicated.
- Patients receiving pharmacotherapy for heart failure require laboratory evaluation of CDB, electrolytes, BUN, and creatinine.

Data from Home Healthcare Nurse Association Panel, 1998.

Box 12-5   SIGNS AND SYMPTOMS OF DIGITALIS TOXICITY

Cardiovascular
Bradycardia; tachycardia; irregular pulse; arrhythmias, including atrial fibrillation

Gastrointestinal
Anorexia, nausea, vomiting, diarrhea, abdominal cramping and pain

Neurological
Headache, drowsiness, confusion, insomnia, muscle weakness

Vision
Double vision, blurred vision, colored vision (usually green or yellow), visual halos

When the patient is experiencing fluid overload, **diuretic therapy** remains a traditional treatment for CHF. Diuretics reduce preload, and this reduction is usually accompanied by a decrease in the patient's weight. Side effects of diuretic therapy include hypokalemia, hyponatremia, hypochloremia, and hypovolemia (see Table 12-1). A record of the patient's weight helps assess the effects of the diuretic. Also, measurement of serum electrolytes is important because electrolyte imbalances may predispose patients to an irregular heart rate and sudden cardiac death. Thiazide diuretics are initially used in cases of mild failure. A potassium-sparing diuretic used in combination with a thiazide or loop diuretic is appropriate for patients who are taking digitalis and who are prone to hypokalemia.

Cardiac glycosides such as digoxin enhance cardiac performance by improving contractility. Electrolyte imbalances such as hypercalcemia, hypokalemia, and hypomagnesemia precipitate

digoxin toxicity, as does compromised renal function. Box 12-5 lists the clinical manifestations of digoxin toxicity. Digoxin levels should be periodically monitored in patients with CHF; therapeutic levels range from 0.8 to 2 mg/ml.

Although not common in home care, **beta-adrenergic agonists** such as intravenous dobutamine and dopamine may be administered via cassette to patients with CHF who are receiving home infusion services. Many of these patients are candidates for heart transplants. These medications stimulate beta-adrenoreceptors and improve contractility of the heart. Depending on dose and concentration, dopamine can improve renal blood flow or cause peripheral vasoconstriction and increased myocardial contractility.

Venodilator therapy generally reduces preload. Venodilators such as nitrates increase venous capacity, redirecting blood flow from the pulmonary vasculature into the systemic vessels.

Arterial dilators or vasodilators reduce systemic vascular resistance and afterload, resulting in reduced force against which the heart must pump to circulate blood. Arterial dilators are also frequently used in the treatment of hypertensive or valvular disorders that reduce cardiac output. Angiotensin-converting enzyme (ACE) inhibitors have become the vasodilators of choice in the patient with mild to severe CHF because of their ability to improve cardiac function and reduce blood pressure with minimal or

Table 12-2 Oral medications used to treat CHF in the home

Medication	Dosage range	Adverse effects
Angiotensin-converting enzyme inhibitors		
Benazepril (Lotensin)	20–40 mg qd	Chronic dry cough; hyperkalemia: renal
Captopril (Capoten)*	50–100 mg tid	dysfunction; hypotension; angioedema;
Enalapril (Vasotec)*	5–20 mg bid	neutropenia
Fosinopril (Monopril)*	20–40 mg qd	
Lisinopril (Prinivil, Zestril)*	20–40 mg qd	
Moexepril (Univasc)	15–30 mg qd	
Quinapril (Accupril)*	10–20 mg bid	
Ramipril (Altace)*	2.5–5 mg bid	
Trandolapril (Mavik)*	2–4 mg qd	
Angiotensin II receptor blockers		
Candesartan (Atacand)	16–32 mg qd	Hypotension; hyperkalemia; renal dysfunction
Irbesartan (Avapro)	150–300 mg qd	
Losartan (Cozaar)	25–100 mg qd	
Telmisartan (Micardis)	40–80 mg qd	
Valsartan (Diovan)	80–320 mg qd	
Direct vasolidators		
Hydralazine (Apresoline)	50–100 mg tid	Hypotension; reflex tachycardia; headache; lupus
Beta-blockers		
Bisoprolol (Zebeta)	1.25–10 mg qd	Bradycardia; hypotension; glucose intolerance;
Carvedilol (Coreg)*	3.125–25 mg bid	sexual dysfunction; fluid retention; worsening
Metoprolol (Lopressor, Toprol XL)*	12.5–100 mg qd	symptoms of heart failure
Loop diuretics		
Bumetanide (Bumex)*	1–2 mg qd	Hypocalcemia; hypokalemia; hypomagnesemia;
Ethacrynic acid (Edecrin)*	50–100 mg qd	hyponatremia; volume depletion
Furosemide (Lasix)*	40–80 mg qd	
Torsemide (Demadex)*	10–20 mg qd	
Aldosterone antagonist		
Spironolactone (Aldactone)	12.5–25 mg qd	Hyperkalemia; gynecomastia; drowsiness
Nitrates		
Isosorbide dinitrate (Isordil, Sorbitrate)	10–40 mg tid	Headache; dizziness; postural hypotension
Isosorbide mononitrate (Ismo, Monoket)	10–20 mg bid	
Isosorbide mononitrate (Imdur)	60–120 mg qd	
Pentaerythritol tetranitrate (Peritrate)	10–40 mg tid	
Cardiac glycoside		
Digoxin (Lanoxin)*	0.125–0.25 mg qd	Cardiac arrhythmias; nausea; vomiting; confusion; visual disturbances

*FDA approved for the treatment of CHF.

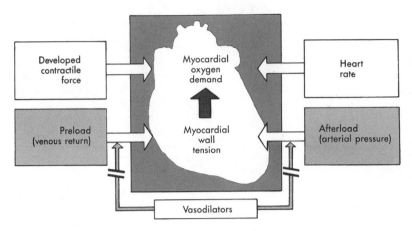

Figure 12-1 Mechanism of vasodilator action in the therapy of chronic congestive heart failure. (From Brody TM and others: *Human pharmacology: molecular to clinical,* ed 3, St. Louis, 1998, Mosby.)

no side effects. As vasodilators, nitrates also play a major role in alleviating anginal chest pain.

A **beta-blocking agent** such as Coreg may be used with ACE inhibitors, digitalis, and diuretics in order to block the negative effects of the sympathetic nervous system on the failing heart. Coreg must be started gradually, increasing the dosage slowly every 2 weeks as tolerated by the patient.

Other medications administered to patients with CHF include potassium supplements, antiarrhythmics to control irregularities of heart rate, and anticoagulants to prevent thrombus formation (due to poor activity levels and incidence of atrial fibrillation). Reglan may be helpful with complaints of nausea.

Supplemental oxygen should be available as required and is usually administered via a nasal cannula. Flows greater than 2 to 3 L/min should be avoided in patients with an additional diagnosis of chronic obstructive pulmonary disease because high flows with these patients may remove the respiratory stimulus to breathe (see Chapter 11).

Diet. Diet is a primary component in the treatment of CHF. Sodium restriction alone may be sufficient to control mild fluid retention. If possible, refer the patient to the registered dietitian for assistance with meal planning and specific dietary instructions. The registered dietitian can provide information about alternative ways to season and cook foods. Patients may wish to use the services of Meals-on-Wheels.

Sodium intake is usually limited to 2 to 4 g of salt daily, depending on the severity of fluid retention. Fluid restrictions are not commonly prescribed for patients with mild to moderate CHF. However, in moderate to severe CHF, fluid restrictions of 1 to 1.5 L of fluid per day are usually implemented. To evaluate diet and response to medication, have patients keep a record of their daily intake and output and a log documenting diet recall (see Appendix XII-I).

Activity. Physical activity should be planned to prevent exhaustion and should be determined by the patient's general condition. Identify those household tasks that cause exhaustion or shortness of breath and devise strategies to reduce cardiac workload.[20] For example, frequent rest periods before and after activities or using oxygen while doing chores may reduce fatigue. As available, make a referral to social services for instruction in progressive relaxation techniques and guided imagery to assist patients in coping with the stress and anxiety associated with illness and subsequent changes in lifestyle.

Patient education

Patient education is a cornerstone of any plan of care (Box 12-6). This is particularly true for patients with CHF because lifestyle and habits strongly influence the stabilization of a weakened heart. In a 1994 study by Hagenhoff, patients with

Box 12-6   PRIMARY THEMES OF PATIENT EDUCATION

- Congestive heart failure: signs and symptoms of disease process to report to the case manager and physician
- When to call 911
- Anginal pain: recognition and treatment
- Medications: purpose, action, dosage, side effects, and methods of administration
- Diet: caloric, fluid, and sodium restriction to prevent fluid overload
- Activity: exercise and rest program
- Home oxygen therapy: operation and maintenance of equipment
- Positive coping mechanisms to use when living with a chronic disease
- Importance of following the medical regimen in order to prevent exacerbation of CHF
- Socioeconomic resources
- Community service available for people with CHF
- General self-care strategies

CHF ranked medication as the most important category of information to learn, followed by anatomy/physiology and then risk factors for exacerbation of CHF.[12]

The disease process and pathophysiology of CHF should be explained in such a way that patients understand the importance of taking prescribed medication and following dietary restrictions to prevent fluid retention. For example, patients should be able to name foods high in salt and should eliminate items such as potato chips, canned meats, and beer from their diet. Instruct patients to determine sodium content by reading food labels.

Avoidance of dusty and humid environments will make breathing easier for patients with CHF. Because smoking increases the demands on the heart, patients should be encouraged to stop. Using extra pillows or a foam wedge (available from the HME vendor) under the head at night can ease breathing and promote rest. If patients should suddenly become short of breath, instruct them to use their oxygen and sit up with their legs and arms in a dependent position to decrease preload and increase oxygenation.

Instruct patients to weigh themselves at the same time each day using the same scale. They should notify the physician's office if more than 2 pounds are gained in 1 day. Patients who are recording intake and output can measure their fluids in standard household measuring cups. Calibrated plastic liners that fit inside the toilet to collect and measure urine can be purchased at most medical supply centers.

When evaluating patients, home care nurses may see signs of noncompliance or confusion with medication. When this occurs the purpose, action, and side effects of *all* medications should be reviewed with the patient. Using charts, coordinating medications with meals, using medication boxes or placing the week's supply of medications in separate envelopes marked for each day and stored in a shoebox for convenience may help remind patients to take their medications. As appropriate, patients should be provided instructions for home oxygen therapy (see Chapter 11). Patients should understand why it is important to take a potassium supplement if they are taking Lasix and should know the signs and symptoms of hypokalemia. They should be instructed to use their nitroglycerin tablets at the onset of anginal pain. Patients taking digoxin should be shown how to take their own pulse. If their pulse is lower than 60 beats/min or higher than 110 beats/min, patients should consult with their physician before taking their digoxin.

If taking warfarin (Coumadin) or anticoagulant therapy, patients should be instructed to avoid over-the-counter medications high in vitamin K. They should be instructed on basic bleeding precautions (i.e., avoidance of using razor or sharp object that may cause bleeding) and to immediately report signs of inappropriate bleeding (e.g., nosebleeds, red or black stools, unusual vaginal bleeding, spontaneous bruising) to the physician.

Home care nurses can use patient education to heighten patient awareness and assist with the stabilization of patients' cardiac status by reviewing conditions or situations that place extra workload on the heart, such as obesity, anemia, infection, or stress. Strategies related to these conditions should be incorporated into the plan of care. For example, instruct patients to avoid or limit physical activities that are excessively fatiguing. Patients with CHF should be aware of signs and symptoms of progressing failure such as clothes or belts suddenly

---

Box 12-7   INTERNET RESOURCES FOR CARDIAC INFORMATION

- The Agency for Healthcare Research and Quality (AHRQ) has published guidelines for the treatment of CHF and other cardiac disorders: http://www.ahrq.gov/clinic
- The American Heart Association publishes recent research and educational materials on heart disease: http://www.americanheart.org
- The Heart Failure Society of American (HFSA) provides information regarding the managment of heart failure and related pharmaceutical hotlinks: http://www.hfsa.org/

---

becoming tight, increases in weight or fatigue, chest pain, unusual congestion of the lungs, and increased frequency of shortness of breath or coughing. They should also receive instruction regarding when to seek immediate medical attention. In addition, information and health care resources on the Internet are also available for patients with CHF (Box 12-7).

SUMMARY

The treatment of CHF is aimed at reducing cardiac workload and fluid retention, improving oxygenation, and decreasing patient anxiety associated with changes in lifestyle. To live at home with CHF and prevent rehospitalizations, patients are encouraged to learn to manage their disease and to cope with necessary changes of habits in a positive manner. These adjustments may be particularly difficult for patients with CHF because periods of illness are interspersed with frequent periods of wellness. As patients begin to feel better, the temptation to return to old habits is great and may precipitate fluid retention. Home care nurses can provide patients with scientific explanations of the disease process, as well as psychological support to foster a sense of responsibility for self-care and positive coping mechanisms. This is important, because it is recognized that no plan of care or medicine can take the place of concern for one's own health.

REFERENCES

1. Agency for Health Care Policy and Research: *Heart failure: evaluation and care of patients with left-ventricular systolic dysfunction.* Clinical practice guideline No 11, Washington, DC; 1994, Agency For Health Care Policy and Research.
2. Agency for Healthcare Policy and Research: *Management of chronic heart failure,* Clinical practice guideline, No 12, Washington, DC; 1996, Agency for Health Care Policy and Research.
3. American Heart Association website: http://www.american heart.org, March 15, 2000.
4. Anderson MA and others: Home care utilization by congestive heart failure patients: a pilot study, *Public Health Nurs* 15(2):146, 1998.
5. Bates B: *A guide to physical examination and history taking,* ed 7, Philadelphia, 1999, JB Lippincott.
6. Borsody JM and others: Using self-efficacy to increase physical activity in patients with heart failure, *Home Healthc Nurse* 17(2): 113, 1998.
7. Cohn JN: Prevention of heart failure, *Cardiology* 92(Suppl 1):22, 1999.
8. Dantone JJ: Medical nutritional therapy—congestive heart failure. In Rice R, editor: *Manual of Home Health Nursing Procedures,* ed 2, St. Louis; 2000, Mosby.
9. Fisher ML and others: Therapeutic options in advanced heart failure, *Hosp Pract* 32:97, 1997.
10. Foote M: Innovations in the management of heart failure in the home health care environment, *Home Health Care Manage Prac* 9(4):35, 1997.
11. Friedman EH: Respiratory patterns and chronic heart failure, *Circulation* 98(4):377, 1998.
12. Hagenhoff B and others: Patient education needs as reported by congestive heart failure patients and their nurses, *J Adv Nurs* 19:685, 1994.
13. Helberg J: Patients' status at home discharge, *Image J Nurs Sch* 23(2):93, 1993.
14. Helberg J: Use of home care nursing resources by the elderly, *Public Health Nurs* 11(2):104, 1999.
15. Home Healthcare Nurse Association Practice Group: Summary of the nursing practice guidelines for the cardiac home care patient, *Home Healthc Nurse* 16(11):743, 1998.
16. Jackson G and others: ABC of heart failure-pathophysiology, *BMJ* 320(7228):167, 2000.
17. Johnstone D and others: Diagnosis and management of heart failure, *Can J Cardiol* 10(6):613, 1994.
18. Knox D: Implementing a congestive heart failure disease management program to decrease length of stay and cost, *J Cardiovasc Nurs* 14(1):55, 1999.
19. Laing G, Behrendt D: A disease management program for home health care patients with congestive heart failure, *Home Health Care Manage Prac* 10(2):27, 1998.
20. Lazarre M, Ax S: Patients, chronic heart failure, and home care, *Caring,* 20, June 1997.
21. McCormick S: Advanced practice nursing for congestive heart failure, *Crit Care Nurs Q* 21(4):1, 2000.
22. Medical Economics Co: *Physicians' desk reference,* Oradell, NJ, 1999, Medical Economics.
23. Mehra MR and others: The unique management of refractory advanced systolic heart failure, *Heart Lung* 26(4): 280, 1999.
24. Rodeheffer RJ and others: The incidence and prevalence of congestive heart failure in Rochester, Minnesota, *Mayo Clin Proc* 68:1143, 1993.
25. Yamani M, Massie BM: Congestive heart failure: insights from epidemiology, implications for treatment, *Mayo Clin Proc* 68:1, 1993.

Medical Nutrition Therapy: Congestive Heart Failure

PURPOSE

- To provide education to the patient/caregiver about the prevention and treatment of congestive heart failure (CHF)
- To stabilize and improve the patient's body weight
- To stabilize and improve the patient's cardiac output through manipulation of sodium and fluid intake
- To promote self-care in the home

GENERAL INFORMATION

CHF occurs when the heart cannot circulate blood to the body tissues in a sufficient manner. This mechanical inadequacy can result in the following signs and symptoms:

- Congestion from edema, especially in the lungs, liver, legs, and bowel
- Shortness of breath
- Fatigue and poor tolerance to exercise
- Rapid pulse rate
- Abdominal fullness with discomfort and loss of appetite
- Mental confusion

Severe weight loss and malnutrition are documented with advanced CHF and are possibly a result of the following:

- Increased metabolism
- Nausea, vomiting, and/or anorexia resulting from digitalis toxicity or congestive enlargement of the liver and abdominal fullness
- Intestinal malabsorption related to venous congestion and edema of the bowel
- Protein-losing intestinal disease

From Dantone JJ: Nutritional care in the home. In Rice R: *Manual of Home Health Nursing Procedures,* ed 2, St. Louis, 2000, Mosby.

EQUIPMENT

1. Scales
2. Cloth measuring tape
3. Calculator
4. Food models or packages with food labels of sodium content
5. Measuring cup and pint-size and quart-size containers or examples of common containers of the same sizes
6. Blood pressure cuff, stethoscope, and thermometer

PROCEDURE

1. Explain the procedure to the patient/caregiver.
2. Consider implementing the following:
   a. Assessing vital signs and evaluating for edema each visit; pay close attention to abnormal changes in blood pressure or adventitious lung sounds; report findings to the physician as necessary
   b. Setting nutritional requirements for the patient; see Nursing Consideration on p. 213 and Box XII-I and Table XII-I; see also Appendix V-I.
   c. Obtaining a measurement of the serum albumin or prealbumin level; it is recommended this be done every 3 months to assess for protein-energy malnutrition; obtain physician's orders for laboratory evaluation
   d. Obtaining a measurement of the serum sodium level, which is necessary to determine the need for a fluid restriction; obtain physician's orders for laboratory evaluation
   e. Calculating the fluid requirement for the patient; patients with CHF normally need approximately 25 ml of fluid per kilogram of actual body weight; fluids may be re-

211

Box XII-I   LOW-SALT DIET (2 G SODIUM)

Reason for the Diet

To lower blood pressure levels and help you lose fluid that may cause complications with blood pressure problems. To decrease ascites (fluid buildup in the body cavity), which may occur if you have heart, kidney, or liver problems. Normal blood pressure in persons younger than 65 years is 120/80 mm Hg. In persons 65 years or older, blood pressure is considered high if it is greater than 160/95 mm Hg.

How Much and/or What to Eat

Breakfast	Lunch and dinner (same)
Fruit or juice	Low-salt meat
Low-salt cereal	Low-salt starch
Egg with little salt	Low-salt vegetable
Toast or biscuit	Low-salt salad with low-salt dressing
Margarine	Bread
Jelly	Margarine
Milk	Dessert
Coffee	Coffee or tea
	Milk (at dinner only)

Do Not Eat These Foods

- **Seasonings:** raw salt, garlic salt, onion salt, celery salt, seasoned salt, soy sauce, Worcestershire sauce, barbecue sauce
- **Beverages:** buttermilk, instant cocoa mix
- **Meats:** canned, cured, processed, or smoked meats, such as ham, bacon, sausage, salt pork, fat back, luncheon meat, bologna, Vienna sausage, potted meat

- **Snacks:** regular crackers, chips, Nabs, pretzels, salted nuts, dips, olives, pickles, regular canned soups, popcorn, sauerkraut
- **Fats:** bacon drippings, fat back, regular salad dressings

You May Eat These Foods

- **Seasonings:** garlic powder, onion powder, herbs, spices, salt substitute (if approved by physician); it is better for you to use herbs and spices to season foods than salt substitute
- **Beverages:** whole, low-fat, or skim milk (up to 2 cups a day)
- **Meats:** fresh pork chops, pork roast, beef, chicken, turkey, fish, lamb, or veal
- **Snacks:** low-salt crackers, crackers with unsalted tops, unsalted popcorn, unsalted nuts, homemade soups with no salt added, any fresh fruits and vegetables, canned fruits and vegetables with no added salt
- **Fats:** margarine, mayonnaise, low-salt salad dressings

Special Instructions

If you wish to use a salt substitute make sure it is approved by your physician first. Use fresh or frozen vegetables and meats instead of canned or cured ones. Use seasoning powders instead of seasoning salts, such as garlic powder instead of garlic salt. Read labels on foods carefully—watch for words such as sodium or salt in the ingredients list.

Modified from Dantone JJ: *Bridging the gap diet manual,* Grenada, Miss, 1997, Nutrition Education Resources.

stricted if hyponatremia occurs; in cases of mild CHF, 1500 to 2000 ml of fluid is recommended, in severe cases of CHF, a restriction of 1000 ml or less is common; demonstrate to the patient/caregiver the correct volume of fluid recommended for the patient to consume daily by using a measuring container familiar to the patient

f. Recording a 24-hour recall of the patient's nutritional intake on the food diary form; analyze the calories, sodium, and fluid content of the diet intake

g. Instructing the patient/caregiver on the low-salt diet instruction sheet and menu (Box XII-I and Table XII-I); use food labels to demonstrate sodium content in various foods (just 1 teaspoon of common table salt contains about 2 g of sodium); use measuring cups familiar to the patient to demonstrate proper fluid amounts to consume

h. Comparing the patient's 24-hour diet recall to his or her prescribed diet order as instructed; make appropriate recommendations to the patient/caregiver for modifying any nutrients found to be inappropriate on the food intake record

Table XII-I   Menu for low-salt diet (2 g sodium)

	Sunday	Monday	Tuesday
Breakfast	Juice of choice **1s** cereal **1s** Eggs of choice **1s** Turkey sausage Biscuit or toast Margarine Jelly Milk Coffee	Juice of choice **1s** Cereal **1s** Eggs of choice Biscuits or toast Margarine Jelly Milk Coffee	Juice of choice **1s** Cereal **1s** Eggs of choice **1s** Turkey sausage Biscuits or toast Margarine Jelly Milk Coffee
Lunch	**1s** Fried chicken **1s** Dried beans or peas **1s** Greens Buttered cornbread Banana Tea	Sandwich with: **1s** Hamburger/**1s** cheese Bun Lettuce/tomato/onion Mayonnaise **1s** Mustard **1s** Oven fries Apple cobbler Tea	**1s** Roast turkey **1s** Giblet gravy **1s** Cornbread dressing **1s** English peas Buttered roll Cranberry sauce Angel food cake Tea
Dinner	**1s** Pork steak **1s** Potato salad **1s** Green beans Buttered roll Pineapple tidbits Milk	**1s** Beef tips **1s** Gravy **1s** Rice **1s** Buttered broccoli Buttered biscuit Stewed prunes Milk	**1s** Potato stew **1s** Tuna salad sandwich Sliced tomatoes **1s** Crackers Mayonnaise Fresh orange Milk

ls = One serving.
From Dantone JJ: *Bridging the gap diet manual,* Grenada, Miss, 1997, Nutrition Education Resources.

3. Clean and replace equipment. Discard disposable items according to standard precautions.

NURSING CONSIDERATIONS

If the patient is taking a potassium-depleting diuretic, a potassium supplement may be necessary. If the patient is taking a potassium-sparing diuretic and an angiotensin-converting enzyme (ACE) inhibitor, the patient should be cautioned about the use of salt substitutes and light salts. Salt substitutes generally contain 2500 to 2800 mg of potassium per teaspoon. Light salt contains 1100 mg of sodium and 1500 mg of potassium per teaspoon. If salt substitutes and/or light salts are used, an increased potassium blood level may result. Make the physician aware of any salt substitute product that the patient is using. Furosemide therapy greater than 80 mg per day for more than 3 months can result in a thiamin deficiency, which causes high-output cardiac failure and impaired cardiac performance.

Studies indicate that thiamin supplementation of 200 mg per day orally for 6 weeks improves left ventricular function, diuresis, and sodium excretion in patients with CHF.

Dysrhythmias and/or increased heart rates can be caused by use of caffeine-containing beverages or medications.

Energy requirements for patients with CHF can be 30% to 50% higher than for healthy individuals because of increased metabolic rates from cardiac and pulmonary expenditures.

The following nutrition intervention guidelines should be monitored by the nurse:

*   Ensure that the patient's intake of calories and protein is adequate

- Restrict sodium to 3 g daily in cases of mild CHF; if large doses of diuretics are required (greater than 80 mg of furosemide daily), restrict sodium to 2 g daily
- Limit excessive fluid intake; restrict fluids in patients with hyponatremia
- Limit alcohol intake to no more than 1 drink per day of 30 ml of liquor or the equivalent of beer or wine
- Encourage smoking cessation
- Encourage exercise as tolerated by the patient and allowed by the physician
- Recommend thiamin supplementation for patients taking large doses of diuretics
- Weigh the patient on each visit; report to the physician a weight gain of 2 pounds in 1 day or 5 pounds between visits
- Obtain vital signs
- Observe the patient for increased difficulty in breathing or shortness of breath

DOCUMENTATION GUIDELINES

Document the following on the visit report:

- The procedure and patient toleration
- Vital sign measurements

- Weight—a 3- to 5-pound weight gain may suggest fluid retention sufficient to cause heart failure; report any weight change to the physician
- Appetite—analyze the intake of calories, sodium, and fluid
- Laboratory data (serum sodium and albumin levels are of special significance)
- Observance of any changes in breathing (e.g., shortness of breath)
- Tolerance of activities such as limited exercise; level of fatigue
- Any patient/caregiver instructions and response to teaching, including answers to feedback questions
- Physician notification, if applicable
- Standard Precautions
- Other pertinent findings

Update the plan of care.

THE VENTILATOR-DEPENDENT PATIENT

Robyn Rice

Clinical applications of advances in medical technology continue to have favorable influences on home care. Patients with debilitating respiratory disease and/or respiratory insufficiency who were previously maintained in intensive care units or chronic care facilities are now being discharged on home mechanical ventilation. Initially used as a lifesaving procedure, mechanical ventilation has evolved into either a life-support or augmenting procedure for patients unable to be "weaned," or taken off the ventilator[27]; hence the term *ventilator-dependent patient* (VDP). Once stabilized on ventilatory support, these patients will continue to require varying degrees of caregiver assistance with their health care needs.

Ensuring safe and competent care for these technology-dependent patients at home presents many challenges for the home care agency. With the assistance of home care nurses and the multidisciplinary team, VDPs and their families can return home and begin to rebuild their lives and renew relationships. Reasons for home treatment and the philosophies of home mechanical ventilation are well documented in the literature.[16,29]

One argument for home mechanical ventilation is that it improves the quality and length of life. Patients who return to their homes can benefit from nurturing environments that relieve the psychological and physiological stressors of hospitalization.[6] Independence and socialization are promoted as patients resume interactions with family and friends in the community and frequently in the workplace or school setting. In additional, cognitive and psychosocial development advances when ventilator-dependent children leave the restrictive hospital environment and experience the richness of the world around them.[2]

As mental health is optimized, improvements in physical health often follow.[20] The home affords ventilator-dependent patients a sense of privacy and allows them to resume normal sleeping and eating patterns. Physiological well-being is further enhanced as these patients are removed from potential sources of nosocomial, or hospital-acquired, infections that can be fatal. In addition, studies of the VDP family caregivers demonstrate that they do not perceive home placement to be a negative experience, and most are unwilling to consider other placement alternatives for their family member.[8,19,25,28]

Cost-effectiveness of home ventilator care is less clear. Many studies have documented that for the VDP home care is less expensive than care in other settings[16,22,27] Sivak and others surveyed costs of home care for 10 ventilator-dependent patients for a 38-month period and estimated the savings from the use of home care (as opposed to hospitalization) at $2.8 million.[27] Today monthly home care costs for direct care of VDPs may vary from $6411 to $38,607, whereas acute care costs can exceed $40,000 per month.[20,24] However, research suggests that many home cost analysis of the VDP do not account for indirect costs of care, which include costs associated with home remodeling, increased utility (i.e., electric, gas, and water) bills, lost caregiver income from work, transportation, and the value of the caregiver's time.[24,31] Hence when proposing home care of the VDP health care providers should make families aware of the financial impact of caring for the VDP at home. In addition, documented disadvantages of home mechanical ventilation include family stress related to long-term patient physical care needs, special transportation needs, lack of equipment support, and costs not covered by third-party payers, including supplies and utility bills.[7,10,20]

Therefore advantages must be carefully weighed against disadvantages when considering home mechanical ventilation. These patients typically require a great deal of emotional and physical support in order to successfully make the transition from the hospital to the home. Before patients are allowed to go home on mechanical ventilation, safety factors (including a home environmental assessment) must also be considered. Most important, to qualify for home discharge, ventilator-dependent patients must be physiologically stable. In addition, their caregivers must be *willing* and *able* to accept the sometimes awesome responsibility of self-care management for these technology-dependent patient at home.[16,20,30]

With these stipulations in mind, the home care nurse should give attention to the following:

- Reinforcing self-care management with patient/caregiver education; identifying patient/caregiver needs as a part of discharge planning and continued service
- Patient assessment and procedural skills
- Socioenvironmental assessment to ensure cost-effective and safe patient care
- Assessment of the ventilator and the availability and functioning of related supplies and equipment to maintain the patient's well-being
- Caregiver and/or family appraisal and support

The following sections of this chapter focus on the clinical management of VDPs in the home setting.

PATHOPHYSIOLOGY

The concepts underlying mechanical ventilation relate to respiration and the mechanics of breathing. The lungs assist cellular metabolism by providing body tissues with oxygen while removing carbon dioxide. The respiratory centers in the brain (pons and medulla) control involuntary respiratory function, and the cerebral hemispheres are responsible for voluntary respiration. Breathing is primarily an automatic process regulated by arterial blood levels of oxygen and carbon dioxide, ex-

---

Box 13-1   NORMAL ARTERIAL BLOOD GAS VALUES

- pH 7.35–7.45 (expression of hydrogen ion concentration, measures acidity of the blood)
- $Paco_2$ 35–45 mm Hg (partial pressure of carbon dioxide)
- Pao_2 60–100 mm Hg (partial pressure of oxygen)
- HCO_3 22–26 mEq/L (amount of bicarbonate dissolved in the blood)
- Sao_2 95% to 100% (oxygen saturation; if Pao_2 is between 60 and 95 mm Hg, Sao_2 should be greater than 90% with a normal pH, temperature, etc.)

---

pressed as the partial pressure of arterial oxygen (Pao_2) and the partial pressure of arterial carbon dioxide ($Paco_2$) (Box 13-1).

Rhythmic patterns of breathing vary according to tissue oxygen needs and metabolic demands of the body. For example, breathing is slower during sleep and relaxed states and is faster with activity or any condition that increases metabolism. Concurrently certain pulmonary, neurological, disease, or drug-induced states may inappropriately speed or slow respiration.

The process of breathing involves two phases: (1) ventilation, which consists of inspiration-expiration (the movement of air between the environment and alveoli), and (2) respiration, the gaseous exchange of oxygen (O_2) and carbon dioxide (CO_2) between alveoli and blood circulating through the lungs and other body tissue.[13] The actual mechanics of ventilation occur because of pressure differences between the lungs (intrathoracic pressure) and the external environment (atmospheric pressure). Contraction of the respiratory muscles and descent of the diaphragm, associated with inhalation, decrease intrathoracic pressure in relation to atmospheric pressure. This causes air to flow from the environment (high pressure) into the lungs (low pressure). At the end of inspiration, as respiratory muscles relax with exhalation, the diaphragm rises to its resting position, increasing intrathoracic pressure in relation to atmospheric pressure. This causes air to flow passively from the lungs into the environment.

Bronchitis or emphysema, bronchopulmonary dysplasia, cystic fibrosis or kyphoscoliosis (structural defects), poliomyelitis, muscular dystrophy, obstructive sleep apnea, central apnea, and trauma (neuromuscular origins) are conditions known to predispose certain patients to respiratory failure or insufficiency.[7] Whatever the cause, patients require ventilatory support when respiration is insufficient to meet the demands of metabolism.

Specific equipment used to assist respiration depends on individual patient needs to balance ventilatory effort (the need for tissue oxygenation) with metabolic demands (the need to eliminate carbon dioxide as a by-product of metabolism) and to conserve respiratory muscles by preventing the fatigue of breathing. Therefore equipment for ventilatory support may be used continuously or intermittently (e.g., during the day or night).

PRINCIPAL EQUIPMENT USED FOR HOME RESPIRATORY SUPPORT

Devices used to assist respiration and ventilatory effort in the home may be classified as positive pressure ventilators for invasive or noninvasive support or as negative pressure ventilators for non-invasive support and are frequently accompanied by a variety of supplies needed to sustain home mechanical ventilation.

Ventilator-dependent patients are often advised to rent equipment because care and maintenance is then provided by the HME vendor. Most HME vendors rent out ventilators for a monthly fee. As a part of the equipment rental package, HME vendors typically provide 24-hour service for equipment malfunction, deliver medical supplies such as tracheostomy tubes and suctioning equipment, and provide educational resources. Medicare now pays 80% of the rental cost for most home mechanical ventilation equipment if the need is well documented and is supported by a physician's order.[11] Medicare also reimburses for home care nurse visits if the need for a skilled service (e.g., monthly tracheostomy tube changes) is documented and the service is ordered by a physician.[11] When considering equipment issues, clarify cost and medical insurance reimbursement issues with the patient/caregiver.

Positive pressure ventilators

With positive pressure mechanical ventilation, air is forced into the lungs by application of positive pressure to the airway. In other words, positive pressure ventilation is accomplished by pushing air

into the chest. At the end of inspiration, positive pressure to the airway is removed and the diaphragm passively ascends, allowing for exhalation. The exception is application of positive end-expiratory pressure (PEEP) with positive pressure ventilation. PEEP maintains positive pressure at the end of exhalation to keep alveoli open and improve oxygenation and ventilatory function. PEEP is becoming more commonly prescribed for use in the home setting. However, PEEP usually requires more complex monitoring and equipment because it may be associated with an increased incidence of hypotension and trauma to the lungs.[16]

Mechanical ventilators are classified according to how the inspiratory phase ends: (1) volume-cycled—a preset volume ends inspiration, (2) pressure-cycled—a preset pressure attainment ends inspiration, (3) flow-cycled—the decrease in patient inspiratory flow requirement ends inspiration, and (4) time-cycled—a preset time interval ends inspiration.

Piston-driven volume-cycled ventilators are commonly used in home care today because they easily compensate for changes in lung compliance and resistance. Many of the current models are microprocessor controlled, which augments the device's precision in delivering consistent breathing patterns. Easy to use and lightweight, these ventilators are readily transported under wheelchairs and require a minimum level of preventive maintenance to ensure long-term, safe operation. Examples of volume-cycled positive pressure ventilators seen in home care today include the LP6PLUS, LP10, and Achieve series, which now have modems for office checks (Mallinckrodt Medical, Inc); the PLV100 and 102 (Respironics); the LTV900, 950, and 1000 (Pulmonetics); and the Bird Legacy02. Although these ventilators differ in size and design, many have basic features that are quite similar (see Appendix XIII-I).

Invasive support. Frequently, positive pressure ventilators in the home setting are used with patients who cannot maintain ventilation for any length of time and who often require continuous mechanical ventilation.[16] Under these circumstances a backup respiratory support system must be placed in the home in the form of a self-inflating manual ventilator (Ambu-bag) and a second ventilator to ensure patient safety and adequate ventilation.

Noninvasive support. Patients whose conditions or disease do not require continous support can frequently be ventilated via a mouthpiece, oral/nasal mask, nasal mask adaptor or pneumobelt in place of a tracheostomy tube. This noninvasive delivery by the volume ventilator meets the needs of patients who typically have neuromuscular dysfunction or early-stage respiratory insufficiency type of diseases who cannot maintain a normal Po_2 or Pco_2 with only spontaneous respirations. Augmenting their spontaneous breathing (respite ventilation), which generally occurs at night, allows the patient daytime freedom.

Negative pressure noninvasive support. Another form of noninvasive ventilatory support in the home may be accomplished with negative pressure ventilators, or rocking beds, or by use of continuous positive airway pressure (CPAP), or by use of a bilevel pressure device (BiPAP). This equip-

ment also does not require a tracheostomy and is typically used with patients who have neuromuscular dysfunction and require ventilatory support at night or periodically during the day. Home care nurses should consult the respiratory therapist from the patient's HME vendor with any questions or concerns regarding the operation and use of this equipment.

Oxygen therapy

Supplemental oxygen may not be necessary for VDPs who require assistance with breathing but do not need additional oxygen to maintain an appropriate Pao_2. As a general guideline, supplemental oxygen should be added to the ventilator circuit to maintain a Pao_2 at or above 60 mm Hg.[21] Oxygen concentrators are frequently used as the primary source of supplemental oxygen for ventilator-dependent patients. An oxygen cylinder and regula-

---

Box 13-2   PRINCIPAL EQUIPMENT AND SUPPLIES USED FOR HOME MECHANICAL VENTILATION

A. Primary ventilator
1.   Ventilator circuits
2.   Ventilator filters
3.   Heated humidifier or cascade
    a.   Sterile or distilled water (optional), or tap water boiled for 15 minutes
    b.   Condensation drainage bags
    c.   Heat and moisture exchangers (optional)
4.   External 12-volt battery with power cord
5.   Volume bag (optional)
6.   Disinfectant
B. Secondary ventilator
1.   Identical backup ventilator (optional)
2.   Ambu-bag (manual resuscitator)
C. Oxygen and related supplies
1.   Oxygen source (optional): oxygen concentrator with backup compressed gas cylinder (tank)
2.   Oxygen connecting tubing: pressure-compensated flowmeters are recommended with the use of 50 feet of connecting tubing
3.   Air compressor and aerosol tubing for nebulizer treatments (optional)
D. Tracheostomy equipment and related supplies
1.   Extra tracheostomy tube(s)—keep a tube one size smaller in home

2.   Dressings (absorbent and lint-free)
3.   Extra tracheostomy tube ties, Velcro collar, or twill tape
4.   Water-soluble lubricant
5.   Syringes
6.   Sterile and nonsterile gloves
7.   Cotton swabs
8.   Stoma ointment (as prescribed by physician)
9.   Sterile unit-dose and bottled normal saline (optional)—may use tap water to rinse suction catheter *after* suctioning is completed
10. Hydrogen peroxide
11. Suction machine
    a.   Extra collection bottles
    b.   Suction catheters (Yankauer catheter—optional)
    c.   Extension tubing
E. Durable medical equipment
1.   Hospital bed (optional)
2.   Patient communication aid
3.   As needed, equipment to assist with patient bowel/bladder management and personal care
4.   Wheelchair/walker/cane

tor are usual backup reserves and improve patient mobility when traveling. Liquid oxygen systems are an alternative for those patients who consume high liter flows of oxygen and are also ambulatory (e.g., students with bronchopulmonary dysplasia). (Review Chapter 11 for further information on home oxygen therapy.)

Adjunct equipment

Additional ancillary equipment and supplies used for home mechanical ventilation are listed in Box 13-2.

Their use varies with patient needs. The HME vendor will deliver requested supplies on a monthly basis or as needed. Be aware that telehealth trends in home ventilator management include incorporating modems into the ventilator that enable personnel to use computers to check on equipment functioning from the office or nurse's car.

Tracheostomy tubes. Tracheostomy tubes are artificial airways made of silver, stainless steel, and plastic or other synthetic materials (Figure 13-1). Costs for tracheostomy tubes range from approximately $18 to $100. Many are reusable. Oxygen, communication needs, and comfort level are critical determinants when selecting a tracheostomy tube to meet specific patient requirements.

Tracheostomy tubes may be cuffed or uncuffed. A cuffless tracheostomy tube or fenestrated tracheostomy tube (which has an opening in the outer cannula above the cuff) allows the patient to talk as air moves upward and over the vocal cords. Patients who require continuous ventilation, for whom aspiration may be a problem, generally benefit from the Bivona FOME-CUF tracheostomy tube or one of the high-volume, low-pressure cuffed tracheostomy tubes made by Shiley/Portex. The cuffs on these types of tracheostomy tubes prevent occlusion of tracheal capillary blood flow, which can cause tissue necrosis. Pediatric tracheostomy tubes are usually uncuffed.

A tracheostomy tube is basically composed of three parts: the outer cannula, the inner cannula, and the obturator. The outer cannula is the main part of the tracheostomy tube and essentially holds the stoma open while the tube is fitted into the tracheostomy and downward into the trachea. The outer cannula is held in place with tracheostomy ties or a Velcro collar (Figure 13-2). Tracheostomy ties are recommended to secure the tracheostomy tube in pediatric or highly mobile patients because

Velcro ties can pop open. Tracheostomy ties should be secured by a double knot at the side of the neck with room for only one finger to slip between the ties and the patient's neck. Change tracheostomy ties daily to prevent irritation to the neck and to maintain good hygiene of the patient.

The inner cannula fits inside the outer cannula and locks into place. The inner cannula is easily removed from the outer cannula. To prevent buildup of secretions, the inner cannula should be removed and cleaned at least daily. Be aware that not all tracheostomy tubes have inner cannulas.

The obturator is a stylet with a smooth, rounded end that fits inside the outer cannula and is used to insert the outer cannula. The tip of the obturator extends beyond the end of the outer cannula and is designed to protect the tracheostomy and trachea from damage during insertion of the outer cannula. The obturator completely occludes the airway when in place. Therefore it is *essential* to remove the obturator as soon as the outer cannula is inserted.

Communication devices. There are numerous communication devices currently available. These include reusable tracheostomy speaking valves that direct exhaled air upward over the vocal cords, an electronic larynx held by hand against the outside of the neck, electronic resonators that are activated by a small tube placed in the mouth and do not require functional upper extremities, typewriters, keyboards, computer terminals, and simple pen and paper.[26] All of these devices encourage ventilator-dependent patients to communicate their needs and feelings. More specialized equipment may be either rented or purchased from the HME vendor.

HOME DISCHARGE PLANNING

Predischarge planning should begin at least 2 weeks before discharge. The HME vendor and professional staff from the hospital usually provide initial patient and caregiver instruction sessions regarding ventilator management and related care to ensure a safe transition from hospital to home.

The home care nurse, home care aide, clinical nurse specialist, respiratory therapist or designated home care coordinator, and physician (the multidisciplinary team) should attend as many of these patient instruction sessions as possible. Doing so enables them to later reinforce previous instruction and also helps to identify any potential problem areas or special patient/caregiver concerns that should be addressed before discharge. It

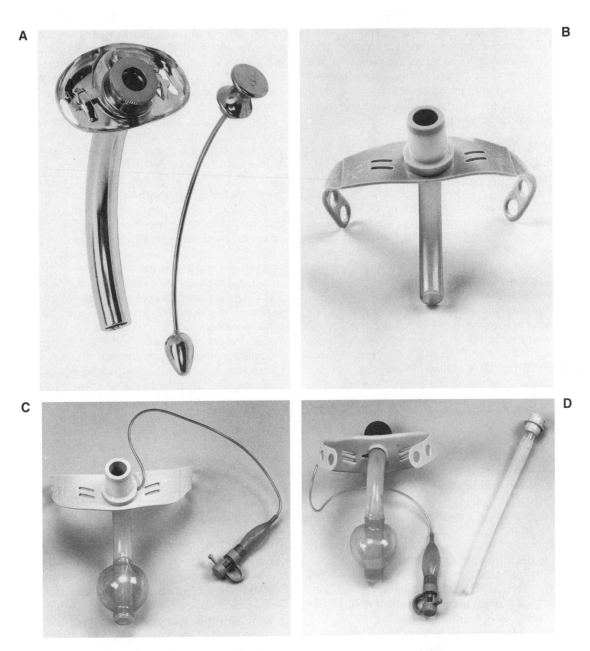

Figure 13-1 A, Silver tracheostomy tube and obturator. **B,** Cuffless tracheostomy tube. **C,** Cuffed tracheostomy tube: anterior view. **D,** Cuffed tracheostomy tube: posterior view and inner cannula. **E,** Cuffed fenestrated tracheostomy tube, inner cannula, and obturator. **F,** Neonatal and pediatric tracheostomy tubes and obturators. **G,** FOME-CUF tracheostomy tube. **H,** DPRV tracheostomy tube, inner cannula, and obturators. (**A,** Photo courtesy Pilling Company, Fort Washington, Pa; **B–D,** photo courtesy Concord/Portex, Inc, Keene, NH; **E, F, H,** photos courtesy Pfizer/Shiley, Inc, Irvine, Calif; **G,** photo courtesy Bivona, Inc, Gary, Ind.)

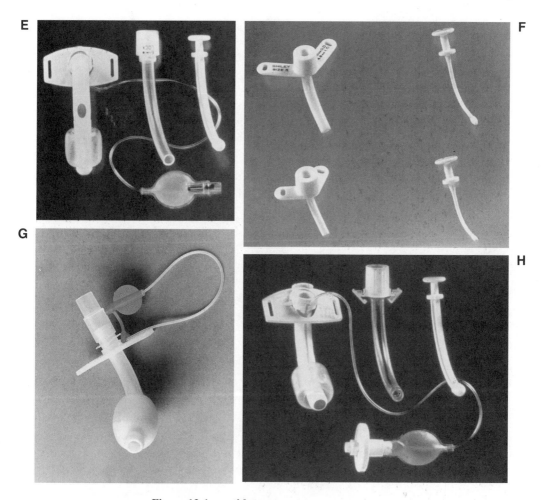

Figure 13-1, cont'd For legend see opposite page.

also provides home care personnel with realistic goals in developing the plan of care for these patients. For example, prior to discharge the home care nurse should establish who will be responsible for changing the outer cannula of the patient's tracheostomy tube and frequency of changes. Any concerns with this procedure should be brought up at this time.

An environmental evaluation of household structural needs and considerations, before patient discharge, further ensures a safe and practical return to the home. For example, patients' rooms should have appropriate electrical outlets for the ventilator and related equipment and afford easy access to the bathroom and kitchen. Widened doors, walkways, and ramps may need to be installed if the patient uses a wheelchair. The bathroom may need to be modified or have special equipment installed for patient use and convenience. A working telephone, running water, and adequate heating and air-conditioning are other household features that support discharging ventilator-dependent patients to their homes. The local electric company should be notified of the patient's electrically powered life-support equipment. These patients are usually placed on a priority list for service. These patients would certainly be priority cliente in the home care agency's disaster plan.

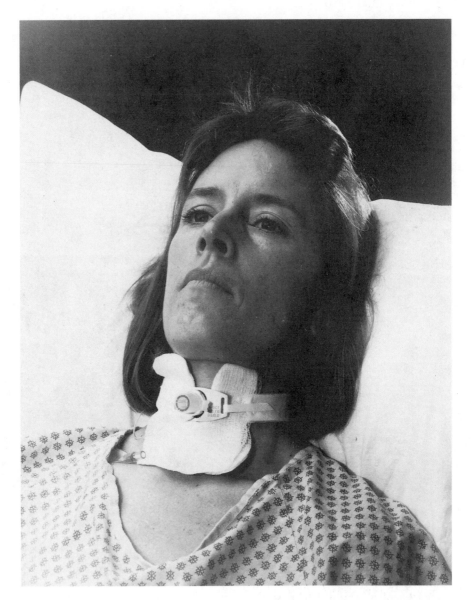

Figure 13-2 Using a Velcro collar to secure the tracheostomy tube. (Photo courtesy Dale Medical Products, Inc.)

Patient/caregiver needs to consider before discharge

Findeis and others,[8] Smith and others,[28] and Thomas and others[33] report that caregivers' most immediate self-perceived needs are to learn essential survival knowledge and skills of home ventilator management such as handling equipment, techniques for suctioning and tracheostomy care, and correct responses to emergency situations.[8,28,33] In planning for discharge, understanding everyday patient physical care needs appears to be more essential information for caregivers than pathophysiological content. Patient perceptions of immediate discharge planning needs commonly reflect those of caregivers; physical care and safety needs appear to overshadow knowledge of lung disease.[34] In addition, knowledge of financial and other matters, including insurance coverage, how to fill out forms, money for supplies, utility bills, oxygen equipment, and transportation to the physician, appear to be primary concerns of patients/caregivers and should be addressed as a part of discharge planning.[34]

Ideally patients/caregivers should be able to administer the majority of required procedural care with little intervention from professional staff before patient discharge (Figure 13-3). This capability helps to reduce patient/caregiver anxiety caused by separation from continuous hospital support.

HOME CARE APPLICATION

Home care agencies should regard patients discharged to the home setting on ventilators as being at high risk for potential problems with equipment and complications with care. The following conditions of acceptance should be considered as policy when admitting VDPs to home care agency services:

- A working telephone in the home
- An HME vendor on call 24 hours a day, 7 days a week, for equipment malfunction and support
- An alternate ventilatory support system and (as appropriate) an additional oxygen source in the home
- A patient support system (caregivers) *willing* and *able* to assist with patient care
- A safe and clean home environment

These conditions of acceptance support patient safety and ensure that home care nurses have reasonable resources to work with.

Visit frequency

The HME vendor installs equipment and plays a major role in establishing the VDP at home. The home care nurse should make an initial visit along with the respiratory therapist from the HME vendor to review equipment and to mutually decide learning needs and outcomes of patient care.

For the first week the home care nurse often makes daily visits to assess the patient's cardiopulmonary status and patient/caregiver progress with procedural aspects of care. The frequency of visits after this period depends on patient needs. During the first 2 weeks, 24-hour private duty care may be requested because this is a very anxious time for patients/caregivers who are developing independ-

ence from the hospital setting. As the VDP and the caregivers settle into their routine and become comfortable with equipment and related care needs, visit frequency typically is decreased to monthly visits for procedural requirements such as tracheostomy tube changes and PRN need.[20] Visits by the respiratory therapist from the HME vendor essentially follow the same pattern as home care nurse visits, eventually occurring monthly to evaluate the patient, deliver supplies, and check equipment.[20] In addition, office ventilator modem checks and other telecare services can be used to supplement care.

Developing the plan of care and patient education

Although the respiratory therapists from the HME vendor are routinely responsible for instructing patients and caregivers in procedural aspects of care, home care nurses should reinforce instructions and evaluate compliance with teaching during their visits. The VDP's care can be complicated and requires sound thinking. An important part of the home care nurse's role in patient/caregiver education is to provide a basis for sound decision making and to foster a sense of competency and good judgment (Box 13-3 and Box 13-4).

The HME vendor typically leaves a patient care manual outlining equipment management and procedural aspects of care in the patient's home. The home care nurse should review this manual as an additional resource for patient education. In addition, ventilator manufacturers should be available to conduct in-service training or problem solve telehealth implementation of ventilator care with staff.

When developing a plan of care, no matter how much equipment surrounds the VDP, home care nurses should never let technology take precedence over basic physical and psychological assessment of the patient. In other words, pay attention to the patient *before* paying attention to the machines.

A holistic assessment of VDPs should include the following:

- Baseline vital signs and cardiopulmonary status as a standard for future evaluation
- Physiological factors that relate disease process and issues involving ventilator dependence
- Patient/caregiver educational needs (includes physical aspects of self-care management and ongoing issues with finances and insurance)

Patient's Name:_____   Caregiver's Name:_____

	Met	Not Met

1. Verbalize phone numbers to post by ventilator:
   - Home care agency _____ _____
   - Home medical equipment (HME) company _____ _____
   - Physician _____ _____
   - 911/Local emergency room _____ _____
   - Local power company (notify the power company
     that the patient is ventilator-dependent and
     request priority service) _____ _____
   - Fire department _____ _____
2. Demonstrate operation of ventilator
   (See manufacturer's manual, equipment varies):
   A. Identify parts of the tubing circuit
      - inspiratory and expiratory tubing _____ _____
      - patient pressure tubing and port
        on rear panel of ventilator _____ _____
      - exhalation valve tubing and port
        on rear panel of ventilator _____ _____
      - exhalation valve _____ _____
      - trach adapter _____ _____
      - air inlet on rear panel of ventilator _____ _____
      - DC power hookup _____ _____
      - Modem hook-up, as applicable _____ _____
   B. Identify location and demonstrate replacement of fuse _____ _____
   C. Check/adjust ventilator setting as ordered
      - mode _____ _____
      - rate _____ _____
      - inspiratory time _____ _____
      - flow _____ _____
      - high-pressure alarm _____ _____
      - low-pressure alarm _____ _____
      - PEEP/CPA _____ _____
   D. Verbalize/demonstrate cleaning, storage and/or
      replacement of equipment _____ _____
   E. Verbalize/demonstrate how to troubleshoot alarms _____ _____
3. Verbalize/demonstrate what to do in case
   there is a power or equipment failure:
   - Manual resuscitation of the patient _____ _____
   - Use of backup home ventilator, if available _____ _____
   - Call and notify the power company _____ _____
   - Call the respiratory therapist, from
     the HME company, for assistance _____ _____
   - Call the home care agency for assistance _____ _____
   - Consider 911 for emergency situations _____ _____
4. Verbalize/demonstrate tracheostomy care (refer
   to manufacturer guidelines as tracheostomy
   tubes vary in use/cleaning):
   - Changing the tracheostomy tube _____ _____
   - Cleaning the tracheostomy site
     and changing ties _____ _____
   - Suctioning the patient _____ _____
   - Cleaning and storage of equipment _____ _____

Comments:

_____Passed   _____Needs to repeat

Professional's Signature:_____   Date:_____

Figure 13-3 Discharge patient/caregiver checklist for home mechanical ventilation.

Box 13-3 PRIMARY NURSING DIAGNOSIS/PATIENT PROBLEMS

- Impaired verbal communication
- Ineffective breathing pattern
- Fluid volume overload
- Risk for infection: respiratory
- Knowledge deficit: for example, disease process and risk complications, socioeconomic resources, troubleshooting and operation of equipment, procedural care, medications, diet, infection control, available community services
- Altered nutrition: potential for less than body requirements
- Activity intolerance:_____ Ambulation, _____ ADLs, _____ Other (*Specify*)
- Self-care deficit:_____ ADLs, _____Grooming, _____ Toileting, _____ Other (*Specify*)
- Risk for pain: stress ulcers
- Risk for injury: tracheostomal trauma
- Risk for impaired skin integrity
- Body image disturbance
- Risk for loneliness
- Powerlessness
- Spiritual distress
- Ineffective individual coping
- Risk for caregiver role strain
- Ineffective family coping

Box 13-4 PRIMARY THEMES OF PATIENT EDUCATION

- The use of alternative speech methods
- Disease process: signs and symptoms to report to the case manager and physician
- When to call 911
- Socioeconomic resources
- What to do in case of equipment or power failure (manual resuscitation of the patient, who to call, etc.)
- Operation and maintenance of equipment
- Procedural care
- Medications
- Diet
- Positive coping strategies to use when living with a chronic illness (positive lifestyle adaptations to school, work, the home milieu, or family role changes)
- Strategies to promote patient ties to religion, family, friends, and community
- Caregiver/family respite alternatives
- General self-care strategies
- Community services available for ventilator-dependent patients and their caregivers/families

- Psychosocial concerns related to ventilator dependence and caregiving
- Spiritual concerns and needs
- Availability of community resources to facilitate self-care management

Asessment of primary complications and nursing management

When conducting the assessment, home care nurses should observe for the following complications and concerns associated with ventilator dependence.[32]

Ineffective breathing pattern. **Assess** for overventilation or underventilation due to inadequate ventilator settings or trauma to lung tissue (for example, as a result of positive pressure from the ventilator producing a rupture in alveolar or pulmonary structures, such as a pneumothorax). Primary signs and symptoms of respiratory distress are patient complaints of unrelieved shortness of breath, a change in the patient's level of consciousness or mentation (the patient may suddenly become combative), and changes in baseline vital signs or skin color. Assess for leaks or cracks in the ventilator circuit tubing, which may cause suspected hypoxia.

Assess for mucous plugs or for very thick tracheal secretions, particularly in children. Mucous plugs can block the airway and cause respiratory distress. Very thick secretions or yellow-green secretion may indicate either insufficient humidity or a possible infection.

Interventions include reporting signs and symptoms of respiratory distress to the physician. Duct tape can be temporarily used to seal circuit air leaks until tubing is replaced. As appropriate, recommend that patients go to a hospital emergency department for further evaluation, and administer supplemental oxygen until emergency medical services arrive. Techniques for cardiopulmonary resuscitation (CPR) should be reviewed with caregivers during the first home visit.

A source of humidity is essential for routine tracheostomy care because the tube bypasses the nose and mouth, which normally humidify inspired air. A tracheostomy collar, vaporizer, room humidifier, or in-line ventilator humidifier can be used to prevent the drying of secretions and formation of mucous plugs.[14]

Risk for infection: respiratory. **Assess** for an elevated temperature, increased heart rate, or changes in the color, consistency, and amount of mucus produced. Be aware that infection in these patients can arise from many different sources, including the environment; evaluate accordingly.

Interventions include reporting an elevated temperature to the physician, who may request a sputum specimen for laboratory evaluation. The patient/caregiver should be instructed to routinely initiate antibiotic therapy at the first signs of respiratory infection. Teach infection control procedures to ventilator-dependent patients and their caregivers, focusing on handwashing and proper techniques for draining tubing and cleaning humidifiers and related equipment.

Fluid volume overload. **Assess** the lungs for increased wheezes, increased lung sounds, or deviations from baseline status. Palpate extremities for edema, and if possible, weigh the patient to evaluate fluid overload. In ventilator dependence, edema originates from the following:

- Heart failure
- Hypoalbuminemia
- Unchanged body position; dependent edema (poor venous return)
- Rebreathing moisture that is normally lost with exhalation (The ventilator-dependent patient may gain as much as 300 to 500 ml of extra water within 24 hours.)
- Positive pressure ventilation (Increases in intrathoracic pressure cause decreased venous return to the heart. This produces a low cardiac output, resulting in a backup of fluid in the extremities. In addition, a low cardiac output stimulates antidiuretic hormone [ADH] production, which conserves fluid in response to the body's false assumption of a dehydrated or hypovolemic state.)
- Renal failure as a consequence of congestive heart failure (CHF) or related disease process

Interventions include diuretics as part of the medication regimen to treat fluid overload. In addi-

tion, blood should be drawn for evaluation of electrolytes (particularly sodium and potassium levels because ventilator-dependent patients are prone to hyponatremia and hypokalemia), blood urea nitrogen (BUN), and creatinine levels to evaluate renal function.[12] Dependent edema can be managed by encouraging mobility and periodically elevating extremities. Chest physiotherapy is helpful to clear the airway of excess secretions (see Chapters 11 and 12).

Altered nutrition: less than body requirements. **Assess** patients for inappropriate weight loss. Malnutrition is frequently associated with chronic obstructive pulmonary disease (COPD) and is caused by poor intake, infection, and increased work of breathing.[12,17]

Interventions include recommending a diet in which half the patient's caloric requirements are met by a fat source (this limits CO_2 production and excess ventilatory demands.[4,12] As possible, initiate a referral to the dietitian for further evaluation. Patients with malnutrition may require enteral feedings or parenteral alimentation (see Chapter 18).

Pain: stress ulcers. **Assess** patient complaints of nausea, abdominal pain, and vomiting. Assess for black, tarry stools, which usually indicate an upper gastrointestinal (GI) bleed. Bright red blood in the stool usually indicates lower GI bleeding. Be aware that ventilator-dependent patients are prone to stress ulcers and gastrointestinal hemorrhage.

Interventions include antacid therapy. Stools should be tested for occult blood when possible. Request ventilator-dependent patients to report blood in their stool or abdominal discomfort to their nurse or physician. Consult with the physican regarding treatment for pain control because some medications may exacerbate gastrointestinal hemorrhaging.

Risk for injury: tracheostomal trauma. **Assess** for signs and symptoms of bleeding from the stoma. Tracheostomal trauma can be caused by the following:

- Too vigorous suctioning
- Overinflation of the tracheostomy tube cuff
- Strictures and adhesions of tissue to the tracheostomy tube

Interventions include teaching the patient and caregiver techniques of tracheostomy care. Tracheostomy tubes should be routinely changed to prevent adhesions and should never be forced into the patient's neck.

Risk for impaired skin integrity. **Assess** for signs/symptoms of skin breakdown caused by immobility or incontinence. Ventilator-dependent patients may become afraid to move from their beds for fear of losing their breath or disrupting the ventilator. This can progress to an essentially bedridden state, although it should be noted that many ventilator patients are not bedbound.

Interventions include obtaining a hospital bed for the patient. This will ease the patient's ability to make transfers. Some patients may require wheelchairs, walkers, or a hoyer lift to improve mobility. In order to prevent skin breakdown, it is important to keep the patient as mobile as possible. Consider a referral to rehabilitation services for a home exercise program (see chapter 17). Also, review wound care in Chapter 14 and incontinence care in Chapter 16.

Risk for patient and caregiver stress: inability to cope. **Assess** the integrity of the caregiver/family unit, in particular their ongoing ability to care for the patient and the patient's response to care (see Chapter 4).

Interventions include utilizing the services of the social worker or psychiatric home health nurse for support with patient/caregiver stress management. Also, see the discussion of psychosocial issues at the end of this chapter.

Medication regimen and procedural care

Medications and treatments for ventilator-dependent patients are similar to those for patients with COPD (see Chapter 11). Bronchodilators, diuretics, steroids, electrolyte supplements, cardiotonic medication, and chest physiotherapy are used to enhance respiration and to control edema. In addition, ventilator-dependent patients are occasionally given antibiotics because they are susceptible to pulmonary infections.

Tracheostomy tube care. Tracheostomy tube changes are a primary skilled service provided by home care nurses for uncomplicated ventilator-dependent patients. Because of potential problems with bleeding and unknown patient response, the first outer cannula exchange should be done by the patient's physician in the medical office or hospital.

The patient's tracheostomy tube should be changed at least monthly to reduce the incidence of infection and esophageal strictures. Infants and children will require more frequent outer cannula changes because of growth and development factors. For complicated cases, a joint visit by two home care nurses may be required for this procedure. Changing the tracheostomy tube in a calm, reassuring, and expedient manner is important because any interruption of the airway can be a frightening and anxious experience for patients and their caregivers.

Tracheostomy tube changes are frequently done with the patient supine. A towel is placed between the shoulder blades to expose the stoma. Although this is a traditional position and useful with infants and children, many adult patients may tolerate this procedure best when sitting up. An upright position may give patients some feeling of control during the procedure and decrease the risk for aspiration and a choking sensation. In addition, instructing the patient to look upward and swallow during the procedure opens the airway to a correct anatomical position for tube insertion and may facilitate insertion. This may also provide a mental focus that distracts the patient from some of the anxiety caused by the procedure and decrease the risk of aspiration.[20]

If possible, caregivers should be taught the fundamentals of changing the tracheostomy tube and encouraged to assist the home care nurse with this procedure. If the tube should become dislodged in the middle of the night or when the patient is away from home, the family is then prepared to handle the situation—without emergency intervention from the ambulance service—until evaluation by the physician or home care nurse is possible.

If the tracheostomy tube accidentally comes out and the caregivers cannot reinsert it or reinsert a tracheostomy tube one size smaller, they should be advised to make a tight seal over the patient's stoma with their hand and manually ventilate the patient with the Ambu-bag via a face mask until the nurse, the respiratory therapist from the HME vendor, or the emergency medical service arrives to provide assistance.[5]

The inner cannula should be cleaned and replaced at least daily. Some inner cannulas are disposable for one-time use only. If reusable, extra outer and inner cannulas may be cleaned with soap and water, rinsed with tap water, air dried, and stored in plastic bags. A 50% hydrogen peroxide solution followed by a tap water rinse may help remove crusted material on the tracheostomy tube. Pipe cleaners or small brushes can be used to clean the inside of the tracheostomy tube. Do not use bleach or bleach products to clean or disinfect respiratory equipment.

Metal tracheostomy tubes may be washed with soap and water, boiled for 5 minutes, and then air dried for storage. Do not use hydrogen peroxide with metal tracheostomy tubes because it will corrode the metal.

Tracheostomy tube cuff management. A tracheostomy cuff is useful for precise oxygen and air volume administration. In additional, a tracheostomy cuff minimizes aspiration in patients with poor ability to swallow. A standard Luer syringe is used to inject air into the cuff via the pilot balloon for most cuffed tracheostomy tubes. An exception is the FOME-CUF tracheostomy tube, which requires a 60-ml syringe to deflate the cuff before insertion and upon removal.

Cuffed tracheostomy tubes should be periodically deflated to prevent tissue damage and promote communication. The syringe should be inserted into the Luer valve, and air should be withdrawn until resistance is felt. When the cuff is deflated, the pilot balloon becomes flat.

Cuff inflation varies according to patient comfort levels and the minimal amount of air required to seal the tracheostomy. The minimal-leak technique is commonly used to reduce the incidence of tracheostomal wall necrosis. As the ventilator gives the patient a breath, the cuff is slowly inflated until it presses against the tracheostomal wall and prevents auscultated air leaks when the patient inhales and exhales. Air is then withdrawn from the cuff until a small air leak is auscultated the next time the ventilator gives a breath. Usually 5 ml of air is required to achieve a minimal occluding volume. The Bivona FOME-CUF is designed to passively inflate until it meets the tracheal wall, providing good occlusion with minimal pressure against the tracheal wall.

Stoma care. The stoma should be cared for daily and as needed. When making a visit, home care nurses inspect the skin surrounding the tracheostomy for signs of redness or infection and report findings to the physician as appropriate. The stoma should be gently cleaned with soap and water. Avoid the use of hydrogen peroxide and Betadine, if possible, as they may enhance skin breakdown.[15,23] After cleaning, apply an absorbent, lint-free dressing around the stoma.

Suctioning. Suctioning should be done whenever the patient's secretions build up in the airway and before and after the tracheostomy tube is changed. Hyperoxygenate and hyperinflate the patient's lungs before and after suctioning to help minimize complications such as hypoxia. Suctioning in children should be approximately ¼ to ½ inch beyond the tip of the artificial airway[23] and approximately 3 to 5 cm, or as tolerated, in adults.[5,21] Of note, data suggest that instillation of normal saline before suctioning has an adverse effect on oxygen saturation and should not be used routinely in patients receiving mechanical ventilation.[1]

Although home care nurses should perform all procedures in as aseptic a manner as possible, in most cases suctioning, like stoma care and routine inner cannula changes, can be done by caregivers using clean technique.[9] Instruct caregivers to irrigate suction catheters with distilled or tap water and to store them in a clean paper towel between uses. Suction catheters should be discarded within 24 hours, or they may be cleaned with a 50% hydrogen peroxide solution and then boiled in water for 10 minutes, air dried, and stored in a new plastic bag for reuse.[21] The suction canister should be emptied and cleaned daily with soap and hot water. Suction tubing should also be cleaned daily with soap and hot water per home health agency policy or per HME vendor guidelines.[21]

Ventilator assessment

The home care nurse should become familiar with the ventilator dials and settings, circuit maintenance, and proper responses to equipment alarms. Box 13-5 provides troubleshooting guidelines. Ventilator settings are primarily determined by patient comfort levels.[16] Ventilator assessment should become a routine part of the home health nurse's visit (see Appendix XIII-I).

Infection control

Typically ventilator setups (tubing) and the humidifier should be changed 2 or 3 times a week or per HME vendor guidelines for disinfection. Tubing and the humidifier reservoir may be washed in soapy water, soaked in a 1:3 white vinegar/tap water solution for 15 to 20 minutes, and then rinsed thoroughly with tap water and air dried.[21] When tubing is dry, it can then be stored in a new plastic bag. The exterior of the ventilator should be cleaned with a common disinfectant. Do not clean or disinfect respiratory equipment with bleach. (Review Chapter 6 for infection control guidelines.)

Box 13-5   PROBLEM SOLVING HOME MECHANICAL VENTILATOR ALARMS

Low-Pressure Alarms

1. Check the circuit for leaks; change circuit tubing as needed.
2. Check the tracheostomy cuff for a leak; inflate per comfort level.
3. Check exhaled air with volume bag. If range is unacceptable, call HME vendor. Manually ventilate the patient with the Ambu-bag until the respiratory therapist from the HME vendor arrives.

Alarms as Patient Experiences Cardiopulmonary Distress

1. Take vital signs.
2. If unsure whether patient is getting sufficient oxygen, disconnect from the ventilator and ventilate the patient with the Ambu-bag.
3. As time allows, suction and administer bronchodilator treatment.
4. Alert the physician. Stay with the patient until the emergency medical service arrives.
5. Administer cardiopulmonary resuscitation as appropriate.

High-Pressure Alarms

1. Suction; use saline to thin mucous plugs.
2. Check tubing for obstructions or collapse. Change circuit tubing as needed.
3. Drain excess water in tubing into drainage receptacle.
4. Administer bronchodilator treatment as ordered.

Note: These are general guidelines. Specific interventions should be based on individual patient assessment and circumstance and home care agency policy and procedures.

Psychosocial and spiritual assessment

Psychosocial and spiritual needs related to ventilator dependence are well documented.[6,7] Depression, fear, and a profound sense of loss are common feelings experienced by ventilator-dependent patients. These feelings can be caused by a restrictive lifestyle, problems with communication and finances, and a high dependency on others for basic needs.[10]

Fear is usually related to equipment malfunction and the possibility of not being able to breathe.[6] Patients with these fears often become very fixated on their immediate surroundings and the length of their tubing. These fixations can progress to complete activity intolerance and magnify problems caused by immobility.

Encourage patient mobility and activity in order to foster healthy mood and outlook. Most wheelchairs can be set up with a ventilator attached to the back, thus allowing the patient opportunities for travel. In addition, disposable heat and moisture exchangers can be added to the patient circuit so cumbersome humidifiers are not needed when traveling.

Fear of equipment and alarms can be managed by patient education. Review the use of alternate ventilatory support systems and help the patient and caregiver identify circumstances when the HME vendor and home care agency should be called. The family may wish to tape the telephone number of the HME vendor on top of the ventilator, along with their physician's number, the home care agency's number, and the local emergency service's number.

Communication should be encouraged. Most VDPs are quite capable of directing their own care. In the home setting this can restore a sense of control and self-esteem. Home care nurses or speech therapists may help the patient choose a communication system that is easy to use and fits within the household budget.

When assessing the integrity of the patient's support system, be aware of problems that can result from constant care needs. Caregivers may become stressed when coping with continuous patient demands.[33,34] In addition, preexisting conflicts that may have temporarily abated with acute illness may resurface when the patient comes home. The impact of illness and the finality of ventilator dependence may not be experienced by patients and their caregivers until they are home, where lost routines and changes in role and body image are poignantly felt.[6]

Caring, listening, being available to encourage communication, and providing information and support as needed are probably the best ways to assess and promote the integrity of the household and the intactness of the family system. Once a feeling is expressed and a problem verbalized, it can then be dealt with realistically as a part of interpersonal relationships. As mentioned earlier, a referral to the psychiatric home health nurse, social worker, the patient's religious leader, or respite services may be necessary to alleviate acute patient and caregiver stress or burnout.

PEDIATRIC ISSUES

Pediatric tracheostomy tubes less than a size 4 are usually cuffless and do not have an inner cannula. These tubes should be changed at least 1 to 2 times a week. Parents with infants should be taught that if the tracheostomy tube accidentally comes out and they cannot reinsert it, they should try to reinsert a tracheostomy tube one size smaller.[2] If this tube cannot be inserted, a suction catheter can be placed in the stoma, and breaths given through the catheter. When the infant relaxes, instruct parents to attempt to reinsert the tracheostomy tube. If problems persist, emergency medical services (EMS) should be contacted immediately and the infant transported to the hospital.

The use of a positive pressure volume ventilator has become common practice for ventilating pediatric home care patients. This type of ventilator provides cardiopulmonary support through the delivery of a preset volume at a guaranteed minimum rate and is protected from barotrauma by a high-pressure cycle control. However, the ventilator configuration is commonly modified to accommodate the pediatric patient's small lung capacity and variable leak. (Note: The cuffless tracheostomy tubes that are traditionally used for the pediatric population allow variable leaks.) Two types of modifications commonly used are (1) pressure limiting of the volume to preset levels for the duration of the inspiratory phase to prevent lung injury and to promote adequate oxygenation and (2) supplying a continuous gas flow to ease the work of spontaneous respirations.

Caregivers should pay special attention to cleaning and handling equipment because children and infants are frequently subject to respiratory infections and other infectious disease related to their young age and immature immune systems. Diet and exercise are essential features of care to increase strength, endurance, and growth. Communication development is a concern for children with tracheostomies. However, extensive cooing and babbling does not appear necessary for later speech development.[26] Sibling adjustment and family coping with long-term ventilatory care will need to be evaluated. Quint and others[19] report that the family's ability to cope with the many needs of the ventilator-dependent child may decline with a longer duration of home ventilatory care.

Coming home to a familiar, busy, and interesting environment will have special importance for pediatric patients, for whom growth and development are essential tasks. There should be an emphasis on feeding and oral stimulation in the plan of care. The use of rehabilitation services is highly recommended. Seek additional resources when caring for pediatric ventilator-dependent patients; their needs are quite different from those of adults.

SUMMARY

The technical focus of this chapter highlights issues involving safe and competent management of VDPs in the home setting. This is not to say that home care nurses should let technology and procedural requirements dominate the plan of care. A holistic and sensitive approach to patient care is the basic foundation of all nursing practice. When working with equipment, never forget to look at the patient; a grimace or a smile can say a lot.

Home mechanical ventilation can offer VDPs much richer and more fulfilling lives than the institutional setting of the hospital. The home environment affords patients the noises, sights, and smells of life and living where relationships and friendships begin anew. Sitting on the porch on a warm summer's day, shopping at the mall, visiting friends, going to church, or returning to work or school restores a sense of self for ventilator-dependent patients and offers hope for a good tomorrow. This is the ideal, and with proper encouragement from home care nurses, it is certainly possible.

As with most things, however, a darker side exists. Home care nurses may work with patients who have essentially become part of the bed, neither moving nor talking, as if in a comatose state.[33] As one family asked, "When is Dad going to die? When we brought him home, they said he wouldn't last long, and that was 4 years ago."

Home care nurses should always assess the intactness of the family as caregivers, as well as the biopsychosocial integrity of the patient. When the patient is without purposeful thought or function and is merely being aerated by the ventilator, the family as the patient's support system *will* show signs of disintegration. In addition, the literature supports a decline in the caregiver's/family's ability to cope with a longer duration of home ventilatory care.[8,18,33] In these circumstances, home care of VDPs becomes more complex and confronts highly sensitive issues. Home care nurses can best meet these challenges by encouraging communication between the household and the patient's physician. If the patient can no longer be cared for at home, other choices (including placement in an extended care facility) should be considered.

At its best, home mechanical ventilation allows patients a rewarding life in a loving environment. At its worst, home mechanical ventilation becomes nothing more than the beeps and hisses of machines. It is critical that home care nurses recognize the vast difference between the two and intervene as is best for both patients and their families.

REFERENCES

1. Ackerman M, Mick D: Instillation of normal saline before suctioning in patients with pulmonary infections: a prospective randomized controlled trial, *Am J Crit Care* 7(4):261, 1999.
2. Aday LU and others: *Pediatric home care: results of a national evaluation of programs for ventilator-assisted children,* Chicago, 1988, Pluribus Press.
3. Beard B, Monaco F: Tracheostomy discontinuation: impact of tube selection on resistance during tube occlusion, *Respir Care* 38(3):267, 1993.
4. Cane R, Green S: Nutritional support of the ventilator-dependent patient, *Nutr Support Serv* 1:51, 1985.
5. Carroll P: Closing in on safer suctioning, *RN,* p 22, May 1998.
6. Clark K: Psychosocial aspects of prolonged ventilator dependency, *Respir Care* 31(4):329, 1986.
7. Elpern E and others: Long-term outcomes for elderly survivors of prolonged ventilator assistance, *Chest* 96(5):1120, 1989.
8. Findeis A and others: Caring for individuals using home ventilators: an appraisal by family caregivers, *Rehabil Nurs* 19(1):6, 1994.
9. Harris R, Hyman R: Clean vs sterile tracheostomy care and level of pulmonary infection, *Nurs Res* 33(2):80, 1984.
10. Haynes N and others: Discharging ICU ventilator-dependent patient to home healthcare, *Crit Care Nurs* 10(7):39, 1990.
11. Health Care Financing Administration: *Health insurance manual,* Pub No 11, Washington, DC, 1995, US Department of Health and Human Services.
12. Irwin M, Openbrier D: A delicate balance: strategies for feeding ventilated COPD patients, *Am J Nurs* 3:274, 1985.
13. Kreit J, Eschenbacher W: The physiology of spontaneous and mechanical ventilation, *Clin Chest Med* 9(1):11, 1988.
14. Law J and others: Increased frequency of obstructive airway abnormalities with long-term tracheostomy, *Chest* 104:136, 1993.
15. Linneaweaver W and others: Topical antimicrobial activity, *Arch Surg* 120:257, 1985.
16. O'Donohue W and others: Long-term mechanical ventilation: guidelines for management in the home and at alternate community sites, *Chest* 90(1):15, 1986.
17. Pingleton S: Nutritional support in the mechanically-ventilated patient, *Clin Chest Med* 9(1):101, 1988.
18. Purtilo R: Ethical issues in the treatment of chronic ventilator-dependent patients, *Arch Phys Med Rehabil* 67(9):718, 1986.
19. Quint R and others: Home care for ventilator-dependent children, *Am J Dis Child* 144(9):1238, 1990.
20. Rice R: *Working with ventilator-dependent patients: case study analysis involving 15 years of field experience.* Paper presented at the National Home Care Association conference, Chicago, 1998.
21. Rice R, editor: *Manual of home health nursing procedures,* ed 2, St. Louis, 2000, Mosby.
22. Rosen R, Bone R: Economics of mechanical ventilation, *Clin Chest Med* 9(1):163, 1988.
23. Runton N: Suctioning artificial airways in children: appropriate technique, *Pediatr Nurs 18(2):*115, 1999.
24. Sevick MA, Bradham D: Economic value of caregiver effort in maintaining long-term ventilator-assisted individuals at home, *Heart Lung,* p 148, March/April 1997.
25. Sevick MA and others: Home-based ventilator-dependent patients: measurement of the emotional aspects of home caregiving, *Chest* 109:1597, 1997.
26. Simon BM and others: Communication development in young children with long-term tracheostomies, *Int J Pediatr Otolayngol* 6:37, 1983.
27. Sivak ED and others: Home care ventilation: the Cleveland Clinic experience from 1977 to 1985, *Respir Care* 31(4):294, 1986.
28. Smith C and others: Caregiver learning needs and reactions to managing home mechanical ventilation, *Heart Lung* 23(2):157, 1994.
29. Splaingard ML: Home positive-pressure ventilation: twenty years experience, *Chest* 84(4):376, 1983.
30. Splaingard ML and others: Home negative pressure ventilation: report of 20 years experience in patients with neuromuscular disease, *Arch Phys Med Rehabil* 66:239, 1988.
31. Stone R, Short PF: The competing demands of employment and informal caregiving to the disabled, *Med Care* 28(6):513, 1990.
32. Strieter R, Lynch J: Complications in the ventilated patient, *Clin Chest Med* 9(1):127, 1988.
33. Thomas V and others: Caring for the person receiving ventilatory support at home: caregivers' needs and involvement, *Heart Lung* 21(2):180, 1992.
34. Thompson C, Richmond M: Teaching home care for ventilator-dependent patients: the patient's perception, *Heart Lung* 19(1):79, 1990.

Appendix XIII-I

Home Ventilator Management

PURPOSE

- To define the responsibilities of the home health nurse caring for the ventilator-dependent patient.
- To provide guidelines for home ventilator management.
- To maximize high-tech quality patient care in the home setting.
- To promote self-care in the home

GENERAL INFORMATION

Defining the roles of the HME vendor respiratory therapist and the home care nurse regarding care of the ventilator patient in the home is the responsibility of the discharge planning team. Weeks prior to the patient's discharge, the patient's home care team, including the caregiver, should be given instructions about actual and potential patient care needs. Caregivers who are *willing* and *able* to assist with patient needs are necessary for home discharge.

The home care nurse is advised to review the patient care manual from the HME vendor, which should outline ventilator management in the home and serve as an additional instructional guide for the patient/caregiver. It is important to refer to individual manufacturers' recommendations to ensure safe and efficacious use of all equipment, including any office modem checks on ventilator function (Figure XIII-I, *C*).

Although the respiratory therapists from the HME vendor are responsible for instructing the patient/caregiver in procedural aspects of care, home health nurses should reinforce instructions and **evaluate** compliance with the plan of care during visits. The patient/caregiver should be familiar with ventilator alarms, know what they mean, and how to take appropriate action. An important role of the home care nurse in patient/caregiver education regarding home ventilator management is to provide a basis for sound decision making and to foster a sense of competency and good judgment.

EQUIPMENT (Figure XIII-I)

1. Ventilator
   a. Ventilator circuits, filters
   b. Heated humidifier or cascade
      i. Sterile or distilled water, tap water if boiled 15 minutes
      ii. Condensation drainage bags
      iii. Heat and moisture exchanger (optional)
   c. External 12-volt battery with power cord
   d. Volume bag (optional)
   e. Disinfectant
   f. Manual self-inflating resuscitation bag
2. Oxygen and related supplies
   a. Oxygen source (optional): oxygen concentrator with backup compressed gas cylinder (tank)
   b. Oxygen connecting tubing: pressure-compensated flowmeter is recommended with the use of 50 feet of connecting tubing
   c. Air compressor and tubing for aerosol treatments (optional)
3. Tracheostomy equipment and related supplies
4. Durable medical equipment
   a. Hospital bed (optional)
   b. Patient communication aid
   c. As needed: equipment to assist with

Modified from Rice R: *Manual of home health nursing procedures,* ed 2, St. Louis, 2000, Mosby.

A

Front Panel

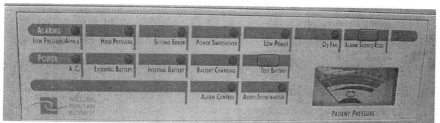

Top Alarm Panel

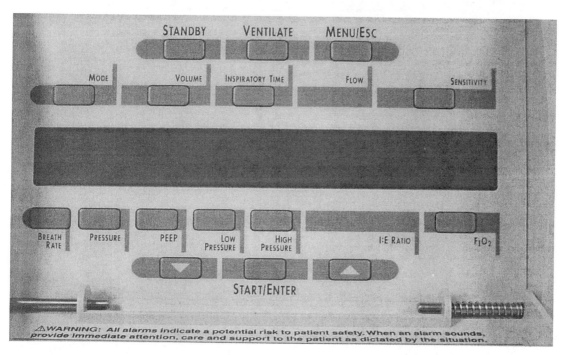

Bottom Door Panel

Figure XIII-I Example of a ventilator commonly found in home care today. Model shown is a Puritan-Bennett Achieva model. **A,** Front panel. (Photos and drawing courtesy Mallinckrodt, Minneapolis, Minn.)

Continued

B

Rear Panel

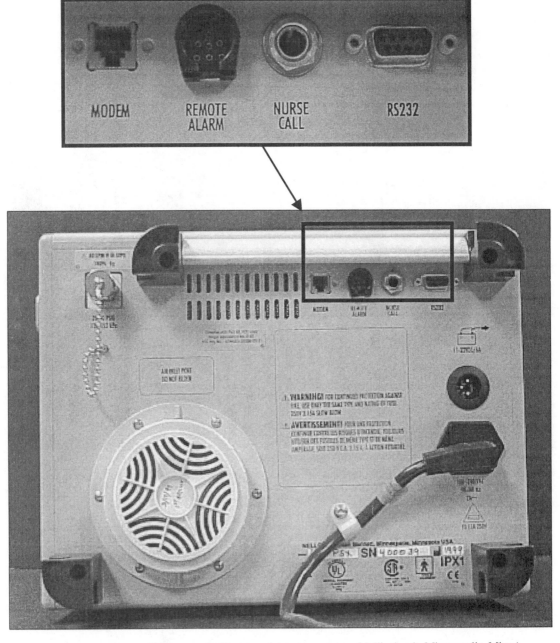

Figure XIII-I, cont'd B, Rear panel. (Photos and drawing courtesy Mallinckrodt, Minneapolis, Minn.)

C

Events Log Report

Each line details either an alarm or parameter change, including an event description, date, time and duration.

Alarm indications include the vent settings at the time of the alarm as well as measured inspiratory, expiratory, peak inspiratory and minimum expiratory pressures.

Parameter changes list the parameter setting before (Pre) and after (Post) the change.

Event Summary Report

The information contained in the Event Log Report is also summarized in the Event Summary Report.

Breath-to-Breath Data

Up to eight hours of waveform data is displayed, representing the peak pressure volume, peak flow and breath rate from each breath. The data can be more closely examined on the computer screen by zooming in and scrolling through the data.

Waveform Plot Graph

A 25-second snapshot of real time flow, volume and pressure waveforms is available at any time the Achieva is ventilating.

Usage Graph and Usage Summary Report

Up to 31 days of ventilator usage data can be collected and displayed.

Shaded bars indicate time the ventilator was ventilating (usage graph only).

Figure XIII-I, cont'd C, Example of report generator software available for use with Achieva line of ventilators. (Photos and drawing courtesy Mallinckrodt, Minneapolis, Minn.) *Continued*

D

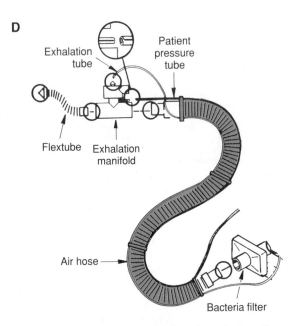

Figure XIII-I, cont'd D, Drawing of a typical ventilator circuit. (Photos and drawing courtesy Mallinckrodt, Minneapolis, Minn.)

patient bowel/bladder management and personal care

d. As needed: cane, walker, wheelchair

PROCEDURE

1. Explain the procedure to the patient/caregiver.
2. Maintain a copy of the most recent plan of care to ensure that all orders are being implemented correctly. When faced with questions that fall outside of the established care plan,contact the HME respiratory therapist and physician for answers. If available, consult with the pulmonary clinical nurse specialist or discharge planning coordinator from the referring hospital.
3. Perform physical assessment to include:
    a. Subjective assessment based on, but not limited to, patient/caregiver comments on shortness of breath, color change, mucus production, fever, and machine or equipment concerns.
    b. Objective assessment of physiological data, such as blood pressure, pulse, respiratory rate, breath sounds, and oxygen saturation.
    c. Assess for complications of ventilator dependence such as skin breakdown, infection, fluid/electrolyte imbalance, malnutrition, and depression.
4. Assess patient/caregiver ability to manage ventilator dependence at home, concerns regarding equipment, resources, psychosocial, spiritual and teaching needs, etc.
5. Perform safety check of all equipment to include:
    a. Patient circuit (Figure XIII-I, *D*):
        i. Drain all tubing of water. Excess water should be considered contaminated and disposed of accordingly.
        ii. Inspect the circuit for wear and cracks.
        iii. Check all connections for tightness.
        iv. Make sure tubing is routed to prevent excess water from draining into the patient's airway or back into the humidifier or ventilator.
    b. Inspect all equipment for proper function and wear, including battery level and operational hours of the ventilator.
    c. Confirm that equipment is being cleaned and changed as ordered or per manufacturer's recommendations.
6. Assess the mode of delivery:
    a. Control mode—delivers a preset tidal volume at a fixed rate. The patient cannot initiate breaths or change the ventilatory pattern.
    b. Assist control volume or rate (ACV)—allows patients to initiate breaths so they can breathe at a faster rate than the preset number of breaths per minute generated by the ventilator. Each breath is delivered at the same preset tidal volume.
    c. Intermittent mandatory ventilation (IMV)—delivers a preset number of mechanical breaths at a preset tidal volume, but also allows patients to breathe with no assistance (positive pressure) from the ventilator at their own tidal volume.
    d. Synchronized intermittent mandatory ventilation (SIMV)—the ventilator senses the patient's spontaneous breath and synchronizes the timed breath with

the patient's breath. This synchronization reduces competition between machine-delivered breaths and patient-spontaneous breaths.

7. Assess the breath rate (ventilator plus patient) Approximate range 1 to 38 breaths per minute.

8. Assess the tidal volume (VT) that the ventilator is giving the patient. VT is 10 to 15 cc/kg. The dial setting of the tidal volume may be compared with results obtained by use of a volume bag.

   a. The HME vendor may provide a clear, plastic sleeve called a volume bag that is used to measure the VT. Attach the volume bag to the exhalation valve or gas collection head on the tubing. Count the number of breaths it takes to completely fill the bag. On the back of the volume bag, a diagram shows total number of breaths taken to fill the volume bag with corresponding tidal volume.

   b. Dial settings from the tidal volume should be similar to what is obtained with the volume bag measurement; if discrepancies are noted, inform the HME vendor's respiratory therapist for follow-up.

9. Assess low-pressure alarm limit setting (when the pressure falls below the set rate, the alarm will sound. For example, if the patient becomes disconnected from the ventilator, the low pressure alarm will be triggered). Approximate range: 2 to 32 cm H_2O.

10. Assess high-pressure alarm limit setting. When the pressure rises above the set rate, the alarm will sound. For example, mucous plugs, excessive secretions, coughing, and lying on ventilator exits will increase pressure, inhibiting the ventilator effort to deliver oxygen and triggering the high-pressure alarm). Approximate range: 15 to 90 cm H_2O.

11. Assess patient pressures by observing low and high limits as the patients breathes.

12. Assess the FiO_2 (fraction of inspired oxygen: room air is 21%) or amount of prescribed oxygen being delivered. Approximate range: 24% to 40% FiO_2 greater than 40% is rarely used in home care.

13. Assess positive end-expiratory pressure (PEEP) if used. High levels of PEEP (>5 cm H_2O) may cause barotrauma. PEEP is rarely used in home care.

14. Instruct the patient/caregiver to post the following phone numbers by the telephone: the HME vendor, the physician's number, the home health agency's number, local power/electricity service number, and local emergency service number for emergencies or problems with equipment. Help the patient/caregiver identify circumstances when emergency numbers should be called.

15. Notify the local power/emergency services of patient's home address and arrange for priority service.

16. Provide patient comfort measures.

17. Clean and replace equipment. Discard disposable items according to standard precautions.

NURSING CONSIDERATIONS

Instruct the patient/caregiver in the use of alternate ventilatory support systems.

Have the patient/caregiver demonstrate the use of the manual self-inflating resuscitation bag.

The ventilator-dependent patient is at risk for respiratory failure, and care should be planned accordingly. Make the initial visits with the respiratory therapist from the HME vendor to review equipment and to mutually assess the needs of the patient/caregiver.

For the first week, daily visits are advised. The frequency of visits after this period depends on the progress of the patient/caregiver with procedural aspects of care. Twenty-four hour private duty care may be required during the first week, which is an anxious time for patient/caregiver, who is developing independence from the hospital setting.

Be aware that, with any modem technology, actual throughput depends on line quality and the presence of quantization noise. Any interference from nearby electrical devices can introduce error into the signal; consult with HME vendor regarding modem technology and applications.

DOCUMENTATION GUIDELINES

Document the following on the visit report:

- The procedure and patient toleration of ventilator dependance

- Cardiopulmonary status
- Teaching, intervention, or procedures implemented (for example, suctioning) and response to teaching
- Ventilator settings or any changes or pertinent findings, such as mode, breath rate, high- and low-pressure alarm limit settings, the patient's high and low pressure reading, V_T, Fio_2, and PEEP (if used)
- Multidisciplinary services and care coordination (physical therapy, occupational therapy, speech therapy, social worker, or home care aide may be involved)
- Any patient/caregiver concerns such as home environment, equipment, resources, or psychosocial needs
- Physician notification, if applicable
- Other pertinent findings
- Standard precautions

Update the plan of care

THE PATIENT WITH CHRONIC WOUNDS

Robyn Rice

Although there are a variety of different types of wounds, home care nurses commonly visit and plan care for those patients who have wounds that do not easily heal. These are referred to as chronic wounds. How do chronic wounds differ from acute wounds such as incisions? Chronic wounds tend to result from an underlying disease process such as vascular insufficiency as opposed to acute wounds, which begin with a stab injury that disrupts vasculature, resulting in hemostasis and activation of the inflammatory response.[9] Because the inflammatory response drives the wound-healing cascade, its absence or suppression may help explain the delayed wound healing seen in chronic wounds.

Chronic wounds commonly seen in home care include pressure or decubitus ulcers, arterial ulcers, diabetic ulcers, and venous stasis ulcers. In a recent survey of four home care agencies, patients with chronic wounds represented an average of 37% of the open cases.[32] Home care may become the most cost-effective and patient-preferred way to manage these disorders, although there is a continued need for research in this area.

The purpose of this chapter is to provide current information about wound healing to assist home care nurses in developing a plan of care for patients with chronic wounds. In additional, the information is presented in such a manner that it may be applied to management of acute and surgical wounds.

ETIOLOGY AND PATHOPHYSIOLOGY OF CHRONIC WOUNDS

Cells join and network to form all body tissues, including the skin. The skin, which is composed of many different kinds of cells, provides support and protection for underlying structures (Box 14-1).

The skin depends on adequate circulation to meet its metabolic needs. Blood transported by arteries and arterioles into capillary beds delivers the oxygen and nutrients that are vital for cellular growth and function. Deoxygenated blood containing toxic by-products of cellular metabolism moves out of the capillary beds and is transported away by venules and veins.

When circulation to the skin is insufficient or disrupted for significant periods of time, cells become essentially oxygen starved and die. Cellular death and necrosis of the skin are manifested by wounds, areas of breakdown, or lesions. The following etiologies of cellular necrosis and delayed wound healing are multifactorial but are primarily related to impaired circulation and a loss of skin integrity.[2,3,8,16,31]

Disease states

Certain diseases are related to circulatory impairment and tissue necrosis. For example, congestive heart failure and peripheral vascular disease contribute to edema and tissue ischemia. Diabetes mellitus, trauma, and neurological or neoplastic disorders can produce losses in sensation and mobility that may cause tissue deterioration and delayed wound healing.

In addition, hyperglycemic-induced leukocyte dysfunction and valvular dysfunction predispose diabetic patients to infection and gangrene. This is why wound management of diabetic patients must include not only measures to maximize tissue perfusion, but also measures to control blood glucose levels.

Box 14-1   THE SKIN

The skin is the largest organ of the body, comprising about 15% of the normal body weight. An acid pH of 4.2 to 5.6 regulates and balances the skin's own natural flora of microorganisms. This flora is unique to each person and, under normal circumstances, serves as a complex line of defense against other potentially pathogenic microorganisms.

The skin is composed of three adjoining layers: the epidermis, the dermis, and the subcutaneous tissues. The outer layer of the skin, the epidermis, is about 0.04 mm thick and without blood supply. The amount of melanin (a dark brown or black pigment) in the epidermis determines the color of the skin.

The epidermis is composed of many layers. Of particular note are the horny layer (stratum corneum) and the basal layer. The basal layer (stratum germinativum) is the basement membrane of the epidermis and depends upon the underlying dermis for nutrition. Epithelial cells at the basement membrane of the epidermis slowly migrate to the outer surface of the skin, the stratum corneum. In this process, called *keratinization,* upwardly migrating epithelial cells lose their nuclei, becoming flat and densely packed. Keratinization occurs at a constant rate, ensuring that cells naturally sloughed off at the surface are regularly replaced. Dry and tough in character, the stratum corneum permits evaporation of water from the skin (insensible loss). The permeability of the stratum corneum allows for the delivery of topical medication into the underlying tissues and systems. Hair follicles, sebaceous glands, and sweat glands are a part of the epidermis and extend downward into the dermis.

The dermis is well supplied with blood and is about 0.5 mm thick. Containing blood vessels, nerve endings, lymphatics, and connective tissue, the dermis is elastic and hardy. The major cell type of the dermis is the fibroblast, which is responsible for the production of collagen and elastin. Collagen gives the skin its tensile strength whereas elastin provides the skin with its elastic recoil. The dermis supports the epidermis and is composed of two layers, the papillary layer and the reticular layer. The dermis merges with the third layer of the skin, the subcutaneous tissues.

The subcutaneous layer, also referred to as the hypodermis, connects the dermis to underlying structures. It contains fat, connective tissue, and nerve endings in addition to blood and lymph vessels. The subcutaneous layer of the skin protects and insulates underlying structures from injury and also provides caloric reserves for the body.

The function of the skin is to provide protection, thermoregulation, and sensation. All three layers of the skin play a role in wound healing. The epidermis is responsible for resurfacing of the wound; however, it is the dermis and subcutaneous tissues that regulate wound repair and tissue regeneration.

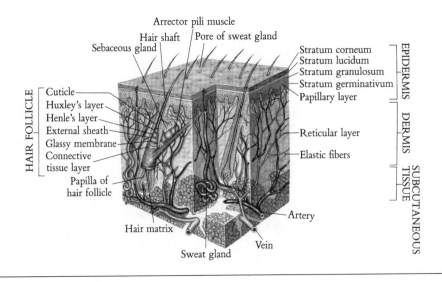

Nutrition

Anemia and poor nutritional status affect the amount of oxygen and nutrients delivered to the cells and impair wound healing. For example, vitamin C and iron are necessary for fibroblast proliferation and subsequent tissue granulation.[12,30] B complex vitamins, copper, and zinc are needed for collagen formation.[6,15] Furthermore, although undernourished patients with protein deficiencies may have defects in leukocyte (white blood cell) function, obese patients are especially hard to heal because of poor vascularization of fatty tissue. In addition, hemoglobin levels below 12 g/100 ml slow healing because oxygen is required for collagen synthesis.[16]

Oxygen and nutrients are the building blocks of a healthy metabolism and tissue generation. In a study of 232 nursing home patients, there is a positive correlation between the development of pressure ulcers and nutritional deficiencies.[30] Consequently a deficient caloric intake, especially a deficient protein intake, is associated with open and chronic, draining wounds.[12,16,30]

Wound contamination

Wound contamination due to moisture, incontinence, and other sources of infection complicates and delays healing. This can be related to inadequate skin care in which patient hygiene is neglected.

Chemical irritants

The presence of chemicals on the skin may cause damage and wound formation. For example, solutions of povidone-iodine (Betadine), improper use of products (tape, skin sealants), and drainage of bodily fluids will erode the epidermis.[26]

Cognitive status, self-neglect, and dependent elder abuse

Certain mental, cognitive, or behavioral states such as confusion, lack of education, or self-neglect may contribute to skin breakdown. For example, smoking reduces the amount of oxygen delivered to cells for metabolic needs. In a study by Guralnik and others, smokers were shown to be 2.9 times more likely than nonsmokers to develop pressure sores.[16] In addition, caregivers who essentially leave the patient to lay in his or her stool or urine place the patient at risk for tissue breakdown and

should be reported as appropriate. See Chapters 8 and 23 for dependent elder abuse guidelines.

Medications

Medications have been shown to influence tissue destruction and repair.[21] For example, steroids delay wound healing. Fibroblast production and tissue generation, discussed in Box 14-1, are slowed with topical administration of steroids onto the wound.[9] Systemic or topical administration of vitamin A can offset the antiinflammatory effects of steroids; however, vitamin A does not appear to speed wound repair in and of itself.[24,35]

Tranquilizers and analgesics can depress sensation and mobility, predisposing the patient to further tissue breakdown. Although topical antimicrobials can enhance healing of contaminated wounds, systemic antibiotics may have little effect on chronic wound healing because of poor circulation and disbursement of the medication.[21,22]

Mechanical forces

Among the primary causes of tissue destruction are prolonged pressure over weight-bearing bony prominences and external forces that interrupt or block circulation. The internal capillary blood pressure, referred to as the capillary closing pressure, is estimated to be about 25 to 32 mm Hg.[22] When external forces and prolonged pressure exceed capillary closing pressure, the vessels collapse and thrombose. They are then unable to assist in meeting the metabolic demands of tissue. This results in ischemia and cellular death with subsequent tissue breakdown and the formation of the wound.

In addition to pressure, forces such as friction and shearing disrupt circulation and damage skin integrity. Abrasion and erosion of the epidermis occur when the skin rubs against another surface, causing friction. Such defects in the skin can become infected and promote ulcer formation. Sacral ulcers are largely attributed to the forces of shearing.[8,21] A common situation that results in shearing occurs when the patient sits with the head of the bed elevated, placing the majority of pressure on the sacral area. As the patient slides down toward the foot of the bed, sacral skin sticks to the sheets and essentially remains in the same place. However, the deep, underlying tissue and muscle are pulled downward, resulting in stretching and tearing of integument and vessels. Consequently, ischemia and a shear ulcer with undermining usually develops. Improper techniques of turning and repositioning the patient also contribute to shearing and friction with resultant skin breakdown.

Age

A failing immune system and reduced mechanical strength of the skin (both associated with aging) place the elderly at risk for skin breakdown. In addition, problems with circulation, diet, elimination, and mobility that are more common in the elderly may complicate the course of wound healing.

CLASSIFICATION OF CHRONIC WOUNDS

Classification and treatment of chronic wounds rests on an understanding of the pathophysiology of tissue destruction and wound repair. For purposes of this chapter, chronic wounds are classified on the basis of cause as pressure or decubitus ulcers, venous ulcers, arterial ulcers, and diabetic or neuropathic ulcers.

Pressure or decubitus ulcers

Pressure ulcers, also referred to as bedsores or decubitus ulcers, result from excessive, unrelieved pressure or from external forces such as shearing or friction. Pressure ulcers are likely to occur over weight-bearing, bony prominences or where the body is exposed to a firm, unyielding surface for varying lengths of time.[3] The patient's position determines the anatomical site at risk for ulceration. However, most pressure ulcers occur on the lower half of the body. The relationship among pressure, time, and body position appears to be a critical determinant in the formation of pressure ulcers. Studies have shown that application of pressure to tissue in excess of 32 mm Hg for 1 to 2 hours is sufficient to cause tissue ischemia and breakdown resulting in pressure sores.[22,24]

Venous ulcers

Venous ulcers result from chronic venous insufficiency (often resulting from a valvular defect) and are characteristically found on the lower extremities. Normally, venous flow is enhanced by exercise, during which contracting leg muscles create pressures that augment blood return to the heart. Factors such as obesity, poor circulation, heart failure, or aging of the veins can contribute to venous valvular incompetence.[36] Valvular incompetence and poor mobility further predispose blood flow to back up into the venous system, leaking out of the capillaries and into tissue. Deprived of oxygen, this edematous tissue becomes ischemic and highly susceptible to breakdown with resultant ulcer formation.

Venous stasis ulcers are associated with firm but edematous extremities that often are stained reddish-brown. This is referred to as "hard" or brawny edema. Cellulitis may accompany these ulcers, which are characteristically shallow and have ragged, uneven edges with copious drainage. A green or yellow wound bed indicative of infection is commonly seen in these ulcers as related to poor circulation to the area.[36] They may be painless to moderately painful.

Fibrin cuffs may also play a role in venous ulcer formation and delayed wound healing. It has been postulated that fibrinogen, leaking into tissue as a result of incompetent valves, may accumulate around capillaries and form a fibrin cuff. These cuffs are believed to block the exchange of oxygen into the cell and prevent capillaries from dilating in response to increased metabolic demands of the tissue. The role of fibrin cuffs in venous ulcer formation and treatment is still under investigation.

Arterial ulcers

Arterial ulcers develop as a result of a constricted or blocked artery. They are often associated with peripheral vascular disease and atherosclerosis.[9] Blood flow to the cells is impaired, producing ischemia and tissue breakdown that results in an ulcer. Arterial ulcers usually develop on the toes or heel of the foot.

The affected extremity is usually pale and hairless with a weak or questionable pulse that reflects the ischemic state. Typically a dry ulcer, the arterial ulcer has well defined edges and is usually deep with a necrotic and black wound base. Arterial ulcers are extremely painful.

Diabetic or neuropathic ulcers

Diabetic patients may exhibit an ulcer on the foot with both circulatory and neurological origins. Impaired circulation and neurological sensation occur as a result of a chronic hyperglycemic state.[25] Ulcerations can also develop in diabetic patients as a consequence of painless trauma in the presence of peripheral neuropathy and a depressed inflammatory response. Diabetic ulcers often look like arterial ulcers. They may or may not be painful and are associated with osteomyelitis. As discussed in Chapter 15, diabetic patients are at significant risk for ulcer formation with resultant lower extremity amputation.

To summarize, when capillary blood flow to the skin is impaired, the cells become ischemic and die. Consequently, necrotic wound formation occurs. The patient's overall health and a number of other factors cited in this section will also reflect the course of tissue breakdown and wound healing.

MECHANISMS OF WOUND HEALING

Wound healing is a very intricate and complex process that may be classified into three primary phases: (1) the inflammatory phase, (2) the restoration phase, and (3) the remodeling phase. All three phases occur in sequence but may overlap. The duration of each phase varies with the extent of tissue damage, any concomitant disease state, and patient lifestyle and self-care factors.

Inflammatory phase

In the inflammatory phase, initial tissue damage and bleeding cause vasoconstriction and the formation of a fibrin-platelet clot. The injured tissue releases histamine and bradykinin, which cause capillary dilatation. Intracellular fluid, proteins, and plasma components leak into the extracellular spaces, causing local increases in skin temperature, swelling, and redness (erythema). This leakage creates a moist environment that attracts different kinds of leukocytes (white blood cells) to the injured area. The leukocytes then begin to debride and cleanse the wound by phagocytizing bacteria, dead cells, and necrotic tissue, eventually becoming part of the wound exudate. Additionally, leukocytes stimulate wound healing. For example, macrophages, a type of leukocyte, not only clean up the wound but also release a protein that stimulates the formation of fibroblasts. Fibroblasts, major components of the dermis, are responsible for collagen synthesis and connective tissue reconstruction, which occur in the next phase.

Restoration phase

Wound repair in the restoration phase (sometimes referred to as the proliferative or fibroblastic phase)

progresses at a rate dependent on the depth of the wound. If the wound is deep with significant loss of dermis and underlying tissue (full thickness wounds), angiogenesis (capillary growth) and granulation of lost tissue must precede the regeneration of the epidermis (epithelization). Superficial tissue loss (shallow or partial thickness wounds) may only need regeneration of the epidermis for repair.

In full thickness wounds, tissue regeneration and granulation begins with angiogenesis. Angiogenesis, the formation and budding of new capillary beds that nourish cellular growth, is thought to be stimulated by macrophages and tissue hypoxia.

During the restoration phase, the wound bed forms granulating tissue that is beefy red, highly vascular, and shiny in appearance. At this point, contraction of the wound bed may also occur, pulling the edges of the wound together and decreasing the area that needs to be filled by new tissue.

Epithelization takes place over a moist, vascular bed of tissue and often accompanies connective tissue repair of the dermis. The wound bed takes on a pink color (especially around the edges), characteristic of the newly formed epithelial cells. Drawn to a moist substrate, epithelial cells migrate from the wound edges onto the red granulating tissue. Epithelial cells may also emerge from intact hair follicles, forming dots of pink tissue in the red wound bed. These epithelial cells advance until they meet other epithelial cells. Once contact between epithelial cells is made, migration stops—a phenomenon referred to as contact inhibition. The defect in the skin is then closed, producing a scar.

A moist wound, free of contamination, promotes leukocyte migration and subsequent wound repair.[20,24] Dried, hard scabs and thick eschar have been shown to retard wound healing because epithelial cells must tunnel underneath the scab to close the wound.

Remodeling phase

During the remodeling phase, collagen (a fibrous protein that lends strength to all body tissues) is resynthesized and reorganized into increasingly tighter and stronger patterns. The collagen fibers are primarily remodeled by fibroblasts, forming the many layers of the epidermis and subsequent scar.

With the formation of the epidermis, the metabolic demands of the skin eventually slow down. When oxygen requirements lessen, capillary networks shrink and retreat, giving scars their characteristically white and bloodless appearance. Scars of full thickness or deep wounds are typically hairless because the hair follicles, a part of the epidermis, do not regenerate if destroyed. Scar tissue has about 80% of its previous strength and is very susceptible to future tissue breakdown.

The preceding review of the causes of tissue destruction and the mechanisms of wound repair leads to some general conclusions about treatment. Wound healing is enhanced by the following:

- A moist wound environment (this means that dead space or the wound cavity must be moisturized and not allowed to dry out)
- A wound bed free of necrotic tissue, eschar, and environmental contamination or infection
- An adequate blood supply to meet metabolic demands for tissue generation
- Sufficient oxygen and nutrition for cellular metabolism and tissue generation
- Elimination of causative factors of tissue breakdown
- Patient/caregiver participation in the plan of care

HOME CARE APPLICATION
Developing the plan of care

Several points should be considered when implementing wound care in the home. The patient/caregiver will have a very active role in wound care because the home care nurse's exposure to the wound will be periodic and intermittent. Therefore, although the plan of care is guided by the physician, the home care nurse and the patient/caregiver must come to some agreement regarding its appropriateness (Box 14-2). Even the best interventions are useless unless the patient/caregiver is willing and able to comply with specific wound care protocols and recommendations. See Chapters 2 and 7 for further information on patient self-care and educational strategies.

A patient referral to the registered dietitian may be helpful in reinforcing the importance of diet in wound healing. For example, patients with open and draining wounds may need to increase their caloric intake to as much as 3000 to 4000 calories/day with the recommended daily protein intake of approximately 2 g/kg[12,15] (see Appendix XIV-I). A referral for home care aide services may be re-

quired for those patients who have limited functional ability and require assistance with activities of daily living (ADLs). Consult with rehabilitation services to evaluate any problems with immobility or functional disability. In addition, the social worker may be able to identify community resources to assist with patient financial needs for wound care products, special beds, etc.

Wounds, like the patients who have them, are capable of dynamic changes. As the condition of the wound shifts, for better or worse, treatments and planned visits should be adjusted accordingly. Documentation on the visit report should validate the visit frequency and subsequent need for treatment.

Visit frequency

The frequency of planned home visits is based on the assessment of patient/caregiver education needs, the condition of the wound, related comorbidities, and provider coverage for care. Home care nurses, as case managers, should be aware of all of these factors when developing the plan of care.

In view of Medicare regulations for reimbursement of home visits, daily or bid visits for usually 1 or 2 weeks may be done for infected, heavily draining, or complex wounds that are overwhelming for the patient/caregiver.[17] Thereafter, visits to the home should decrease as the wound heals and the patient/caregiver becomes comfortable and adept in dressing changes. Eventually the home care

Box 14-2 PRIMARY NURSING DIAGNOSIS/PATIENT PROBLEMS

- Impaired skin integrity
- Pain
- Risk for infection
- Knowledge deficit: for example, disease process and risk complications, medications, operation of home medical equipment, procedural care, diet, infection control, socioeconomic resources, available community services
- Altered nutrition: less than body requirements
- Body image disturbance
- Self-care deficit:__ADLs,__Feeding,__Toileting,__Other (*Specify*)

nurse would then visit the patient 1 or 2 times a week to evaluate the wound's progress toward healing and the patient's readiness for discharge from home care services. See Chapter 9 for tips to secure visits when working with health maintenance organizations (HMOs).

Patient education

Self-care management of the wound is encouraged through patient/caregiver education. When devising the plan of care, initial assessment should determine whether the patient is able to learn wound care. If not, a designated caregiver or family member should be identified who is willing and able to assist with care plan implementation; this is the person who should observe initial dressing changes and learn the wound care regimen (Box 14-3).

When teaching wound care in the home, it is important to be sure that the "why" and "how" aspects of care are understood. Consequently the patient/caregiver will require a great deal of instruction on wound assessment and when to call the physician and case manager regarding complications in care, dressing changes, proper use of any equipment, and lifestyle habits influencing tissue breakdown and wound healing. Routine skin care will also be an important part of health teaching. If the patient or caregiver is doing the dressing change, clean technique is usually taught.

Box 14-3   PRIMARY THEMES OF PATIENT EDUCATION

- Wound assessment: when to call the case manager and physician
- When to call 911
- Medications: purpose, action, dosage, side effects, and methods of administration
- Use, operation, and maintenance of home medical equipment
- Dressing changes and related procedural care
- Diet
- Infection control
- Lifestyle habits that influence wound repair
- Socioeconomic resources
- Community services or alliances available for people with chronic and debilitating illness
- General self-care strategies

It may be worthwhile to write up guidelines for specific dressing changes and post them in a convenient place in the patient's home (such as on the refrigerator) as a way of ensuring that everyone is correctly following treatment regimens (Box 14-4).

Medications

Patients with infected wounds are often placed on antibiotics. Patients should be taught the appropriate use of their antibiotic in order to successfully treat the wound and reduce the emergence of antibiotic-resistant pathogens. It is important to emphasize to the patient that he or she must take the full course of the antibiotic therapy in order for the medication to be effective. If oral therapy is ineffective, consider placing the patient on intravenous (IV) antibiotic therapy.[35] See Chapter 18 for IV antibiotic guidelines. Recommended alternative antibiotics for the treatment of serious wound infections that are caused by resistant organisms are vancomycin for methicillin-resistant *Staphylococcus aureus* (MSRA), ceftriaxone (Rocephin), cefotaxime (Claforan), or vancomycin for vancomycin-resistant enterococci (VRE); and combined beta-lactam and aminoglycoside therapy for VRE.

Infection control

Wound infection prolongs the inflammatory phase and delays healing. *Bacteroides* is the most common anaerobe, and *Pseudomonas* and *Staphylococcus* are the most common aerobes cultured. A green color or fruity odor often indicates *Pseudomonas,* whereas a fetid odor is often associated with an anaerobic infection. Assess the wound for infection and culture when appropriate.

When culturing the wound, gently cleanse with a physiological solution (such as normal saline) to remove debris before obtaining the culture. Using a swab, obtain the culture by moving across the wound bed using a zigzag motion (Figure 14-1). Consult with the physician; some form of antibiotic may be required (see discussion of medications).

Home care nurses should perform dressing changes using an aseptic technique when possible, especially with diabetic patients because of risk of infection and lower extremity amputation. Likewise, dressing changes should be done so that part of the dressing does not get lost in the patient's wound or overlooked in subsequent changes. Such an occurence can create a serious infection and cer-

---

Box 14-4   PATIENT/CAREGIVER EDUCATION GUIDELINES: WOUND CARE

1. Always wash your hands before and after changing your dressing because good hand-washing will help keep your wound clean and prevent the spread of germs.
2. Keep all your medical supplies in a clean area; boxes of dressings, gloves, and other medical supplies may be stored in a clean plastic trash-bag.
3. Discard wound care solutions after 1 week or sooner if you see particles forming in the container or if the solution changes color or becomes cloudy.
4. Notify the home health organization if you are running out of supplies.
5. Gather up your supplies. Prepare a plastic bag for disposal of dirty dressings and supplies.
6. Prepare your new dressing as your case manager has instructed you. All caregivers should wear gloves when assisting you with your dressing changes.
7. Carefully remove your old dressing and look at your wound. Any noticeable differences in size, color, or drainage should be reported to your case manager or home health aide at the next visit.
8. Apply your new dressing as the case manager has shown you. Follow the instructions below for specific steps to put on your new dressing. Your dressing should be changed according to schedule or if it comes off or becomes wet or moist. Seal and dispose of the bag in your family trash.
9. Call your case manager if you have an elevated temperature or problems with pus or excessive wound drainage or if swelling or pain occur with your wound.

Specific Steps to Clean Your Wound and Change Your Dressing:

Patient/caregiver signature: _____ Date: _____
Case manager signature: _____ Date: _____
Care path #: *1-Skin/Integumentary*
White copy-patient's home record; Yellow copy-medical record
Copyright 2000; American Nursing Development, Maryville, Ill.

---

tainly delay wound healing. Nurses should recognize the potential for this when packing a wound and make sure the wound is packed in a manner so that old dressings are easily detected and removed.

Patients/caregivers are usually taught clean technique in the home. It is important to explain to the patient/caregiver the idea that infection slows healing. Potential sources or circumstances promoting infection in the wound should be identified and discouraged. If the home is unclean or has dirt floors, ask the patient always to wear socks and shoes to protect the skin from germs. Medical supplies can be kept fairly clean if stored in a plastic trash bag and kept off the floor.

Wound assessment and evaluation of healing

Although there is much information on wound management, nationally there is some disagree-

Start

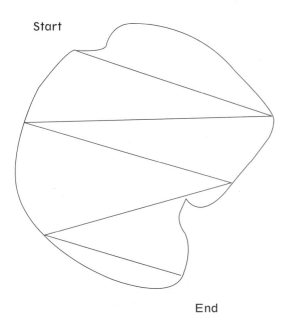

End

Figure 14-1 Using a zigzag method to culture the wound.

ment on uniform standards of evaluation. A variety of classification systems and measurement techniques exist in the literature. Classification methods that include staging and the red, yellow, black system are popular. Photography, tracings, molds, and linear measurement techniques are also used. Although it is recognized that trends among many practitioners are now focusing more on an objective assessment, staging of pressure sores and other chronic wounds continues to remain an acceptable method of classification. Additionally, a critique of the red, yellow, and black system of wound measurement is that it does not systematically account for the depth of the wound, which certainly impacts the type of dressing used. In the *Clinical Practice Guidelines on Pressure Ulcers in Adults* by the Agency for Health Care Policy and Research (AHCPR)*, staging of pressure ulcers (Figure 14-2) reflects recommendations from the National Pressure Ulcer Advisory Panel (NPUAP) and others:[18,28,29]

---

*Note: Name has been changed to Agency for Healthcare Research and Quality (AHRQ)

Stage I: Nonblanchable erythema of intact skin; the heralding lesion of skin ulceration. Note: Reactive hyperemia can normally be expected to be present for one half to three fourths as long as the pressure occluded blood flow to the area; it should not be confused with a stage I pressure ulcer.

Stage II: Partial thickness skin loss involving epidermis and/or dermis. The ulcer is superficial and presents clinically as an abrasion, blister, or shallow crater that is often red; painful.

Stage III: Full thickness skin loss involving damage or necrosis of subcutaneous tissue that may extend down to, but not through, underlying fascia. The ulcer presents clinically as a deep crater with or without undermining of adjacent tissue. Undermining and copious drainage of exudates may be present; usually painless. These wounds often have yellow, green, or black wound beds.

Stage IV: Full thickness skin loss with extensive destruction, tissue necrosis, or damage to muscle, bone, or supporting structures (for example, tendon or joint capsule). Copious drainage of exudates, undermining, and sinus tracts may be present; usually painless. These wounds often have yellow, green, or black wound beds.

Be aware that staging has limitations, which include (1) difficulties in staging pressure ulcers in patients with darkly pigmented skin, (2) difficulties in accurately staging the wound until the eschar has sloughed or the wound has been debrided, and (3) difficulties in problems with subjective interpretation among field staff when staging.

In order to overcome some of these problems, the author recommends that wounds should be measured at least weekly by the case manager (the same nurse) to ensure consistency in documentation. In addition, irrigate the wound before assessing it to get an accurate measurement. Finally, the home care agency should have uniform policies regarding wound measurement, evaluation, and management in order to promote quality care and uniform documentation.

The visible portion of the wound may represent only a fraction of actual tissue necrosis (undermining). Therefore when assessing depth and size of the wound, explore the wound base with a sterile swab for signs of undermining or sinus tract formation.

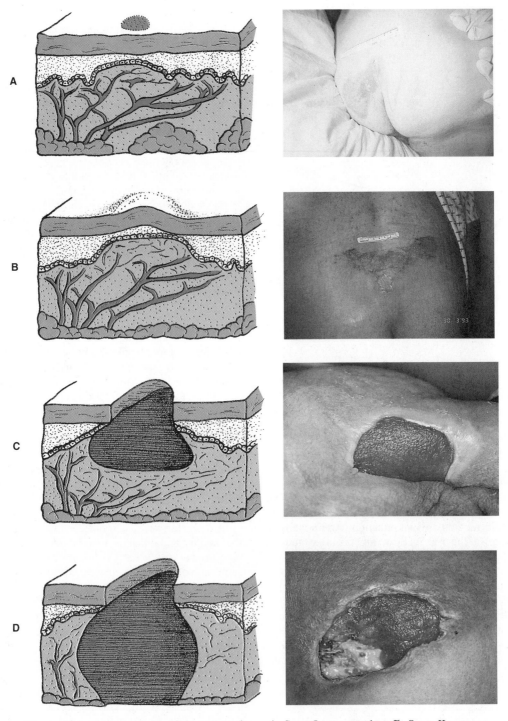

Figure 14-2 Diagram of stages of pressure ulcers. **A,** Stage I pressure ulcer. **B,** Stage II pressure ulcer. **C,** Stage III pressure ulcer. **D,** Stage IV pressure ulcer. (From Lewis SM and others: *Medical-surgical nursing: assessment and management of clinical problems,* ed 5, St. Louis, 2000, Mosby.)

Skin assessment and measurement of wounds should include the size and extent of the wound along with any potential areas of breakdown. Black patients may not show typical reddened areas over affected tissue; however, heat and swelling can easily be palpated over tissue subjected to pressure. The author recommends using staging with a combination of descriptive wound assessment parameters, including the following:

- All measurements in centimeters
- Anatomical location (where is the wound located)
- Length, width, and depth of wound
- Description of wound bed (color, appearance of tissue)
- Presence/absence of undermining (consider a clock with the patient's head being at the 12 mark and the feet being at the 6 mark; note where the undermining is deepest according to its position in relation to hands on a clock)
- Presence/absence of odor (avoid subjective descriptions of odors; simply note a yes or no according to findings)
- Color and amount (small, moderate, large) of drainage or wound exudate
- Wound stage according to AHRQ recommendations
- Condition of surrounding skin
- Associated risk factors predisposing patient to skin breakdown

Current trends in wound care

Wound care products. Many wound management products are noteworthy. As described earlier, leukocyte migration and epithelization are enhanced when a moist substrate is present. Current trends in many wound products suggest that use of a moist dressing to loosely fill dead space within the wound cavity fosters a healing environment, in addition to providing protection from contamination.[10,11,40] There is a vast array of wound care products on the market.[19] Some of these products currently available are listed in Appendix XIV-II. Topical moisturizers, foams, gels, transparent adhesive dressings, hydrocolloid dressings, and impregnated gauze dressings (to name a few) are now being used to moisturize the wound and protect it from secondary infections. Occlusive dressings such as hydrocolloids should not be used on wounds with excessive purulence, deep sinus

tracts, bone or tendon exposure, or in severely immunocompromised patients because of incidence of anaerobic infections.[20] In these cases, a moist gauze dressing is recommended.

Calcium alginate dressings are useful in controlling drainage.[7,37] Do not use calcium alginate dressings in wounds with minimal or no drainage because they will further dry out the wound bed. Remember, you want a moist wound bed and not one that is flooded with infectious drainage or one that is dried out.

Research in chronic wound care is exploring the use of growth factors.[34] Growth factors are small proteins, secreted as intercellular messengers, that regulate the growth of different cell types. Addition of exogenous growth factors could be a new therapeutic approach to management of chronic non-healing ulcers.

Cleansing and debridement. There also have been recent developments in wound cleansing and debriding.[5,38] Along with the use of heat lamps, historically wounds were essentially scrubbed with solutions such as povidone-iodine (Betadine) or acetic acid until they bled. It is now known that just as the removal of eschar, pus, and exudate promotes healing, abrasive cleansing and irrigation of healthy, pink granulating tissue destroys the fibroblasts responsible for collagen synthesis.

Antiseptic solutions, such as povidone-iodine (Betadine), acetic acid, and Dakin's have been shown not only to kill bacteria, but to destroy fibroblasts and viable tissue.[26] The same holds true for several aseptic solutions such as hydrogen peroxide. Therefore physiological or detergent solutions (normal saline or water-based) are recommended for wound cleansing and irrigation.[23] There are always exceptions to the rule. If antiseptic or aseptic solutions *must* be used on an infected wound, apply a dilute concentration of 25% (one-fourth strength) or less.[14,26]

Plan cleansing and debriding treatments on the basis of wound bed assessment. For example, do not use wet-to-dry dressings on clean, granulating tissue as this will erode a healthy wound bed. Such tissue will only require gentle irrigation with a physiological solution and topical moisturizing. Yellow, green, or black wound beds will likely require debridement as discussed below.

Mechanical debridement can be achieved by hydrotherapy (whirlpool or Water Pik), normal saline wet-to-dry dressing changes, irrigation with a

35-ml syringe attached to an 18- or 19-gauge needle, or gently cleansing the wound with soap and water.[9,13,38] If using home whirlpool therapy, the patient may wish to purchase a plastic trash can solely for whirlpool therapy. Bathtubs can be difficult for the elderly to move around in and often do not prevent oversplash of water created by the whirlpool. Instruct the patient/caregiver to clean the trash can after each use with a 10% bleach solution, rinse it out with tap water, and allow it to air dry. Emphasize that the trash can is to be used solely for the patient's whirlpool therapy.

Chemical debridement involves application of one of the numerous topical debriding agents now on the market. Topical debriding agents have enzymatic qualities that liquefy eschar, facilitating its removal. Chemical debridement should be done by home care nurses who have received in-service training on the technique and should be discontinued once eschar is removed. Product instructions must be followed carefully, avoiding application of the enzymatic compound to healthy tissue. When using a chemical debriding agent, consider encircling the wound with a hydrocolloid dressing during the procedure as an additional safety measure to prevent potential destruction of healthy tissue. Enzymatic preparations are not active in a dry environment and should not be used on dry eschar. Crosshatch eschar with a scalpel and keep the wound surface moist for optimal effects.

When surgical debridement with a sharp instrument is needed for thick, black eschar, consult the physician.

Negative pressure wound therapy, also known as vacuum-assisted closure (VAC) is a new treatment in which controlled negative pressure is used to evacuate wound drainage, stimulate granulating tissue, and decrease the potential for wound infection.[27] The device is composed of a pump and sponge and essentially converts an open wound into a controlled closed wound. Consult with the local medical supplier for more information on VAC.

Current trends in pressure management

Although the role of pressure in wound formation has been well described, pressure management continues to be redefined and improved. Patients at risk for wound formation, as well as those with open wounds, should be placed on a regimen of skin care that controls exposure to forces of friction, shearing, and pressure. The use of elbow/heal protectors, socks, or a sheepskin may be helpful to relieve friction and prevent excessive pressure on soft tissues. If pressure is not relieved, all other interventions are relatively ineffective.

Minimize moisture from urine or stool, perspiration, or wound drainage to prevent chemical irritation. When moisture cannot be controlled, consider use of (1) pads or briefs that absorb urine and have a quick-drying surface that keeps moisture away from the skin, (2) a cream or ointment to protect the skin from urine, stool, or wound drainage, and (3) a rectal pouch to control incontinence of feces.

Emphasize proper seating position for chair-bound patients. In the presence or likelihood of skin breakdown on the ischia, sacrum, or coccyx, a correct upright sitting position is even more important to address. Sitting has many benefits (including improved breathing, circulation, mobility, and independence), which improve the healing process and overall health of the patient. (Refer to Chapter 17 for proper positioning techniques to seat chair-bound patients.)

Wrinkle-free sheets, simple schedules for turning from side to back to side, and techniques of correct body positioning continue to be effective interventions in pressure management. Placing the patient in a 30-degree oblique position almost totally prevents forces of shearing and can usually be done by family members using a couple of pillows. Turning schedules should be individualized to meet the patient's needs or coordinated with care activities (Box 14-5).

Not all patients have available caregivers to assist with a turning schedule or skin regimen. It may be necessary to recommend various types of medical equipment that can be purchased or rented from the home medical equipment (HME) vendor to prevent the deleterious effects of excessive pressure on soft tissue. At present, equipment is recommended for pressure management based on the degree of patient mobility and is classified as either a pressure reduction or pressure-relief device.[1,39]

Pressure reduction devices. Pressure reduction devices are recommended for patients who are able to assist with turning and have some degree of mobility. Trapeze bars and side rails may also be used to aid in turning and moving. Pressure reduction devices do not consistently maintain pressure below capillary closing pressure but have been

---

Box 14-5   RECOMMENDATIONS FOR PRESSURE ULCER PREVENTION IN ADULTS

Skin care

1. All individuals at risk for pressure ulcers should have a systematic skin inspection daily.
2. Skin cleansing should occur at the time of soiling and at routine intervals.
3. Minimize environmental factors leading to skin drying such as low humidity (less than 40%) and exposure to cold. Dry skin should be treated with moisturizers.
4. Avoid massage over bony prominences.
5. Minimize skin exposure to incontinence, perspiration, or wound drainage.
6. Minimize the forces of shearing and friction through proper positioning, transferring, and turning techniques. In addition, friction injuries may be reduced by the use of lubricants (such as cornstarch and creams), protective films (such as transparent film dressings and skin sealants), protective dressings (such as hydrocolloids), and protective padding.
7. Encourage good nutrition.
8. Consider rehabilitation referral for problems with immobility.

Mechanical loading and support surfaces

1. All individuals in bed who are assessed to be at risk for developing pressure ulcers should be repositioned at least every 2 hours if consistent with overall patient goals. Use a written turning schedule.
2. For individuals in bed, positioning devices such as pillows or foam wedges should be used to keep bony prominences (for example, knees or ankles) from direct contact with one another.

3. Individuals in bed who are completely immobile should have a care plan that includes the use of devices that totally relieve pressure on the heels. *Do not use donut-type devices.*
4. When the side-lying position is used in bed, avoid positioning directly on the trochanter.
5. Maintain the head of the bed at the lowest degree of elevation consistent with medical conditions and other restrictions. Limit the amount of time the head of the bed is elevated.
6. Use lifting devices such as a trapeze or bed linen to move (rather than drag) individuals in bed who cannot assist during transfers and position changes.
7. Any individual assessed to be at risk for developing pressure ulcers should be placed (when lying) on a pressure-reducing device, such as foam, static air, alternating air, gel, or water mattresses.
8. Any person at risk for developing a pressure ulcer should avoid uninterrupted sitting in a chair or wheelchair. The individual should be repositioned, shifting the points under pressure at least every hour or be put back to bed if consistent with overall patient management goals. Individuals who are able should be taught to shift weight every 15 minutes.
9. For chairbound individuals, the use of a pressure-reducing cushion is recommended. *Do not use donut-type rings.*
10. Positioning of chairbound individuals in chairs or wheelchairs should include consideration of postural alignment, distribution of weight, balance and stability, and pressure relief.

Modified from National Panel for the Prediction and Prevention of Pressure Ulcers in Adults: *Pressure ulcers in adults: prediction and prevention.* Clinical practice guideline No 3, AHCPR Pub No 92-0047, Rockville, Md, 1992, Agency for Health Care Policy and Research, Public Health Services, U.S. Department of Health and Human Services.

---

shown to be effective in preventing tissue necrosis with patients who are able to turn or move. This category includes water mattresses, gel pads, foam mattresses or pads, air support mattresses, and a variety of seated cushions.[29]

In recommending a cushion for the seated patient, correct wound care protocol dictates that the cushion should remove pressure from and ventilate the wound site. Therefore the ischials should be suspended in air, not encased in foam, gel,

rubber, or vinyl. In addition, when considering what type of pressure reduction device to use, evaluate the appropriateness of the product as related to the patient's weight. For example, a high-density foam mattress may work well with a patient of normal weight but may be useless for an extremely obese patient. The HME vendor should be able to provide patient weight guidelines and product information. Avoid the use of donut rings; these generally do more harm than good.[28]

Pressure-relief devices. Pressure-relief devices are useful for patients with complete immobility and limited caregiver assistance. Pressure-relief devices (for example, air-fluidized therapy) maintain pressures below capillary closing pressures. The patient essentially floats on a fluid medium that distributes pressure evenly.[1] The patient's home must have appropriate electrical outlets and structural support because these beds are electric and may weigh 2000 pounds or more. Additional costs of these surfaces should also be a consideration because the continued use of electrical service will be realized in the patient's electric bill. Air flotation beds may render patient management at home easier for elderly caregivers who have difficulty meeting the demands of a frequent turning schedule, and may be more cost-effective in wound management for certain patients.[1,4] Patients on air-fluidized therapy should be well hydrated because this treatment can cause dehydration by increasing water loss through the skin and respiratory tissues.

Current philosophies of wound care blend the new with the old. Frequent position changes, use of medical equipment, application of cornstarch-based powder on the bed, use of transparent adhesive films or hydrocolloid dressings over areas at risk for breakdown, limiting the head of the bed position to 30 degrees to prevent shearing, incontinence management, and good nutrition all promote wound healing. However, the question of what dressing is appropriate for what wound is necessary to consider.

Specific therapy: matching wounds to treatments and products

Treatment for all types of wounds should primarily be guided by four goals:[10]

1. Prevention of further tissue destruction by reducing or controlling predisposing causes of tissue destruction
2. Prevention of infection
3. Planning treatments as appropriate for (a) the type of chronic wound (pressure, venous, arterial) and (b) the condition and size of the wound (stage, amount of drainage, and related factors)
4. Patient/caregiver preferences for care and abilities for self-care

Recommendations for specific therapy of chronic wounds first begin with a discussion of as-

sessment findings and treatment options with the patient/caregiver, and physician. Decide among all what will work best in order to mutually determine a plan of care, including wound treatment protocols that the patient/caregiver is willing and able to follow. Specific treatment guidelines are as follows:

Stage I: Nonblanchable erythema of intact skin
Interventions and specific treatment: prevention. Use pressure reduction techniques along with application of transparent adhesive films to protect "reddened" areas of skin at risk for breakdown (Box 14-6). Institute skin care regimen for stages I to IV. Condition is reversible with prompt intervention.

Stage II: Partial thickness wound
Interventions and specific treatment: clean/protect. Gently cleanse/irrigate the wound bed with physiological or detergent solution. Application of a hydrocolloid dressing, transparent adhesive film, foam, topical moisturizer, or impregnated gauze dressing will maintain a moist environment for healing and protect the wound from environmental contamination.

Stage III: Full thickness wound: shallow
Interventions and specific treatment: debride/absorb/protect. Filled with eschar, slough, and copious exudate, these wounds are often infected. Use a physiological solution to cleanse and irrigate. A diluted concentration of an antiseptic or aseptic solution may be useful when working with highly infected wounds. However, as healthy tissue (red) appears, the home care nurse is strongly urged to switch to a physiological solution for cleansing and irrigation because antiseptic and aseptic solutions are cytotoxic.

Debride the wound as ordered by the physician. Eliminate dead space in the wound with an absorber (foam or granules or light packing with moistened gauze dressing) and cover with a secondary protective dressing. Calcium alginate dressings may help control excessive drainage.[7] Avoid solitary use of transparent adhesive films or hydrocolloid dressings; these will not fill dead space. Consult with the physician; antibiotic therapy—either systemic or topical (silver sulfadiazine cream)—may also be useful. In addition, negative pressure wound therapy may be helpful to control copious drainage that does not respond to other therapies.[27]

**Box 14-6   APPLICATION OF HYDROCOLLOID DRESSINGS AND TRANSPARENT
ADHESIVE FILMS**

Purpose

- To promote wound healing
- To minimize pain and infection
- To protect the skin

General information

Hydrocolloid dressings and transparent adhesive films are useful to protect excoriated, reddened, or blistered areas of skin. They are used on partial thickness wounds. Transparent adhesive films are semipermeable dressings that are commonly used to protect skin against friction.

Equipment

1. Hydrocolloid dressing and transparent adhesive film (see Appendix XIV-II)
2. Hypoallergernic tape
3. Plastic sheet or towel
4. Disposable nonsterile and sterile gloves, protective apron (see Chapter 6)

Procedure

1. Explain procedure to the patient/caregiver.
2. Assemble equipment in a convenient work area.
3. Assist the patient to a comfortable position to expose the wound. Place a plastic sheet or towel under the patient to prevent soiling of linen. Drape the patient for privacy.
4. Gently remove old tape and dressing. Assess the drainage on the old dressing; then discard in a plastic trash bag and secure.
5. Clean and irrigate the wound as prescribed by the physician. Clean from least contaminated area to the most contaminated area.
6. Inspect the wound, and evaluate it for healing.
7. Pat wound edges dry with a gauze pad, making sure surrounding skin is free of oily or greasy substances. Consider use of a skin prep to anchor the dressing.
8. Prepare dressing (hydrocolloid dressings and adhesive films are sterile and should be handled appropriately) in the following manner:
   a. Cut and prepare the dressing so that it covers a 1 1/2 inch margin of healthy skin.
   b. Carefully remove the paper backing from the dressing to prevent contamination of the sterile adhesive side.
9. Apply hydrocolloid dressing and adhesive film in the following manner:
   a. Gently *roll* the dressing over the wound (avoid stretching).
   b. Shape and mold the dressing into place, securing it around the wound edges; shape, mold, cut, and taper the dressing for hard-to-fit areas.
10. Secure the hydrocolloid dressing and adhesive film with hypoallergenic tape as needed.
11. Change the hydrocolloid dressing and transparent adhesive film about every 3 to 7 days or as required for leakage. (The hydrocolloid dressing may leave a gel residue in the wound bed; irrigate the wound with a normal saline solution; then apply a new dressing.)
12. Provide patient comfort measures.
13. Clean and replace equipment. Discard disposable items in a plastic trash bag and secure.

Nursing considerations

Perform wound care using sterile technique, unless ordered otherwise by the physician. Instruct the patient/caregiver in the clean technique as approved by the physician.

Documentation guidelines

Document the following on the visit report:
- The treatment and condition of the wound (each visit)
- Appearance of the wound bed (black, yellow, green, tan, red, or pink)
- Wound measurements (at least weekly), including the length, depth, and width of the wound in centimeters
- Depth and location of undermining in centimeters
- Inflammation or erythema of the skin around the wound
- Color, odor, and estimated amount of drainage
- Stage the wound weekly, and compare the progress with the goals of therapy
- Any patient/caregiver instructions on wound care and patient's adherence to instructions, including ability to change dressings
- Physician notification, if applicable
- Standard precautions as applicable
- Other pertinent findings
Update the plan of care.

Modified from Rice R: *Manual of home health nursing procedures,* ed 2, St. Louis, 2000, Mosby.

Stage IV: Full thickness wound: deep

Interventions and specific treatments: essentially same as for stage III.

VENOUS STASIS ULCERS. Treatment should control edema and promote healing. Underlying medical and nutritional disorders should be corrected. For example, congestive heart failure should be controlled to reduce lower-extremity edema. If obesity is present, a weight reduction program should be initiated.

Periodically elevating the legs above the level of the heart with the use of compression therapy will control edema. Examples of compression therapy include compression stockings, elastic wraps, and the Unna boot. Instruct the patient to put compression stockings or Ted Hose on before getting out of the bed in the morning. Compression stockings are to be worn all day. Elastic wraps or bandages should be placed on the leg when edema is minimal in order to maximize compression and venous return. Likewise, the application of a compression dressing such as the Unna boot is helpful to control edema (Box 14-7).

A hydrocolloid dressing over the ulcer in combination with an impregnated gauze dressing or a hydrocolloid-based elastic bandage may also prevent edema and promote healing. In addition, calcium alginate–based compression dressings have been shown to be beneficial, because they pick up exudates and absorb drainage yet maintain a moist environment for wounds that are at risk for maceration. Follow suggested interventions for stage II wounds.

ARTERIAL AND DIABETIC ULCERS. Arterial and diabetic ulcers are difficult to treat because of their relatively ischemic state. Wound management should be directed toward the following:

- Avoiding excessive pressure to the area by total non–weight-bearing or corrective shoes/inserts
- Cleansing/debriding the wound (consult with the physician regarding debriding agent; debridement is contraindicated in the presence of gangrene because removal of eschar results in an open wound with impaired blood flow and susceptibility to infection; in this case surgical intervention is strongly recommended)[9]
- Preventing infection
- Supporting the patient (encourage good nutrition, control edema, and control disease process—blood glucose and blood pressure)

Compression therapy is generally contraindicated in patients with an ischemic injury. Tight, restrictive clothing or ill-fitting shoes should also be avoided.

Because diabetic patients tend to lose sensation in the feet, improper weight distribution and subsequent tissue destruction may occur. Orthotics are specially fitted shoes designed to prevent such traumatic ulceration. In addition, total contact casts or below-the-knee plaster casts with minimal padding over bony prominences may be used to reduce forces of shearing and pressure in noninfected ulcers. Trauma must be avoided.

Activities will likely be limited for patients with peripheral vascular disease if the ulcer is to receive maximal perfusion. Patients with diabetes should never use hot water bottles or foot soaks to "warm up" the feet because warmth increases the demand for blood. If neuropathy is present with arterial insufficiency and this increased demand for blood cannot be met, tissue injury results. (Refer to Chapter 15; pay close attention to recommendations for diabetic foot care.) Utmost emphasis should be placed on teaching the patient to seek care for even the smallest wound.

The use of topical antibacterials and systemic antibiotics to treat an ischemic ulcer varies among practitioners. Although a topical antibacterial may help control infection, systemic antibiotics may not reach the wound bed because of poor circulation.[35] Topical medications that contain steroids are not recommended because they trigger vasoconstriction.

Patients with ischemic ulcers are at tremendous risk for gangrene and lower extremity amputation. Aseptic technique in dressing changes is advised and often difficult for the patient/caregiver to learn. Therefore the physician should be encouraged to order dressing changes to be done only by the home care nurse until the wound is sufficiently healed to prevent the risk of gangrene.

Infected diabetic ulcers require immediate surgical excision of eschar and necrotic tissue. In addition, vascular surgery may be required when the blood flow is significantly impaired or treatment fails.

Documentation

Services planned and medical equipment and supplies ordered by the physician are the basis for Medicare reimbursement of wound care at home. Appropriate documentation of the patient's condi-

---

Box 14-7   APPLICATION OF MEDICATED COMPRESSION DRESSING

Purpose
- To promote healing of venous stasis ulcers and to minimize cellulitis
- To minimize pain and infection

General information

The medicated dressing or Unna boot is used to control edema and to promote healing of poorly vascularized areas of the leg and foot. The Unna boot is often used to treat venous stasis ulcers.

Equipment

1. Medicated compression dressing or Unna boot (see Appendix XIV-II)
2. Gauze or elastic bandage
3. Hypoallergenic tape
4. Plastic sheet or towel
5. Disposable nonsterile and sterile gloves, protective apron (see Chapter 6)

Procedure

1. Explain the procedure to the patient/caregiver.
2. Assemble the equipment at a convenient work area.
3. Assist the patient to a comfortable position to expose the lower leg. Place a plastic sheet or towel underneath the leg to prevent soiling the linen or the floor. Drape the patient for privacy.
4. Gently remove the old tape and dressing. Assess the drainage on the old dressing; then discard the dressing in a plastic trash bag.
5. Clean and irrigate the wound as ordered by the physician. Clean from the least contaminated area to the most contaminated area.
6. Inspect the wound and evaluate it for healing versus signs of infection.
7. Apply medicated compression dressing or Unna boot by wrapping the dressing from above the toes to below the knee to control edema.
8. Cover the heel with oblique turns.
9. Make circular, figure-of-eight turns around the leg, overlapping each turn by half the width of the medicated dressing.
10. Cover the entire area 2 to 3 times. Do not make reverse turns, because such turns cause unnecessary creases and pressure.

11. Cut and smooth the dressing to avoid creases or pleats.
12. Apply gauze or elastic bandage over the medicated dressing for support and to absorb copious drainage; then secure the gauze or elastic bandage with hypoallergenic tape.
13. Change the dressing 1 or 2 times a week. Remove the medicated compression dressing or Unna boot in the following manner:
    a. Remove the elastic bandage or gauze wrap.
    b. Carefully cut and remove the dressing from the leg (soaking the dressing loose decreases the debriding effect).
14. Provide patient comfort measures.
15. Clean and replace the equipment. Discard disposable items in a plastic trash bag and secure.

Nursing considerations

Perform wound care using sterile technique, unless ordered otherwise by the physician.
    Clean technique is often used with leg ulcers.

Documentation guidelines

Document the following on the visit report:
- The treatment and condition of the wound (each visit)
- Appearance of the wound bed (black, yellow, green, tan, red, or pink)
- Wound measurements (at least weekly), including the length, depth, and width of the wound in centimeters
- Depth and location of undermining in centimeters
- Inflammation or erythema of the skin around the wound
- Color, odor, and estimated amount of drainage
- Stage the wound weekly, and compare the progress with the goals of therapy
- Any patient/caregiver instructions on wound care and patient's adherence to instructions, including ability to change dressings
- Physician notification if applicable
- Standard precautions as applicable
- Other pertinent findings

Update the patient care plan.

Modified from Rice R: *Manual of home health nursing procedures,* ed 2, St. Louis, 2000, Mosby.

tion is crucial. Medicare views the following nursing skills as basic to wound care[17]:

- Direct hands-on wound care treatment (procedural)
- Skilled observation and assessment of the wound
- Patient/caregiver education regarding treatment and interventions

On each visit, the home care nurse should document the treatment and procedural care and evaluate the wound for signs of healing versus infection. As discussed previously, measure and stage wounds weekly. Focus documentation of wound management on complicated procedural dressing changes, the need for patient education, and evaluation of wound healing along with any comorbidity status that requires the services of the skilled nurse. Wound care is covered by Medicare as long as the need for skilled care and the need for treatment are clearly and precisely documented.[17] As case managers, home care nurses should be aware of other provider guidelines for documenting wound care.

Despite everyone's best efforts, healing may not always occur, and the patient may require hospitalization for more intensive therapy.

SUMMARY

Home care nurses have a powerful influence over wound healing. Although the physician directs and guides the treatment, it is the home care nurse who orchestrates the plan of care. As case manager, the nurse's role is collaborative with patients/caregivers and physicians. Changes in the plan of care and home visit frequency rely heavily on nursing assessment and recommendations for treatment. It is not uncommon for patients and physicians to seek advice from the nurse regarding which products work best with different types of wounds and when treatment should be modified.

Such a powerful voice must be informed. Home care nurses best meet this challenge by being knowledgeable about current trends and products for wound care and by being sensitive to the unique relationship between patient, wound, and home environment.

REFERENCES

1. Allman R and others: Air-fluidized beds or conventional therapy for pressure sores, *Ann Intern Med* 107:641, 1987.
2. Anthony D and others: An evaluation of current risk assessment scales for decubitus ulcer in general inpatients and wheelchair users, *Clin Rehabil* 12(2):136, 1998.
3. Barczak CA and others: Fourth national pressure ulcer prevalence survey, *Adv Wound Care* 10:18, 1997.
4. Barnes S, Rutland B: Air-fluidized therapy as a cost-effective treatment for a "worst case" pressure necrosis, *J Enterostomal Ther* 13(1):27, 1986.
5. Barr JE: Principles of wound cleansing, *Ostomy/Wound Manage* 41:155, 1995.
6. Bobel L: Nutritional implications in the patient with pressure sores, *Nurs Clin North Am* 22(2):379, 1987.
7. Bpharm T: Use of a calcium alginate dressing, *Pharm J* 8:188, 1985.
8. Braden B: Preventing pressure sores, *Home Health Focus* 4(1):6, 1997.
9. Bryant R: *Acute and chronic wounds,* ed 2, St. Louis, Mosby, (in press).
10. Cuzzell J: Choosing a wound dressing, *Geriatr Nurs* 18(6):260, 1997.
11. Cuzzell J: Wound care across the continuum, *Home Health Focus* 4(11):84, 1998.
12. Dantone JJ: Medical nutrition therapy: the patient with pressure sores. In Rice R, editor: *Manual of home health nursing procedures,* ed 2, St. Louis, 2000, Mosby.
13. Diekmann J: Use of a dental irrigating device in the treatment of decubitus ulcers, *Nurs Res* 33(5):303, 1984.
14. Doughty D: A rational approach to the use of topical antiseptics, *Ostomy Wound Manage* 40(6):50, 1995.
15. Flanigan K: Nutritional aspects of wound healing, *Adv Wound Care* 10(2):48, 1997.
16. Guralnik J and others: Occurrence and predictors of pressure sores in the national health and nutrition examination survey follow up, *J Am Geriatr Soc* 36(9):807, 1988.
17. Health Care Financing Administration: *Home health insurance manual,* Pub No 11, Washington, DC, 1995, US Department of Health and Human Services.
18. Henderson CT and others: Draft definition of stage I pressure ulcers: inclusion of persons with darkly pigmented skin, *Adv Wound Care* 10:16, 1997.
19. Hess C: Wound care products: a directory, *Ostomy Wound Manage* 40(3):70, 1994.
20. Hutchinson J: Prevalence of wound infection under occlusive dressings: a collective survey of reported research, *Wounds* 1(2):123, 1989.
21. Kosiak M: Etiology and pathology of ischemic ulcers, *Arch Phys Med* 40(1):63, 1959.
22. Kosiak M: Etiology of decubitus ulcers, *Arch Phys Med* 42(1):19, 1961.
23. Kucan J and others: Comparison of silver sulfadiazine, povidone-iodine and physiologic saline in the treatment of chronic pressure ulcers, *J Am Geriatr Soc* 19(5):232, 1981.
24. Kurzuk-Howald G and others: Decubitus ulcer care: a comparative study, *West J Nurs Res* 7(1):58, 1985.
25. Laing P: Diabetic foot ulcers, *Am J Surg* 167(1A):31S, 1994
26. Linneaweaver W and others: Topical antimicrobial toxicity, *Arch Surg* 120:257, 1985.
27. Mendes-Eastman S: Negative pressure wound therapy, *Plast Surg Nurs* 18(1):27, 1999.

28. National Pressure Ulcer Advisory Panel: *Pressure ulcers in adults: prediction and prevention.* Clinical practice guideline No 3, AHCPR Pub No 92-0047, Rockville, Md, 1992, Agency for Health Care Policy and Research, Public Health Service, US Department of Health and Human Services.

29. National Pressure Ulcer Advisory Panel: *Treatment of pressure ulcers.* Clinical practice guideline No 15, AHCPR Pub No 95-0652, Rockville, Md, 1994, Agency for Health Care Policy and Research, Public Health Service, US Department of Health and Human Services.

30. Pinchcofsky-Devin G, Kaminiski M: Correlation of pressure sores and nutritional status, *J Am Geriatr Soc* 34(6):435, 1986.

31. Pontieri-Lewis V: The role of nutrition in wound healing, *Med Surg Nurs* 6:187, 1997

32. Rice R: Wound prevalence and cost in home care: a survey of one community based home care agency and three hospital-based home care agencies—case study presentation. Paper presented at the National Association for Home Care, San Diego, October 1999.

33. Rice R: Dermatological care. In Rice R, editor; *Manual of home health nursing procedures,* ed 2, St. Louis, 2000, Mosby.

34. Robson MC: The role of growth factors in the healing of chronic wounds, *Wound Repair Regeneration* 5:12, 1997.

35. Robson MC and others: The efficacy of systemic antibiotics in the treatment of granulating wounds, *J Surg Res* 16:299, 1974.

36. Rudolph DM: Pathophysiology and management of venous ulcers, *J Wound Ostomy Continence Nurs,* 25(5):248, 1998.

37. Scurr JH and others: A comparison of calcium alginate and hydrocolloid dressings in the management of chronic venous ulcers, *Wounds* 6(1):1, 1994.

38. Thomas S: Assessment and management of wound exudate, *J Wound Care* 6(7):327, 1997.

39. Thomason S and others: Specialty support surfaces: a cost containment perspective, *Decubitus* 6(6):32, 1993.

40. Williams RL, Armstrong DG: Wound healing: new modalities for a mew millenium, *Clin Podiatr Med Surg* 15(1):117, 1998.

Medical Nutrition Therapy: Pressure Ulcers

PURPOSE

- To educate individuals who are at risk of developing pressure ulcers (PUs) by identifying nutrition risk factors and biochemical markers
- To provide instruction on appropriate nutritional measures to prevent PUs
- To offer nutritional interventions for treatment of existing PUs
- To promote self-care in the home

GENERAL INFORMATION

The following factors are associated with PU development:

- Progressive dependency on others to meet activities of daily living (ADLs)
- Low body weight, low body mass index, or small triceps skinfolds
- Low serum albumin level
- Low serum cholesterol level
- Low hemoglobin and hematocrit levels

Extrinsic variables include shearing forces and friction. Intrinsic variables include malnutrition; anemia; reduced oxygen delivery to tissue, which already may be ischemic; both increased and decreased body weight; elevation of temperature; skin moisture—particularly incontinence and dehydration—either from low fluid intake or high fluid loss from excessive wound drainage; diuretic therapy; diarrhea and vomiting; acute blood loss; or uncontrolled diabetes. The etiology of pressure ulcers appears to be multifactorial and often the result of multiple pathologic processes. The common thread of treatment of all of these conditions is improvement of the patient's nutritional status. With the use of the proper medical nutrition therapy (MNT), clinical and functional outcomes will be positively affected.

From Dantone JJ: Nutritional care in the home. In Rice R: *Manual of home health nursing producers,* ed 2, St. Louis, 2000, Mosby.

EQUIPMENT

1. Cloth measuring tape
2. Scales or recent weight history
3. Calculator
4. Food labels
5. Food models
6. Measuring cups and spoons commonly used by the patient
7. Blood pressure cuff, stethoscope, thermometer, and glucose meter

PROCEDURE

1. Explain the procedure to the patient/caregiver.
2. Consider implementing the following:
   a. Assessing vital signs on each visit; weigh the patient at least weekly; report abnormal findings to the physician
   b. Assessing the patient's skin and wound; report abnormal findings to the physician
   c. Setting nutritional requirements for patient

      or

      Identifying the calorie, protein, and fluids required by the patient, using the following guidelines (discuss with the patient/caregiver the importance of the patient meeting the following nutrient requirements):
      - **Calories**—minimum of 30 to 35 kcal/kg body weight
      - **Protein**—1.2 to 1.5 g protein/kg body weight
      - **Fluids**—minimum of 1500 ml (unless medically contraindicated) or 30 ml/kg body weight per day
   d. Recording a 24-hour recall of the patient's nutritional intake on the food diary form; analyze the total calories and protein content of the diet intake
   e. Instructing the patient/caregiver on the diet instruction sheet and menu for wound

Box XIV-I   WOUND HEALING DIET (High Protein, High Iron, High Vitamin C)

Reason for the Diet

To help you learn which foods are needed to correct iron deficiency and anemia and to heal skin problems, pressure sores, surgery, broken bones, and/or burns.

How Much and/or What to Eat

Breakfast	Lunch and dinner (same)
Orange, grapefruit, or tomato juice	3-4 oz meat or meat substitute
Cereal	Starch
2 eggs	Vegetable
Bacon, ham, or sausage	Salad with dressing
Toast, biscuit, or muffin	Bread
Margarine	Margarine
Jelly, syrup, or gravy	Dessert
Milk	Milk (both meals)
Coffee or tea	

Do Not Eat These Foods

There are no foods you cannot eat on this diet. But if your appetite is poor, do not drink a lot of coffee, tea, or soft drinks with caffeine, which will make your appetite even worse.

Special Instructions

It is important that you eat at least one serving from each of the basic four food groups at each meal. This combination of foods will increase the iron in your blood and keep it normal. The basic four food groups are listed below. The foods high in protein, iron, or vitamin C are listed for each food group. The foods in italic type and followed by an asterisk are highest in iron.

Meat or Meat Substitutes

beef *	*oysters* *	turkey	peanut butter
pork *	*dried beans, peas* *	lamb	nuts
liver *	*red meats* *	veal	
eggs *	chicken	fish	

Milk

whole milk	nonfat instant milk	cheese	pudding
buttermilk	milk shakes	yogurt	chocolate milk
ice cream	cottage cheese		

Breads and Cereals

"instant" cream of wheat *	*bran cereal* *
"Total" dry cereal *	*fortified or enriched cereal* *

Fruits and Vegetables

Dried fruits (e.g., prunes, raisins, apricots, apples, dates, figs) *		*Greens (e.g., turnips, mustards, collard,*	
spinach *	oranges	*chard, kale)* *	
grapefruit juice	tomatoes	orange juice	grapefruit
broccoli	white potatoes	tomato juice	V-8 juice

Other

Molasses * (the darker the better)

For wound healing, it is suggested that your diet intake include zinc and vitamin C. The recommended amounts to heal a wound is zinc sulfate 220 mg (or zinc 50 mg) once a day and vitamin C 500 mg twice a day. Zinc should be taken only if a deficiency exists. Your physician will notify you of such a deficiency, based on the results of a blood test. Any vitamin/mineral supplement should be approved by the physician first. Also drink plenty of water—1 to 2 quarts per day as tolerated, according to your weight. A vitamin or mineral supplement pill should be taken with a citrus juice, such as orange juice, to increase the absorption of iron.

Modified from Dantone JJ: *Bridging the gap diet manual,* Grenada, Miss, 1997, Nutrition Education Resources.

Table XIV-I Menu for wound diet (High protein, high iron, high vitamin C)

	Sunday	Monday	Tuesday
Breakfast	Orange juice	Grapefruit juice	Tomato juice
	Total cereal	Instant cream of wheat	Total cereal
	2 Eggs of choice	2 Eggs of choice	2 Eggs of choice
	Sausage	Bacon	Sausage
	Biscuit or toast	Biscuits or toast	Biscuit or toast
	Margarine	Margarine	Margarine
	Dark molasses	Dark molasses	Dark molasses
	Milk	Milk	Milk
	Coffee	Coffee	Coffee
Lunch	Fried chicken livers	Sandwich with:	Roast turkey
	Dried black-eyed peas	Cheeseburger	Giblet gravy
	Seasoned greens of choice	Bun	Cornbread dressing
	Buttered cornbread	Lettuce/pickle/onion	English peas
	Banana	Mayonnaise/mustard	Cranberry sauce
	Coffee	Baked potato	Coconut cake
		Margarine/sour cream	Milk
		Apple cobbler	
		Milk	
Dinner	Ham	Beef tips	Potato salad
	Potato salad	Gravy	Tuna salad sandwich
	Seasoned green beans	Rice	Sliced tomatoes
	Buttered roll	Buttered broccoli	Crackers
	Pineapple tidbits	Buttered biscuit	Mayonnaise
	Milk	Stewed prunes	Fresh orange
		Milk	Milk

From Dantone JJ: *Bridging the gap diet manual,* Grenada, Miss, 1997. Reprinted with permission Nutrition Education Resources.

healing (Box XIV-I and Table XIV-I); use food models, measuring utensils, and food labels to demonstrate calorie and protein content of different foods

f. Comparing the patient's 24-hour diet recall to his or her prescribed diet order as instructed; make appropriate recommendations to the patient/caregiver for modifying any nutrients found to be inappropriate on the food intake record

g. Discussing with the patient the importance of accurately measuring the foods as listed on the diet instruction sheet; illustrate correct measurement using standard measuring cups and spoons; in the home setting, identify utensils that can be used to measure foods

h. Discussing with the patient the times of the day he or she usually eats meals; compare those times to the times indicated on the diet instruction sheet; work with the patient to establish a regular eating pattern, due to the importance of food and medication timing in controlling the patient's disease process

i. Discussing the following nutrition risk factors for PUs with the patient/caregiver:
- Significant weight loss
- Significantly low weight for height
- Poor appetite, not meeting nutritional requirements
- Significant change in functional status (ADLs)
- Deficient biochemical markers—albumin, prealbumin, hemoglobin, hematocrit, cholesterol
- Vitamin/mineral deficiency
- Dehydration

- Presence of disease management processes (e.g., diabetes, Alzheimer's)
- Presence of factors that reduce dietary intake (e.g., dysphagia, depression)

j. Discussing with the patient/caregiver the importance of prevention of PUs; the key in preventing PUs is routine assessment of nutritional status and estimation of the patient's nutritional intake; food preference and consistency tolerances must be individualized to each patient; instruct the patient/caregiver how to be creative with food preparation methods, seasonings, types of foods to keep the menu selections appetizing and yet sufficient in nutrients; continual reassessment of the patient's food intake through logging of a food intake diary is helpful

k. Supplementing vitamins/minerals; the importance of each should be taught to the patient/caregiver; because of possible toxicity and nutrient interactions, vitamin/mineral supplementation in high doses is not recommended unless the patient is suspected of being deficient; the physician should order any vitamin/mineral; consider the following:

- Vitamin C—helps make collagen, promotes healing, helps build resistance to infection; requirements are increased in acute stress, malnutrition, and with smoking
- Stage I to II: patients may require 100 to 200 mg vitamin C daily
- Stage III to IV: patients may require 1000 to 2000 mg vitamin C daily
- Vitamin A—helps body make new skin cells
- RDA is 800 to 1000 μg RE for adults
- Zinc—promotes wound healing, improves immunity; assess the patient's serum zinc level for deficiency before administering a zinc supplement; 15 to 25 mg of zinc per day may be beneficial in healing PUs; zinc is not recommended in quantities of more than 50 mg per day because of the possibility of causing a copper deficiency, leading to anemia
- Iron—helps carry oxygen to nourish cells
- RDA is 10 to 15 mg for adults

3. Clean and replace equipment. Discard disposable items according to standard precautions.

NURSING CONSIDERATIONS

Treatment depends on the stage of the pressure ulcer. Pressure ulcers are classified, or staged, according to the degree of tissue damage.

The literature on treating pressure ulcers with MNT emphasizes increasing protein intake. Before increasing protein intake, assess total energy intake first. The body's first priority is adequate energy intake.

DOCUMENTATION GUIDELINES

Document the following on the visit report:

- The procedure and patient toleration
- Vital signs
- Calorie, protein, and fluid requirements of the patient
- Medical treatment used for PUs
- Nutrition interventions/treatments used for PUs
- Analysis of the patient's food intake and the modifications suggested
- Patient/caregiver instruction and response to teaching, including understanding of the diet and adherence to nutritional recommendations
- Answers to feedback questions
- Physician notification, if applicable
- Standard precautions
- Other pertinent findings

Update the plan of care.

Dermal Wound Care Products

Product	Manufacturer	Comments
PHYSIOLOGIC SOLUTIONS		Isotonic solutions used in wound irrigation and mechanical debridement; no chemical or antiseptic action
Normal saline	Generic	
Ringer's lactate	Generic	
ANTISEPTIC SOLUTIONS		
Acetic acid	Generic	Known to inhibit growth of *Pseudomonas aeruginosa*, *Trichomonas* vaginalis, and *Candida albicans;* strong concentrations may destroy fibroblasts; dilute to 0.25%
Alcohol/ethanol	Generic	Use only on iodine-sensitive patients
Povidone-iodine	Generic	Can be absorbed through any body surface except adult intact skin; dries skin; may destroy fibroblasts unless properly diluted to <1%
Dakin's (diluted sodium hypochlorite)	Generic	Controls odor; may interfere with coagulation; solution unstable; replace every day
ASEPTIC SOLUTIONS		
Hydrogen peroxide	Generic	Use only on wounds with necrotic debris; can separate new epithelium from underlying tissue; do not use in abdominal cavity because gas may invade capillaries and lymphatics; slightly warms wound, enhancing vasodilation and decreasing inflammation; in strong concentrations, shown to destroy fibroblasts; dilute to <3%
Zephiran Chloride (benzalkonium)	Generic	Inactivated by soaps; rinse wound thoroughly with normal saline solution before use; reported to enhance growth of some *Pseudomonas* species; do not cover with occlusive dressings
DETERGENT SOLUTIONS		Isotonic solutions used in wound irrigation and mechanical debridement; no antiseptic action
Cara Klenz	Carrington Labs	
Safclens	Calgon-Vestal-Merck	
Constant-Clens	Sherwood Medical	
COTTON DRESSINGS (GAUZE)		
Fine-mesh gauze	Generic	Approximately 41 to 47 thread count in a 4- × 4-inch pad; capillary beds rarely grow into the interstices of fine mesh and are not damaged when dressing is removed
Wide-mesh gauze	Generic	Approximately 30 to 39 thread count in a 4- × 4-inch pad; used in mechanical debridement because coarse weave allows necrotic debris to adhere to dressing for removal
COTTON DRESSINGS (IMPREGNATED)		Drying out adversely affects wound healing
Adaptic	Johnson & Johnson	
Melolite	Smith-Nephew	
Mesalt	Scott Health Care	
Scarlet-Red	Cheesbrough-Ponds	
Zeroform	Sherwood Medical	
Vaseline gauze	Cheesbrough-Ponds	

From Rice R: *Manual of home health nursing procedures,* ed 2, St. Louis, 2000, Mosby.

Product	Manufacturer	Comments
COMBINATION DRESSINGS		Provide nonadherent, absorbent layer within a transparent membrane
Viasorb	Cheesbrough-Ponds	
Polymen	Ferris	
Nu-Derm	Johnson & Johnson	
COTTON DRESSINGS (PASTE BANDAGE)		Cotton mesh, impregnated with zinc oxide, calamine (Unna boot), and gelatin; dries to provide extremity with compression and support; no gaps should be left in bandage, otherwise edema will accumulate
Unna boot	Miles Pharmaceuticals	
Viscopaste	Smith-Nephew	
EXUDATE ABSORPTIVE DRESSINGS		Absorb and wick up bacteria and exudates
Bard Absorption	Bard Home Health	
Debrisan	Johnson & Johnson	
DuoDerm Granules	ConvaTec	
DuoDerm Paste	ConvaTec	
Hydra-Gran	Baxter	
Hydron	Bioderm Sciences	
Algosteril	Johnson & Johnson	
Kaltostat	Calgon-Vestal-Merck	May be used in conjunction with prescribed solution for copious-draining wounds; is not the treatment of choice for wound management because gauze may leave particles and fibers in the wound
Sorbsan	Dow Hickman	
Wound Exudate	Hallister	
Absorber Gauze	Generic	
FOAM DRESSINGS		Avoid using in wounds with dry eschar
Allevyn	Smith-Nephew	
Epi-Lock	Calgon-Vestal-Merck	
Lyofoam	Ultra Labs	
Primaderm	Absorbent Cotton Corporation	
Synthaderm		
HYDROCOLLOID DRESSINGS		Dressing change required about every 4 to 7 days or PRN for leakage; relatively impermeable to gas and vapor exchange; use with caution in deep, full thickness wounds because it may foster anaerobic infection
Comfeel Pressure Relief Dressing	Kendall	
Comfeel Ulcer Care Dressing	Kendall	
Cutinova Hydro	Beiersdorf Medical	
Duoderm and Duoderm CGF	ConvaTec	
Hydropad	Baxter	
Intact	Bard Home Health	
Johnson & Johnson Ulcer Dressing	Johnson & Johnson	
Restore	Hollister	
Tegasorb	3M	
Ultec	Sherwood Medical	
HYDROGEL DRESSINGS		Available in gel or sheet gel form; normalize wound humidity; sterile as packaged
Intrasite gel	Smith-Nephew	
Vigilon	Bard Home Health	
Geliperm	E. Furgera & Co.	
Nugel	Johnson & Johnson	
Elastogel	Southwest Technologies	

Product	Manufacturer	Comments
HYDROPHILIC POWDER DRESSINGS		Hydrophilic powder dressing that becomes a gel when contact is made with the wound surface
Chronicure	ABS LifeScience	
Miltidex	Lange Medical Products	
TOPICAL DEBRIDING AGENTS		Absorb wound drainage and bacteria
Debrisan	Johnson & Johnson	
DuoDerm Paste	ConvaTec	Physiologic debrider
Elase	Parke-Davis	Indicated for slough and eschar
Santyl	Knoll	Indicated for slough and eschar
Silvadine Cream	Marion Labs	Physiologic debrider with antimicrobial properties; bacterial and fungicidal action maintained for about 12 hours; change twice each day
Travase	Flint Labs	Indicated for eschar; moisten only with sterile water or saline; not appropriate for pregnant women
TOPICAL MOISTURIZERS		Available in gel, granulate, or sheet form
Carrington Gel	Carrington Labs	
Dermagran	Dermasciences	
DuoDerm Paste	ConvaTec	
Geliperm Wet	E. Furgera & Co.	
Second Skin	Spence	
TRANSPARENT FILM (ADHESIVE)		Semipermeable; dressing change required about every 4 to 7 days or PRN; may be used to protect skin against friction
Acuderm	Acme United	
Bio-Occlusive	Johnson & Johnson	
Ensure	Deseret	
Opraflex	Professional Medical Products	
Op-Site	Smith-Nephew	
Polyskin	Kendall	
Tegaderm	3-M	
Uniflex	Acme United	
TRANSPARENT FILM (NONADHESIVE)		Clings to superficial open wounds without the need of adhesive; topicals may be applied to the dressing; removal—when the dressing falls off or by flushing with normal saline solution
Jobskin	Jobst	
Omiderm	Dermatological Research Laboratories (D.R. Labs)	
MISCELLANEOUS (TRADITIONAL)		
Karaya	Generic	Absorbent, adhesive, and hydrophilic properties; promotes wound bed
Insulin	Generic	Enhances protein synthesis by skin; observe for hypoglycemia; apply at mealtimes
Stomahesive	ConvaTec	Useful in debriding thick, hard necrotic tissue
Sugar	Generic	Hypertonic sugar solutions absorb moisture and debris, which may enhance wound healing; use with caution because sugar may provide a medium for bacterial growth
MISCELLANEOUS (CONTEMPORARY)		
Biobrane	Woodruff Labs	Silicone membrane coated with collagen and hydrophilic peptide; drying and sticking to wound bed may damage healthy tissue; often used for burns
Procurren	Curatec	Platelet-derived formula containing growth factors to increase healing of severe and chronic wounds

THE PATIENT WITH DIABETES

Susan Heady

Diabetes mellitus is a disorder characterized by chronic hyperglycemia resulting from defects in insulin secretion, insulin action, or both. The deficiency of insulin leads to marked abnormalities in carbohydrate, protein, and fat metabolism. These disturbances are associated with the development of microvascular and macrovascular complications in persons with diabetes, including retinopathy, nephropathy, neuropathy, and cardiovascular, peripheral vascular, and cerebrovascular disease.[20] The prevalence of diabetes and its long-term complications result in high levels of morbidity and mortality, as well as tremendous personal, social, and economic costs to affected persons and society.[25]

About 10 million people in the United States are known to have diabetes, and there are also large numbers of people with undiagnosed type 2 diabetes. The prevalence of diabetes has been increasing (particularly in the older age groups) and is expected to continue to increase. The incidence is highest in those over age 64 and is increasing in this group. African-Americans, Mexican-Americans, and Native Americans are at increased risk for diabetes and its complications. People with diabetes have an excess risk of mortality from cardiovascular disease even when other risk factors are adjusted.[25]

Diabetes management and education are essential to reducing the incidence and severity of long-term complications.[8] Findings of the Diabetes Control and Complications Trial (DCCT) provide evidence that intensive therapy significantly delays the development and progression of retinopathy, nephropathy, and neuropathy in type 1 diabetes.[19] The results of the United Kingdom Prospective Di-

abetes Study (UKDPS) also suggest similar benefits of near normalization of blood glucose levels in type 2 diabetes.[41]

Home health nurses encounter a wide variety of patients with diabetes and play a significant role in helping them to achieve improved glycemic control and effective self-management of their health care needs. Typical home care patients are elderly adults who may be in poor glycemic control and who may already have complications. This chapter focuses on adult home care patients. Although some of the information also applies to patients who are children or adolescents, information addressing their specific needs is beyond the scope of this chapter.

PATHOPHYSIOLOGY AND CLASSIFICATION OF DIABETES

Diabetes is a group of metabolic diseases with various forms having differing etiologies and clinical characteristics. New recommendations for the classification and diagnosis of diabetes include the preferred use of the terms "type 1" and "type 2" instead of "insulin dependent (IDDM)" and "noninsulin dependent (NIDDM)" to designate the two major types of diabetes. The revised criteria are for diagnosis and not treatment criteria or goals of therapy.[20] Because most home care patients with diabetes have either type 1 or type 2, this chapter focuses on these two types.

Type 1

In type 1 diabetes (formerly referred to as IDDM or juvenile-onset diabetes), there is an absolute deficiency of insulin secretion. This type includes those cases in which an autoimmune pathological process destroys pancreatic islet beta cells. Serological markers of this destruction include autoantibodies (islet cell, insulin, and/or others). The disease also has strong human leukocyte antigen (HLA) associations. The etiology includes both genetic and environmental factors. The rate of beta cell destruction is variable, usually rapid in some (children and adolescents) and slow in others (mainly adults). As a result some are prone to ketoacidosis, whereas others have moderate fasting hyperglycemia, which can rapidly change to severe hyperglycemia and/or ketosis in the presence of infection or other stress. Although type 1 diabetes commonly occurs in children and adolescents, it can occur at any age.[20]

Type 2

Type 2 diabetes (formerly known as NIDDM or adult-onset) is the most prevalent form of diabetes, with 90% of those diagnosed having type 2.[25] This type results from insulin resistance with an insulin secretory defect, or a relative insulin deficiency. There is no evidence of autoimmune beta cell destruction. Most patients are obese and insulin resistant. Ketoacidosis seldom occurs except with a stress situation such as infection.[20]

Type 2 diabetes may go undiagnosed for years because the hyperglycemia develops slowly and may not be severe enough to cause noticeable symptoms, although pathological changes are already occurring in target tissues. Complications may be present at the time of diagnosis. Type 2 is also commonly associated with a strong genetic disposition,[20] older age, positive family history of the disease, minority ethnicity, lower socioeconomic status, obesity, and physical inactivity.[25]

ACUTE COMPLICATIONS

Two hyperglycemic conditions, diabetic ketoacidosis and hyperosmolar nonketotic state, are associated with hospital admission and mortality in persons with diabetes.[30]

Diabetic ketoacidosis

Diabetic ketoacidosis (DKA) consists of the triad of hyperglycemia, ketosis, and acidemia. Insulin deficiency, elevated counterregulatory hormones, and dehydration contribute to the development of DKA. Patients may become drowsy, stuporous, or comatose, with classic symptoms including polyuria, polydipsia, weight loss, vomiting, abdominal pain, Kussmaul respirations, dehydration, acetone odor on the breath, and signs of vascular shock. Precipitating factors include infection, intercurrent illness, and omission of or inadequate insulin therapy.[30]

Hyperglycemic hyperosmolar nonketotic state

Hyperglycemic hyperosmolar nonketotic state (HHNS) is defined by extreme hyperglycemia, increased serum osmolarity, and severe dehydration without significant ketosis or acidosis. Hyperglycemia is usually more severe (greater than 600 mg/dl), dehydration is more pronounced, there is greater incidence of depressed sensorium, and the prognosis is poorer than in DKA. Hyperglycemic hyperosmolar nonketotic state occurs more frequently in the elderly and in patients with newly diagnosed diabetes and often has an insidious onset. Acute illness is the precipitating factor in many cases.[30]

Other common causes of DKA and HHNS are stress and ethanol abuse.[16] Treatment consists of fluid and electrolyte replacement and administration of insulin. Determination and elimination of precipitating factors is essential.[30]

Infection

Infection is the most common precipitating factor for diabetic ketoacidosis or coma, especially in the older person with newly diagnosed diabetes. The occurrence of infection complicates the management of diabetes. Whether the incidence of infection is higher in persons with diabetes remains debatable; however, those with diabetes appear to be at increased risk for infection at specific sites and due to certain organisms. Increased susceptibility to the following has been noted: urinary tract infection (in women only), complications of respiratory infection, bacterial infection of the skin or soft tissues (furuncles and carbuncles, infections of the extremities, necrotizing infections, postoperative wound infection), osteomyelitis, malignant external otitis, vaginitis or vulvitis, phycomycetes infection, and periodontal infection. Poor metabolic control, vascular and neurological abnormalities, and the increased performance of invasive medical procedures are associated with infection in patients with diabetes.[34]

CHRONIC COMPLICATIONS

Long-term macrovascular and microvascular complications occur in both type 1 and type 2 diabetes.[25]

Macrovascular disease

Macrovascular disease accounts for the majority of deaths in those with diabetes. Atherosclerosis involving the coronary, cerebrovascular, and peripheral vessels tends to occur prematurely and with greater severity in persons with diabetes than in the nondiabetic population.[12]

Cardiovascular disease

Coronary heart disease is the leading cause of death in people with diabetes.[25] Since diabetes may be a significant independent risk factor for coronary disease, the importance of modifying other risk factors such as hypertension, hyperlipidemia, weight, and smoking is magnified.[40]

Cerebrovascular disease

Stroke occurs twice as frequently in the diabetic population. Hypertension is a major risk factor and should be adequately controlled.[35]

Peripheral vascular disease

Peripheral vascular disease, peripheral neuropathy, infections, and inadequate foot care increase the risk for lower extremity amputation in individuals with diabetes.[24] More in-hospital days are spent treating problems involving the lower extremities than any other complication of diabetes.[33]

Microvascular complications

Changes in the smaller vessels characterized by thickening of the capillary basement membrane associated with hyperglycemia lead to retinopathy, nephropathy, and neuropathy.[29]

Retinopathy. Diabetic retinopathy is a leading cause of blindness. Retinopathy occurs frequently in both type 1 and type 2 diabetes. The development is related to the duration of diabetes. Characteristic lesions include nonproliferative and proliferative retinopathy.[4]

Nephropathy. Nephropathy is a common complication of both type 1 and type 2 diabetes. Diabetes is the most common cause of end-stage renal disease in the United States.[8] Persistent microalbuminuria indicates the earliest stage of diabetic nephropathy and is a significant risk marker for cardiovascular disease. Untreated hypertension can accelerate the progression of renal disease.[3,8]

Neuropathy. Distal symmetric sensorimotor neuropathy is an important predictor of ulcers and amputation. Loss of sensation and altered foot structure resulting from neuropathy lead to increased risk of foot trauma and diabetic ulcers.[7]

Autonomic neuropathy can affect gastrointestinal, cardiovascular, and genitourinary function.[8] Cardiac autonomic neuropathy may result in resting tachycardia and postural hypotension. Impotence is the most common clinical manifestation of autonomic neuropathy, affecting more than 50% of men with diabetes. Gastrointestinal effects include diarrhea and gastroparesis, which may not only cause symptoms but also alter the absorption of meals and impair glycemic control.[36]

HOME CARE APPLICATION

Specific goals of treatment in the home are to achieve normalization of blood glucose levels and to prevent complications. Therapy for diabetes focuses on diet, exercise, and (for some patients) insulin or oral blood glucose–lowering agents. The emphasis of therapy varies according to the type of diabetes and the severity of the disease. For persons with type 1 diabetes, insulin therapy is essential for survival, but oral blood glucose–lowering agents are ineffective. Some of those with type 2 diabetes may be treated with diet only, whereas others require insulin or oral blood glucose–lowering agents to control hyperglycemia. Nutritional management is a major priority for both types. Exercise is also an important factor in achieving metabolic balance.

The overall goal of home care is for patients/caregivers to acquire the knowledge and skills needed for accurate monitoring and effective self-management of diabetes and complications. This goal is achieved through assessment and education of the patient/caregiver.

Thorough diabetic assessment is essential regardless of the duration of diabetes. Assessment includes the interview integrated with the physical examination and evaluation of the patient's/caregiver's practices. A complete physical examination is usually performed, but only those areas related to diabetes will be presented here.

Physical assessment

General assessment. Check the patient's height and weight on the initial visit and the weight on each subsequent visit to assess nutritional status and hydration. Monitor blood pressure to assess for hypertension, which contributes to complications, and for postural hypotension, which may result from autonomic neuropathy. Observe the skin for general hygiene and signs of infection. Check for heat intolerance and excessive sweating of the face and body, which may indicate autonomic dysfunction.[15]

Cerebrovascular. Check for symptoms of cerebrovascular disease, including intermittent dizziness, transient loss of vision, slurring of speech, and paresthesia or weakness of one arm or leg. Carotid bruits may be heard.[39]

Eyes/vision. Assess functional vision by noting whether the patient is able to do the following: (1) read printed materials, (2) compare blood or urine test strips with color chart accurately, and (3) draw up the dose of insulin correctly. If vision is blurry, is this associated with hyperglycemia? Note any report of seeing "floaters" or "cobwebs," which may indicate retinal bleeding; or sudden, painless loss of vision, which may occur with a major retinal hemorrhage.[32] Refer patients to an ophthalmologist for evaluation if (1) blurry vision persists for more than 1 to 2 days and is not associated with a change in blood glucose level, (2) sudden loss of vision in one or both eyes occurs, or (3) black spots, cobwebs, or flashing lights appear in the field of vision.[39]

Cardiovascular. Assess for typical symptoms of coronary heart disease such as chest pain, shortness of breath, or congestive heart failure. Since neuropathy may mask chest pain, myocardial infarction should be suspected in unexplained congestive heart failure or diabetic ketoacidosis.[8]

Gastrointestinal. Assess for symptoms of autonomic neuropathy. Anorexia, early satiety (a sense of fullness or bloating), and nausea after meals may indicate gastroparesis. Diarrhea that is nocturnal, is not accompanied by pain or cramps, is intermittent at first, and is associated with fecal incontinence may be related to autonomic neuropathy. Ask whether the patient is taking metoclopramide or other appropriate medications.[15]

Genitourinary/renal. Assess for neurogenic bladder, which is characterized by decreased urinary frequency, and urinary tract infection. Later, difficult or incomplete bladder emptying may occur. Test the urine for nitrite (which may indicate infection) and for protein (which may indicate nephropathy). In the elderly, the classic symptoms of urinary tract infection may be absent, with change in mental status being the only manifestation.[15]

With impotence, careful history and evaluation are essential to distinguish between psychogenic and organic erectile dysfunction. Organic impotence is gradual in onset and partner nonspecific. Early morning erection is absent. A referral to a physician may be needed to test for neurogenic impotence by monitoring nocturnal penile tumescence and rigidity.[15]

Lower extremities. Assess the feet for proper foot care. Guidelines appear in Box 15-1. Check for signs and symptoms of peripheral vascular disease, including intermittent claudication, cold feet, and decreased or absent pulses in the lower extremities.[20] Typical symptoms of neuropathy include spontaneous uncomfortable sensations, contact paresthesias, impaired balance, diminished proprioception and position sense, absent or reduced vibratory sensation, numbness, and unnoticed injuries. An early sign is diminished deep tendon reflexes, especially of the Achilles tendon. Pain may be described as superficial or deep, burning, shooting, stabbing, aching, or tearing and is often more intense at night. The majority of patients report minimal or no symptoms, with deficits being noted on routine examination or because complications are present.[11]

With neuropathic ulcers the foot is typically warm with easily palpable dorsalis pedis pulses. Note areas of local edema and warmth, which are at risk for tissue breakdown.[11]

Diabetes management and patient education

Each aspect of management should be reviewed to determine the plan of care and priorities. Patient education should be directed toward the knowledge and skills needed for competent self-management (Boxes 15-2 and 15-3).

Insulin. Insulin is necessary for carbohydrate, protein, and fat metabolism.[5] Normally the hormonal system is remarkably efficient in maintaining blood glucose levels within a narrow range despite alterations in periods of food intake and

---

Box 15-1   PATIENT EDUCATION GUIDE: FOOT CARE

The nurse should provide the patient with the following instructions:

Inspection
- Look at your feet each day in a place with good light; use a mirror if you can't bend over to see the bottom of your feet.
  - Look for dry places and cracks in the skin, especially between the toes and around the heel; check for ingrown toenails, corns, calluses, discoloration, swelling, or sores.
- If looking carefully at your feet is difficult for you, have a friend or family member help.
- If corns, calluses, or other problems persist, see a foot doctor.

Bathing
- Wash your feet daily in warm (not hot) water; always test the water temperature with your wrist or a bath thermometer to prevent burning yourself.
  - Do not soak your feet, because it will dry your skin.
  - Use a mild soap and rinse well; dry feet with a soft towel, making sure to dry between the toes.
- To soften dry feet and keep the skin from cracking, use a cream or lotion such as Nivea, Eucerin, or Alpha Keri; do not put lotion between your toes.
- If your feet sweat alot, lightly dust with foot powder; wear cotton socks and change them several times a day.

Toenails
- Trim your toenails only after bathing, when they are soft and easy to cut.
- Always cut or file nails to follow the natural curve of your toe.
- Avoid cutting nails shorter than the ends of your toes.
- File sharp corners and rough edges of nails with an emery board so they do not cut the toes next to them.
- Do not use sharp objects to poke or dig under the toenail or around the cuticle.
- See a podiatrist for treatment of ingrown toenails and nails that are thick or tend to split when cut.

Corns and calluses
- Control corn and callus buildup; after washing your feet, gently rub with a pumice stone.
- Pad corns to reduce pressure.

- Avoid using do-it-yourself corn or callus removers; they are caustic and may hurt healthy skin.
- Never cut your corns and calluses with a razor blade; no bathroom surgery.

Socks
- Wear clean, soft cotton or wool socks.
  - Socks should fit well and be free of seams and darns.
- Never wear round garters or hose with elastic tops that might reduce the blood supply to your feet.

Shoes
- Always wear shoes or slippers to cover and protect your feet.
- Wear shoes that fit well. Shoes that do not fit well can cause sores, blisters, and calluses, but shoes that feel good have room for all the toes to be in their natural place; avoid pointed shoes that pinch the toes. The top part of the shoe should be soft and pliable; the lining should not have ridges, wrinkles, or seams; the toe box should be round and high to allow space for toe deformities; you may need to see an orthotic specialist for special shoes or to have your shoes adapted to your feet.
  - When you buy shoes, make an outline of each foot from stiff paper to insert in shoes.
- Before you put on your shoes, carefully check for stones or rough spots that might hurt your feet.

Improve your circulation
- Try to quit smoking if you smoke.
- Exercise every day; take a brisk daily walk for 1/2 to 1 hour; if you are not able to walk or move about easily, ask your nurse or doctor what types of exercises are best for you.
- Avoid being in the cold for long periods; wear wool socks.

Treatment of injuries
- Look at your feet if you stumble or bump a hard object.
  - If your foot is hurt, do not keep walking on it, since that can cause more damage.
  - Cuts and scratches should be treated right away; wash with soap and water and apply a mild antiseptic such as Bactine or Johnson & Johnson First Aid Cream; never use strong chemicals such as boric acid.
- Notify physician or podiatrist of any blisters or sores on your feet.

From Fain JA: Nursing management of adults with diabetes mellitus. In Beare PG, Myers JL, editors: *Adult health nursing,* ed 3, St. Louis, 1998, Mosby.

Box 15-2 PRIMARY NURSING DIAGNOSIS/PATIENT PROBLEMS

The following nursing diagnoses may be appropriate for the patient with diabetes mellitus:

- Knowledge deficit: diabetes care, prevention of complications
- Ineffective individual coping
- Alteration in nutrition: more than body requirements (if obese)
- Ineffective management of therapeutic regimen
- Risk for fluid volume deficit related to hyperglycemia
- Risk for injury related to neuropathy
- Risk for hypertension
- Risk for altered urinary elimination related to renal failure
- Activity limitation or intolerance related to diabetic complications

Box 15-3 PRIMARY THEMES OF PATIENT EDUCATION

- Diabetes self-care management
- Diet, importance of modifying fat
- Exercise
- Medication/insulin administration
- Blood glucose monitoring
- Foot care
- Sick-day management
- Hypoglycemia: recognition and interventions
- Hyperglycemia: recognition and interventions
- Infection: recognition and interventions
- Importance of self-care management in prevention/reduction of complications
- General self-care strategies

fasting.[27] The physiological secretion of insulin to control blood glucose is timed precisely to meet the body's needs. In persons with diabetes, insulin therapy attempts to duplicate this.[38]

Insulin regimens. Numerous patterns of insulin administration may be prescribed based on the needs of the individual. A commonly used regimen consists of two injections per day of an intermediate-acting insulin with the first dose given before breakfast and the second before supper or at bedtime. When the injection is given before meals, regular insulin may be added when necessary to reduce postprandial hyperglycemia. More intensive regimens with multiple injections may be needed if the goal is to restore blood glucose levels to nondiabetic values throughout the day.[38]

Insulin preparations. Human insulin is manufactured by recombinant DNA technology, whereas animal insulin is obtained from beef or pork pancreas. Human insulin has a more rapid onset and shorter duration of action than pork insulin. Most patients currently beginning therapy are given human insulin.[5]

Insulin is available in rapid-, short-, intermediate-, and long-acting forms. A rapid-acting insulin is lispro. Short-acting insulins include regular (R) and semilente. Intermediate-acting insulins are NPH and lente. Long-acting insulin is ultralente.[1] Action times for insulins are listed in Table 15-1. Concentrations available in the United States are U-100 and U-500, with U-100 used most frequently and U-500 used only in rare cases of extreme insulin resistance.[5]

Storage and appearance. Insulin may be stored at room temperature for about a month. Extreme temperatures should be avoided. Insulin should be at room temperature and inspected before use. Rapid- and short-acting regular insulin should be clear, and all other forms should be uniformly cloudy.[5]

Mixing insulins. Premixed insulin is useful in patients who may not be able to master mixing of insulins and whose diabetes is stable on this combination. The most typical commercially available mixture is 70% NPH and 30% regular insulin.[1]

In mixtures of regular and lente, the binding of the regular insulin by the zinc is associated with blunting the effects of the regular insulin. When using mixtures of insulin, patients need to time the injection based on the types of insulin and keep their procedures for injection standardized.[5]

Syringes. Insulin syringes are available in 0.25-, 0.3-, 0.5-, and 1-ml capacity.[5] Syringes must match the concentration of the insulin being used (e.g., U-100 syringe for U-100 insulin).[39] Local guidelines for syringe disposal should be followed. Syringes

Table 15-1 Insulin action curves

Insulin type	Onset	Peak (hours)	Usual effective duration (hours)	Usual maximum duration (hours)
Animal				
Regular	0.5-2.0 hours	3-4	4-6	6-8
NPH	4-6 hours	8-14	16-20	20-24
Lente	4-6 hours	8-14	16-20	20-24
Ultralente	8-14 hours	Minimal	24-36	24-36
Human				
Lispro	<15 minutes	0.5-1.5	2-4	4-6
Regular	0.5-1.0 hour	2-3	3-6	6-10
NPH	2-4 hours	4-10	10-16	14-18
Lente	3-4 hours	4-12	12-18	16-20
Ultralente	6-10 hours	?	18-20	20-24

Source: American Diabetes Association: 1999 Buyer's guide to diabetes products, *Diabetes Forecast* 51(10):32, 1998.

that will not be reused should be placed in a punctureproof container for disposal.[5,8]

SYRINGE REUSE. Syringes should never be shared with another person. Manufacturers recommend that disposable syringes be used only once; however, syringe reuse by an individual is safe and practical with certain precautions. Syringes should be discarded when the needle becomes dull, is bent, or has touched any surface other than skin. Because of the increased risk of infection, those with poor personal hygiene, an acute concurrent illness, open wounds on the hands, or decreased resistance to infection should not reuse syringes. For reuse the needle must be recapped after each use. To be capable of safely recapping a syringe for reuse, patients must have adequate vision, manual dexterity, and no obvious tremor. Skin around the injection sites should be inspected periodically for unusual redness or sign of infection.[5]

Injection sites. Insulin may be injected into the subcutaneous tissue of the upper arm, the anterior and lateral aspects of the thigh, the buttocks, and the abdomen (avoid a 2-inch radius around the umbilicus). Rotation of sites is important in preventing lipohypertrophy or lipoatrophy. To obtain consistency in action of insulin, varying sites within the same anatomical region rather than between regions is recommended.[5] Using only abdominal sites may improve the consistency of insulin and glucose profiles in many cases.[39]

Absorption. Absorption of insulin may be affected by many factors. Speed of absorption varies with the site of injection, with the abdomen having the fastest rate of absorption, followed by the arms, thighs, and buttocks. The absorption rate may be increased by exercise. Injection depth affects insulin absorption, with intramuscular injection resulting in more rapid absorption than subcutaneous injection.[5]

Insulin administration. Home care nurses should observe the patient's/caregiver's techniques in preparing and injecting insulin. Patients with hyperglycemia without identifiable cause have been noted to be unaware of errors in their injection technique.

Several important deficits have been observed in patients' ability to measure and prepare insulin in a syringe. Inability to calculate total amount of regular and NPH insulin (due to difficulty with basic arithmetic involving addition), not rolling the NPH vial to mix it properly, not eliminating air bubbles from the syringe, and contaminating the regular insulin with the NPH insulin were noted. Factors associated with errors include age, arthritis of the hands, visual acuity, and education.[37]

Steps for preparation and injection of insulin are as follows:

1. Before each injection, the hands and the injection site should be clean.

2. For all insulin preparations except short-acting, gently rotate the vial in the palms of the hands (do not shake) to resuspend the insulin.

3. Draw up and inject an amount of air equal to the dose of insulin into the vial to avoid creating a vacuum. For a mixed dose, put sufficient air into both bottles.

4. Draw up the insulin. When mixing short-acting insulin with intermediate- or long-acting insulin, the clear short-acting insulin should be drawn into the syringe first.

5. Inspect the syringe for and eliminate air bubbles, which could cause the injected dose to be decreased.

6. Lightly grasp a fold of skin and inject at a 90-degree angle. Thin individuals may need to inject at a 45-degree angle to avoid intramuscular injection.[5]

PREFILLED INSULIN SYRINGES. To promote independence in those who are capable of injecting insulin but are unable to draw it up, prefilled syringes may be appropriate. Home care nurses should use the following guidelines when using prefilled syringes:

- Keep all prefilled single or mixed insulin syringes refrigerated and use within 30 days.
- Store syringes vertically with the needle up so that particles do not settle and clog the needle.
- Instruct patients to resuspend the preparation before injection by rolling the syringe.
- The interval between mixing and injecting should be standardized based on the specific types of insulin mixed because of the variation in rates of binding.[5] For example, if the patient has been using syringes filled days ahead, when the home health nurse visits and fills syringes, the patient should use a syringe filled on a previous visit, not a freshly mixed syringe.

ASSISTIVE DEVICES. Numerous devices designed to make giving an injection easier are available, including spring-loaded needle insertion aids, syringe magnifiers, dose gauges, needle guides, and vial stabilizers. These products may be especially helpful for people who are visually impaired or who have slight dexterity problems. Before a device is purchased, it should be tested by the user to determine whether it meets the individual's needs. One assistive device for those who are visu-

ally impaired is the Becton Dickinson Magni-Guide, which magnifies the entire length of the syringe and holds both the syringe and insulin vial, assisting the user to insert the needle into the vial properly. "The Buyer's Guide" in *Diabetes Forecast* describes many diabetes products that may assist persons to be independent in insulin administration.[1]

Complications of insulin therapy. Hypoglycemia is by far the most frequent complication in patients treated with insulin.[38] Severe hypoglycemia may result in seizures, coma, long-term cognitive deficits, or death.[45]

As a general rule, hypoglycemia is defined as a blood glucose level below 50 mg/dl.[18] In patients receiving insulin, hypoglycemia most often occurs because of a mismatch between the timing of insulin, meals, and exercise. Hypoglycemia may be caused by increased intensity or frequency of exercise, omission of meals, decreased caloric intake, weight loss, use of alcohol,[38] and sulfonylurea therapy.[18]

Symptoms of hypoglycemia vary and include sweating, trembling, weakness, visual disturbance, hunger, pounding heart, difficulty with speaking, tingling around the mouth, dizziness, headache, anxiety, nausea, difficulty concentrating, tiredness, drowsiness, and confusion.[28] Patients often have certain symptoms that are typical for them. Individuals and their significant others need to learn to recognize the symptoms of developing hypoglycemia that are most reliable for them.[14] Hypoglycemic unawareness (lack of classic symptoms) is common in those with type 1 and increases their susceptibility to the adverse effects of hypoglycemia.[45]

Initial treatment of hypoglycemia for those who are able to swallow consists of consuming 15 g of carbohydrates such as orange juice (4 oz); sugar-containing cola (5 oz); honey, maple syrup, or corn syrup (1 tablespoon); candy (8 Lifesavers); sugar (4 teaspoons dissolved in water); cake icing (1 small tube); or glucose tablets or gel.[45] Monitor the patient's response, check the blood glucose level, and follow with food to maintain the blood glucose level.[18]

If the patient is unable to swallow, the nurse or caregiver should administer glucagon, 1.0 mg, intramuscularly or subcutaneously. After recovery from a hypoglycemic episode, every effort should be made to prevent recurrence by identifying the cause and correcting the treatment plan accordingly.[38] Assess the patient's/caregiver's knowledge of the causes, symptoms, and treatment of hypoglycemia and instruct as needed. Make sure the patient/caregiver understands the need to always carry a source of rapid-acting carbohydrate whenever leaving home.

Other complications of insulin therapy include lipoatrophy, lipohypertrophy, insulin edema, insulin antibody development, and insulin allergy. Lipoatrophy, loss of fat at the injection site, is usually relieved by using purified insulin. In lipohypertrophy, the subcutaneous tissue becomes swollen or fibrous as a result of repeated injections at the same site, leading to poor or irregular absorption of insulin. Treatment consists of rotating injection sites.[38]

Oral blood glucose–lowering agents. Several types of oral blood glucose–lowering agents are used to treat hyperglycemia in patients with type 2 diabetes. These include sulfonylureas, metformin, and acarbose, an alpha glucosidase inhibitor. Sulfonylureas stimulate the pancreatic beta cells to secrete insulin. Metformin lowers blood glucose primarily by reducing hepatic glucose production. Acarbose lowers blood glucose by retarding intestinal glucose absorption.[26] Oral agents and their doses are listed in Table 15-2.

The major adverse effects of sulfonylureas are hypoglycemia and weight gain.[26,44] Severe hypoglycemia is associated with the use of long-acting forms (such as glyburide and chlorpropamide); age (over 65); inadequate nutrition; intercurrent illness; chronic renal, hepatic, or cardiovascular disease; and concomitant use of other drugs that cause hypoglycemia or potentiate sulfonylureas.[31] Side effects other than hypoglycemia are infrequent and include nausea, vomiting, abdominal discomfort, and skin rashes. Hematologic disorders and liver disease are rare. The use of chlorpropamide may result in water retention, hyponatremia, and alcohol-induced flushing.[32]

Metformin is often used for its effect on insulin resistance. Side effects reported with metformin, which are usually self-limiting and transient, include abdominal bloating, nausea, cramping, a feeling of fullness, diarrhea, a metallic taste, and a reduction in vitamin B_{12} levels.[44]

Acarbose may be used in patients to lower postprandial hyperglycemia. The most common side

Table 15-2 Oral blood glucose–lowering agents

	Initial dose (mg)	Maximum total daily dose (mg)
Sulfonylureas		
Tolbutamide	500	2000
Glibenclamide	2.5	15
Glipizide	2.5	20
Glicazide	80	240
Glimepiride	1	6
Metformin	500	3000
Acarbose	50	600

Modified from Hein RJ, and others: Optimal control of Type 2 diabetes:current and future prospects. In Betteridge DJ, editor: *Diabetes:current perspectives,* London, 2000, Martin Dunitz.

effects of acarbose are dose-related gastrointestinal complaints (flatulence, diarrhea, and abdominal pain). Acarbose should be avoided in patients with intestinal disorders.[44]

Have the patient/caregiver describe the action and side effects of the medication and how and when it is taken. Make sure the patient/caregiver understands the factors that may contribute to hypoglycemia.

Diet. Diet is regarded as both an essential component of treatment and one of the greatest challenges in diabetes management.[6] Although the dietitian ordinarily calculates the diet and develops the plan for diet management with input from the home care team, home health nurses have ongoing responsibility for instructing patients and assessing metabolic control. Nurses should be knowledgeable about the current dietary recommendations and rationale to assist the patient/caregiver in understanding this aspect of diabetes care.

Currently there is no one diabetic or American Diabetes Association (ADA) diet. The recommended diet is defined as a dietary prescription based on individual nutrition assessment and treatment goals.[3] General nutrition recommendations for people with diabetes, many of which are the same as for the general population, appear in Table 15-3. For individuals using insulin therapy, it is important to eat at consistent times synchronized with the action times of the insulin preparation used. In type 2 diabetes, emphasis is on achieving glucose, lipid, and blood pressure goals. Although weight

Table 15-3 Summary of nutrition recommendations

Calories	To achieve or maintain reasonable body weight
Protein	10%-20% of total calories 10% with nephropathy
Fat and carbohydrate	80%-90% of total calories
Saturated fat	<10% of total calories
Cholesterol	≤ 300 mg/day
Fiber	20-35 g from a variety of sources
Sodium	<3000 mg/day ≤2400 mg/day with mild to moderate hypertension

From: American Diabetes Association: Nutrition recommendations and principles for people with diabetes mellitus, *Diabetes Care* 23(Suppl 1):S43, 2000.

loss is desirable, traditional dietary strategies have not been very effective in achieving long-term weight loss; therefore the emphasis needs to expand beyond weight loss to improvement in blood glucose levels.[6]

In adults, a diet with adequate calories for maintaining or attaining reasonable body weight is recommended. Reasonable weight is the weight an individual and health care provider acknowledge as achievable and maintainable, both short- and long-term. This may not be the same as the desirable or ideal body weight.[6]

Improvement in food choices using general nutritional guidelines such as Dietary Guidelines for Americans[42] and the Food Guide Pyramid[43] is an initial strategy. The Diabetes Food Guide Pyramid is more specific for those with diabetes.[10] A nutritionally adequate meal plan with reduction of total fat, especially saturated fats, can be used. Moderate weight loss (10 to 20 pounds) has been shown to improve diabetes control, even if desirable body weight is not achieved. Weight loss is best attempted by a moderate decrease in calories (250 to 500 calories less than average daily intake) and an increase in caloric expenditure.[6]

Nonnutritive sweeteners (saccharin, aspartame, and acesulfame-K) are safe to consume by all people with diabetes. Nutritive sweeteners (sucrose, fructose, corn syrup, fruit juice or fruit juice concentrate, honey, molasses, dextrose, maltose, sorbitol, mannitol, and xylitol) may be consumed when accounted for in the meal plan. Patients with dyslipidemia should avoid consuming large amounts of fructose. Excessive intake of sorbitol, xylitol, and mannitol may have a laxative effect.[6]

Precautions regarding alcohol use that apply to the general public also apply to people with diabetes. Alcohol in moderation will not ordinarily affect blood glucose levels when diabetes is well controlled. Because of the increased risk for hypoglycemia in those treated with insulin or blood glucose–lowering agents, if alcohol is consumed it should be ingested with a meal. For those using insulin, two or fewer alcoholic beverages can be ingested with and in addition to the regular meal plan. Reduction or abstention from alcohol may be advisable for people with diabetes and other medical problems such as pancreatitis, dyslipidemia, or neuropathy. Calories from alcohol need to be calculated as part of the total caloric intake and substituted for fat exchanges or fat calories (1 alcoholic beverage = 2 fat exchanges).[6]

Diets should be individualized based on what patients are able and willing to do, their usual eating habits, and other lifestyle factors. Cultural, ethnic, and financial considerations are also very important.[6]

In the home, have the patient/caregiver record intake for 3 days, including the time, type, amount/portion size, and preparation (e.g., baked, fried). Observe the food available in the home. Is it consistent with the patient's needs? Ask the dietitian to review the diet record with the patient's diet prescription. Are there limitations due to inability to purchase, obtain, or prepare appropriate foods? If glycemic control is inadequate, consult with the dietitian to determine an appropriate plan for teaching and regimen adjustment.

Exercise. Many diabetic patients are homebound or unable to exercise because of complications. For those whose condition may improve or who have no contraindications for exercise, understanding the importance and effects of exercise is essential.

Benefits resulting from exercise include improvement in cardiovascular and pulmonary health, sense of well-being, and ability to cope with stress.[22] For type 2 patients with insulin resistance, obesity, blood lipid abnormalities, and cardiovascular disease, the potential benefits of exercise are obvious and the risk of serious hypoglycemia relatively low. In patients with type 1 diabetes, the risk of serious hypoglycemia or worsened hyperglycemia and ketosis consequent to exercise merits caution. Attention must be given to balancing insulin, diet, and exercise so that the consequences of hypoglycemia do not outweigh the benefits of exercise.[23]

Before patients start an exercise program they should have a complete medical examination, including assessment of diabetic complications and blood glucose control. Exercise programs must be individualized to reduce risk. For many patients, precautions regarding exercise of the feet are needed.[2]

Assessment of glycemic control. Monitoring glycemic control is essential to assessing the need for adjustments in the therapeutic regimen and to evaluating diabetic control. In the home, glycemic control is evaluated by using devices for self-monitoring of blood glucose (SMBG) and by urine testing.

Self-monitoring of blood glucose. SMBG is widely accepted as an important tool in diabetes management. SMBG in the home makes it possible to prevent many avoidable hospitalizations due to hypoglycemia and hyperglycemia, to evaluate the response to insulin replacement, to reveal the effects of overeating to those with type 2 diabetes,[17] and to reinforce the benefits of exercise and medication.[13]

SMBG procedures involve obtaining a drop of capillary blood by finger stick using a lancet, applying the blood to a reagent strip (or with some new meters, to the glucose sensor), and reading the results at a specified time. Some strips can be read visually, whereas others can only be read by meters. Accuracy of results depends on following the manufacturer's instructions precisely.

Times and frequency of testing should be based on the individual's needs and goals. Until stabilized or with intensive therapy, many patients test 4 times a day: before each meal and at bedtime. Once a pattern is stabilized, the frequency of testing may be decreased. The frequency of testing should be increased during illness. For patients who are not willing to or who cannot afford to test frequently, establishing a realistic schedule is important.

Blood glucose target goals are 80 to 120 mg/dl before meals and 100 to 140 mg/dl at bedtime. Individual glycemic target goals should be set based on the patient's ability to understand and carry out the treatment regimen, the risk for severe hypoglycemia, and other factors that may increase risk or decrease benefit.[8]

Assess the accuracy of SMBG by observing the patient's/caregiver's technique. Evaluate the present level of blood glucose control and teach the patient/caregiver to do so by reviewing the patient's testing record. Ask the patient to state what glucose level is too high or too low and what action should be taken for each.

Glycated protein testing. Periodic measurement of Ghb (glycated hemoglobin, glycohemoglobin, glycosylated hemoglobin, Hb A_1, or Hb A1c) is useful in patients with type 1 and type 2 diabetes. The test provides an accurate estimation of the average blood glucose level during the 2 to 3 months preceding the test. The test should be performed at least 2 times a year in those with stable glycemic control and more frequently in those with therapy changes or who are not meeting their glycemic goals. The goal of therapy is a Ghb of less than 7%.[9]

Urine testing. All patients should test their urine for ketones whenever blood glucose is consistently above 300 mg/dl, with acute illness, stress, or symptomatic hyperglycemia. Urine testing for glucose has been replaced by blood glucose monitoring in most patients with diabetes. One limitation of urine testing is that in a patient with a high renal threshold for glucose, elevated blood glucose levels will not be reflected by urine testing. Hypoglycemia is not detected by urine testing. Because of its simplicity and low cost, urine glucose testing may be useful for those who are unable or unwilling to perform blood glucose monitoring.[9]

Urine testing products are sensitive to light, temperature extremes, and moisture. Patients/caregivers should follow manufacturer's instructions for storage, and keep tablets for urine testing out of the reach of children because they are poisonous.[1]

Hyperglycemia. Assess the patient's/caregiver's knowledge of the causes, symptoms, and treatment of hyperglycemia. Provide instructions regarding the importance of recognition and treatment of infection.

Sick-day management. Illness may disrupt the patient's diabetes management program. Since

---

Box 15-4   PATIENT EDUCATION GUIDE: SICK-DAY MANAGEMENT OF DIABETES MELLITUS

Sick means having fever, vomiting, nausea, diarrhea, or congestion. The nurse should provide the patient with the following instructions:

Insulin

If you take insulin shots, always take your insulin when you are sick, *even if you cannot eat your regular meals.* You may need extra insulin, for example:
1. If BG is 240-400 mg/dl add 2 to 4 units of regular insulin to the usual dose before meals and take the usual dose at bedtime.
2. If BG is 240-400 mg/dl and the urine is moderate to large for ketones, add 4 to 6 units of regular insulin to the usual dose for *every* insulin dose until ketones are no longer moderate.

Medication

If you take a pill for diabetes, be sure to take it when you are sick. If vomiting, contact your physician or diabetes nurse educator.

Diet

If you are unable to eat your usual meals, try to drink fluids containing 10 g of carbohydrates every hour while awake. The following servings contain 10 g of carbohydrates:
1/2 cup ginger ale (not diet)
1/2 cup Coca-Cola (not diet)
1/2 cup chicken soup with noodles
3/4 cup chilled Gatorade
   If you *are able to eat* usual meals, then drink 1/2 cup of calorie-free fluid every hour while awake. The following are calorie-free:
Broth or bouillon
Decaffeinated tea
Sugar-free/caffeine-free soda, such as 7-Up or Sprite
Water

Urine/blood testing

Check your urine for ketones/acetone and check your blood glucose level every 4 hours. Seek professional advice if you have any of the following:
Diarrhea or vomiting for more than 6 hours
Moderate or large levels of ketones (++ or +++) in your urine even after two injections of regular insulin as instructed
Your blood tests for glucose are over 400 or urine tests for glucose are 2% to 5% even after two injections of regular insulin as instructed

From Fain JA: Nursing management of adults with diabetes mellitus. In Beare PG, Myers JL, editors: *Adult health nursing,* ed 3, St. Louis, 1998, Mosby.

---

illness is often accompanied by hyperglycemia, the patient/caregiver needs to be instructed on the importance of continuing medication, maintaining adequate fluid and caloric intake on sick days, and seeking professional advice regarding temporary adjustment of the treatment program. Guidelines appear in Box 15-4.

SUMMARY

Living with diabetes presents many challenges. Glycemic control may be difficult to achieve even in an ideal situation. Many home care patients have numerous barriers confronting them daily. Assessment of the individual's particular situation and practical, appropriate education and intervention are crucial to promoting adherence to the plan of care. The unique privilege of direct observation of the person's real-life situation may enhance the home health nurse's ability to tailor the treatment regimen to the individual's lifestyle. The mutual

establishment of realistic goals and plans will demand the creativity of the home care nurse and the perseverance of the patient, but it is the best way to increase adherence and improve clinical outcomes.

REFERENCES

1. American Diabetes Association: 1999 Buyer's guide to diabetes products, *Diabetes Forecast* 51(10):32, 1998.
2. American Diabetes Association: Diabetes and exercise, *Diabetes Care* 23(suppl 1):S50, 2000.
3. American Diabetes Association: Diabetic nephropathy, *Diabetes Care* 23(suppl 1):S69, 2000.
4. American Diabetes Association: Diabetic retinopathy, *Diabetes Care* 23(suppl 1):S73, 2000.
5. American Diabetes Association: Insulin administration, *Diabetes Care* 23(suppl 1):S86, 2000.
6. American Diabetes Association: Nutrition recommendations and principles for people with diabetes mellitus, *Diabetes Care* 23(suppl 1):S43, 2000.
7. American Diabetes Association: Preventive foot care in people with diabetes, *Diabetes Care* 23(suppl 1):S55, 2000.

8. American Diabetes Association: Standards of medical care for patients with diabetes mellitus, *Diabetes Care* 23 (suppl 1):S32, 2000.

9. American Diabetes Association: Tests of glycemia in diabetes, *Diabetes Care* 23(suppl 1):S80, 2000.

10. American Diabetes Association and the American Dietetic Association, *The first step in diabetes meal planning,* Alexandria, Va, 1997.

11. Broadstone VL and others: Diabetic peripheral neuropathy: sensorimotor neuropathy, *Diabetes Educ* 13(1):30, 1987.

12. Chait A, Bierman EL: Pathogenesis of macrovascular disease in diabetes. In Kahn CR, Weir GC, editors: *Joslin's diabetes mellitus,* ed 13, Philadelphia, 1994, Lea & Febiger.

13. Cooppan R: General approach to the treatment of diabetes. In Kahn CR, Weir GC, editors: *Joslin's diabetes mellitus,* ed 13, Philadelphia, 1994, Lea & Febiger.

14. Cryer PE and others: Hypoglycemia, *Diabetes Care* 17(7):734, 1994.

15. Cyrus and others: Diabetic peripheral neuropathy: autonomic neuropathies, *Diabetes Educ* 13(2):11, 1987.

16. Davidson JK: Diabetic ketoacidosis and the hyperglycemic hyperosmolar state. In Davidson JK, editor: *Clinical diabetes mellitus: a problem-oriented approach,* ed 2, New York, 1991, Thieme.

17. Davidson JK, Russo G: Monitoring of blood and urine glucose and ketone levels. In Davidson JK, editor: *Clinical diabetes mellitus: a problem-oriented approach,* ed 2, New York, 1991, Thieme.

18. Davidson JK and others: Insulin therapy. In Davidson JK, editor: *Clinical diabetes mellitus: a problem-oriented approach,* ed 2, New York, 1991, Thieme.

19. Diabetes Control and Complications Trial Research Group: The effect of intensive treatment of diabetes on the development and progression of long-term complications in insulin-dependent diabetes mellitus, *N Engl J Med* 329:977, 1993.

20. Expert Committee on the Diagnosis and Classification of Diabetes Mellitus, American Diabetes Association: Report on the expert committee on the diagnosis and classification of diabetes mellitus, *Diabetes Care* 23(suppl 1):S4, 2000.

21. Fain JA: Nursing management of adults with diabetes mellitus. In Beare PG, Myers JL, editors: *Adult health nursing,* ed 3, St. Louis, 1998, Mosby.

22. Giacca A and others: Exercise and stress in diabetes mellitus. In Davidson JK, editor: *Clinical diabetes mellitus: a problem-oriented approach,* ed 2, New York, 1991, Thieme.

23. Goodyear LI, Smith RJ: Exercise and diabetes. In Kahn CR, Weir GC, editors: *Joslin's diabetes mellitus,* ed 13, Philadelphia, 1994, Lea & Febiger.

24. Habershaw G: Foot lesions in patients with diabetes: cause, prevention and treatment. In Kahn CR, Weir GC, editors: *Joslin's diabetes mellitus,* ed 13, Philadelphia, 1994, Lea & Febiger.

25. Harris ME: Diabetes in America: epidemiology and scope of the problem, *Diabetes Care* 21(suppl 3):C11, 1998.

26. Hein J and others: Optimal control of type 2 diabetes: current and future prospects. In Betteridge DJ, editor: *Diabetes: current perspectives,* London, 2000, Martin Dunitz.

27. Henquin J: Cell biology of insulin secretion. In Kahn CR, Weir GC, editors: *Joslin's diabetes mellitus,* ed 13, Philadelphia, 1994, Lea & Febiger.

28. Hepburn DA: Symptoms of hypoglycemia. In Frier BM, Fisher BM, editors: *Hypoglycemia and diabetes,* London, 1993, Edward Arnold.

29. King GI, Banskota NK: Mechanisms of diabetic microvascular complications. In Kahn CR, Weir GC, editors: *Joslin's diabetes mellitus,* ed 13, Philadelphia, 1994, Lea & Febiger.

30. Kitabchi AE and others: Diabetic ketoacidosis and the hyperglycemic hyperosmolar nonketotic state. In Kahn CR, Weir GC, editors: *Joslin's diabetes mellitus,* ed 13, Philadelphia, 1994, Lea & Febiger.

31. Lebovitz HE, editor: *Physician's guide to non-insulin dependent (type II) diabetes: diagnosis and treatment,* ed 2, Alexandria, Va, 1988, American Diabetes Association.

32. Lebovitz HE: Oral antidiabetic agents. In Kahn CR, Weir GC, editors: *Joslin's diabetes mellitus,* ed 13, Philadelphia, 1994, Lea & Febiger.

33. Logerfo FW, Gibbons GW: Vascular disease of the lower extremities in diabetes mellitus: etiology and management. In Kahn CR, Weir GC, editors: *Joslin's diabetes mellitus,* ed 13, Philadelphia, 1994, Lea & Febiger.

34. McGowan JE: Infections in diabetes mellitus. In Davidson JK, editor: *Clinical diabetes mellitus: a problem-oriented approach,* ed 2, New York, 1991, Thieme.

35. McKenna MJ and others: Cerebrovascular diseases. In Davidson JK, editor: *Clinical diabetes mellitus: a problem-oriented approach,* ed 2, New York, 1991, Thieme.

36. Nathan DM: Relationship between metabolic control and long-term complications of diabetes. In Kahn CR, Weir GC, editors: *Joslin's diabetes mellitus,* ed 13, Philadelphia, 1994, Lea & Febiger.

37. Newman KD, Weaver MT: Insulin measurement and preparation among diabetic patients at a county hospital, *Nurs Pract* 19(3):44, 1994.

38. Rosenweig JL: Principles of insulin therapy. In Kahn CR, Weir GC, editors: *Joslin's diabetes mellitus,* ed 13, Philadelphia, 1994, Lea & Febiger.

39. Sperling MA, editor: *Physician's guide to insulin-dependent (type I) diabetes: diagnosis and treatment,* Alexandria, Va, 1988, American Diabetes Association.

40. Steiner G: Hyperlipidemia and atherosclerotic cardiovascular disease. In Davidson JK, editor: *Clinical diabetes mellitus: a problem-oriented approach,* ed 2, New York, 1991, Thieme.

41. United Kingdom Prospective Diabetes Study Group: Intensive blood-glucose control with sulphonylureas or insulin compared with conventional treatment and risk of complications in patients with type 2 diabetes, *Lancet* 352:837, 1998.

42. US Department of Agriculture, US Department of Health and Human Services: *Nutrition and your health: dietary guidelines for Americans,* ed 3, Hyattsville, Md, 1990, USDA's Human Nutrition Information Service.

43. US Department of Agriculture: *The food guide pyramid,* Hyattsville, Md, 1992, USDA's Human Nutrition Information Service.

44. White JR: The pharmacological reduction of blood glucose in patients with type 2 diabetes mellitus, *Clin Diabetes* 16(2), 1998.

45. Widom B, Simonson DC: Iatrogenic hypoglycemia. In Kahn CR, Weir GC, editors: *Joslin's diabetes mellitus,* ed 13, Philadelphia, 1994, Lea & Febiger.

THE PATIENT WITH BLADDER DYSFUNCTION

Kathryn A. Houston

Bladder dysfunction resulting in altered urinary elimination is a clinical problem frequently encountered by home care nurses. Bladder dysfunction affects all age groups, is a major cause of disability and dependency, and is a source of significant stress for caregivers. Home care nurses play a vital role in helping patients/caregivers manage bladder dysfunction in the home. This chapter provides an overview of the pathophysiology and manifestations of bladder dysfunction and details nursing assessment and interventions for patients with urinary retention or urinary incontinence.

DEFINITION OF THE PROBLEM

Bladder dysfunction is a general term that refers to the failure of the bladder either to store urine or to empty urine properly. Although the underlying causes of the problem vary, bladder dysfunction is manifested symptomatically as urinary retention, urinary incontinence, or both.

Urinary retention is defined as the inability to void and empty the bladder spontaneously.

Urinary incontinence is defined as the involuntary loss of urine in an amount or with a frequency sufficient to constitute a social or health problem.[24]

PREVALENCE

Urinary incontinence increases with age, is more common in women, and is significantly more prevalent in persons with cognitive or functional impairments.[48] Incontinence is most prevalent in long-term care settings,[34,35,55] however, among community-dwelling elderly, prevalence rates range between 10% and 55%.[20,21,42,53] The preva-

lence of incontinence in elderly persons cared for by family members has been reported to be as high as 53%.[30,50]

Urinary incontinence ranks among the 10 principal diagnoses in patients using home health agency services and fourth in total Medicare charges for home health services.[44] The direct medical cost of urinary incontinence in the United States has been estimated at more than $16 billion each year.[55]

One survey of patients receiving home care services found that 22% of the sample were incontinent.[30] Only 5% of those who were incontinent had received a formal evaluation of the problem. Management strategies to deal with incontinence most commonly consisted of the use of protective pads and garments (56%), a toileting schedule or habit retraining (38%), indwelling catheters or external collection devices (24%), and adaptive equipment (19%).

With rapid discharge of patients from acute care settings who have unresolved bladder dysfunction and with a growing amount of acute and long-term care being provided in the home, home care nurses are in a key position to identify bladder dysfunction and to initiate interventions aimed at continence restoration and incontinence management.

PHYSIOLOGY OF THE LOWER URINARY TRACT

Bladder storage occurs under control of the sympathetic nervous system, whereas bladder emptying is a parasympathetic nervous system function. The sympathetic nervous system facilitates urine storage primarily by inhibiting the contractile effects of the parasympathetic system on the bladder. In addition, the sympathetic system is responsible for maintaining outlet resistance by stimulating alpha-adrenergic receptors in the bladder base and proximal urethra.

Bladder function is regulated by means of an involuntary spinal cord reflex involving sacral spinal cord segments S2 to S4. As the bladder fills, stretch receptors located in the detrusor muscle are stimulated and carry impulses by way of parasympathetic nerves to the sacral spinal cord, where these nerves synapse with motor fibers that innervate both the pelvic ganglia and the bladder musculature. Stimulation of motor fibers results in detrusor contraction. This reflex can be voluntarily inhibited or facilitated through higher cerebral cortical control. Generally between 150 and 350 ml of urine can be stored in the bladder before bladder pressure begins to increase and the initial urge to void is perceived. Normal bladder capacity is between 300 and 600 ml.[24]

ABNORMALITIES OF MICTURITION
The uninhibited neurogenic bladder

Damage to the brainstem or any portion of the spinal cord that interrupts the pathways transmitting inhibitory impulses to the bladder can result in an uninhibited neurogenic bladder. This condition is characterized by frequent, uncontrolled voiding that occurs whenever the micturition reflex is initiated. Conditions most commonly associated with this abnormality include cerebrovascular accidents, brain tumors or trauma, demyelinating disease such as multiple sclerosis, dementia, and Parkinson's disease.

The atonic bladder

Lesions, damage, or deterioration of sensory or motor components of the sacral spinal cord can interfere with initiation or completion of the voiding reflex. The bladder fills to capacity, and urine leakage occurs as the bladder becomes overdistended. If sensory fibers are intact but motor nerves are involved, the individual is able to perceive bladder fullness but cannot voluntarily initiate voiding. If destruction of sensory nerve fibers is the cause of the atonic condition, stretch signals from the bladder cannot be transmitted and initiation of the micturition reflex is prevented. Common causes

of an atonic bladder include infection, immobility, diabetes, pelvic surgery, medications, tumors, and injuries to the sacral region of the spinal cord (such as injuries that occur with vertebral compression fractures or trauma).

The automatic bladder (reflex bladder)

If the spinal cord is damaged above the level of the sacral region and anatomical components of the voiding reflex remain intact, reflex or automatic bladder dysfunction results. With this abnormality, voluntary inhibition of the micturition reflex is lost. The bladder can be emptied spontaneously, though, with elicitation of the micturition reflex by external cutaneous stimulation or other mechanisms. Reflex bladder is most commonly seen in individuals with upper motor neuron spinal cord injuries and multiple sclerosis.

CLASSIFICATION OF URINARY INCONTINENCE

Several nosologies are used to classify the various types of urinary incontinence.[55] These classifications are based on a combination of symptoms and underlying etiology (see Table 16-3). It is helpful to understand the different subclasses of urinary incontinence because nursing management interventions are specific for each one.

- Urge incontinence: involuntary loss of urine associated with a strong desire to void. It is often associated with involuntary bladder contractions.
- Stress incontinence: involuntary loss of urine during coughing, sneezing, or other activities that increase intraabdominal pressure. In this condition, the urethral sphincter is unable to generate enough resistance to retain urine in the bladder.
- Overflow incontinence: involuntary loss of urine associated with overdistention of the bladder.
- Functional incontinence: involuntary loss of urine related to chronic physical or cognitive limitations that impair bladder function awareness or physical ability to toilet independently.
- Reflex incontinence: involuntary urine loss that occurs without warning or sensory awareness.

EFFECTS OF AGING ON BLADDER FUNCTION

Although aging itself is not necessarily a cause of bladder dysfunction, certain anatomical and physiological changes associated with aging can predispose elderly individuals to develop problems with urine storage and emptying.

Degeneration and fibrosis of the bladder wall tissues result in a decline in bladder capacity as individuals age.[24] This reduction in bladder capacity may result in more frequent trips to the bathroom. In addition, the kidneys' ability to concentrate urine diminishes with age. Larger volumes of urine along with a smaller bladder capacity give rise to nocturia.

Changes in bladder contractility with advanced age can also alter bladder function. Decreased bladder contractility results in increased residual urine remaining in the bladder after voiding. Urinary residuals have been implicated as contributing to the higher prevalence of bacteriuria in the elderly population. Detrusor instability associated with changes in the neuromuscular threshold to bladder stretch causes the prevalence of involuntary bladder contractions to increase with age. It has been estimated that approximately 15% of healthy elderly men and women have uninhibited bladder contractions in the absence of an underlying pathological condition.[24]

In women the decline in estrogen production after menopause greatly reduces urethral resistance and urethral closure pressure. Urethral mucosal changes resulting from estrogen loss disrupt oxygenation, tissue integrity, and the normal flora, predisposing the tissues to inflammatory and infectious states such as atrophic vaginitis and urethritis.[15,26,27] Childbirth, gynecological surgery, and obesity further weaken the pelvic floor muscles, placing elderly women at greater risk for the development of stress incontinence. In men prostatic hypertrophy can obstruct the bladder outlet, resulting in urinary retention or overflow incontinence.

The higher prevalence of cognitive dysfunction in the elderly places them at greater risk for developing urinary incontinence. Dementias, depression, and delirium can interfere with the ability to recognize toileting needs and carry out the necessary psychomotor activities involved in toileting.

HOME CARE APPLICATION

Home care nurses caring for patients with bladder dysfunction must first assess the status of the patient. The information obtained is then used as a basis for initiating appropriate patient education and for choosing and implementing suitable interventions.

Health history and assessment

Despite the fact that many individuals with bladder dysfunction will benefit from assessment and treatment, studies indicate that a large proportion of them do not undergo any type of evaluation.[49] Patients are often embarrassed or reluctant to report bladder problems, and many elderly persons may consider loss of urine control part of the normal aging process. Therefore home care nurses should include an assessment of bladder function in the overall assessment of the patient.

Nursing assessment should be geared toward determining the underlying factors contributing to the bladder dysfunction so that potentially reversible factors can be corrected and management strategies appropriate for the particular condition can be instituted. A thorough assessment of bladder function should include a health history, with emphasis on bladder habits and bowel function; a physical assessment, including bedside urodynamic testing; functional, cognitive, and environmental evaluations; and collection of laboratory test results for further evaluation, particularly a urinalysis and determination of serum glucose level.[28]

The history. Key aspects of the continence history are summarized in Box 16-1. Onset and duration of the problem, frequency of accidental urine loss, and volume of leakage should be ascertained. Characteristics that delineate the type of incontinence the individual may be having should be determined. For example, it is important to note whether urine loss is associated with a sudden sense of urgency (urge incontinence) or whether leakage occurs with exertional activities such as exercise, bending, coughing, or laughing (stress incontinence). Hesitancy, straining to void, frequent dribbling, constant leakage of small amounts of urine, and a sensation of incomplete bladder emptying are symptoms of urinary retention (overflow incontinence). Associated symptoms such as burning on urination, frequency, urgency, hematuria, or fever may indicate a urinary tract infec-

<table>
<tr><td>

**Box 16-1   ESSENTIAL ELEMENTS
OF THE HISTORY**

- Onset, duration, frequency of accidental urine loss
- Volume of urine loss
- Characteristics of bladder dysfunction: urgency, hesitancy, straining, dribbling, urine loss on exertion or with coughing, sneezing, or bending
- Associated symptoms of bladder dysfunction: dysuria, frequency, nocturia, lack of sensation, vaginal discharge or itching, hematuria
- Pattern of urine loss: times, activity at time of leakage, relationship to fluid or medication consumption
- Past and current medical problems: neurological disorders, diabetes, strokes, congestive heart failure, venous insufficiency
- Past genitourinary/gynecological history: childbirths, surgery, dilatations, radiation, recurrent urinary tract infections
- Medications
- Fluid intake: amount, type, times
- Bowel habits: frequency, consistency

</td></tr>
</table>

tion, although these classic symptoms may be absent in elderly patients. Vaginal discharge, itching, dyspareunia, and recurrent urinary tract infections are signs of atrophic vaginitis, which is often associated with stress incontinence.

The pattern of urine loss should be elicited. Morning incontinence may be related to daily use of a diuretic. Nocturia may be caused by the consumption of alcohol, caffeine, or other fluids near bedtime. Incontinence that occurs only when away from home might indicate a functional loss that results from the inability to find toileting facilities when needed (functional incontinence).

Relevant medical history should be reviewed during the assessment because many medical problems can result in bladder dysfunction. Diabetic patients may experience incontinence as a result of polyuria associated with elevated blood glucose levels or because of diabetic neuropathy rendering the bladder hypotonic. Neurologic disorders such as strokes, Parkinson's disease, dementia, and multiple sclerosis are frequently associated with detrusor instability, which when coupled with the functional disabilities of these medical conditions can result in urinary incontinence. Patients with con-

gestive heart failure or venous insufficiency may experience frequency, urgency, and nocturia as a result of postural diuresis associated with assuming a horizontal position during sleep.

Past genitourinary and gynecological history in women should ascertain the number of vaginal births, bladder or abdominal surgeries, and urethral dilatations. In men, prostate surgery and radiation therapy are important to note. In both men and women the frequency of urinary tract infections should be determined because recurrent infections may necessitate referral to a urologist.

A careful review of medications that the patient is taking should be conducted, because many medications can alter bladder function (Table 16-1).

Assessing fluid intake is another important aspect of the patient's history.[14] Amount, type, and times of fluid consumption should be determined. Fluid consumed close to bedtime may contribute to nocturia or nighttime incontinence. Beverages containing alcohol, caffeine, or aspartame (Nutrasweet) can cause urinary frequency and urgency and often have prolonged effects on elderly individuals.

Assessment of bladder habits. Description of the patient's bladder habits is also useful in determining appropriate nursing interventions. A bladder record (Figure 16-1) is a good way to establish the patient's bladder habits and pattern of incontinence.[40,55] The bladder record can be kept by the patient, family, or formal caregiver. The patient is checked for wetness every 2 hours for several days, and a log is filled out describing the times and volumes of successful voids, incontinent episodes, and fluid intake. The bladder record not only helps assess the type and pattern of accidental urine loss, but also is used to establish behavioral interventions and protocols for managing incontinence.

Assessment of bowel function. Constipation may be a major factor contributing to incontinence because stool mass in the rectum obstructs the bladder outlet. In addition, fecal incontinence may coexist with urinary incontinence and often will improve with use of the same treatment modalities employed to manage bladder problems.

Patients/caregivers should be questioned to determine the frequency and consistency of bowel movements; when the last bowel movement occurred; whether or not patients have problems with

Table 16-1 Medications that can potentially affect continence

Type of medication	Potential effects on continence
Diuretics	Polyuria, frequency, urgency
Anticholinergics	Urinary retention, overflow incontinence, fecal impaction
Psychotropics	
Antidepressants	Anticholinergic actions, sedation
Antipsychotics	Anticholinergic actions, sedation, rigidity, immobility
Sedatives and hypnotics	Sedation, delirium, fecal impaction
Narcotic analgesics	Urinary retention, fecal impaction, sedation, delirium
Alpha-adrenergic blockers	Urethral relaxation
Alpha-adrenergic agonists	Urinary retention
Beta-adrenergic agonists	Urinary retention
Calcium channel blockers	Urinary retention
Alcohol	Polyuria, frequency, urgency, sedation, delirium, immobility

constipation, fecal incontinence, or impactions; what types of foods are eaten; how much fluid is consumed on a daily basis; and whether laxatives are used and if so how often.

Physical assessment. The physical assessment of incontinent patients should include neurologic, abdominal, pelvic, and rectal examinations. A brief evaluation of cranial nerve responses, reflexes, muscle strength, and sensation to the lower extremities and perineal area should be conducted. Abnormalities such as focal and parkinsonian signs suggest that the bladder dysfunction has a neurological component. Integrity of the sacral reflex arc can be determined by testing for the bulbocavernosus reflex. This is done by inserting a gloved finger into the patient's rectum. Gently stroking the glans penis in males and the skin near the clitoris in females should elicit an anal contraction if the reflex is present. Absence of the reflex does not always indicate a pathological condition but can be helpful in further defining problems with neurological innervation if focal findings are present.

The abdomen should be inspected for scars indicating previous abdominal surgeries and for distension. The abdomen should also be palpated to determine the presence of any masses, tenderness, or bladder distension.

The perineum should be examined for redness and skin breakdown. A simple pelvic examination involving inspection of the vaginal canal for atrophic vaginitis or infection and palpation for anatomical abnormalities and masses can be done in the home. During the rectal examination, the rectum should be checked for fecal impaction, masses, prostatic enlargement, and muscle tone. A digital rectal examination is performed by inserting a gloved finger approximately 2 cm past the anus and external sphincter to the internal sphincter. The patient is asked to squeeze around the examining finger to test the contraction strength, then the examining finger is withdrawn to the external sphincter and the patient is asked to squeeze again. If muscle strength and nerve innervation are intact, the patient should be able to contract both sphincters strongly.

Bedside urodynamic testing. Bedside urodynamic testing is a simple screening procedure to determine the cause of persistent urinary incontinence (i.e., urge, stress, or overflow). The procedure and its diagnostic usefulness are outlined in Table 16-2. Ouslander and others compared bedside with standard multichannel cystometry in 171 elderly incontinent patients.[36,37] Bedside testing was reported to have a 75% sensitivity and

BLADDER RECORD

Name_____Date_____

Time	Amount Urinated in Toilet	Urine Leakage Small Amount	Urine Leakage Large Amount	Activity When Leakage Occurred	Leakage of Stool	Fluid Intake
8:00 am	ml					
9:00 am	ml					
10:00 am	ml					
11:00 am	ml					
12:00 pm	ml					
1:00 pm	ml					
2:00 pm	ml					
3:00 pm	ml					
4:00 pm	ml					
5:00 pm	ml					
6:00 pm	ml					
7:00 pm	ml					
8:00 pm	ml					
9:00 pm	ml					
10:00 pm	ml					
11:00 pm	ml					
12:00 am	ml					
1:00 am	ml					
2:00 am	ml					
3:00 am	ml					
4:00 am	ml					
5:00 am	ml					
6:00 am	ml					
7:00 am	ml					

Figure 16-1 Sample bladder record.

Table 16-2 Bedside cystometry procedure

Procedure	Normal finding	Abnormal finding	Diagnostic usefulness
1. Have patient void. Then catheterize.	Catheter passes with ease.	Catheter is difficult to pass.	OVERFLOW INCONTINENCE from mechanical obstruction.
2. Measure postvoid residual (PVR) urine.	<100 ml PVR.	>100 ml PVR.	OVERFLOW INCONTINENCE secondary to retention.
3. Fill bladder slowly with sterile solution. Note volume when initial urge to void is sensed.	Initial urge to void generally sensed when bladder holds 250 ml to 300 ml.	Strong initial urge sensed at <200 ml.	URGE INCONTINENCE related to small bladder capacity.
4. Continue to fill bladder slowly until patient can hold no more.	Normal bladder capacity between 400 ml and 600 ml.	Patient unable to tolerate minimum of 400 ml.	URGE INCONTINENCE secondary to diminished bladder capacity.
5. Note any involuntary bladder contractions.	No contractions or leakage around catheter noted.	Retrograde movement of fluid into syringe. Leakage around catheter, patient expresses sense of urgency.	URGE INCONTINENCE related to uninhibited bladder contractions.
6. With bladder filled to capacity, remove catheter and have patient cough in supine and standing positions.	No leakage.	Leakage of fluid from bladder with stress maneuvers.	STRESS INCONTINENCE associated with pelvic muscle weakness.
7. Have patient empty bladder into measuring "HAT." Observe patient void.	Calculated PVR <100 ml. Strong urine stream.	Calculated PVR >100 ml. Hesitancy, straining, intermittent stream present.	OVERFLOW INCONTINENCE secondary to an obstruction or atonic bladder.

79% specificity for detrusor instability. Diokno compared the provocative stress test (a component of bedside cystometry) with self-reported continence status and incontinence symptoms.[12] The estimated sensitivity of provocative stress testing was 39.5% with a specificity of 98.5%. Bedside urodynamic testing is neither sensitive nor specific for detrusor hyperactivity with impaired contractility or other forms of outlet obstruction.

Although multichannel synchronous pressure flow studies offer the most accurate method of evaluating bladder dysfunction, these studies are also more expensive, invasive, and time-consuming than bedside testing. Bedside testing therefore has value as an initial screening procedure to evaluate bladder dysfunction in the home setting.

Functional assessment. Because many patients suffer from impaired mobility, it is important for home care nurses to determine the extent to which functional disabilities contribute to urinary incontinence. An assessment of gait, balance, and transfer ability can ascertain whether bladder problems have a functional component. Patients should be observed as they rise from a bed or chair. Immediate standing balance, step symmetry, step continuity, speed, stability with movement, and appropriate or inappropriate use of assistive devices should be noted. If patients are confined to a bed or wheelchair, the ability to shift weight while sitting and lying should be assessed because use of a urinal or bedpan will depend on the degree to which patients are able to maneuver themselves.

Assessment of cognitive function. Evaluating cognitive function is an important part of assessing patients with bladder dysfunction because the nursing interventions chosen to treat the problem must be consistent with patients' abilities to learn, remember, and carry out instructions. There are standard instruments available for assessing mental status. Multidisciplinary conferences with the mental health nurse may be helpful during the process of evaluating cognitive function.

Environmental assessment. Environmental factors that should be assessed include distance to the toilet, toilet access, seat height, presence of safety or supportive devices, lighting, safety of floor surfaces, obstacles in the pathway to the bathroom, type of clothing and footwear worn by the patient, ability to manipulate clothing, accessibility of adaptive equipment, and availability of caregiver assistance. Although not used commonly in the home setting, physical and chemical restraints should be recognized as environmental barriers that may interfere with the performance of toileting tasks.

Laboratory tests. Urinary tract infections can cause urinary incontinence and urinary retention. This very treatable source of bladder dysfunction can be ruled out by laboratory evaluation. A postvoid catheterization should be performed on all incontinent patients to check for residual urine. A residual volume of 100 ml or greater indicates urinary retention. The urine sample that is collected should be sent to the laboratory for urinalysis and culture. The accepted definition of significant bacteriuria is the growth of one or more organisms from a clean catch or catheterized specimen with a count of greater than 100,000 colony-forming units (CFUs) per milliliter of urine.[1] The presence of red blood cells in the absence of pyuria or bacteriuria may indicate the need for a urologic evaluation to rule out tumors or calculi. Identification of the infecting organism by culture ensures the choice of appropriate antibiotic treatment.

Dipstick testing is an acceptable screening technique for analysis of urine. It has a reported sensitivity rate as high as 90%. Urine that is dipstick positive for leukocytes, red blood cells, or nitrite is generally infected. Often antibiotic therapy is initiated based on dipstick findings alone.

Blood urea nitrogen (BUN) and serum creatinine, end products of metabolism, can be helpful in identifying renal failure. Urea nitrogen rises gradually during acute renal failure, and serum creatinine rises rapidly during chronic renal failure. The BUN may be elevated if the individual is dehydrated, febrile, or receiving increased proteins parenterally or in the diet.

Nursing management and patient education

The plan of care for patients with bladder dysfunction is based on assessment and subsequent determination of the cause of the problem (Box 16-2). A variety of interventions are available for the management of urinary incontinence and retention. Therapies most appropriate for each type of bladder dysfunction are outlined in Table 16-3 and are discussed in detail in the following sections.

Interventions for patients with bladder dysfunction should be directed toward goals of care that are realistic and achievable, reflecting patients'/caregivers' physical, psychological, and intellectual capabilities (Box 16-3).

Box 16-2   PRIMARY NURSING DIAGNOSIS/PATIENT PROBLEMS

- Urinary elimination, alteration in pattern related to prostatic hypertrophy, retention, urethral sphincter weakness, infection, detrusor hyperreflexia, and functional impairment
- Bowel elimination, alteration in: constipation or fecal impaction related to immobility, decreased fluid intake, medication side effects, and decreased gastrointestinal motility
- Potential for urinary tract infection related to chronic indwelling catheter use
- Self-care deficit: toileting
- Potential for skin breakdown secondary to incontinence
- Self-concept/self-esteem alteration related to urinary incontinence

Table 16-3 Types, causes, and treatments of persistent urinary incontinence

Classification	Definition	Characteristics	Causes	Treatment options
Stress	Loss of urine with intraabdominal pressure	Small-volume urine loss Common in women Urine loss with coughing, laughing, bending, lifting, sneezing, or when standing up	Pelvic muscle relaxation secondary to decreased estrogen production, childbirth(s), trauma, surgery, and obesity Damage to urethral sphincter from surgery, radiation treatment, or trauma	Pelvic floor exercises Suspension surgery Artificial urinary sphincter Alpha-adrenergic agonist Estrogen replacement Electrical stimulation Vaginal pessary Penile clamp Biofeedback
Urge	Sudden loss of urine associated with sense of urgency to void	Large-volume urine loss Loss of urine in any position Frequency Urgency Nocturia	Detrusor instability secondary to a neurological condition or bladder irritation, e.g., infection, cancer, foreign body Idiopathic bladder instability	Anticholinergics, antispasmodics, or antibiotics Biofeedback Behavioral training procedures Electrical stimulation Surgical removal of irritating lesion
Reflex	Sudden urine loss when the spinal cord reflex arc is completed	Large-volume urine loss May or may not sense need to void	Spinal cord injury Multiple sclerosis	Cutaneous stimulation Credé's maneuver Behavioral training Bladder relaxants
Overflow	Leakage of urine from an overdistended bladder secondary to mechanical obstruction of the urinary outlet or an atrophied state of the detrusor muscle	Frequent or continuous dripping of urine Urine loss in small volumes Hesitancy or straining to void Diminished urine stream	Bladder outlet obstruction due to enlarged prostate, urethral stricture, cancer, pelvic prolapse Atonic detrusor muscle due to medications or neurological involvement, e.g., diabetes, multiple sclerosis, or trauma	Surgery to relieve obstruction Intermittent catheterization Cholinergic Temporary use of indwelling catheter
Functional	Urinary leakage associated with inability to toilet because of cognitive impairment, physical disability, psychological unwillingness, or environmental barriers	Large-volume urine loss Normal muscle and sphincter function Voiding at inappropriate times	Impaired mental status as with dementia, head injury, depression, psychosis Physical disabilities that slow down or impair motor function, e.g., arthritis, strokes, Parkinson's disease Unfamiliar environment Environmental barriers such as restraints, distance to the toilet	Habit training Scheduled training Adaptive equipment Absorbent pads and pants Environmental manipulation

Box 16-3   PRIMARY THEMES OF PATIENT EDUCATION

- Complications from disease process: when to call the physician and case manager
- Catheter management
- Medications: purpose, action, dosage, side effects, and methods of administration
- Urinary tract and bladder infection: recognition and treatment
- Diet: fluid intake (volume, types, scheduling); dietary measures for managing constipation
- Infection control
- Skin care
- Toileting schedules
- General self-care strategies

Behavioral training procedures. Behavioral interventions aim to improve bladder function by providing a patient/caregiver-initiated stimulus and reinforcer to establish continent behavior.

Pelvic floor exercises. Pelvic floor (Kegel) exercises are used to treat stress incontinence in men and women with intact cognitive function. These exercises involve repetitive contraction and relaxation of the periurethral muscles to help strengthen them so that tighter urethral closure can be achieved[60] (Box 16-4). Success rates of 70% or more have been reported with the use of Kegel exercises.[55] Although the optimal number and frequency of pelvic floor exercises required to achieve urine control have not been established, several training times per day are generally suggested. Anywhere from 6 to 12 weeks of continued exercise will be necessary before patients begin to see results. Ongoing exercise to maintain muscle tone will be necessary once the desired results are achieved. Having patients perform these exercises during a digital rectal or vaginal examination provides feedback to ensure that the correct muscles are being tightened. Instruct patients to practice starting and stopping the flow of urine when voiding to become familiar with the muscles that need to be targeted. These exercises should be practiced frequently. Patient motivation and compliance are essential for the success of this treatment.

Vaginal weights for pelvic floor training. Pelvic floor exercises should be taught with some

Box 16-4   KEGEL EXERCISES

Kegel exercises are a technique used to strengthen the pelvic floor muscles to prevent loss or leakage of urine that can occur when these muscles are weak. Here's how you do Kegel exercises:

- Sit or stand. Without tensing the muscles of your legs, buttocks, or abdomen, imagine that you are trying to control the passing of urine by squeezing the muscles of the vagina together. Hold one hand on your stomach to make sure the abdominal muscles are not moving as you slowly squeeze the sides of the vagina together.
- As you do this, the ring of muscles around the rectum will also squeeze together. This is normal.
- Practice squeezing the vagina together, counting to three as you squeeze tightly. Give one last extra squeeze on the count of four, and then relax the muscle for three counts.
- Do a series of 10 exercises 4 times per day. Count one, two, three, extra squeeze, relax. Two, two, three, extra squeeze, relax. Three, two, three, extra squeeze, relax, and so on up to a total of 10 Kegel exercises.
- Good times to practice Kegel exercises are in the morning before getting up, in the evening at bedtime, and during the day when you go to the bathroom. When you are passing urine, practice stopping the urine flow and then restarting it again.

It is important to do your Kegel exercises daily. It will take about 6 to 8 weeks of *daily* exercising before you begin to notice any results.

form of evaluation to ensure correct muscle contraction. One means of providing both biofeedback and a training stimulus is the vaginal weight. A set of vaginal weights consists of five weights of identical shape and volume varying from 20 g to 100 g. The weight is inserted into the vagina above the pelvic floor muscle and worn for 15 minutes twice a day while the user is ambulatory. Once the person can retain the lightest weight for the specified time period, she progresses to the next heaviest weight. The weights help to increase muscle tone and pelvic support by sustaining a low-intensity prolonged muscle contraction.[39]

Bladder training. Bladder training involves progressive lengthening or shortening of toileting intervals to correct the negative habit of frequent voiding or waiting too long to void. This improves the patient's ability to suppress the urgency caused by bladder instability. Bladder training incorporates adjunctive techniques such as triggering and emptying techniques, intermittent catheterization, and the use of a bladder record to identify a voiding schedule and adjust the amount and timing of fluid intake.

Bladder training is applicable to patients with a neurogenic bladder or patients who have had an indwelling catheter.[22,41] Adequate cognitive function, mobility, and motivation are necessary for bladder training to be successful.

Scheduled toileting. Scheduled toileting assists patients to void at fixed intervals, usually every 2 hours during the day and every 4 hours at night. The goal of scheduled toileting is to reduce the number of wet episodes. Scheduled toileting should be used when the patient does not respond to caregiver feedback about wetness checks and verbal prompts to use the bathroom but is still able to use the toilet or commode. Because this intervention is caregiver dependent, its potential success relies heavily on the availability and motivation of caregivers to implement the procedure. Scheduled toileting is useful for managing urge and functional incontinence.

Habit training and patterning. Habit training, as opposed to scheduled toileting, consists of a flexible toileting schedule based on the patient's pattern of incontinence. Colling and others found that 82% of an individual's voiding episodes occurred daily during the same hourly blocks of time.[9] When habit training is used, a bladder record is documented for several days and then examined for patterns of voiding episodes. A program of toileting is then developed based on the patient's voiding pattern.

Positive reinforcement for continent behaviors is an important component of habit training. The goal of habit training is to avoid incontinent episodes. Generally adjustment in the timing and volume of fluid intake is necessary to achieve the desired goal. Habit training can be used to manage functional and urge incontinence but is largely caregiver dependent.

Prompted voiding. Prompted voiding is recommended for patients with urinary incontinence who are cognitively impaired or unable to void without assistance. Prompted voiding involves four major components.[22] The caregiver is taught to (1) physically check the patient for wetness every 2 hours, (2) ask the patient if he or she is wet or dry and give corrective feedback based on the physical check, (3) ask the patient if he or she would like toileting assistance, and (4) socially reinforce the patient for requesting assistance or for staying dry. The patient is toileted only if the response to the prompt is affirmative. Prompted voiding has been found to significantly reduce wet episodes and increase toileting requests by the patient; however, it is also more expensive in terms of labor costs than standard continence care.[10,38,45,46]

Prompted voiding is most successful in patients who have some awareness of bladder fullness or the need to void, who ask for assistance or respond when prompted to void, who can discern whether they are wet or dry, who have a functional bladder capacity of 150 ml or more, who void when assisted to the toilet, and whose frequency of urination is not more than 4 times during a 12-hour period.[22,51] The goal of prompted voiding is to increase the patient's awareness of the need to void and thereby initiate toileting before the incontinence occurs.

Credé's maneuver. In the Credé's maneuver, bladder emptying is aided by manually exerting pressure over the lower abdomen to express urine. This method can be used for patients with urinary retention secondary to a neurogenic bladder or with reflex incontinence. It should not be performed if an abdominal mass or aneurysm is present. Patients should be instructed to sit upright on the toilet and place hands flat—one on top of the other—on the abdomen just below the umbilicus. They should press down firmly toward the perineum 6 or 7 times until urine starts flowing. Once the urine stream begins, they should maintain light pressure until it stops. After relaxing for 2 minutes, patients should repeat the maneuver until urine can no longer be expressed.

Catheters and catheter care

Several types of catheters and catheterization procedures are used in the home setting to manage urinary incontinence. These include indwelling catheters, intermittent catheterization, and external catheters or collection devices. Indications and nursing management practices for each type of catheter or catheterization procedure are discussed in the following sections.

Indwelling catheters. Chronic indwelling catheterization for the management of bladder dysfunction should not be regarded as a routine nursing intervention. It should be limited to the following situations: (1) when urinary retention is present and cannot be corrected either surgically or medically and intermittent catheterization is traumatic or impractical, (2) when skin wounds or pressure sores are present and need to be protected from urine contamination, (3) when patients are terminally ill or debilitated and bed or clothing changes are uncomfortable or disruptive, and (4) when it is the preference of patients/caregivers after all other treatments have failed.[24,55]

Both short- and long-term urethral catheterization are associated with a high risk of urinary tract infection. Other complications include renal and bladder stones, hydronephrosis, bladder carcinoma, epididymitis, pyelonephritis, prostatic and urethral abscesses, and urethral fistulae. Trauma, discomfort, leakage of urine, and encrustation causing blockage of the catheter lumen are problems that have been identified with chronic indwelling catheters.[43] For these reasons, catheters should be avoided unless absolutely necessary.

Selecting the catheter. Plastic and latex catheters are recommended for short-term use of 1 to 3 weeks.[43] Urethral pain and bladder spasms are more common with the less flexible plastic catheters, and a higher incidence of encrustation has been noted with latex catheters. Catheters with hydrogel-bonding, teflon, and silicone coatings should be used for long-term purposes, because lower incidences of encrustation and catheter bypassing (i.e., leakage of urine around the catheter) have been reported with their use.[25] Bonded catheters may last longer than silicone catheters because this coating prevents bacterial adherence and reduces mucosal friction. However, if the patient is sensitive to latex, a silicone catheter should be used.

Catheter size depends on the individual, how long the catheter will be in place, and the purpose for inserting the catheter. In general a small catheter size is recommended because large-diameter catheters have been associated with more complications.[43] The catheter should be small enough to pass with ease through the external meatus to ensure its passage through the rest of the urethra. A 14 to 16 French (Fr) catheter is recommended in most instances. Catheter lumen sizes increase by 2 Fr increments. Each gradation of 1 Fr equals 0.33 mm. Two catheter lengths are currently available: the male length (41 cm) and the shorter female length (23 cm).

Balloon size is also a factor to consider in choosing a catheter. Urinary catheters come with balloon volumes of 5, 10, or 30 ml and can be inflated with water or air. The 30-ml balloon is often used after transurethral prostatectomy to prevent hemorrhage. Smaller balloon sizes of 5 or 10 ml should be used in most cases, since they take up less space, cause less mucosal irritation, and are less often associated with bladder spasms and bypassing of urine.

Inserting the catheter. Using sterile technique, home care nurses should insert indwelling catheters according to policy and procedure guidelines of their agency. Resistance may be encountered during insertion when the catheter tip reaches the internal sphincter. Pausing for a few seconds to allow the sphincter to relax may help overcome this problem. Prostatic hypertrophy and urethral strictures cause greater resistance to catheter passage. Using a smaller lumen or a coudé tip (curved tip) catheter may make insertion easier. Force should never be used to overcome resistance, since edema or urethral perforation can occur. A physician should be notified if resistance continues and gentle manipulation of the catheter fails to allow insertion. With male patients, it is important to retract the foreskin back over the head of the penis once catheterization is completed.

The patient should not experience pain when the balloon is inflated. If pain occurs, the balloon is in the urethra instead of the bladder. In this case, the balloon should be immediately deflated and then reinflated once the catheter is advanced farther.

Bladder decompression. Misconceptions surrounding the proper procedure for emptying the overdistended bladder continue to abound despite lack of scientific evidence. The prevailing belief is that rapid bladder emptying can result in hemorrhage, hypovolemic shock, or bladder collapse and therefore catheter clamping should occur after drainage of 500 to 750 ml of urine.

More recent reviews of the literature suggest that these beliefs are unfounded.[6,51] Bristol and others compared rapid versus slow bladder decompression in randomly assigned groups. Patients were monitored for pain, diaphoresis, frank hematuria, and changes in blood pressure and pulse during bladder emptying. No statistically significant changes were found between the two groups.[6]

On rare occassions, postobstructive diuresis may occur in patients with long-term bladder neck obstruction.[4] These patients can experience hypotension secondary to excessive losses of sodium and water in the urine and may require intravenous fluid replacement and sodium supplementation. However, the majority of patients with chronic retention experience no ill effects after rapid bladder decompression.[23,51,54]

Maintaining the catheter and drainage system. A closed catheter system should be the standard of care for patients requiring indwelling urethral catheters. However, even with a closed system, bacteriuria will occur. It is possible to delay the onset of bacteriuria with maintenance of a closed system.

The drainage system chosen should be suited to the patient's individual needs so that, once intact, disconnection of the system is unnecessary. For example, if the patient is fairly mobile, a leg bag can be used and a special drainage system can be connected to the distal part of the leg bag at night. In this manner, the closed system does not have to be interrupted to change drainage bags. The drainage system should also have a one-way valve between the bag and the catheter tubing to prevent reflux of urine back into the bladder. The collection bag should always be kept below the level of the patient's bladder.

The catheter should never be disconnected from the collection tubing to obtain urine samples. Aspiration of urine with a sterile needle and syringe from a port on the tubing for this purpose is the appropriate mechanism for obtaining a urine specimen.

Routine catheter care. Handwashing by the nurse, patient, or family caregiver before and after handling the catheter and drainage system is essential. Periurethral care includes cleansing the perineum with soap and water each day and after each bowel movement, using care to wipe from the urethra toward the anus. Application of antiseptic agents such as Betadine to the periurethral area has not been proven effective in reducing bacteriuria. The catheter should always be secured to the upper thigh to help reduce movement in and out of the urethra, which can cause inflammation. Catheter drainage bags should be emptied at least every 4 hours in order to avoid prolonged urine stasis and bacterial migration intraluminally along the inside of the catheter.[32]

Changing the catheter. No data are available on how frequently catheters should be changed. Typically insurance reimbursement allowances drive the standard practices. Recommendations for frequency of catheter changes vary from every 4 weeks to only when obstruction or malfunction occurs. The catheter material will partly determine how often it will require changing. Some silicone catheters can be left in place for up to 6 months. Many institutional protocols stipulate that catheters be changed every 4 weeks unless problems necessitate changing more frequently. It is accepted that Foley catheters should never be reused once they are removed.

Home care nurses should always use sterile technique when changing catheters in order to reduce the chances of introducing microorganisms to which the patient has no resistance. However, frail, debilitated, and elderly patients develop infections whether clean or sterile technique is used. Therefore, because clean technique is easier and more practical for caregivers in the home setting, caregivers who learn to change the catheter may use clean technique.

Bladder irrigation. The effectiveness of routine bladder irrigation in preventing infection and obstruction remains unclear. Evidence suggests that routine bladder irrigation does not prevent infection,[3] and both open and closed bladder irrigation methods have been reported to cause urinary tract infections.[18]

In the home, bladder irrigation is usually indicated for catheter obstruction or to instill medication. Bladder instillation is similar to intermittent bladder irrigation except that the catheter is clamped after the fluid is instilled to allow the solution to remain in the bladder for a specified time period. The flow rate of the irrigant must be controlled, and the patient must be observed closely for signs of bladder retention.

Solutions commonly used for bladder irrigation are sterile normal saline or sterile 0.25% acetic acid. Normal saline is isotonic and reduces the chance of hemolysis or fluid overload that can occur with the use of sterile water. Acetic acid acidifies the urine and prevents debris formation, which can lead to encrustation around the catheter tip.

Little evidence exists to support the efficacy of catheter clamping prior to discontinuation.[58] To remove an indwelling catheter, deflate the balloon by attaching a syringe to the balloon lumen and aspirating the fluid. The catheter is then withdrawn slowly. If the balloon does not deflate, the physician should be contacted immediately. Caregivers should be instructed to notify the home health agency of any problems with the indwelling catheter such as leakage, a lack of urine, patient complaints of abdominal pain or tenderness, change in urine color, or fever. They should be taught how to discontinue the catheter if problems arise during the night or when the home care nurse is not available. Simple instructions regarding discontinuation of the catheter may save an unnecessary and expensive trip to the emergency department. Ideally home care agencies should have after-hours service managers taking calls to help patients and their caregivers troubleshoot problems with Foley catheters or to help them make decisions regarding questionable situations.

Treating infections. Even with the use of aseptic technique, by the end of 30 days of catheterization, 78% to 95% of patients will be bacteriuric.[19] However, the majority of patients with long-term urethral catheters and bacteriuria are asymptomatic. Routine surveillance cultures are not necessary in the chronically catheterized patient. The use of antimicrobial agents for prophylaxis or treatment of asymptomatic bacteriuria is not recommended because this practice may lead to the development of more resistant organisms and/or drug toxicity.[8,33]

Two thirds of febrile episodes in elderly, long-term catheterized patients are related to urinary-tract infections. Therefore temperatures of patients with indwelling catheters should be closely monitored. Mental status changes, diaphoresis, abdominal pain, tachycardia, hypotension, nausea and vomiting, and restless or agitated behaviors are other symptoms that may indicate the presence of a urinary tract infection or bacteremia. It is important to monitor the patient's response to antibiotics and correlate the laboratory sensitivity findings with the medical treatment because many strains of bacteria in long-term catheterized patients are resistant to commonly used antimicrobial agents. If symptomatic urinary tract infections recur frequently, patients should be referred to a urologist to rule out an underlying pathological condition.

Encrustation and obstruction. Encrustation refers to accumulation of debris around the catheter tip that blocks the drainage holes. One way of preventing obstruction from encrustation is to change the catheter more frequently. In addition, maintaining an acidic urinary pH helps reduce encrustation. This can be achieved with dietary measures. Cranberry juice and an acid-ash diet make the urine more acidic. It is recommended that the patient drink 5 to 8 oz of cranberry juice 3 times a day and incorporate meat, whole grains, eggs, prunes, and plums in the diet.[13]

Since encrustation occurs more frequently when the urine is concentrated, patients should be encouraged to maintain a fluid intake of 2000 to 3000 ml per day. Adequate fluid intake will ensure a steady stream of urine in the catheter tubing, reducing the possibility of catheter obstruction.

Silicone catheters should be used whenever possible because this material is less susceptible to encrustation. Milking the catheter tubing several times a day can help maintain catheter patency. If the catheter does become obstructed, catheter replacement is recommended.

Leakage. Although leakage of urine around the catheter can occur if the catheter is obstructed, it may also occur if the patient is having bladder spasms. Bladder irritability and spasms may result from a variety of causes. Urinary tract infection, constipation or fecal impaction, bladder stones, or an oversized catheter balloon are possible sources of bladder irritability.

When leakage occurs, measures should be taken to alleviate the irritating condition. If such measures fail to maintain dryness, an antispasmodic agent such as oxybutynin can be used to relax the bladder muscle.

Odor. Physical cleanliness is important in controlling urine odor. Perineal care with soap and water should be carried out daily. Odor from drainage bags and appliances is caused by bacteria, and reduction of bacterial growth in drainage bags has been found to eliminate odor.[7]

Drainage systems should be changed whenever the catheter is changed. Camasso[7] recommends adding 10 ml of sterile hydrogen peroxide through the drainage porthole each time the drainage bag is emptied. This allows maintenance of a closed system and reduces odor. Drainage bags can be deodorized by filling them with a solution of 2 parts vinegar to 3 parts water and soaking for 20 minutes. Because this method does not maintain a closed system, it is best used for cleansing external collection devices and associated drainage systems.

Intermittent catheterization. Intermittent catheterization is usually implemented in the home care setting for problems associated with persistent urinary retention. The goal of intermittent catheterization is to avoid high intraluminal pressure and overdistension, which decrease blood flow to the bladder muscle and make it susceptible to bacterial invasion. Intermittent catheterization should be performed frequently enough so that the bladder is not allowed to accumulate more than 500 ml of urine.

Generally, clean technique is recommended when intermittent catheterization is done at home. Clean technique has not been found to significantly increase the overall incidence of urinary tract infections and is reported to decrease the overall incidence of urinary tract complications.[57] Patients/caregivers should be taught to wash their hands before the procedure. Procedural guidelines outlined by agency protocols should be followed. After the procedure the catheter should be washed with soap and water and allowed to dry thoroughly. Catheters can be stored or carried in plastic bags. They may be reused but should be discarded when they begin to crack or develop an odor.

Suprapubic catheterization. A suprapubic catheter is inserted percutaneously through the abdominal wall into the bladder and is sometimes used after gynecological and urological surgery. As with indwelling urethral catheters, infection is a primary concern. Other complications of suprapubic catheters include cellulitis, leakage, hematoma near the insertion site, and obstruction. These catheters are maintained much like an indwelling urethral catheter.

External catheters. External catheters and collection systems are used to manage rather than prevent or resolve the symptoms and problems associated with bladder dysfunction. These devices should be used only on patients who have not responded to other measures to correct problems with incontinence or on patients who are extremely physically dependent.

External catheters for men consist of either a penile funnel that is held to the pubic area by waist straps or a condom that is attached to the penis with adhesive and elastic straps. Condom catheters are the most common external device for men. Although many believe external catheters are quite safe, symptomatic urinary tract infections are more prevalent among men who wear condom catheters than among those who do not.[35] Complications of condom catheters include edema, skin breakdown, penile constriction, penile ischemia, and urethral diverticula.[29]

The penis should be cleansed with soap and water and allowed to dry before application of an external device. For greater comfort and adherence, it may be necessary to shave the pubic hair. The condom should fit snugly but not tightly. If tissue swelling and color change occur, the condom is too tight and should be discontinued immediately. Condoms should be removed daily or every other day to wash and evaluate the skin. Every 3 to 4 days the condom should be left off to allow the skin to be exposed for 24 hours. If skin irritation occurs, the condom should be removed until the area is completely healed.

If the penis is retracted, a condom catheter will not be useful. Special pouches, similar to ostomy bags, are available that fit over the penis and attach to the pubic area. These pouches need to be sized appropriately, and the pubic area must be shaved for them to fit properly. Their disadvantage is that the penis is not protected from urine contact.

External catheters for females are commercially available, but their safety and efficacy have not been established. Problems that have been encountered with the use of female external catheters include displacement, leakage, labial pressure sores, and erosion of soft tissues of the vulva.

Environmental manipulation and supportive measures

Because many environmental factors can contribute to functional urine loss, adjustments in the environment may be necessary. These adjustments consist of removing environmental barriers or adding supportive devices.[5]

Environmental barriers to toileting include such factors as inadequate lighting, distance to the toilet, clutter, the type of clothing the individual is wearing, and physical or chemical restraints. Bathroom lighting should be adequate at all times, especially at night. Night-lights in bathrooms not only help patients identify the location of the toilet but are also an important safety measure to prevent falls. Distance to the toilet should be no more than 30 to 40 feet from the living area. Making toilet access easier by moving the bed or chair closer or by providing a toilet substitute may help the patient with impaired mobility maintain dryness. Walkways to the bathroom should be kept clean and clutter-free, and throw rugs on bathroom floors should be removed. Clothing must be nonconstrictive and easy to remove. If buttons or zippers are difficult for the patient to manage, elastic-waisted pants or Velcro fasteners may be substituted. In some cases, underwear and stockings may need to be eliminated to allow independent toileting. Patients should always wear supportive, nonskid shoes or slippers when going to the bathroom. Physical restraints and pharmacological agents that alter mental status should be avoided.

Supportive devices consist of mobility-enhancing adaptive equipment and toilet substitutes. Equipment to enhance mobility includes bathroom wall rails, toilet railings, canes, walkers, wheelchairs, electric chair raisers, trapeze bars, and elevated toilet seats. Toilet substitutes consist of bedside commodes, overtoilet chairs for transporting the patient to the toilet, bedpans, and urinals.

Absorbent pads and pants. Protective undergarments and pads are designed to absorb urine and provide a moisture barrier to protect clothing, bedding, and furniture. Absorbent products are either disposable or reusable and are the most widely used aid for managing urinary incontinence.[49] A catalogue of incontinence products can be obtained from an organization called Help for Incontinent People (PO Box 544, Union, SC 29379).

It is important that diapers and other absorbent products be prescribed only after a thorough evaluation of the bladder dysfunction. When used prematurely, these products simply obscure the problem.

Skin care. Because there is a strong association between skin disorders and urinary incontinence, interventions for promoting skin integrity are an essential component of the care of the patient with bladder dysfunction. The goal of skin care is to maintain an environment that best approximates continent, dry skin conditions. These conditions include maintenance of an acidic pH, minimization of skin hydration, and alleviation of exposure to

feces and urine. Since most soaps tend to be alkaline, skin cleansing with soap should be reserved for the removal of feces. At other times cleansing with water alone is sufficient.

Moisture-barrier products that contain a mixture of silicone, bentonite, zinc oxide, and petrolatum have been found to be superior to pure petrolatum and allantoin-based protectants in their ability to inhibit the passage of water-soluble tracers into the skin.[56]

Medication and fluid modification. Home care nurses can help patients modify medications and fluid intake to facilitate normal bladder function. Several types of medication can aggravate incontinence. Diuretics should be taken early in the morning to prevent patients from having to void frequently during the night. If the diuretic is being given for blood pressure maintenance but is considered a significant cause of incontinence, the nurse should discuss this problem with the physician. In many cases another antihypertensive agent can be prescribed in place of the diuretic. If the patient is receiving sedatives, tranquilizers, or narcotic analgesics, the nurse should be aware of the effects of these drugs on cognition. Caregivers will need to be alerted to the fact that patients will require assistance to the bathroom or a reminder to toilet themselves. In some cases a voiding schedule will be necessary.

Adequate oral fluid intake is important for establishing healthy voiding patterns and should be planned in conjunction with a toileting schedule. Poor fluid intake leads to concentrated and low-volume urine production such that the bladder is never fully expanded. Chronic low-volume voiding reduces bladder capacity and decreases detrusor muscle tone, making incontinence more likely.[14] Voiding upon awakening, after meals, once between meals, and at bedtime is a schedule that works well, since most individuals drink the bulk of their fluids with meals. A daily fluid intake of 2000 to 3000 ml should be consumed between breakfast and supper with fluids limited to 150 ml after the evening meal. Consumption of alcohol and beverages containing caffeine (such as coffee, tea, and colas) should be avoided.

Cranberry juice. For many years folk wisdom has suggested that cranberry juice can be used to prevent the occurrence of urinary tract infection. One study found that cranberry juice reduced bacteriuria and pyuria by 50% in elderly women who drank 300 ml daily over a 6-month period.[16] It is thought that cranberry juice inhibits adherence of bacteria to the epithelial cells lining the mucosal surface of the urinary tract. Another study reported a reduction of 6.7 cases of urinary tract infections per month after nursing home residents began receiving 4 ounces of cranberry juice per day at a cost of $0.13 per resident per day.[11] Although additional research must be conducted, it does appear that cranberry juice may be clinically useful in the prevention and management of urinary tract infections.[31]

Pharmacological treatment for bladder dysfunction. Drug therapy for bladder dysfunction can be implemented alone or in conjunction with other therapeutic modalities. The pharmacological agents used most commonly are those that improve bladder emptying, decrease bladder hyperactivity, and increase or decrease resistance of the bladder outlet.[17,59] These drugs are summarized in Appendix XVI-I. The medications that appear in this table are those that are recommended in the clinical practice guidelines established for urinary incontinence management by the Agency for Healthcare Research and Quality (formerly the Agency for Health Care Policy and Research).[55]

Bowel management. Nursing measures to restore or maintain normal bowel function include dietary modification, increasing fluid intake, and increasing the patient's level of activity. Adequate amounts of fluid and fiber, both of which are important in preventing constipation, are often lacking in the diets of homebound individuals. Between 4 and 6 g of fiber per day are recommended to facilitate normal bowel function.[2]

Increasing fluid intake to between 2000 and 3000 ml per day in the absence of cardiovascular disease, and to approximately 1500 ml daily if the patient has a history of congestive heart failure, will help reduce the incidence of constipation. Popsicles or ice chips are helpful alternatives to water and juices. Intravenous fluids may be necessary to prevent dehydration and bowel complications in patients with nausea and vomiting.

Increasing the level of physical activity may be a seemingly impossible task for the debilitated homebound patient. However, even extremely frail individuals can benefit from the increased motion afforded by position changes (such as sitting in a chair) and by active or passive range of motion exercises. Wheelchair-confined patients may receive motivation from music or exercise tapes, which are available through local libraries or specialty organizations such as the Arthritis Foundation.

SUMMARY

Home care nurses frequently care for patients with bladder dysfunction, a potentially debilitating condition that adversely affects the physical, psychological, and social well-being of patients and their families. Home care nurses can have a tremendous impact on patients' efforts to improve urinary control. Through assessment, planning, and implementation of strategies to achieve continence, home care nurses can significantly enhance patients' dignity and quality of life.

REFERENCES

1. Abrams WB, Berkow R: *Merck Manual of Geriatrics.* Rahway, NJ, 1990, Merck, Sharp & Dohme Research Laboratories.
2. Behm RM: A special recipe to banish constipation, *Geriatr Nurs* 6:216, 1985.
3. Bergener S: Justification of closed intermittent urinary catheter irrigation/instillation: a review of current research and practice, *J Adv Nurs* 12:229, 1987.
4. Bishop MC: Diuresis and renal functional recovery in chronic retention, *Br J Urol* 57:1, 1985.
5. Brink CA, Wells TJ: Environmental support for geriatric incontinence, *Clin Geriatr Med* 2:829, 1986.
6. Bristoll SL and others: The mythical danger of rapid urinary drainage, *Am J Nurs* 89:344, 1989.
7. Camasso JA: Peroxide to prevent odor in drainage bags, *Geriatr Nurs* 5:284, 1985.
8. Childs SJ, Egan RJ: Bacteriuria and urinary infections in the elderly, *Geriatr Urol* 23:3, 1996.
9. Colling J and others: The effects of patterned urge response toileting (PURT) on urinary incontinence among nursing home residents, *J Am Geriatr Soc* 40:135, 1992.
10. Creason NS and others: Prompted voiding therapy for urinary incontinence in aged female nursing home residents, *J Adv Nurs* 14:120, 1989.
11. Dignam RR and others: The effects of cranberry juice on urinary tract infection rates in a long-term care facility, *Ann Long Term Care* 6:163, 1998.
12. Diokno AC: Diagnostic categories of urinary incontinence and the role of urodynamic testing, *J Am Geriatr Soc* 38:300, 1990.
13. Dolan M: *Community and home health care plans,* Philadelphia, 1990, Springhouse Corp.
14. Dowd TT, Campbell JM: Fluid intake and urinary incontinence in older community dwelling women, *J Community Health Nurs* 13:179, 1996.
15. Elia G, Bergman A: Estrogen effects on the urethra: beneficial effects in women with genuine stress incontinence, *Obstet Gynecol Surv* 48: 509, 1993.

16. Fleet JC: New support for a folk remedy: cranberry juice reduced bacteriuria and pyuria in elderly women, *Nutr Rev* 52:168, 1994.

17. Ghoniem GM: Pharmacologic therapy for urinary incontinence, *Urol Nurs* 16:55, 1996.

18. Gilbert V, Gobbi M: Making sense of bladder irrigation, *Nurs Times* 85:40, 1989.

19. Hardyck C, Petrinovich L: Reducing urinary tract infections in catheterized patients, *Ostomy Wound Manage* 44:36, 1998.

20. Heavner K: Urinary incontinence in extended care facilities: a literature review and proposal for continuous quality improvement, *Ostomy Wound Manage* 44:46, 1998.

21. Herzog AR, Fultz NH: Prevalence and incidence of urinary incontinence in community-dwelling populations, *J Am Geriatr Soc* 38:273, 1990.

22. Hiser V: Nursing interventions for urinary incontinence in home health, *J Wound Ostomy Continence Nurs* 26:142, 1999.

23. Hryntschak T: Sudden and complete decompression versus slow emptying of the distended urinary bladder, *J Urol* 61:545, 1949.

24. Kane RL, and others: *Essentials of clinical geriatrics*, ed 3, New York, 1993, McGraw-Hill.

25. Liedberg H, and others: Refinement in the coating of urethral catheters reduces the incidence of catheter-associated bacteriuria: an experimental and clinical study, *EurUrol* 17:236, 1990.

26. Maloney C: Estrogen in urinary incontinence treatment: an anatomic and physiologic approach, *Urol Nurs* 17:88, 1997.

27. Maloney C: Hormone replacement therapy in female nursing home residents with recurrent urinary tract infections, *Ann Long Term Care* 6:77, 1998.

28. McDowell JB: Basic elements of continence assessment, *Urol Nurs* 14:120, 1994.

29. Melekos M, Asbach HW: Complications from urinary condom catheters, *Urology* 27:88, 1986.

30. Mohide EA, and others: Prevalence of urinary incontinence in patients receiving home care services, *Can Med Assoc J* 139:953, 1988.

31. Nazarko L: The therapeutic uses of cranberry juice, *Nurs Stan* 9:33, 1995.

32. Newman DK; Managing indwelling urethral catheters, *Ostomy Wound Manage* 44:26, 1998.

33. Nguyen A and others: Does your elderly patient have asymptomatic bacteriuria or urinary-tract infection? *Ann Long-Term Care* 5:97, 1997.

34. Ouslander JG, Schnelle JF: Incontinence in the nursing home, *Ann Intern Med* 6:438, 1995.

35. Ouslander JG and others: External catheter use and urinary tract infections among incontinent male nursing home patients, *J Am Geriatr Soc* 35:1063, 1987.

36. Ouslander JG and others: Simple versus multichannel cystometry in the evaluation of bladder function in an incontinent geriatric population, *J Urol* 140:1382, 1989.

37. Ouslander JG and others: Simplified tests of lower urinary tract function in the evaluation of geriatric urinary incontinence, *J Am Geriatr Soc* 37:706, 1989.

38. Ouslander JG and others: Predictors of successful prompted voiding among incontinent nursing home residents, *JAMA* 273:1366, 1995.

39. Perkins J: Vaginal weights for assessment and training of the pelvic floor, *J Wound Ostomy Continence Nurs* 25:206, 1998.

40. Pfister SM: Bladder diaries and voiding patterns in older adults, *J Gerontol to Nurs* 25:36–41, 1999.

41. Publicover C, Bear M: The effect of bladder training on urinary incontinence in community-dwelling older women, *J Wound Ostomy Continence Nurs* 24:319, 1997.

42. Roberts RO and others: Urinary incontinence in a community-based cohort: prevalence and healthcare-seeking, *J Am Geriatr Soc* 46:467, 1999.

43. Roe BH, Brocklehurst JC: Study of patients with indwelling catheters, *J Adv Nurs* 12:713, 1987.

44. Ruther M, Helbing C: Health care financing trends: use and cost of home health agency services under medicare, *Health Care Financ Rev* 10:105, 1989.

45. Schnelle JF: Treatment of urinary incontinence in nursing home patients by prompted voiding, *J Am Geriatr Soc* 38:356, 1990.

46. Schnelle JF and others: A cost and value analysis of two interventions with incontinent nursing home residents, *J Am Geriatr Soc* 43:1112, 1995.

47. Schnelle JF and others: Skin disorders and moisture in incontinent nursing home residents: intervention implications, *J Am Geriatr Soc* 45:1182, 1997.

48. Skelly J, Flint AJ: Urinary incontinence associated with dementia, *J Am Geriatr Soc* 43:286, 1995.

49. Starer P, Libow LS: Obscuring urinary incontinence: diapering the elderly, *J Am Geriatr Soc* 33:842, 1985.

50. Steeman E, Defever M: Urinary incontinence among elderly persons who live at home, *Nurs Clin North Am* 33:441, 1998.

51. Sueppel C: Rapid or slow bladder decompression? *Urol Nurs* 15:64, 1995.

52. Sullivan DH, Lindsay RW: Urinary incontinence in the geriatric population of an acute care hospital, *J Am Geriatr Soc* 32:646, 1984.

53. Thom D: Variation in estimates of urinary incontinence prevalence in the community: effects of differences in definition, population characteristics, and study type, *J Am Geriatr Soc* 46:473, 1998.

54. Upson C, Kirby KA: Catheter clamping after catheterization and rapid urine loss, *Urol Nurs* 15:63, 1995.

55. *Urinary incontinence in adults: acute and chronic management.* Clinical practice guideline No 2, AHCPR Pub No 96-0682, Rockville, Md, 1996, Agency for Health Care Policy and Research. Public Health Service, US Department of Health and Human Services.

56. Vinson J, Proch J: Inhibition of moisture penetration to the skin by a novel incontinence barrier product, *J Wound Ostomy Continence Nurs* 25:256, 1998.

57. Webb RJ and others: Clean intermittent self-catheterization in 172 adults, *Br J Urol* 65:20, 1990.

58. Weber EM and others: Protocol for indwelling bladder catheter removal in the homebound older adult, *Home Healthc Nurse* 16:604, 1998.

59. Wein AJ: Pharmacologic treatment of incontinence, *J Am Geriatr Soc* 38:317, 1990.

60. Wells TJ: Pelvic (floor) muscle exercise, *J Am Geriatr Soc* 38:333, 1990.

Drugs Used to Treat Urinary Incontinence

Drug	Dosage	Mechanism of action	Type of incontinence	Adverse effects
Anticholinergic and antispasmodic agents				
Oxybutynin	2.5–5 mg bid or tid	Increase bladder capacity; decrease involuntary contractions	Urge incontinence with detrusor instability	Dry mouth, blurred vision, constipation, delirium, elevated intraocular pressure, postural hypotension
Propantheline	7.5–30 mg tid or qid	Increase bladder volume to the first involuntary contraction, decrease contraction amplitude, increase total bladder capacity	Urge incontinence with detrusor instability	Dry mouth, blurred vision, drowsiness, tachycardia, constipation
Tolterodine	1–2 mg bid	Increase bladder capacity; decrease involuntary contractions	Urge incontinence with detrusor instability	Dry mouth, blurred vision, constipation, delirium, elevated intraocular pressure, postural hypotension
Alpha-adrenergic agonists				
Pseudoephedrine	15–30 mg bid or tid	Increase urethral smooth muscle contraction	Stress incontinence with sphincter weakness	Elevation of blood pressure, headaches, tachycardia
Phenylpropanol-amine	75 mg bid or tid	Increase urethral smooth muscle contraction	Stress incontinence with sphincter weakness	Headaches, tachycardia, anorexia, elevation of blood pressure
Tricyclic agents				
Imipramine	10–25 mg qd to tid	Decrease involuntary bladder contractions and increase urethral smooth muscle contraction	For mixed stress and urge incontinence	Nausea, dry mouth, dizziness, postural hypotension, blurred vision, constipation
Estrogen therapy				
Premarin (oral)	0.3–1.25 mg qd	Restore urethral mucosal integrity and tone, increase alpha-adrenergic responsiveness of the urethral muscle	Stress incontinence Urge incontinence associated with atrophic vaginitis	Breast tenderness, endometrial hyperplasia
Topical	2 g or fraction/day			
Alpha-adrenergic antagonists				
Terazosin	1–10 mg qd	Relax smooth muscle in bladder neck and prostate	Overflow incontinence associated with prostate enlargement	Postural hypotension, headaches, dizziness, syncope, tachycardia, palpitations
Doxazosin	1–10 mg qd	Same as above	Same as above	Dizziness, headaches, fatigue, tachycardia, edema, hypotension

The Patient Receiving Home Care Rehabilitation Services

Robyn Rice

Rehabilitation is an important and increasingly used service of the home care industry. The availability of rehabilitation services has increased greatly over the past decade.[6] Rehabilitation as described in this chapter is a restorative process to help ill, physically impaired, or handicapped persons regain their maximum physical, mental, and vocational usefulness following disease or injury.[2,3,8]

The specific rehabilitation professionals referred to include physical therapists, occupational therapists, and speech language pathologists. Effective rehabilitation for patients with impaired mobility is an educational process involving the coordinated efforts of patients, caregivers, physicians, home health nurses, and various health specialists. The ultimate goal for patients with impaired mobility is to maximize their independence and daily functioning within their home environment.

As the average life expectancy for Americans increases, so does the incidence of illness, disease, and physical disability, resulting in an increased need for rehabilitation. In addition, since the onset of the prospective payment system, patients are being discharged from hospitals much sooner than in the past. When first seen at home, patients are frequently in the acute phase of their disease process or injury and often have received only initial instructions and an abbreviated version of the rehabilitation program.

Patients are frequently treated at home because of insurance coverage limitations for inpatient stay or a lack of available beds for admission into a rehabilitation unit or facility. Skills learned in a rehabilitation center may not apply to the patient's home setting or may not be carried over by the patient into the home very easily. Oftentimes, a few visits by the rehabilitation professional will accelerate the patient's ability to adapt skills to the home setting.

As is the case with any service related to home, financial coverage for rehabilitation services is provided by private, state, and federal government insurance programs. Patients receiving home care rehabilitation under their hospitalization Medicare benefit (Medicare Part A) must be homebound; that is, they must need the assistance of another person or device to leave their home.[5] This is not the case when receiving services billed under the supplemental medical insurance (Medicare Part B). Payment under Medicare Part B reimburses at a rate of 80%, whereas reimbursement of 100% is provided under Medicare Part A.[5]

To receive the Medicare home care benefit, a patient must have a signed order from a physician for treatments and services to be rendered.[5] Rehabilitation treatments must require the skills of a professional physical therapist, occupational therapist, or speech and language pathologist.[5] The patient must have the expectation of improved physical mobility or at least have a reasonable rehabilitation potential.[5] The exception to this requirement is for home visits to instruct and educate a caregiver regarding transfer and positioning techniques, range of motion exercises, and establishment of a home exercise program for patients with chronic disabilities or patients with no apparent rehabilitation potential.[5] Medicare will not, however, reimburse for maintenance therapy.[4]

INDICATIONS FOR REHABILITATION SERVICES

Nurses new to home care may experience difficulty in determining the appropriateness and need for rehabilitation services. This difficulty is largely due to a lack of working experience with patients who could benefit from physical, occupational, or speech therapy and unfamiliarity with each discipline's area of expertise. Case management strategies for home care nurses would be to learn principles of rehabilitation therapy and build a collaborative practice with the home care team.

To ensure patients' maximal recovery or restoration of function or to prevent further dysfunction, a multidisciplinary approach is essential. Open and ongoing communication among the nurse, the physician, and all rehabilitation professionals regarding the establishment of goals and the plan of care will result in an overall improvement in the quality of patient care. Likewise, coordination of patient care with the home health aide and/or social services may be needed.

When establishing a plan of care for any patient, it is important that home care nurses take a holistic approach to assessing needs related to the patient's illness, injury, or disease process. These include, but are not limited to, physical, emotional, social, and economic needs.[3,4] The home care nurse will assume an important role in helping patients adjust to and accept alterations in body image secondary to disease or illness by addressing loss, anxiety, and depression.[3]

When home care nurses assess patients to determine the appropriateness of rehabilitation services, it is important that they assess patients' overall mobility levels and functional status. Asking seated patients if they have difficulty ambulating is frequently inconclusive. It is important to have patients demonstrate their abilities, rather than focusing on their subjective complaints of disability. By observing patients' abilities or assisting them to ambulate, home care nurses can quickly assess many areas of physical functioning and thus are able to determine the need for other services. For example, difficulty understanding or following commands may be indicative of speech or cognitive deficits. Prior to ambulating, patients must come to a standing position. When they are doing so, home care nurses can assess such things as

balance and coordination deficits, the ability or inability to move forward and rise from a seated position, and the paralysis or dysfunction of any extremity. Patients may have an unawareness of body parts or a lack of perception or spatial orientation, making these tasks nearly impossible. Observing patients ambulate will help to determine their gait ability and possibly the need for additional equipment or gait devices. At this point, home care nurses can also identify those patients at risk for falls.[6,7]

During the initial visit, the home care nurse should note if the patient has specific difficulties, such as maneuvering around the kitchen for meal preparation or cleanup or using the bathroom facilities safely. Any details in these areas will assist the rehabilitation professional in determining if a referral is appropriate and which discipline should be involved.

Equally important in determining the need for rehabilitation services is a knowledge and understanding of the patient's prior functional status. It is unlikely that patients with chronic disabilities who have not ambulated in several years will be appropriate candidates to receive physical therapy for gait training. It is also beneficial to investigate whether patients have previously received physical, occupational, or speech therapy for the same or similar conditions or problems and the degree of patient/caregiver compliance. It is also important to recognize that patients occasionally are not accepting of their disability or dysfunction and are therefore not amenable to receiving therapy services.

The majority of patients referred for rehabilitation services generally have a diagnosis that implies impairment of the neuromuscular and/or musculoskeletal systems. Box 17-1 lists common conditions and diagnoses that may assist home care nurses to make appropriate referrals for specific rehabilitation services. Conditions and diagnoses must be acute or represent a recent exacerbation of a chronic disease. Patients who suffer from several of the conditions and diagnoses listed in the box may have multiple deficits and thus need services from any or all of the three rehabilitation disciplines (physical, occupational, and speech therapy).

Frequently patients may appear to need skilled therapy because of weakness or impaired mobility.

Box 17-1   COMMON CONDITIONS AND DIAGNOSES APPROPRIATE FOR HOME CARE REHABILITATION REFERRALS[4,7]

- Patients who have sustained fractures or dislocations
- Patients who have undergone orthopedic surgeries, including joint replacements or reconstructive surgeries
- Patients suffering from degenerative joint or disk disease
- Patients suffering from rheumatoid arthritis
- Patients who have undergone amputations or require prosthetic training
- Patients who have sustained burns with joint involvement or have physical impairment with an associated decrease in function
- Patients who have suffered cerebral vascular accidents
- Patients who have suffered head injuries or spinal cord injuries
- Patients with multiple sclerosis
- Patients with amyotrophic lateral sclerosis
- Patients with Parkinson's disease
- Patients with a decrease in function as a result of neuropathies and/or myopathies
- Patients with chronic obstructive pulmonary disease who require postular drainage and teaching
- Patients with cardiac impairment requiring cardiac rehabilitation
- Patients with severe immobility as a result of any disease process requiring instruction to the caregiver in Hoyer lift transfers or any assistive device
- Patients suffering from newly diagnosed blindness
- Patients with head/neck cancer resulting in partial or total laryngectomies or glossectomies
- Patients whose underlying disease process, illness, or injury has resulted in dysphagia
- Patients suffering from a hearing loss

Data from: Guzelaydin SK: Treading the path of interdisciplinary boundaries: a community health care approach to rehabilitation services in the home, *J Home Health Care Pract* 4(4):24, 1992; Kauffman DD: Physical therapy interaction in the home, *Caring* 11(8):16, 1992.

However, before making an interdisciplinary referral, home care nurses must consider the available reimbursement sources. Payment for rehabilitation services for patients experiencing weakness or immobility from prolonged hospitalization secondary to medical complications may be denied by Medicare. Fiscal intermediaries often view this as a weakness or temporary loss of function that will improve spontaneously and does not warrant the intervention of a skilled therapist. When assessing patients' needs for additional services, it is important that home care nurses not concentrate solely on the medical diagnosis, because the therapist treats loss of function and not the specific disease or illness.

Chapter 9 describes clinical indicators for a rehabilitation referral. In all phases of health care, as well as in the exploding home care arena, there is a severe shortage of qualified speech, occupational, and physical therapists. Often the home care nurse will have to fill the needs of the patient in the absence of a qualified therapist. Community resources may include the home medical supply dealer, representatives from manufacturers, and literature from journals. If a therapist is available, a consultation or an evaluation with instruction may be all that is necessary to maximally benefit the patient.

HOME CARE APPLICATION

Home care nurses can serve as an important link in the restoration of patients' function or in the prevention of further dysfunction. Their ability to assist patients with transfers, gait training, or range of motion exercise programs established by the rehabilitation professional hastens the recovery process. Spiritual and emotional support will also be needed by patients/caregivers in adjusting to and accepting changes in body image resulting from disease and disability (Box 17-2 and Box 17-3). Home care nurses may also help patients to recognize that they gain new skills to replace ones that have been lost. In this manner, many patients who recover with rehabilitative care experience a form of health within illness as human senses and abilities are reshaped and redefined. Nursing and therapist support of patient efforts towards recovery or independence are critical to this process.

Of note, when faced with the patient's many needs, caregivers may experience role strain and require respite services. Signs of caregiver role strain are discussed in Chapter 4 . The home care aide and social worker may be of assistance in

Box 17-2   PRIMARY NURSING DIAGNOSES/PATIENT PROBLEMS

- Knowledge deficit: lack of information about condition and care
- Activity intolerance: _____ Ambulation, _____ ADLs, _____ Other *(Specify)*
- Self-care deficit: _____ ADLs, _____ Feeding, _____ Toileting, _____ Other *(Specify)*
- Body image disturbance
- Impaired physical mobility
- Risk for trauma
- Risk for caregiver role strain

Box 17-3   PRIMARY THEMES OF PATIENT EDUCATION

- Disease process: when to call the case manager or physician
- When to call 911
- Medications: purpose, action, dosage, side effects, and methods of administration
- Body mechanics regarding lifting and transfers
- Gait training and strength endurance
- Range of motion exercises
- Operation and function of mobility aids (walkers, canes, crutches, or wheelchairs)
- Operation and function of home medical equipment and assistive devices (hospital beds, hoyer lifts, sliding boards, bedside commodes, bathtub seats, tub transfer benches, button hooks, dressing sticks, communication aids)
- ADL self-care management
- Home environmental safety
- Positive coping mechanisms to improve body image adaptation
- Socioeconomic resources
- Available community services for people experiencing stroke or problems with immobility
- Caregiver respite services
- General self-care strategies

helping patients/caregivers adjust and adapt to physical disability or change.

Identifying patient needs for care and home independence

Most rehabilitation therapy intervention plans require a complete assessment. Everyone should understand what the patient can do when building the bridge to what the patient wants or needs to do. In addition, the patient should be asked if he or she wants information about all of the available options or just assistive equipment that will be funded. In general the home care nurse should be aware that the treating therapist does the following[1,2,9]:

- Performs a functional abilities evaluation.
  ADLs
  Transfers
  Mobility (e.g., assisted ambulation, manual wheelchair, power wheelchair)
  Communication (verbal, manual board, augmentative system)
  Perceptual and cognitive skills
  Feeding
  Vision
  Leisure skills
- Performs a physical evaluation.
  Joint mobility
  Neurological evaluation
  Skin inspection
  Response to gravity in the sitting position

  Hands-on simulation
  Status of present secondary devices (e.g., orthotics, augmentative devices)
- Conducts a home assessment.
  Environmental fit of equipment
  Use patterns (e.g., bathroom transfers)
- Synthesizes evaluation findings.
  Determines needs for equipment.
  Outlines treatment plan including outcomes of care.

The following sections are primarily designed to provide home care nurses with a basic knowledge of techniques pertinent to rehabilitation. Working with patients experiencing loss and depression is discussed in Chapter 22. Many of the following techniques (such as body mechanics for moving and lifting, transfer training, gait training, and range of motion exercises) and assistive devices may be incorporated in the nursing care plan. In addition, proper seating techniques are extremely important in order to prevent skin breakdown (see Appendix XVII-I).

Body mechanics/patient transfer training

An awareness and understanding of good body mechanics is essential for home care nurses to prevent injury to themselves and patients. By applying the principles of body mechanics when lifting or moving patients, home care nurses take advantage of the body parts best suited to lifting: the legs.[9] When moving or lifting a patient, it is important to maintain balance with the feet spread slightly apart to increase the base of support. The nurse's back should be kept in alignment, with the spine staying as erect as possible. When reaching over a patient in bed, it is beneficial to advance one foot forward and under the bed if possible, to allow the trunk to remain reasonably erect. Stooping or bending at the waist should be avoided. To prevent strain on the back muscles, it is important to squat, bending the hips and knees while keeping the back straight and in proper alignment. When returning to the standing position, the muscles in the legs should be allowed to do the actual lifting. Movements should be smooth and steady, never jerky or sudden. Turning while lifting should be accomplished by moving the feet rather than by twisting the trunk or waist.

When transferring the patient from a bed to a chair, it is important to place the bed at a moderate and comfortable height if possible. Place the chair parallel or at a slight angle to the bed, closest to the patient's uninvolved side if possible. Instruct the patient to assist with whatever movements he or she is capable of doing safely. Assist the patient to a sitting position on the edge of the bed; the patient's feet should be flat on the floor. If possible, have the patient push up with the hands on the bed while the nurse or therapist grasps around the waist or gait belt. Assist the patient to a standing position by straightening the patient's hips and knees. Block the patient's knees when paralysis or weakness exists.[9,10] Either turn slowly, sidestep, or pivot the patient one quarter turn until the backs of the legs rest against the chair. Have the patient reach for the arm of the chair, if able, to achieve a sitting position. This method of stand-pivot transfer is generally used with patients who can offer some assistance or who do not need transfers with the use of

mechanical devices, such as hoyer lifts or sliding boards.[8,9,10]

Range of motion exercises

The prevention of joint contractures and adhesions and the maintenance of joint mobility are essential aspects of any patient's care. These goals are accomplished through joint range of motion exercises, which can be performed by home care nurses and patients following instructions in basic range of motion techniques (Table 17-1 and Figure 17-1). Range of motion can be described in four ways:

Passive range of motion. This is range of motion in which patients offer no assistance. The movements are performed completely by another person.

Active-assistive range of motion. This is range of motion in which patients assist with the movements but still require assistance from another person.

Active range of motion. This is range of motion in which the patients perform all movements unassisted.

Resistive range of motion. This is range of motion in which movements are performed with weights or against physical resistance.

Caregiver education regarding range of motion exercises is important and should be done on an ongoing basis. This is especially true for patients who are bedridden, who are susceptible to skin breakdown, or who have an abnormality in muscle tone.

Gait training and mobility aids

Patients' abilities to function within the home are largely controlled by their gait ability or ability to manage a wheelchair. Gait safety is a primary concern with all patients. Older patients often have impaired vision, mild balance disturbances, or decreased sensation. Patients' lack of knowledge of safety measures frequently contributes to falls and further injury. All efforts should be taken to ensure maximal safety at home. Home care nurses can assist with this by reinforcing safety precautions and noting environmental hazards or barriers. Rearranging furniture allows for ease of maneuverability. Removing throw rugs, telephone wires, and electric cords will contribute to increased safety within the home.

Table 17-1 Range of motion exercises

Body part	Type of joint	Type of movement	Body part	Type of joint	Type of movement
Neck and cervical spine	Pivotal	Flexion: bring chin to rest on chest Extension: return head to erect position Hyperextension: bend head back as far as possible Lateral flexion: tilt head as far as possible toward each shoulder Rotation: turn head as far as possible to right and left			Internal rotation: with elbow flexed, rotate shoulder by moving arm until thumb is turned inward and toward back External rotation: with elbow flexed, move arm, until thumb is upward and lateral to head Circumduction: move arm in full circle. Circumduction is combination of all movements of ball-and-socket joint
Shoulder	Ball-and-socket	Flexion: raise arm from side position forward to position above head Extension: return arm to position at side of the body Hyperextension: move arm behind body, keeping elbow straight	Elbow	Hinge	Flexion: bend elbow so that lower arm moves toward its shoulder joint and hand is level with shoulder Extension: straighten elbow by lowering hand Hyperextension: bend lower arm back as far as possible
		Abduction: raise arm to side position above head with palm away from head Adduction: lower arm sideways and across body as far as possible	Forearm	Pivotal	Supination: turn lower arm and hand so that palm is up Pronation: turn lower arm so that palm is down
			Wrist	Condyloid	Flexion: move palm toward inner aspect of the forearm Extension: move fingers so that fingers, hands and forearm are in same plane

Table 17-1 Range of motion exercises—cont'd

Body part	Type of joint	Type of movement	Body part	Type of joint	Type of movement
		Hyperextension: bring dorsal surface of hand back as far as possible Radial flexion: bend wrist medially toward thumb Ulnar flexion: bend wrist laterally toward fifth finger	Hip	Ball-and-socket	Flexion: move leg forward and up Extension: move leg back beside other leg
Fingers	Condyloid hinge	Flexion: make fist Extension: straighten fingers Hyperextension: bend fingers back as far as possible			Hyperextension: move leg behind body
		Abduction: spread fingers apart Adduction: bring fingers together			Abduction: move leg laterally away from body Adduction: move leg back toward medial position and beyond if possible
Thumb	Saddle	Flexion: move thumb across palmar surface of hand Extension: move thumb straight away from hand Abduction: extend thumb laterally (usually done when placing fingers in abduction and adduction) Adduction: move thumb back toward hand Opposition: touch thumb to each finger of same hand			Internal rotation: turn foot and leg toward other leg External rotation: turn foot and leg away from other leg

Continued

Table 17-1 Range of motion exercises—cont'd

Body part	Type of joint	Type of movement	Body part	Type of joint	Type of movement
		Circumduction: move leg in circle			Inversion: turn sole of foot medially Eversion: turn sole of foot laterally
Knee	Hinge	Flexion: bring heel back toward back of thigh Extension: return heel to floor	Toes	Condyloid	Flexion: bring heel back toward back of thigh Extension: return heel to floor
					Abduction: spread toes apart Adduction: bring toes together
Ankle	Hinge	Dorsal flexion: move foot so that toes are pointed upward Plantar flexion: move foot so that toes are pointed downward			

Frequently patients live alone or with an elderly spouse or caregiver and are fearful of ambulating in the absence of the nurse or physical therapist. Home care nurses can hasten the recovery process by assisting patients with their established gait programs. Patients may require standby assistance, verbal cueing, or gait devices when ambulating. There are numerous gait devices or mobility aids available. These include standard walkers, wheeled walkers, reciprocating walkers, hemi-walkers, standard canes, quad canes, standard crutches, and loft strand crutches.[1,6]

Walkers are generally used for patients who have lower extremity weight-bearing restrictions and whose balance or strength does not warrant the use of crutches. Walkers are used more often with the elderly, whereas crutches are commonly used with the younger population. Canes are frequently used for patients who have mild weakness or balance disturbances or for patients who have unilateral upper extremity limitation or absence of function and are unable to use devices requiring the use of both upper extremities. Wheelchairs may be the only means of locomotion throughout the house for some patients. Wheelchairs can be customized and adapted to the specific needs and requirements of each patient. Wheelchairs vary, ranging from standard wheelchairs to reclining wheelchairs, hemi-wheelchairs with one-arm drive, and electric wheelchairs. A variety of accessories and options are available.

Home medical equipment and assistive devices

Home medical equipment and assistive devices serve as an adjunct in the rehabilitation process for many patients. Hospital beds, overhead trapeze bars, and bed rails are used to assist patients' mo-

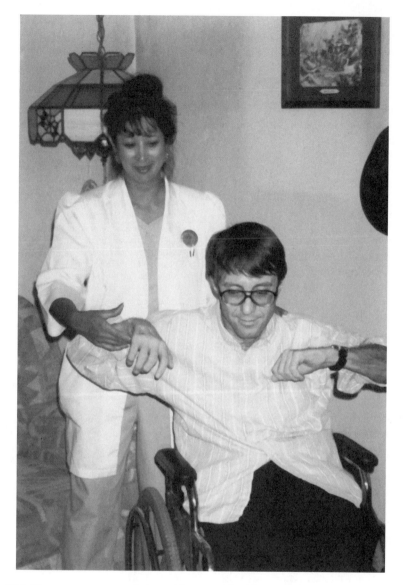

Figure 17-1 Home care nurse assisting with range of motion exercises. (Photo courtesy Home Health Department, Gila Regional Medical Center, Silver City, NM.)

bility and safety in bed. Hoyer lifts and sliding boards ease the transferring of patients with impaired mobility. Raised toilet seats, toilet safety rails, bedside commodes, bathtub seats, tub transfer benches, tub safety rails, and grab bars all promote increased independence in performing such activities of daily living (ADLs) as toileting and bathing. Some of these items are shown in Appendix

XVII-II. Self-help assistive devices used to facilitate independence with dressing, grooming, feeding, and cooking include long-handled reachers, sponges or shoe horns, stocking aids, button hooks, and dressing sticks. Universal cuffs are beneficial for patients who have a loss of motion or strength and need help holding objects when performing basic self-care activities. Built-up handles may be needed on eating and cooking utensils used by patients with diminished hand function or decreased coordination.[6]

Patients with impaired communication or phonation may require augmentative communication devices, cassette talking tapes, or an electrolarynx.

With instruction and careful selection of the proper equipment and/or assistive device, patients have the potential to increase their independence and functional ability within the home. With knowledge of available equipment, home health nurses will have less difficulty in determining the need for physical therapy, occupational therapy, or speech pathology intervention.

SUMMARY

Through the collective efforts of home care nurses, rehabilitation professionals, and all involved caregivers, achieving the primary goal for any patient is possible.[4] For patients requiring home health rehabilitation, that goal is to restore the maximum attainable level of functioning and independence. Likewise, by facilitating and understanding the grieving process, health care professionals can address the loss, anxiety, and depression that this group of patients may experience. Patients are encouraged to emphasize and utilize their assets, to become involved in activities of daily living, and to take pride in themselves and in the mastery of their accomplishments.[3,4]

With proper care and patient education, disabilities can be prevented from becoming handicaps. Consequently team commitment and a knowledge of the care being delivered by each health professional is essential for the effective treatment of all patients receiving home rehabilitation services.

REFERENCES

1. Barnes MR, Crutchfield C: *The patient at home: a manual of exercise programs, self-help devices and home care procedures,* rev ed, Thorofare, NJ, 1984, Slack.
2. Bergen A: Assistive technology, *Caring,* 18, January 1998.
3. Drench M: Changes in body image secondary to disease and injury, *Rehabil Nurs* 19(1):31, 1994.
4. Guzelaydin SK: Treading the path of interdisciplinary boundaries: a community health care approach to rehabilitation services in the home, *J Home Health Care Pract* 4(4):24, 1992.
5. Health Care Financing Administration: *Health insurance manual,* Pub No. 11 -Thru T273, rev March 1995, Washington, DC, 1995, U.S. Department of Health and Human Services.
6. Hieber K. Orthopaedic essentials: mobility health assessment, *Orthop Nurs* 17(4):30, 1998.
7. Kauffman DD: Physical therapy interaction in the home, *Caring* 11(8):16, 1992.
8. Neal LJ: Rehabilitation and activities of daily living, *Home Health Nurse* 14(7):539, 1996.
9. Topp R, and others: Developing a strength training program for older adults: planning, programming, and potential outcomes, *Rehabil Nurs* 19(5):266, 1994.
10. William M, Worthingham C: *Therapeutic exercise for body alignment and function,* Philadelphia, 1957, WB Saunders.

Seating Tips for the Chairbound Patient

The home care patient probably spends a majority of waking hours sitting up in some kind of chair: a wheelchair, a recliner, a couch, or a sofa. While assessing the patient and developing the plan of care, the home health nurse must address the position the patient is supported in when sitting. Proper positioning can reduce contracture formation and skeletal deformities, protect the skin from pressure ulcers, enhance internal organ functioning, improve patient comfort, and put the patient in as functional a position as possible to enhance independence in daily activities. It is healthy to sit correctly.

Standard living room furniture typically is made for generic comfort and is not structured enough to provide positioning support for patients experiencing weakness, paralysis, or contractures. It will be easier to support patients in a more upright chair such as a wheelchair. Many patients have a tendency to sit in a slouched position with their hips placed forward on the seat, back curved, knees lower than the hips, and feet unsupported. Therefore in assisting patients to maintain an upright, neutral body position, the nurse must address patient seat, back, foot, and leg supports.

Seat. Begin by assessing the patient's sitting position by looking at the patient from the side. The keystone in proper positioning is pelvic control. The seat cushion should help hold the hips back on the seat as close to the backrest as the patient's body structure will allow. Securing the pelvis in this position will help the patient sit upright. This prevents a slouched position, which is damaging to the patient's skin and uncomfortable over time. Use a cushion that cradles the ischials and blocks them from sliding forward on the seat.

Back. Back support must be addressed both for comfort and to help keep the pelvis in a neutral position. If the back is allowed to slouch, the hips will tend to push forward away from the backrest, and the pelvic control gained by the seat cushion will be lost. Wheelchairs typically have a sling-type upholstery that encourages a slouched back position. Living room furniture occasionally provides back support. The home health nurse must ensure that the patient's back and lumbar (lower back) curves are supported as upright as the body allows. There is a wide variety of back cushions on the market, from small lumbar pillows to larger pieces that extend from the seat to the shoulders. Consult with the home medical supplier regarding cushion selection. The goal is to use the most economical piece that helps the patient maintain the most upright position the body structure will allow.

Feet. The patient's feet must be supported so that the weight of the legs does not drag the person forward out of position. Be sure that enough foot support is provided so that the knees and hips are on the same level; that is, the thigh is parallel to the floor. This can be accomplished in a wheelchair by raising the footrests, or in the living room by providing a stool of the proper height.

Legs. Now examine the patient from the front. The thighs should be aligned so that they are pointing straight ahead rather than rolling together or falling away from each other. Thigh supports may be needed to keep them properly aligned. Also, trunk support may be needed to help keep the patient from leaning heavily to one side.

Side and front assessment. Assess the patient from the side and front as follows:

1. Assess from the side
   a. Keep the pelvis as close to the backrest as possible by providing a seat cushion that keeps the ischials from sliding forward.
   b. Prevent a slouched back posture and a pelvis that rolls backward by providing

back support to maintain the natural lumbar curve.

c. Bring the patient's knees to the same level as the hips by providing foot support.

2. Assess from the front

a. Maintain the thighs in a flat, straight-ahead position by providing support between or alongside the thighs if needed.

b. Prevent leaning of the trunk to the side by providing side supports.

(Review Chapter 14 for recommendations for seating with skin breakdown.)

Adaptive Equipment Commonly Used in the Home

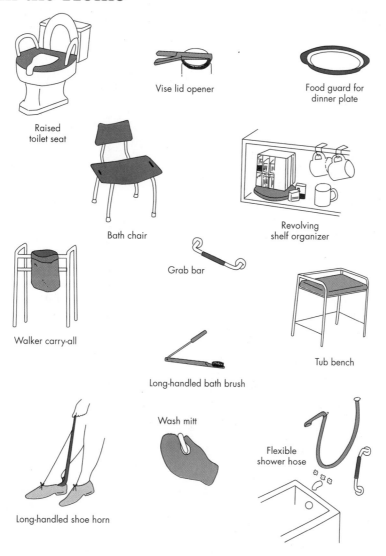

Raised toilet seat

Vise lid opener

Food guard for dinner plate

Bath chair

Revolving shelf organizer

Walker carry-all

Grab bar

Long-handled bath brush

Tub bench

Long-handled shoe horn

Wash mitt

Flexible shower hose

From Bronstein KS and others: *Promoting stroke recovery: a research based approach for nurses,* St. Louis, 1991, Mosby.

18 THE PATIENT RECEIVING HOME INFUSION THERAPIES

Sally C. Adams and Robyn Rice

Overview

Home infusion therapy is no longer new to the home care industry. The first home intravenous (IV) therapy programs appeared with the advent of the prospective payment system in the 1970s. In the 1980s pressure to reduce inpatient length of stay prompted additional growth of the industry. At first payers paid large sums for home infusion services to reduce the inpatient length of stay. Eventually payers realized they at times were paying as much for home infusion as they would have paid for keeping the patient hospitalized. Infusion providers saw new rates being offered from the payers, with much smaller profit margins. Today the home infusion market is highly competitive, with only a few large national providers and many small local providers remaining. The market is being integrated into alternative sites, such as ambulatory infusion centers in order for providers to be more attractive to managed care companies. Over the past 5 years, home infusion has grown 15% to 30% per year.[14] Growth in the home infusion industry is influenced by several factors: the patient population, technology, cost, and consumer awareness.

Patient population

Patients discharged to the home now are often sicker than those who required home care in the past. As patient acuity levels rise, home care services such as home infusion therapies will expand to meet complex health care needs. Home care now includes care for patients with infectious disease and cardiac, prenatal, oncology, transplant, and perinatal patients, all of whom require aggressive treatment.

Technology

Advances in technology have contributed to the safety and feasibility of home infusion therapy. Portable infusion pumps developed over the past 15 years are safer, more accurate, and easier to use (Figure 18-1). Patients no longer have to manipulate bulky and heavy equipment in their homes. A variety of flexible silicone catheters with longer dwell times have replaced large steel needles, improving the reliability and safety of home infusion therapy. For example, the refinement of the central venous catheter has made the infusion of vesicants and high-dextrose fluids safe in the home setting. Because of the growth of home infusion and the decreased margins for profit, several telecommunication technologies have also been introduced. Several ambulatory pumps have the capability to be accessed by the home infusion provider over a telephone line to make changes to a pump's infusion program, monitor a patient's participation in their therapy, and evaluate any alarms that the patient may be experiencing. Other systems under development and/or refinement allow a central monitoring station, usually set up at a hospital or clinic, to actually visualize the patient while recording vital signs, weight, blood glucose level, and breath sounds. This promises to be very helpful in the management of patients with large wounds, allowing the doctor to visualize the status of the wound at any time[5,13] (see Chapter 26).

the recovery process with less disruption to their lifestyles.

Issues such as staffing, safety, patient education, availability of supplies, and clinical expertise to execute IV therapy services must be considered when implementing home infusion therapy. Home infusion therapy is nursing intensive because coordination provided by trained nurses is vital to safely administer these therapies outside of the acute care setting. Services and products used include nursing care and pharmacy services, drugs, nutrients and solutions, supplies and specialized medical equipment, administration and support services, and quality improvement activities.[6]

The most common infusion therapies administered in the patient's home include antibiotic therapy, pain management therapy, chemotherapy, hydration, parenteral nutrition, and enteral nutrition.[15] Home blood transfusion and other therapies described in this chapter are becoming more common. The purpose of this chapter is to present an overview of principles of home infusion management in order to prepare home care nurses to meet the complex needs of this patient population.

ADMINISTRATIVE ISSUES
Reimbursement

One of the key administrative issues in providing home infusion services is ensuring adequate reimbursement for services and supplies. Payment for home IV therapy services varies and should be researched thoroughly with each patient admission. Although services for IV therapy are covered, with the revocation of the Medicare Catastrophic Coverage Act of 1988 there is limited reimbursement for specific IV drugs under the Medicare program. Parenteral nutrition and a selected number of other drugs have coverage under Medicare Part B if they meet the appropriate clinical diagnosis and certain criteria requirements. Part B also provides limited reimbursement for supplies used in conjunction with skilled nursing visits and therapies as long as Medicare guidelines are met. The advent of Medicare HMOs has allowed patients to receive most infusion therapies in the home, which in the past would have necessitated hospitalization or a stay in a skilled nursing facility. Medicaid, a state-administered health care plan, has requirements that vary from state to state.

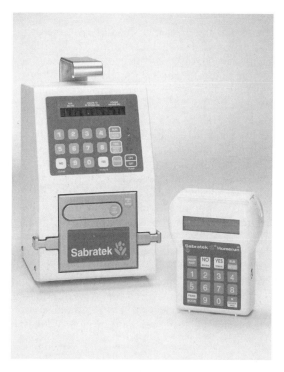

Figure 18-1 The 3030 and 6060 Homerun multitherapy infusion pumps. (Homerun is a registered trademark of Sabratek Corporation. Printed with permission of Sabratek Corporation, Skokie, Ill.)

Cost

Home IV therapy costs substantially less than in-hospital therapy. Cost reductions of $2370 to $3665 per patient per illness have made home IV therapy an attractive option to both payers and patients.[1] The demand for cost-effective health care will continue to fuel a steady growth in the home infusion market.

Consumer Awareness

As educated consumers, patients are taking a more active role in meeting their own health care needs. Many patients prefer to be treated at home, where they feel more in control of their body and the circumstances leading to recovery. In the fast-paced world of work, many people are reluctant to spend time away from careers and other obligations. Often, providing high-technology services at home allows patients and their families to participate in

Referrals and quality care

Once the patient population and potential needs are assessed, policies regarding admission and referrals should be developed by clinical and administrative managers. Most licensing bodies require procedures outlining specific patient admission criteria.[9] As part of quality control, trained personnel (usually nurses) should screen referrals for eligibility and appropriateness. Examples of criteria to be assessed for potential home infusion therapy include the patient's general health status as it relates to the appropriateness of home infusion therapy, patient/caregiver willingness and ability to assist with care, accessibility and licensure of the physician, and adequacy and safety of the home environment (including availability of water, electricity, and telephone service). In addition, patients with Medicare and Medicaid need to be evaluated for homebound status.

It may be possible to correct any deficit(s) before providing home care services. However, referral sources should be informed of admission criteria to avoid confusion and inappropriate referrals.

Agency policies and procedures should be developed in accordance with local guidelines and standards of care (see Chapter 10). For instance, infusion therapy protocols can be developed from the national standards published by organizations such as the Intravenous Nurses Society (INS), the Oncology Nursing Society (ONS), the American Society of Parenteral and Enteral Nutrition (ASPEN), and the National Association of Vascular Access Nurses (NAVAN) and the Center for Disease Control and Prevention (CDC). In addition, local hospitals and physicians may have specific requirements relating to home care that further ensure the delivery of quality patient care. For example, accreditation agencies, such as the Joint Commission on Accreditation of Healthcare Organizations (JCAHO), now require the pharmacist to have a care plan for home IV therapy patients.[9] From a legal/ethical point of view, home care agency policy should provide field staff with clear guidelines to access top level agency administration if problems arise in the field (for example, inadequate response from on-call supervisory staff, or field staff requiring guidance in decision making for problematic situations).

The physician

The role of the physician should be clarified with staff when providing home infusion. Physicians traditionally have been solicited for their referrals by home infusion companies. Gastroenterologists, infectious disease specialists, oncologists, and internal medicine physicians have proven to be sound referral sources. Once the referral is made, the physician acts as the medical case manager by ordering the plan of care and serving as consultant to the pharmacist and home care nurses.

The home infusion department should also have a designated medical director to review the appropriateness of administering certain medications in the home. Many times the medical director will simply request clarification from the patient's physician as to how the infusion will be monitored (e.g., therapeutic blood levels). They can also provide guidance on the safety of providing new therapies, drugs being given for diagnoses not approved by the Food and Drug Administration (FDA), and requests for administration of investigational drugs.

The nurse manager and staffing concerns

The role of the clinical nurse manager is one of coordinator and support person for patients and staff. Nurse managers need to be aware of the staff necessary to provide high-technology services. Ideally nurses providing care should be certified in peripherally inserted central venous catheter (PICC) and chemotherapy. Nursing visits can range from 45 minutes for a follow-up visit to 4 hours for a blood transfusion or intravenous immunoglobulin (IVIG) administration. Taking into account the geographic size of the service area and the type of IV therapy to be provided, the nurse manager calculates the number of full-time equivalent (FTE) staff necessary. Many states and licensing bodies require that agencies provide 24-hour access to nursing care. Because payment by managed care companies for a hospital day ends at midnight, it is becoming more the norm to see patient discharges late in the afternoon or early evening. This requires staff to be available up to 16 hours per day, with on-call services after that.

One staffing model used is coverage from 7:00 AM to 10:00 PM, using 8-hour staggered shifts. A 4-day workweek may make the unattractive shifts more acceptable. A nursing supervisor should be available at all times, especially when a nurse is still out in the field.

The issue of staff safety is of concern. The agency should have provisions to protect staff members making evening or night visits. Contracting with security services, "buddying-up" for visits in potentially dangerous areas, and providing adequate emergency communication systems (car phones, beepers, calling cards) are suggestions. Though some of these mechanisms can add to the cost per visit, they can be well worth their price in terms of staff satisfaction and safety.

The quality of the home care agency can be measured by the quality of its personnel. Another role of the nurse manager is to coordinate continuing education opportunities for the staff. A monthly scheduled in-service program to enhance clinical expertise may include such topics as infection control, new chemotherapeutic modalities, nutritional assessment, and stress management. Often professionals from local agencies are willing to provide such information, as are representatives from the drug manufacturing companies.

HOME CARE APPLICATION

There are numerous reasons for the initiation of home infusion therapy. It is used to replace fluids and correct electrolyte imbalances in dehydrated patients; to replace fluids and electrolytes lost as a result of vomiting, diarrhea, suctioning, wound drainage, or blood loss; to provide caloric value for the malnourished or for those who cannot eat; and to administer IV medications such as antibiotics, chemotherapy, or blood products. Routes of administration used in home infusion therapy include the following[18]:

- Intravenous—into a vein
- Intramuscular—into the muscle
- Intraarterial—into an artery
- Intraventricular—into the ventricles of the brain
- Intraosseous—into the bone marrow
- Subcutaneous—under the skin
- Epidural—into the space just outside the dura, a membrane surrounding the spinal cord and brain
- Intrathecal—into the subarachnoid space that immediately surrounds the spinal cord
- Intraperitoneal—into the free space of the abdominal cavity
- Enteral—into the digestive system

Vascular access devices

Peripheral and central line management. When initiating peripheral IV therapy, consider the size of the vein and the viscosity of the solution. Select the smallest gauge needle or catheter needed for the infusion. On selecting a site, consider the location and condition of the vein (Figure 18-2). Know the purpose of the infusion and the duration of the therapy. It is beneficial to know whether

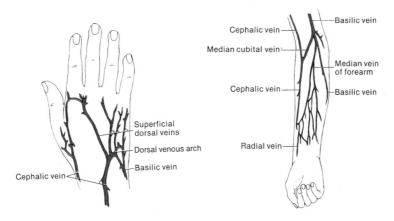

Figure 18-2 Venous anatomy. (From Perry AG, Potter PA: *Clinical nursing skills and techniques,* ed 4, St. Louis, 1998, Mosby.)

patients have previously received IV therapy and their tolerance to it.

Occasionally a patient may have poor peripheral venous access due to numerous IVs while hospitalized and therefore is not a candidate for long-term IV therapy. The administration of subcutaneous fluid or hypodermoclysis may serve as an alternate method of hydrating these patients.

A central venous catheter (CVC) is required for patients with a variety of medical conditions, including cancer and bowel disease. A tunneled CVC is generally a long silicone rubber catheter approximately 1/8 inch in diameter with a cuff to secure it in place once inserted. The cuff also assists with preventing the spread of infection along the tract of the catheter. These catheters are used for long-term venous access and spare the patient repeated venipunctures. Common CVC catheters used in home care are Hickman-Broviac catheters or Groshong catheters. A nontunneled catheter is placed directly into the subclavian vein. Without the cuff to tunnel, this type of catheter is used more for therapies of short duration. Implanted vascular access devices (IVADs) (e.g., Port-a-Cath) and PICC systems are also used (Table 18-1).

The insertion of a tunneled CVC requires a minor operation, but the procedure should cause little discomfort. The patient is given a local anesthetic, and two small incisions are made, one directly above the collarbone and the second to the side of one of the breasts. After the incisions are made, the proximal end of the CVC is inserted into the superior vena cava leading into the right atrium of the heart. The distal end of the CVC is placed beneath the skin and exited through the second incision. A cuff is attached to the CVC, which lies beneath the skin, prevents the catheter from migrating during daily activities or while being used.[6] The CVC may or may not be sutured at the exit site.

The CVC is ready for use immediately after insertion. The patient may feel some discomfort at the incision sites for several days. (Table 18-2 indicates recommended flushing of the CVC.)

Groshong catheter. Unlike traditional open-ended catheters, the Groshong catheter has a rounded closed tip and a patented three-position valve near the closed tip, which opens outward during infusion and inward during blood withdrawal (Figure 18-3). The valve closes automatically when not in use because venous blood pressure is not great enough to spontaneously open the valve inward. If, for example, the catheter accidently becomes disconnected from the infusion, the valve will automatically close and prevent air embolus. This also prevents blood from backing up into the lumen and clotting the catheter. Because of this special valve, heparinization and clamping of the Groshong are unnecessary. (For irrigation instructions, see Table 18-2.)

Implantable vascular access device. The subcutaneous or implantable vascular access device (IVAD) is also used for the delivery of medications, blood products, and nutritional fluids directly into the blood stream. The terms *subcutaneous* and *implantable* refer to the fact that the device is placed in the subcutaneous layer beneath the patient's skin. The device, commonly referred to as a port, is visible as a raised area beneath the skin. Daily care is not required, and thus there is less disruption of the patient's normal activities.

The ports are made from special medical-grade materials designed for safe, long-term use in the body. The ports are small disks about 1½ inches in diameter with a raised center or septum. The septum is made from a self-sealing rubber material. Ports may have a single or double septum. In the double-septum ports there is no communicating flow of fluid between ports. The noncoring needle is inserted into the septum for delivery of IV fluids. The IV fluid is carried from the port into the bloodstream through a small, flexible catheter. The port also provides a simple means for collecting blood samples.

The port is inserted during a minor surgical operation that is usually performed with a local anesthetic. The physician places the port just beneath the skin and inserts the proximal end of the catheter into the vein selected for administration of the IV fluids. The port is frequently placed in the upper chest just below the collarbone, a position convenient for patient treatment.

Once the port is placed, it is ready for use. During the first few days after the insertion of the port, it is important for the patient to avoid heavy exertion. When the incision has healed, the patient may resume normal activities.

The port can be used in two ways. One method, referred to as a bolus injection, delivers the medication or IV fluid all at once with the special needle being left in place for only a short time. In the other method, referred to as continuous infusion, a sterile transparent dressing is placed over the needle and port to secure the needle. Extension tubing is attached to the needle with an injection cap on the distal end of the tubing. If the patient is receiving a continuous infusion or long-term daily IV therapy, the noncoring needle is changed once a week. A blood return should be confirmed each time the port is accessed or before an infusion is started. (For flushing procedure, see Table 18-2.)

Percutaneously inserted central catheter line. Current trends for venous access in the home setting favor a percutaneously inserted central catheter, commonly referred to as a PICC line. A PICC line provides a percutaneously inserted catheter into the basilic, cephalic, or median veins of the antecubital region. It is used for venous access for intermediate-term (7 days) or longer (6 to 8 weeks) infusion therapies.[6,8,16] Final placement is in the central venous corridor (subclavian vein or superior vena cava). The INS is now recommending that all PICC line placements be verified by x-ray examination. This would require a mobile x-ray unit for patients who require placement in the home.

Further definition has been given to catheters that were referred to as PICC lines in the past: the midline and midclavicular catheters. A midline catheter is defined as a "peripherally inserted catheter with the tip terminating in the proximal portion of the extremity."[6] These catheters are usually about 8 inches in length. A midclavicular catheter is defined as a "peripherally inserted catheter with the tip location in the proximal axillary or subclavian veins." If a line intended for the superior vena cava (SVC) location falls short and ends up in the brachiocephalic (innominate) vein, it should be considered midclavicular.[6]

Only registered nurses certified in the insertion technique should place PICC lines.[2] Approval for insertion must be obtained from the physician, who indicates catheter dwell time and placement. PICC lines may be used for antibiotic, pain, hydration and other selected therapies.[2,6]

Mechanical phlebitis may occur within 24 to 72 hours after insertion. Treatment involves application of moist heat 4 times a day and elevation of the arm. If phlebitis persists, consult the physician about possible removal of the PICC line. If catheter sepsis is suspected, the PICC line must be removed. Only a physician or a trained nurse may remove a PICC line.

Hemostats (or any clamp with teeth or sharp edges) should not be used on the PICC line. Blood pressure cuffs or tourniquets should not be placed on the arm where the line is inserted, and blood specimens should not routinely be obtained via a PICC line, unless the catheter is 4 to 5 Fr in size.

When providing central venous catheter or PICC line care, it is important to have a repair kit available in the home and/or to establish at the time of admission which local emergency department can handle the repair of the line if necessary. These lines will crack and leak but can be repaired.

Dressing changes and catheter care. An IV gauze dressing should be changed every 48 hours. A transparent or occlusive IV dressing, commonly used with CVCs, should be changed 1 to 2 times a week.[4,8] The IV catheter should be secured to the patient's arm or chest as appropriate and never allowed to hang loose. (For dressing change, flushing, access port and tubing changes, see Table 18-2.) In response to the Occupational Safety and Health Administration (OSHA) bloodborne pathogen standard, many home care agencies have switched to needleless IV systems.[7] (The reader is referred to individual manufacturer's guidelines for use and maintenance of needleless IV systems.) If used, needles inserted through an injection cap should be 1 inch or less in length. Exit site IV catheter care includes cleansing the site with alcohol and provodone iodine.[4,8] Crusted drainage at the catheter exit site may be cleaned with hydrogen peroxide.

Other access methods for intravenous management used in home care

Continuous subcutaneous rather than intravenous infusion of narcotic therapy may be used for pain management. This has proven to be very beneficial for end-stage cancer patients whose pain is unable to be controlled with PO or transdermal therapy. However, better results in pain managment may be achieved using the intravenous route.

The **epidural** or **intrathecal space** may be also used for pain management. Epidural catheters are for both temporary and long-term use. Temporary catheters are directly placed in the epidural space and are most often used in the hospital until a

Table 18-1 Types of vascular access devices

Characteristics	Insertion site(s)	Tip location	Insertion procedure
Short peripheral	Veins of upper and lower extremities Jugular veins in neck	Close to insertion site	Clean, no-touch Over-the-needle
Midline	Basilic, cephalic, or median veins of the antecubital region	Upper arm level with axilla, distal to the shoulder	Sterile technique Through-the-introducer Polyurethane can be over-the-needle
Midclavicular	Same as midline	Distal axillary or proximal subclavian vein	Same as midline
PICC	Basilic, cephalic, or median veins of the antecubital region	Superior vena cava at the level of the third intercostal space	Sterile technique Through-the-introducer or Seldinger method Maximum barrier precautions recommended
Percutaneous nontunneled central	Distal subclavian, internal or external jugular, femoral veins	Superior vena cava at the level of the third intercostal space If femoral vein is used, tip will be in the inferior vena cava	Sterile technique Seldinger method Maximum barrier precautions recommended
Tunneled	Enters distal subclavian or proximal axillary vein, tunneled in subcutaneous tissue to exit chest wall at a lower site	Superior vena cava at the level of the third intercostal space	Sterile technique in a surgical setting
Implanted port	Enters distal subclavian or proximal axillary vein with port pocket close to this location. Antecubital placement same as PICC Also placed in arterial or epidural locations	Superior vena cava at the level of the third intercostal space	Sterile technique in a surgical setting

From Hadaway LC: Vascular access in home care: 1997 update, *Infusion* 4(1):18, 1997.

long-term catheter can be placed. Temporary catheters should be monitored closely for stability and intact staying sutures. Long-term catheters are placed in the epidural space and tunneled through the subcutaneous tissue to an exit site, usually on the front of the patient. An epidural port catheter is placed in the epidural space, and the port body is placed against a bony prominence on the front side of the patient. The intrathecal space is surrounded by the epidural space and separated from it by the dura matter. This space contains cerebral spinal fluid, which bathes the spinal cord.[5,11]

Indications	Contraindications	Limitations of use
IV fluids for replacement/ hydration Most IV medications (although many cause significant local complications)	Total parenteral nutrition or any solution with a dextrose content over 10 percent	Changes in peripheral veins related to age, disease process, nutrition or fluid balance status, and previous use
IV fluids for replacement and hydration Most IV medications when admixed in an iso-osmotic or near iso-osmotic manner	Total parenteral nutrition or any solution with a dextrose content over 10 percent Continuously infused vesicants	Poor venous access in antecubital region and upper arm Inability to advance catheter to preferred tip location related to presence of venous valves, scarring, and sclerosing
Same as midline	Same as midline	Recently published research now pointing to a higher complication rate with this tip location
All types of IV fluids, medications, and nutrition	Anomalies of central venous structure Thromboses of subclavian, innominate, or superior vena cava	Poor venous access in antecubital region and upper arm Inability to advance catheter to preferred tip location related to venous valves, scarring, and sclerosing
All types of IV fluids, medications, and nutrition Hemodynamic monitoring Primarily seen in acute care settings	Anomalies of central venous structure Thromboses of subclavian, innominate, or superior vena cava Burns, radiation, surgeries in area of insertion	Fluid volume deficit Respiratory diseases Curvatures of the spine Tracheotomy
Long-term, frequent, ongoing need for all types of fluids, medications	Thromboses of subclavian, innominate, or superior vena cava Cardiac tamponade	Patient preferences Septicemia
Long-term, intermittent need for all types of fluid, medications	Thromboses of the subclavian, innominate, or superior vena cava Cardiac tamponade	Patient preferences Septicemia

All medications administered into the epidural or intrathecal space should be preservative free. Medications not preservative free will permanently scar nerve endings when given via the epidural space.[8] Alcohol is contraindicated for site preparation or cleansing of tubing connections because of the potential for migration of alcohol into the epidural space and possible nerve damage. A 0.2-μ filter without surfactant should be used for medication administration.[17]

The epidural catheter can be aspirated, with a physician's order, to ascertain the absence of spinal

Table 18-2 Home infusion practice guidelines

	Flushing	Dressing change	Injection/access port change	Tubing change	Blood sampling	Special considerations
PICC	· 3-5 ml normal saline · 3-5 ml heparin solution 10 u-100 u/ml. · Flush every 12-24 hours. · Use 5 ml syringe or larger.	· Transparent dressing change every 3-7 days. · Gauze dressing, need to secure all edges & change every 48 hours. Gauze under a transparent dressing is a gauze dressing. · Change dressing when damp, loosened or soiled. Also when site inspection necessary.	*Access port change when:* · Removed to start infusion or draw blood. · Unable to flush blood from access port. · Signs of blood precipitate, cracks, leaks or other defects. · Septum no longer intact. · One time weekly to coincide with weekly dressing change.	· Primary/secondary continuous every 24-48 hours. · May consider 72 hours if no increase in catheter related infection. · Primary/secondary intermittent every 24 hours. · Blood/blood component sets changed with each unit. · TPN/lipid tubing changed every 24 hours.	· Recommended for 4.0-5.0 Fr catheters only. · Discard 3-5 ml blood. · Draw labs. · Flush with 10-20 ml saline then 3-5 ml heparin solution 10 u-100 u/ml.	· Do not lift anything over 10 pounds. · Encourage use of arm. · Measure bicep 1×/week. · Monitor upper arm for edema, redness and cording of vein. · If clamp available, clamp when not in use. · When removing PICC, if resistance is met, do not attempt removal. Place warm pack on arm and attempt again. If still unable to remove, wait 24 hours before another attempt.
CVC	· 3-5 ml normal saline. · 3-5 ml heparin solution. 10 u-100 u/ml. · Flush every 24 hours. · Groshong— 5 ml saline only—flush weekly when not in use. · Use 5 ml syringe or larger.	· SAME AS PICC. · May use clean technique for dressing changes in 7-10 days after sutures are removed, for tunnelled catheters.	· SAME AS PICC.	· SAME AS PICC.	· Discard 5 ml blood. · Draw labs. · Flush with 10-20 ml saline then 3-5 ml heparin solution 10 u-100 u/ml.	· Never place toothed clamp on catheter. · Catheter can be repaired by experienced clinician. · Sutures may be removed with physician order on a tunnelled catheter.

Device	Flush/Maintenance	Dressing Change	Tubing	Tubing	Flush/Blood Draw	Comments
Implanted port	· 5-10 ml normal saline. · 5 ml heparin solution 10 u-100 u/ml. · Maintenance flush monthly. · Use 5 ml syringe or larger.	· SAME AS PICC	· SAME AS PICC	· SAME AS PICC	· Flush with 5 ml saline. · Discard 5 ml blood. · Draw labs. · Flush with 10-20 ml saline then 5 ml heparin solution 10 u-100 u/ml.	· If clamp available, clamp when not in use. · Always use non-coring needle to access port. · Needle change every 7 days or as needed
Peripheral	· 1-3 ml normal saline · 1-2 ml heparin 10 u-100 u/ml. · Flush every 12-24 hours.	· Transparent dressing change whenever the device is changed. · Change when damp, loosened, soiled or when site inspection is necessary.	· Every 48-72 hours with restart or as noted above.	· Primary/secondary continuous every 24-48 hours. · May consider 72 hours if <5% phlebitis rate. · All other tubing as above.	N/A	· Rotate site every 48-72 hours. · May leave catheter intact up to 7 days if venous access limited with physician order. Pediatric catheters may remain intact if no signs and symptoms of complications with a physician order. · If clamp is available and catheter not in use, clamp.
Epidural	· Not routinely flushed. · Preservative free saline for flushing only with physician order.	· Transparent dressing change every 3-7 days. Gauze dressing is not recommended. · Change when damp, loosened, soiled or when site inspection is necessary.	· Change should occur when the tubing is changed, not to exceed 7 days.	· Per closed system recommendations, not to exceed 7 days for a continuous infusion.	N/A	· A 0.2 micron filter should be used for medication administration · Never use alcohol for site preparation or when accessing catheter. · Aspiration and flushing under physician order only.

Courtesy Home Parenteral Services, Springfield, Mo.

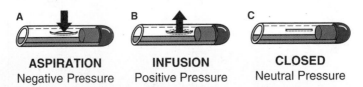

ASPIRATION
Negative Pressure

INFUSION
Positive Pressure

CLOSED
Neutral Pressure

Figure 18-3 Groshong catheter tip with patented three-way valve. **A,** When negative pressure (suction) is applied (usually by a syringe), the valve opens inward, allowing blood to flow through the catheter into the syringe. **B,** When positive pressure is applied, the valve opens outward, allowing fluid to enter the bloodstream. **C,** The valve stays closed when the catheter is not in use and when subjected to normal central venous blood pressures. (Courtesy Bard Access Systems, Salt Lake City, Utah.)

fluid prior to administration of medication. A syringe of preservative-free normal saline is attached to the catheter, which is then aspirated gently using minimal pressure. No fluid or a small amount of blood-tinged or clear fluid is normal. Aspirating blood could be indicative of the catheter migrating in the intravascular space. Larger amounts of clear fluid may be indicative of the catheter migrating into the intrathecal space. In both instances, the infusion should not be started, and the physician should be notified. Epidural catheters do *not* require routine flushing.[5]

Implantable infusion pump technology is now being used with epidural catheters. One type of implanted pump can deliver a set rate of narcotics, or another type can be programmed outside of the body, using a computer with a telemetry device that is placed over the implanted device. This type allows rates of infusions to be changed without having to completely empty the implanted pump. Both types of pumps are filled using a noncoring needle, similar to those used to access an IVAD.[15]

Enteral access is used to administer nutrient solutions into the gastrointestinal tract. A gastrostomy tube is commonly used for long-term therapy. A pump is recommended to ensure accurate flow rates.

Infusion device and pump management

One of the goals of home infusion is to make the patients as independent as possible in the administration of their therapies at home. When that is not possible, devices are chosen that administer all doses of an ordered therapy, and the patient/caregiver is taught to troubleshoot the devices.

As margins continue to decrease in the home infusion market, companies look to administering therapies in the most cost-effective manner. With this in mind, certain antibiotics are being given IV push. This has proven to be a safe and efficient means of delivery that is easy for most patients to learn. This method is used only for select cephalosporins and should not be used for other classes of antibiotics.[10]

The gravity drip system is the next simplest system for home infusion therapy. The solution is hung on a pole above the patient, and the solution follows the forces of gravity. The rate of flow is typically managed by an in-line roller clamp that is adjusted to control a given rate of drops per minute. Because of an inherent inaccuracy and lack of an alarm system to warn of blockage, this is not ideal for all therapies.

Disposable elastomeric devices are pressurized pumps that consist of an elastic sphere containing a small balloon, filled with the drug by the pharmacist. Once activated, the elastomeric membrane contracts, forcing the drug into the catheter and patient. The flow rate is usually accurate, and the pump is easy to use. The primary disadvantage of this system is that because each dose requires a new device, it may not be cost-effective in the long run.

Many patients sent home from the hospital require IV antibiotic, IV nutrition therapy, or IV pain control or cardiovascular medications. These can be administered through ambulatory infusion pumps, which are small, lightweight, and function on battery power, thus enabling the patient to move about freely. The pumps can be worn in a pouch carried over the shoulder or hooked to a belt. Attached to the pump is a reservoir that holds the necessary medication. The reservoir is usually con-

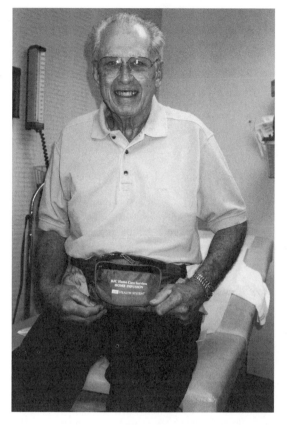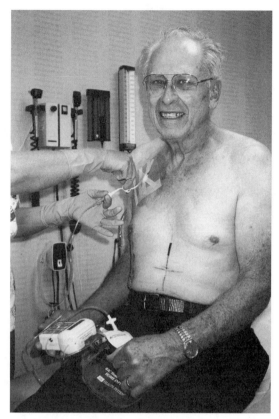

Figure 18-4 Patient wearing an ambulatory infusion pump. (Courtesy BJC Home Infusion Services, St. Louis, Mo.)

nected to extension tubing, which is attached to a needle or catheter (Figure 18-4).

Infusion pumps work in a variety of ways, depending on the patient's needs. The pumps can deliver a constant rate of medication; can deliver doses intermittently (e.g., every 8 hours), can auto ramp up and down when giving an infusion; and can also be programmed in period modes, where the pump will automatically increase rates of an infusion after a certain length of time. Certain pumps are designed to deliver medication only when the patient activates a dose/rate button (e.g., patient-controlled analgesia, or PCA, pump). Pumps are designed to be lightweight and easy for patients to transport, again so they can be as mobile as possible (see Figure 18-1).

Complications of intravenous therapy

Intravenous therapy is not without complications. It is important that the patients/caregivers are instructed on signs and symptoms of complications, so they can monitor their infusion sites when the nurse is not present in the home. A hematoma may develop at the insertion site, resulting in tenderness or bruising. It may be impossible to advance or flush the catheter. The vein may infiltrate, or the needle or catheter may puncture through the vein wall at the time of insertion. When complications occur, nursing actions include removing the IV device, applying pressure and warm soaks to the affected area, and documenting assessment and interventions.[2,8] If resistance is met on venipuncture, do not try to advance the needle further.

Infiltration of the IV occurs when the catheter becomes dislodged from or perforates the vein. The presenting symptoms of an infiltration are swelling and tenderness above the IV site, which may extend along the entire limb. There may be decreased skin temperature around the site. The backflow of blood may be absent, the flow rate may become slower or stop, or fluid may continue to infuse into tissue even if the vein is occluded. For infiltration of vesicant drugs, follow an established extravasation protocol, and document assessment and interventions. Infiltrations can be prevented by frequent assessment of the IV site, securing the IV site with an occlusive clear dressing or arm board, and not constricting the limb above the site with tape.

Phlebitis may occur when hypertonic or viscous medications and solutions are administered. Repeated use of the same vein, movement of the catheter in the vein, and use of a catheter too large or a flow rate too rapid for the size of the selected vein may also cause phlebitis. A thrombophlebitis may occur if there is clotting at the tip of the catheter. The area proximal to the insertion site will become red, tender, and warm; the vein will be hard when palpated. There will be a decrease in IV flow rate, and the patient will experience increased pain or discomfort with the infusion. Prevention of phlebitis includes use of large or central veins for hypertonic solution, use of the smallest IV catheter to accommodate viscosity of fluid and size of vein, and regular IV site rotation every 2 to 3 days or as needed.

Intravenous therapy can also produce site infection. Its presenting symptoms are redness, tenderness, swelling, and warmth at the insertion site, with possible purulent exudate. Site infection may result from failure to maintain aseptic technique during insertion or site care. Site infection can also be caused by insertion of an IV catheter for longer than 3 days or by immunosuppression. The IV catheter should be removed if site infection is present. The home care nurse should obtain a culture of the catheter tip, notify the physician for follow-up, restart the IV at a different site, and document nursing assessment and interventions and the patient's response to care.[8] Site infections can be prevented by using aseptic technique during IV starts, dressing changes, and initiation of medications and solutions. Peripheral IV sites should be rotated at least every 2 to 3 days.[2,6,8]

Clotting of an IV site is another complication of therapy. It is likely to occur when the IV rate is too slow to maintain patency of the catheter or when a heparin lock solution is not routinely used to flush the catheter. The site may be clotted when the IV catheter does not flush easily, the IV flow rate is sluggish, or there is tenderness at the IV site. An attempt should be made to withdraw the clot with a syringe to clear the IV catheter. If the clot cannot be withdrawn, the catheter should be removed and the IV restarted at another site.[15]

As approved by the physician and per agency policy, heparinized saline or a fibrinolytic agent may be used to dissolve a clot that has formed in a CVC.[17] The fibrinolytic agent should be injected into the catheter and the catheter clamped. The home care nurse should wait for 10 minutes, unclamp the catheter, and aspirate the clot. The procedure should be repeated with a 20-minute dwell time if the catheter remains clotted.[2,8] Then the catheter should be irrigated with normal saline. Documentation should include the assessment and interventions. Flushing of the IV catheter routinely with a heparin lock solution and saline solution or maintaining a constant IV flow rate should prevent clotting of an IV site. Home care nurses should be aware that patient position may prevent CVC irrigation and blood sampling. Changing intrathoracic pressure may move the catheter tip away from the wall. This can be accomplished by having the patient breathe deeply or change positions such as turning to one side, lying flat, raising or lowering the arms, or by performing the Valsalva's maneuvers.[5,8]

Serious systemic complications of IV therapy include air embolism and circulatory overload. An air embolism may be caused by an empty solution container, IV tubing that has run dry or has not been properly purged or primed of air, or a disconnected IV. Symptoms may include respiratory distress, a weak and thready pulse, hypotension, loss of consciousness, and diminished or absent breath sounds.

In the event of an air embolism, the IV infusion must be discontinued immediately. The patient should be turned onto the left side with the head down to allow the air to enter the right atrium and disperse through the pulmonary artery. Oxygen should be administered, if available, and emergency services called as soon as possible. The physician should be immediately notified. Nursing assessment and interventions and the patient's response to care should be documented on the visit report. Prevention of an air embolism includes purging or priming the tubing of all air before initiating the infusion and securing all connections with tape. Reflux valves, which are part of the needleless systems, also help prevent the chance of air embolism because they do not require opening the catheter to air except when cap changes are required.

Circulatory overload, another potential complication of IV therapy, is the result of miscalculation of the patient's fluid requirements or a "runaway" IV caused by a loosened roller clamp. The patient's symptoms will include generalized discomfort, neck vein engorgement, hypertension, fluid-filled lungs, shortness of breath, and a fluid intake greater than fluid output. Nursing actions include decreasing the flow rate or stopping the infusion, elevating the patient's head, notifying the physician, and administering medication and oxygen as ordered. Document assessment and interventions and the patient's response to care. The patient may need to be seen by the physician for complications of infusion therapy. Table 18-3 provides steps for troubleshooting IV therapy in the home.

Types of home infusion therapy

Antibiotic therapy. It is recommended that a CVC or PICC line be used for antibiotic therapy lasting longer than 3 weeks.[6] When possible, the patient should receive the initial intravenous dose of the antibiotic in a controlled environment (hospital, clinic, emergency department, or physician's office) to monitor for allergic or anaphylactic reactions. Intravenous home antibiotic therapy is usually administered 1 to 4 times a day depending on the drug and patient-specific factors such as disease severity.[16] Most often gravity is used to infuse antibiotics. If possible, the IV push method is used because it is easy for patients to learn and administer. A pump is recommended for aminoglycoside or vancomycin infusions, when a PICC line is used, and for patients with fluid overload problems. Peripheral IV sites are rotated every 2 to 3 days or as needed.

Patients with diseases involving hepatic, renal, hematopoietic, cardiac, and pulmonary systems must be carefully evaluated for complications of infusion therapy. High doses of penicillin-related drugs can cause seizures and other central nervous system changes. Aminoglycosides and vancomycin require assessment for nephrotoxicity and ototoxicity. Any patient receiving long-term antibiotic therapy, especially an immunosuppressed patient, should be assessed frequently for signs and symptoms of superinfection with resistant organisms. In addition, home care nurses should be aware of appropriate laboratory tests when monitoring antibiotic administration. These tests are outlined in Table 18-4.

Chemotherapy. Qualified nursing personnel may administer oral, intramuscular, or subcutaneous chemotherapeutic agents. Approved chemotherapy for home administration should be listed according to agency policies and procedures and administered under the guidance of the medical director. It is recommended that only chemotherapy-certified nurses carry out home administration of intravenous push (IVP) or infusions of chemotherapeutic agents. Pregnant and lactating women are advised not to administer IV push chemotherapeutic agents. Intravenous push chemotherapeutic agents must be administered through the stopcock of a running IV. They should not be administered into the line containing solution with additives.

Patients should receive the first dose of chemotherapy in the hospital or physician's office.[2] It is recommended that intravenous infusions be administered only via central venous access devices, such as an implanted port or long-term tunneled silicone catheter.[8]

Extravasation kits should be available and must be taken to the patient's home along with written procedures for treating extravasation of vesicant chemotherapeutic agents. Chemotherapy spill kits should be provided by the home care agency for use in the patient's homes in the event of a spill or leakage of the hazardous drug.

Before administering chemotherapeutic agents, home care nurses must be aware of certain baseline information.[15] In addition to a record of the patient's vital signs, they should know the results of a complete blood count (including platelets) performed within 1 week of chemotherapy administration. If white blood cell count is less than 3500 and/or platelet count is less than 100,000, the patient's physician should be consulted before administering chemotherapy.

Table 18-3 Troubleshooting IV therapy in the home: patient/caregiver education

Complication	Action
Infusion slows or stops	Observe for swelling, pain, or hardness around needle/catheter site. If any of these are noted, stop the infusion and immediately notify the home care nurse and/or physician. If the above signs and symptoms are not present: 1. Check for twisted tubing or pressure on tubing. 2. See if the patient has moved or bent his or her arm. If so, return arm to original position. 3. If the flow rate remains slow or stopped, turn regulator off and contact the home care nurse.

Circulatory overload
Occurs when patient has received too much fluid.
Symptoms:
  Coughing, shortness of breath
  Increased respirations
  Headache, facial flushing
  Rapid pulse rate
  Dizziness
	Stop the infusion and immediately call the home care nurse and/or physician.
	Call an ambulance directly if the situation is an emergency.

Air embolism
Air gets into the blood stream.
Symptoms:
  Extreme shortness of breath
  Anxiety
  Lips and nail beds turn blue
  Rapid pulse rate
  Loss of consciousness
	This is a medical *emergency.* Turn patient on left side with head down
	Immediately call an ambulance. Stay with the patient.

Pyrogenic reaction
May occur with exposure to contaminated equipment or solutions.
Symptoms:
  Abrupt temperature, chills
  Complaints of backache, headache
  Nausea and vomiting
  Flushed face
  Dizziness
	Discontinue IV therapy.
	Call home care nurse/notify physician.
	Stay with the patient until arrival of the home care nurse. (If symptoms are severe, take the patient to an emergency department.)
	Save the equipment/IV solution for laboratory analysis.

Severed catheter	Clamp the line and notify the home care nurse/physician.

Table 18-4 Drug classification and suggested laboratory tests

Drug classification	Suggested test and frequency
Aminoglycosides	
Gentamicin	CBC, SMA6, peak and trough twice weekly
Amikacin	Audiogram if therapy greater than 2 weeks
Tobramycin	
Miscellaneous	
Vancomycin	CBC, SMA6, peak and trough weekly
Clindamycin	Audiogram weekly if therapy greater than 2 weeks
Beta-lactam cephalosporins	
Ancef	CBC, SMA6 SGOT/weekly
Ceftriaxone	
Ceftazidime	
Penicillins	
Ampicillin	CBC, SMA6 SGOT/weekly
Pen G	
Pen V	
Antifungals	
Amphotericin B	CBC, SMA6, Mg twice weekly
Fluconazole	CBC, SMA6, SMA12 weekly
Sulfonamides	
Bactrim	CBC, SMA6 weekly
Antivirals	
Ganciclovir	CBC, SMA6 twice weekly
Acyclovir	
Foscavir	CBC, SMA6, Ca, Mg, PO_4 twice weekly fluids
Quinolones	
Ciprofloxacin	CBC, SMA6, SMA12 weekly
Colony-stimulating factors	
GCSF (granulocyte colony-stimulating factor)	CBC weekly
GMCSF (granulocyte-macrophage colony-stimulating factor)	
Erythropoietin	
Blood products	
Packed red blood cells	CBC, platelets before and after transfusion
Platelets	
Gamma globulin	
Antineoplastics	
Refer to each antineoplastic drug to determine relevant clinical monitoring/observations.	CBC, SMA6, Ca, Mg before therapy
Diuretics	
Lasix	SMA6 weekly weight each SNV
Sympathomimetics	
Dobutamine	SMA6 and Mg weekly weight each SNV
Anticoagulants	
Heparin	CBC, protime weekly
Hydration	SMA6, Mg weekly weight each SNV

Home care nurses administering IV push chemotherapeutic agents must wear disposable protective gowns and sized sterile gloves during the procedure. When bubbles are removed from syringes or IV tubing, a sterile alcohol wipe should be placed carefully over the tip of the needle, syringe, or tubing in order to collect any of the drug that may be discharged. In case of skin contact with an antineoplastic drug product, the affected area should be washed thoroughly with soap and water. If the drug gets into the eyes, they should be flushed immediately with a copious amount of water.

Home care nurses should not mix chemotherapeutic agents. All chemotherapeutic agents should be prepared by a pharmacy. Any defective syringe or bag containing chemotherapy should be sent back to a pharmacy for safe disposal.

Home care personnel and caregivers should be cautioned to avoid skin contact with excreta of individuals treated with antineoplastic agents. Hands should be washed thoroughly and gloves worn when disposing of excreta. Institutional guidelines for the treatment of hazardous waste must be followed in disposing of excess portions of the agent or contaminated equipment.[15] Unused portions should not be disposed of down the drain or toilet.

Contaminated needles, IV bags, and syringes are disposed of intact to prevent aerosolization contamination. (These items should be placed in a container with a label specified for chemotherapy waste disposal.)

Pain management. Narcotics can be used for effective intravenous pain management to alleviate severe pain, decrease anxiety, and maximize the patient's best level of functioning. When the epidural route is used, the two main types of drugs that are used are opioids, such as morphine, fentanyl, and Dilaudid, and local anesthetics, such as bupivacaine and ropivacaine.[11] Cancer, neurological, orthopedic, or certain diseases related to acquired immunodeficiency syndrome (AIDS) are conditions that may require pain management in the home. (See Chapter 24 for further pain management guidelines.)

Narcotics can be administered intravenously, intermuscularly, subcutaneously, intrathecally, or epidurally when the patient is no longer responsive to oral, rectal, or transdermal drug administration. Frequency and dosage of administration should depend on the patient's response to the medication.

Narcotics commonly infused in home care include morphine, hydromorphone, levorphanol, and methodone.[11] Patient-controlled analgesia pumps are often appropriate for use with narcotics.

Hemotransfusions. Blood transfusions are most frequently given to restore blood volume and blood components lost as a result of surgery, hemorrhage, or disease. Hemotransfusions maintain and promote the oxygen-carrying capacity of blood by supplying red cells and supplement the coagulation properties of platelets. Red blood cells and blood components may be administered in the home by a qualified registered nurse in accordance with the standards of the American Association of Blood Banks (Box 18-1).

A physician's order must be written for transfusion of blood or blood components. The order should state the type and amount of blood or component, the duration of the infusion, the date of the transfusion, and the pretransfusion and posttransfusion blood work. The physician should be available for consultation by telephone or pager throughout the time of blood or blood component administration in case complications arise.

Informed consent must be obtained from patients receiving hemotransfusions before initiation of therapy. The physician is responsible for initial instructions related to the nature and purpose of the agent to be administered, the risks involved, and

---

Box 18-1   REFERRAL CRITERIA FOR IN-HOME TRANSFUSIONS

The patient must meet the following criteria:
- Resides within the local community
- Has physical limitations that render the patient homebound
- Is alert, cooperative, and able to respond to instructions
- Has a medical condition that allows for safe transfusion therapy at home
- Has available a responsible adult in the home during the procedure to witness verification checks and be available to call for help
- Has adequate peripheral/central venous access as determined by a home IV care nurse
- Has a hemoglobin level of less than 10 g/100 ml (for red blood cell recipients)

the alternatives available for treating the patient's condition. Home care nurses are responsible for reinforcing the physician's instructions, explaining the procedure to the patient, reviewing signs and symptoms of potential transfusion reactions (both immediate and delayed), and obtaining signatures on the consent form. (Blood for typing and crossmatching must be drawn and delivered to the blood bank 24 to 48 hours before the transfusion.)

Nurses administering hemotransfusion must bring an emergency drug kit to the home and keep it readily available during the entire length of the visit (Box 18-2). For a patient with a history of allergic reaction, the physician may order premedication with an antihistamine before hemotransfusion and/or administration of a leukocyte-poor preparation. (The blood bank must be informed of leukocyte-poor needs at the time the request for blood is made.)

A patent IV must be established; 18 gauge or larger is ideal. The signs and symptoms of infusion reaction to observe for include chilling, fever, dyspnea, cyanosis, hives, headache, muscle ache, sharp pain in the lumbar area, a nonproductive cough, itching, vomiting, swelling, pain at the infusion site, dark urine, chest pain, flushing, shock,

hypothermia or hyperthermia, hypotension, hypertension, and tachycardia. Reactions may occur immediately or 24 to 48 hours, 1 to 6 weeks (delayed hemolytic), or 1 to 6 months later (hepatitis, other viral infections).

Blood and blood components should not be piggybacked. Two consecutive units may be administered through one transfusion set by flushing with normal saline after each unit. An *exception* is a sepacell filter (for leukocyte-reduced blood), which may only be used for one unit. Infusion length is determined by the physician order and the patient's condition in accordance with the standards of the American Association of Blood Banks and the home health agency's policies.[2] One unit of packed cells is usually transfused over $1\frac{1}{2}$ hours with a maximum time of 4 hours. A longer infusion time of 2 to 4 hours per unit is considered for the following:

- Infants
- Adults over age 60
- Patients with chronic anemia
- Patients with cardiopulmonary disease
- Debilitated patients

Home transfusion is not recommended for patients with a prior history of transfusion reaction or those with a history of circulatory overload.

Enteral nutrition therapy. Enteral nutrition involves tube feeding into the patient's stomach or intestine. Such therapy is used for patients who are unable or unwilling to swallow or who cannot otherwise ingest food or fluids by mouth, yet who have normally functioning lower gastrointestinal tract functions.

Nasogastric tubes are preferred for short-term use, whereas gastrostomy tubes are preferred for long-term use. Refer to manufacturer recommendations and agency policy for nasogastric and gastrostomy tube management. Complications may arise if the formula is not administered properly and may include aspiration, diarrhea, bloating, pneumonia, and possibly death.

Routine monitoring for therapeutic effectiveness is also a part of enteral nutrition therapy. It is of extreme importance to instruct caregivers to sit the patient up at a minimum 45-degree angle during and for 1 hour after feedings to prevent aspiration.

Total parenteral nutrition. Total parenteral nutrition (TPN) provides nutrition when the alimentary route cannot or should not be used (e.g., pa-

---

Box 18-2   EMERGENCY DRUG KIT CONTENTS

One IV tubing (macrobore)
500 ml of 0.9% sodium chloride
Two prefilled syringes of diphenhydramine hydrochloride, 25 mg each
One 3-ml syringe with 25-gauge 5/8-inch needle
One ampule of epinephrine, 1:10,000 (.1 mg/ml)
Two ampules of epinephrine, 1:1,000 (1 mg/ml)
Two 3-ml Luer's syringes
Two filter needles
Two 23-gauge 1-inch needles
Two 20-gauge 1-inch needles
Povidone-iodine wipes
Alcohol wipes
One adult oral airway
Index card for each allergic reaction procedure
Two ethylenediamine tetraacetic acid (EDTA) tubes
One urine specimen cup
One laboratory requisition
Three labels

tients with malnutrition resulting from Crohn's disease, short-bowel syndrome, cancer, ulcerative colitis, and AIDS-related malnutrition).[5]

Total parenteral nutrition fluids must be prepared in a pharmacy, and glucose concentrations greater than 10% should not be given peripherally.[8] Because of the high electrolyte and glucose concentrations and volumes used, the rate should not be increased or decreased dramatically because this can result in electrolyte imbalance, hyperglycemia, hypoglycemia, or fluid overload. An infusion pump is always used to ensure constant flow rates.

Administration of TPN requires a written physician order, which specifies the frequency of checks of vital signs and blood glucose. For patients with impaired renal function, serum chemistry panels are obtained and recorded weekly or as ordered. These are listed in Table 18-4.

The TPN solution must be refrigerated in the patient's home. The patient/caregiver must be instructed to remove the solution from the refrigerator to allow it to reach room temperature before infusion. Rapid infusion of a cold solution can cause shaking chills and lead to ventricular arrhythmias.[6] A 1.2-μ filter for lipid-containing TPN fluids is recommended, and strict aseptic tubing standards must be met. Tubing changes are done every 24 hours.[2,8]

Blood samples should not be taken from the TPN line. An alternate intravenous route should be used for IV push medications and for intravenous piggybacks (IVPBs).

Other therapy. The following may also be administered in the home setting: hydration therapy, dobutamine or other inotropic agents to improve cardiac contractility for patients with severe congestive heart disease, tocolytic therapy (administration of terbutaline for the treatment of premature uterine contractions in high-risk pregnancies), chelation (or iron overload) therapy for patients suffering from chronic iron overload conditions such as thalassemia, and growth hormone therapy. In addition, infusion therapies may include aerosolized pentamidine (or other medication by inhalation); hemodialysis; hormonal treatments (for multiple sclerosis and organ rejection after a transplant); anticoagulant therapy, such as ". . . heparin, enoxaparin, and dalteparin; alpha₁-antitrypsin therapy . . . (for the treatment of alpha₁-antitrypsin deficiency); and biologicals such as,

filgrastim, epoietin alpha, oprelvekin, and sargramostim."

Stringent home care policies regarding admission, monitoring, and implementation of these therapies are highly recommended in order to ensure safe and efficacious patient care.

Developing the plan of care and patient education

Home infusion therapy patients typically are discharged from the hospital at higher acuity levels than the average home care patient (Box 18-3). The delivery of services and supplies must be coordinated to ensure a safe transition from the hospital to home. As with any high-technology procedure in the home, feasibility of the service must be determined before admission. As described in the beginning of this chapter, the home milieu must be able to support IV therapy equipment and related services.

Although home infusion therapy is a very technical service, patient/caregiver requirements for self-care management are derived from a holistic needs assessment as described in Chapter 2. It should be emphasized that patient/caregiver education and self-determination for self-care is an essential component of successful home infusion therapy.

A major focus of service is to enable patients/caregivers to manage long-term home infusion safely with minimal intervention by home care nurses. Therefore the patient/caregiver *must* be able to demonstrate administration techniques, express a willingness to comply with techniques, understand the signs and symptoms of therapy complications, and be able to identify appropriate interventions (Box 18-4).

Patients/caregivers are taught how to initiate or discontinue the IV therapy, how to flush the catheter, and how to prepare IV fluids for administration. In addition, patients/caregivers are generally taught maintenance and operation of infusion pumps. This includes changing the battery, starting and stopping the pump, and responding appropriately to alarm signals. Finally, patients/caregivers must be taught how to deal with complications of IV therapy. Box 18-4 provides patient education guidelines for troubleshooting IV therapy in the home. In order to meet established outcomes of care, the plan of care is developed to reflect nursing assessments,

Box 18-3 PRIMARY NURSING DIAGNOSES/PATIENT PROBLEMS

- Knowledge deficit: for example, lack of information about home IV therapy and risk complications, medications, operation of home medical equipment, procedural care, diet, activity, socioeconomic resources, available community services
- Altered nutrition: less than body requirements
- Pain
- Risk for infection
- Activity intolerance: _____ Ambulation, _____ ADLs, _____ Other *(Specify)*
- Self-care deficit: _____ ADLs, _____ Feeding, _____ Toileting, _____ Other *(Specify)*

Box 18-4 PRIMARY THEMES OF PATIENT EDUCATION

- Complications of IV therapy or disease process: recognition, treatment, when to call the case manager and physician
- When to call 911
- Medications: purpose, action, dosage, side effects, and methods of administration
- Administration and management of IV therapy
- Operation and maintenance of equipment
- Infection control
- Socioeconomic resources
- General self-care strategies

actions, multidisciplinary collaboration, and ongoing monitoring and evaluation that includes physician and patient/caregiver involvement.

SUMMARY

Medications previously administered in the hospital setting such as amphotericin B, dobutamine, heparin, intravenous immunoglobulins, ganciclovir, and pentamidine now are being administered in the home. As a result, home infusion therapy is possible only in conjunction with standards of nursing practice that stress the importance of staff expertise, systems coordination, and patient education emphasizing active involvement with therapies as fundamental to the plan of care. Such standards may be derived from guidelines published by the CDC and the INS.

In conclusion, home IV therapy offers the promise of high-technology health care services in an environment that is safe, familiar, and cost-effective. With the information presented in this chapter, home care nurses can help to make the potential of home infusion therapy and quality patient care a reality.

REFERENCES

1. Appleby CR: For profits that are not humble, there's no place like the home infusion market, *Healthweek* 3:18, 1990.
2. BJC Home Care Services: *Clinical policy and process manual,* St. Louis, 1998.
3. Cain D: Home infusion practice guidelines: the Show Me State works for standardization, *Infusion* p 42, 1998.
4. Camp-Sorrel D: *Access device guidelines: recommendations for nursing practice and education,* 1996, Oncology Nursing Society.
5. Gorski L: *Best practices in home infusion therapy,* 1999, Aspen Publishers.
6. Hadaway LC: Vascular access in home care: 1997 update, *Infusion* 4(1):18, 1997.
7. Hanchett M, Kung L: Do needleless intravenous systems increase the risk of infection? *J Intraven Nurs,* p 117, June 1999.
8. Intravenous Nurses Society: *Revised intravenous nursing standards of practice,* 1998. The Society.
9. The Joint Commission on Accreditation for Health Care: *1999–2000 Comprehensive accreditation manual for home care,* Oakbrook Terrace, Ill, 1998 The Commission??
10. Nowobilski-Vasilias A, Poole S: Development and preliminary outcomes of a program for administering antimicrobials by IV push in home care, *Am J Health Syst Pharm,* p 76, January 1999.
11. Pasero C: Providing epidural analgesia, *Nursing 99,* 1999.
12. Pearson ML: Guidelines for prevention of intravascular device related infections. *Am J Infect Control,* p 262, 1996.
13. Schlachta L: Leveraging technology: telemedicine in disease management, implications for infusion services, *Infusion,* p 36, November 1997.
14. Stephenson R: *1999 HIDA home care financial performance survey,* 1999, Health Industry Distributors Association.
15. Terry J, and others, editors: *Intravenous therapy: clinical principles and practice,* Philadelphia, 1995, WB Saunders.
16. Tice A: *Handbook of outpatient parenteral therapy for infectious diseases,* New York; 1997, Scientific American.
17. Weinstein S: *Plumer's principles and practice of intravenous therapy,* ed 6, Philadelphia, 1997, JB Lippincott.
18. West V: Alternate routes of administration, *J Intraven Nurs,* p 221, August 1998.

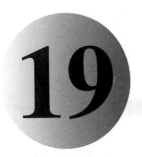

THE PATIENT WITH NEUROLOGICAL DYSFUNCTION

Ellen Barker and Robyn Rice

Individuals with a nervous system disorder must live not only with the effects of the disease, they also experience threats to their very existence in ways that are unlike any other type of illness. A neurological disease may affect cognition (e.g., the ability to think, to learn, and to make judgments). In addition, it may affect the ability to move, ambulate, eat, eliminate, communicate, hear, and even breathe.

This chapter will focus on patients who have been diagnosed with one of the three most significant neurological diseases home care nurses will encounter in the community: cerebrovascular accident (stroke), multiple sclerosis (MS), and dementia, specifically Alzheimer's dementia. Although these diseases are the ones most frequently encountered, others may be seen that require similar care. Nurses may feel that home management of patients with neurological disorders is difficult and demanding; however, a basic review of pathophysiology and a summary of case management guidelines will enable the home care nurse to meet the needs of patients and families. Home care nurses will be personally and professionally rewarded as they strive to improve the quality of life for patients and provide dignity in the face of a neurological illness. Expanded knowledge of the neurological disease process, including its progression and prognosis, is the foundation for providing high-quality home care. Appropriate medication and treatment regimens tailored to the patient's needs in the home setting are necessary to ensure the best possible outcome, whether that be recovery or a peaceful and dignified death.

Family members of patients with neurological deficits may feel particularly frustrated and stressed in their dual role as loved one and 24-hour caretaker. Extensive interaction with families is an integral part of the home care nurse's responsibilities. The home care nurse may need to care for two patients in the home setting—the assigned patient and the spouse or loved one. Often the spouse or loved one is elderly and not in good health, which further complicates the home setting. Enormous support, teaching, and follow-up by the home care nurse are needed to ensure that family members also stay healthy, rested, and able to continue the important role of caretaker for the homebound patient with neurological dysfunction. Ongoing family education and evaluation are an integral part of every home visit. (Refer to Chapter 4, which discusses working with families and caregivers in the home.)

Patients and family members alike will benefit from a home care nurse who is knowledgeable and competent, and who possesses a broad-based understanding of the neurological disease.

CEREBROVASCULAR ACCIDENT

Cerebrovascular disease, or *stroke,* is defined as an abnormal condition of the cerebral blood vessels characterized by an occlusion or hemorrhage that causes ischemia and damage to the brain tissue perfused by the involved vessel. This interruption in the blood supply to specific areas of the brain has been described in the past as "accidents of the vessels," hence the term *cerebrovascular accident* (CVA). Hippocrates provided the first description of stroke as far back as 460 to 370 BC. Despite the long history of this serious and complex disease, it remains a primary cause of disability among adults and is the third leading cause of death in the United States after heart disease and cancer.[1,12]

Incidence

The National Stroke Association reports that 500,000 to 600,000 persons suffer a new or recurrent stroke each year, resulting in 150,000 deaths.[8] Although stroke death rates are declining, the numbers of strokes may be increasing because of the growing elderly population, in which the incidence is higher. Men have a 25% increased risk of stroke because of high rates of hypertension and poorer health risk habits. The risk of stroke among African-Americans is twice that of the white population, primarily because of hypertension.[8,12]

Pathophysiology

There are four types of stroke syndromes: (1) transient ischemic attack (TIA), or temporary interruption of blood flow that lasts an average of 1 minute and no longer than 24 hours with no permanent damage (symptoms may include motor and sensory impairment, speech and visual impairment, and dysphasia), (2) reversible ischemic neurological deficit (RIND), which lasts longer than 24 hours with no symptoms or neurological deficits after 48 hours, (3) stroke in evolution, or progressing stroke, with increasing neurological deficits lasting longer than 24 hours, and (4) completed stroke, in which the symptoms stabilize and the neurological deficits cease to escalate.

Stroke is also divided into two groups or classifications: hemorrhagic and ischemic (or occlusive).

Hemorrhagic stroke. A cerebral hemorrhage can occur within the parenchymal or brain tissue as an intracerebral hemorrhage, or the bleed can be within the spaces surrounding the brain on its surface. For example, bleeding can occur from a subdural hemorrhage, under the dura and above the arachnoid membrane. The bleed can also result from a subarachnoid hemorrhage (SAH), where the bleeding is usually caused by an aneurysm or arteriovenous malformation (AVM). The subarachnoid space, which is between the arachnoid and the pia, is the only "true space" over the brain and is filled with cerebrospinal fluid (CSF). The hemorrhage causes the CSF to become bloody as seen on lumbar puncture (LP). Vessels on the surface of the brain that rupture fill the spaces between the brain and the skull, exerting downward pressure on the surrounding brain tissue and resulting in increased intracranial pressure (ICP).

Aneurysms and AVMs are usually congenital and silent. There is no warning to herald the rupture. The sudden onset of a hemorrhagic stroke is dramatic as the blood enters the area surrounding the ruptured vessel. Headache, often described as "the worst headache of my life," invariably occurs as the blood products break down and irritate the meninges, or brain tissue. Aneurysms can rupture at any time, although it is more often a condition seen in healthy adults between 20 and 50 years of age.[2] After the initial rupture, the vessel constricts, a clot forms to seal the leak, and medical intervention is necessary to prevent a rebleed. Berry (saccular) aneurysms are the most common type. Giant, mycotic, and dissecting aneurysms are seen less frequently.

An SAH from a ruptured aneurysm may range from a small leak to a massive bleed, graded I through V. The symptoms from a grade I reflect only a minimal bleed with no deficits. When the hemorrhage is mild (grade II), the patient may develop a headache. Grade III, described as a moderate bleed, usually results in a change in the level of consciousness (LOC) with or without neurological deficits. Grades IV or V produce life-threatening symptoms as a result of moderate to severe hemorrhage and require intensive care and emergency measures.

When an intracerebral bleed is massive or near vital centers, the outcome can be fatal. This is considered "large vessel disease." If, however, the patient has had a long history of hypertension, the hemorrhage may occur in small penetrating vessels. This is called "small vessel disease," with a potentially more favorable outcome if detected and treated early.

Occlusive stroke. An occlusive or thrombotic stroke results when a cerebral vessel's circulation is decreased or completely obliterated by an infarct or stenosis. When an area of the brain has no blood supply or too little blood supply, focal ischemia from low perfusion pressure will gradually cause symptoms. In a local process (e.g., atherosclerosis), fatty materials called plaque build up in the inner lining of the artery, usually at the bifurcation in the common carotid. Over time, the plaque will enlarge and become irregular and pitted with ulcer craters that bleed or form clots. Platelets aggregate to the ulcer site, enlarging the clot, which eventually will completely fill the lumen of the vessel or break off. Clot fragments or plaque travel distally until they lodge in penetrating branches of vessels, obstructing blood flow and causing ischemia.

Local ischemia over time signals a compensatory response or collateral circulation that may delay stroke symptoms. When the collateral circulation fails or becomes inadequate to perfuse the brain, low perfusion will cause warning signals and symptoms of stroke.

In contrast to the slow progressive disease of thrombotic stroke, embolic strokes occur the instant a fragment or embolus that has traveled from another source (e.g., the diseased heart) enters the cerebral circulation. The blockage causes instant symptoms as the affected vessel becomes occluded. Cerebral edema accumulates around the lesion following the ischemia. The deficits correlate with the vascular territory involved.

Acute complications

The location of the affected blood vessel and the circumscribed cerebral area are dependent on the vessel's blood flow. The area deprived of blood will determine the stroke syndrome (Table 19-1). Damage will be measured by the amount of brain tissue deprived of oxygenated blood. Immediate signs and symptoms may include the following:

- Decreased LOC or coma
- Increased ICP
- Paralysis or decreased motor function
- Sensory loss
- Respiratory problems (e.g., atelectasis and pneumonia)
- Unstable vital signs
- Infection
- Aphasia
- Memory loss
- Dysarthria with impaired communications
- Dysphasia with the potential for choking and aspiration
- Impaired thought patterns
- Headache and/or pain
- Urinary tract infections

Treatment

In the acute phase, once neurodiagnostic studies are completed to determine whether the stroke is hemorrhagic or occlusive, measures are directed toward patient survival with appropriate interventions. The treatment is determined by the patient's age, state of health at the time of stroke, location and extent of the cerebral attack, and the degree of deficit that the patient has suffered. Surgery, angioplasty, or endoscopic procedures to obliterate an aneurysm may correct the hemorrhagic stroke.

Cerebral angioplasty, a newer experimental option available at some centers for "brain attacks" that have occurred within 6 to 8 hours, is showing great promise. A small dose of agents (e.g., urokinase) is injected in the cerebral vessel downstream from the clot via a small catheter threaded into the femoral artery to quickly dissolve the infarct and reopen the artery. Patients treated early with cerebral angioplasty may suffer less brain tissue death and therefore have a more rapid recovery with a much better chance for return of functions.

Surgery can also be an option for prevention of ischemia (e.g., carotid endarterectomy). Traditional modalities with pharmacological treatment to prevent further thrombotic events include agents (e.g., anticoagulation and antiplatelet agents).

Once the patient has recovered from the acute event, rehabilitation and discharge planning are needed to prepare the patient for home recovery.

HOME CARE APPLICATION
Assessment

Patients recovering from a major stroke often require a multidisciplinary home care team to regain activities of daily living (ADLs) and instrumental activities of daily living (IADLs). The nursing care is integrated with other health care professionals to meet patient goals for optimal outcome, with the nurse assuming the role as case manager or team leader. Helping the patient cope with the sequelae following the stroke, adjusting to the home environment, and gaining independence can be hampered by problems with immobility, musculoskeletal function, altered nutrition, altered elimination, skin integrity, and altered sensation. A combination of these problems creates a high risk for injury. Altered cognition compounds the patient's inability for self-care and patient teaching, especially if the patient has residual confusion following the stroke event.

Table 19-1 Stroke syndromes secondary to occlusion or stenosis

Location/vessel	Area of brain infarcted	Signs and symptoms noted
Anterior and central circulation	NOTE: The internal carotid enters the Circle of Willis and supplies the lateral anterior and central portions of the cerebral hemispheres through the middle cerebral artery and the paramedial frontal lobe superior to the corpus callosum through the anterior cerebral artery; penetrating branches serve the deeper layers of the hemispheres.	
Internal carotid	If collateral circulation is intact, there is commonly no infarction; if infarcted, it is in the same area as the middle cerebral artery.	• Arterial pressure may be low in the retina. • Bruits over the internal carotid artery. • Possible retinal emboli. • History of TIAs. • Positive noninvasive studies.
Middle cerebral artery (MCA) (most common area); either stem or branches of MCA	Cortical motor area (face, arm, leg) and/or posterior limb, internal capsule, corona radiata.	• **Motor:** contralateral hemiparesis or hemiplegia, greater in face and arm than leg.
	Cortical sensory area (face, arm, leg) and/or posterior limb of internal capsule.	• **Sensation:** contralateral loss in same distribution as motor loss.
	Broca's area and deep fibers in the dominant hemisphere.	• **Speech:** expressive (motor) disorder with anomia (left hemisphere most commonly affected) with nonfluent aphasia and some comprehension defects.
	Broca's area and deep fibers in the nondominant hemisphere.	• **Speech:** dysarthria.
	Optic radiations deep in the temporal lobe.	• **Vision:** contralateral homonymous hemianopsia or quadrantanopsia.
	Location not known.	• **Motor:** mirror movements. • **Respirations:** Cheyne-Stokes respirations, contralateral hyperhidrosis, occasional mydriasis.
	Posterior limb or internal capsule and adjacent corona radiata.	• **Motor:** pure motor hemiplegia.
	Penetrating branches of MCA (lenticulostriate branches) into the basal nuclei.	• **Motor:** varying degrees of contralateral weakness of face, arm, or leg. • **Sensory:** little or no loss; if present, contralateral following the motor distribution. • **Speech:** transcortical sensory aphasia (communicating pathways are interrupted). • **Perception:** transient visual and sensory neglect on the left if a right lesion.
Anterior cerebral artery (ACA) (least common)	Proximal segment: corona radiata (rarely).	• **Motor:** when present, a mild contralateral hemiparesis, greater in leg; with bilateral occlusion of ACA, cerebral paraplegia in both legs can occur.

Modified from Adams RD, Victor M: *Principles of neurology,* ed 4, New York, 1989, McGraw-Hill; Bronstein KS and others: *Promoting stroke recovery: a research-based approach for nurses,* St. Louis, 1991, Mosby; Kandel ER and others: *Principles of neural science,* ed 3, New York, 1991, Elsevier; and Millikan CH and others: *Stroke,* Philadelphia, 1987, Lea & Febiger. In Barker E: *Neuroscience nursing,* St. Louis, 1994, Mosby.

Continued

Table 19-1 Stroke syndromes secondary to occlusion or stenosis—cont'd

Location/vessel	Area of brain infarcted	Signs and symptoms noted
Anterior and central circulation—cont'd		
Anterior cerebral artery (ACA) (least common)—cont'd	Main stem (complete occlusion is uncommon, thus areas affected differ and collateral circulation may alleviate signs or symptoms); medial aspect of frontal lobes, caudate nucleus, and corpus callosum are supplied by the ACA.	• **Motor:** contralateral paralysis or paresis (greater in foot and thigh); mild upper extremity weakness. • **Sensory:** mild contralateral lower extremity deficiency with loss of vibratory and/or position sense, loss of two-point discrimination. • **Speech:** may have transcortical motor and sensory aphasia if left hemisphere.
Posterior circulation	NOTE: The posterior circulation includes the posterior cerebral artery, the vertebral arteries, and the basilar artery; the anatomical territory covered includes the posterior aspects of the hemispheres, the central areas of the thalamus and midbrain, and the brainstem; occlusion of the vessels is most commonly by emboli; effects of infarct in these vessels and their penetrating vessels can be specific or devastatingly global; many complex syndromes have been identified (see the original sources from which this table is compiled or basic neurology texts [e.g., Kandel] for detailed descriptions).	
Vertebral arteries	Medulla and spinal cord tracts, anterior spinal artery and penetrating branches (medial medullary syndrome).	• **Motor:** contralateral hemiparesis (face spared) and/or impaired contralateral proprioception; flaccid weakness or paralysis of the tongue and/or dysarthria.
Basilar artery (three sets of branches)	Midline structures of pons (paramedian branches); three general areas of infarction are common: (1) medial inferior pontine syndrome, (2) medial midpontine syndrome, and (3) medial superior pontine syndrome.	• **Motor:** contralateral hemiparesis or hemiplegia, ipsilateral lower motor neuron facial palsy, "locked-in syndrome." • **Sensory:** contralateral loss of vibratory sense, sense of position with dysmetria, loss of two-point discrimination, impaired rapid alternating movements. • **Visual:** inferior pontine: diplopia; impaired abduction of ipsilateral eye: internuclear ophthalmoplegia; medial superior: diplopia, internuclear ophthalmoplegia, skewed deviation.
	Corticospinal and corticobulbar tracts in pons, sensory tracts of medial and lateral lemnisci, vestibular nuclei, inferior and middle cerebellar peduncles, cranial nerve nuclei and/or fibers, cerebellar connections in tectum, descending sympathetic pathways, central brainstem, pontine tegmentum (vertebral basilar syndrome).	• **Motor:** upper motor neuron type of weakness: paralysis in combinations involving face, tongue, throat, and extremities; dysphagia, facial weakness, dysmetria, ataxia (either trunk or extremities), weak mastication muscles. • **Sensation:** combinations of impaired sensation (vibratory, two-point, position sense, pain, temperature), facial hypesthesia, anesthesia of cranial nerve V.

Modified from Adams RD, Victor M: *Principles of neurology,* ed 4, New York, 1989, McGraw-Hill; Bronstein KS and others: *Promoting stroke recovery: a research-based approach for nurses,* St. Louis, 1991, Mosby; Kandel ER and others: *Principles of neural science,* ed 3, New York, 1991, Elsevier; and Millikan CH and others: *Stroke,* Philadelphia, 1987, Lea & Febiger. In Barker E: *Neuroscience nursing,* St. Louis, 1994, Mosby.

Table 19-1 Stroke syndromes secondary to occlusion or stenosis—cont'd

Location/vessel	Area of brain infarcted	Signs and symptoms noted
Posterior circulation—cont'd		
Posterior cerebral artery (PCA)	Central territory (thalamic area, dentothalamic tract, cerebral peduncle, red nucleus, subthalamic nucleus, and cranial nerve III).	• **Motor:** contralateral hemiplegia with possible dysmetria, dyskinesia, hemiballism or choreoathetosis, dystaxia, cerebellar ataxia, and tremor; contralateral upper motor neuron palsy; several syndromes are associated: (1) Weber: cranial nerve III palsy and contralateral hemiplegia; (2) thalamoperforate syndrome: superior, crossed cerebellar ataxia or inferior crossed cerebellar ataxia with cranial nerve III palsy (Claude syndrome), (3) decerebrate attacks. • **Sensory:** contralateral sensory loss of all modalities without agraphia. • **Function:** prosopagnosia (inability to recognize familiar faces), topographic disorientation, memory deficits, alexia, inability to read, color anomia. • **Level of consciousness:** in bilateral PCA syndromes, coma with absent doll's eyes or loss of alertness may occur; if tegmentum of midbrain near hypothalamus and third ventricle is damaged, akinetic mutism may occur.
Small vessel disease	NOTE: Small penetrating vessels in brain parenchyma that supply areas near the basal ganglia are most vulnerable to infarction although any small vessels can occlude deep in the brain and cause injury, producing neurological signs or symptoms; such infarcts are commonly called **lacunes** ("small pit or hollow"), a term that is changing in meaning. They can be caused by emboli but are most commonly associated with microatherosclerosis although they can be found in otherwise healthy people, those with concurrent atherosclerosis, hypertension, and/or diabetes have a higher incidence of this type of infarct.	
	Internal capsule, most commonly.	• **Motor:** contralateral hemiparesis on a single side, with equal deficit in face, arm, and leg; often unaccompanied by detectable signs of sensory, visual, and speech loss, depending on location; old term is "pure motor stroke" although evidence suggests that other neurological signs are present but overlooked because of low intensity.
	Thalamus, most commonly.	• **Sensory:** complete or partial loss in face, arm, trunk, and leg that appears exactly midline; may be accompanied by pain, hypesthesias, and uncomfortable sensations.

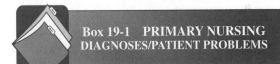

Box 19-1   PRIMARY NURSING DIAGNOSES/PATIENT PROBLEMS

Cerebrovascular Accident (CVA)

- Impaired cognition
- Alterations in behavior
- Impaired physical mobility
- Altered nutrition: less than body requirements
- Incontinence
- Impaired skin integrity
- Altered sensory/perceptual status

Box 19-2   PRIMARY THEMES OF PATIENT EDUCATION

Cerebrovascular Accident (CVA)

- Risk factors for stroke
- Signs and symptoms of stroke
- Aftercare from medical interventions and/or surgery
- Coping strategies
- Community reentry
- Management of neurological deficits
- General self-care strategies

Initial assessment focuses on a complete evaluation of the patient to plan functional restoration modalities or a death with dignity (Box 19-1). This section will review how to preserve the patient's current neurological status and/or help to restore the patient to the highest level of function (Box 19-2).

Components of the neurological assessment, including cranial nerve assessment (Table 19-2), follow with interventions and expected patient outcomes. The home care nurse must maintain a high vigilance to detect a possible second stroke, complications related to the acute stroke, and side effects from medications, especially anticoagulants. Stroke risk factors to monitor for prevention of a recurrent stroke include the following:

- High blood pressure
- Heart disease
- High red cell count
- Cigarette smoking
- Alcohol consumption
- Obesity
- Cholesterol over 200 mg/dl
- Physical inactivity
- Diabetes mellitus (DM)
- Carotid bruit

Nursing interventions

Cognition, behavior, and psychosocial. The home care nurse should determine the premorbid cognitive ability by reviewing the patient's history, interviewing family members, and reviewing the acute care record for results describing the location and degree of brain damage and neuropsychological reports. Initial and frequent serial testing are recommended using the Short Portable Mental Status Questionnaire (SPMSQ) (Figure 19-1) or Mini-Mental State Examination (Figure 19-2). Most stroke victims will regain a significant amount of lost functions within 1 to 2 years; however, individuals who receive consistent stimulation and rehabilitation may continue to recover smaller degrees of function up to 10 years. In working with patients who are cognitively impaired, effective therapy devices include items for a reminder of date, time, and orientation. For example, place the bed near a window to help the patient observe the changes of day and night, daily weather, and seasonal changes. Use verbal comments for emphasis.

Survivors of stroke may suffer from neurobehavioral deficits that range from an inability to adjust to the home environment to frank psychotic disorders. Interventions include first identifying the cause of the unwanted behavior, removing barriers that provoke it, and containing the behavior until it is no longer present. Medications that potentiate confusion should be eliminated or substituted. Pharmacological or physical restraints should not be used if possible.[12]

A consistent routine, a calm approach combined with adequate periods of rest, and an environment with minimal noise and confusion are desirable.[9] If depression, anxiety, and stress persist following discharge to home, consider a psychological referral to the psychiatric home care nurse or social worker for early detection and treatment. Psychosocial concerns may be overwhelming for the patient, the family, and the caregivers.

Table 19-2 Cranial nerves

Cranial nerve	Origin and course	Function
I Olfactory		
Sensory	Mucosa of nasal cavity; only cranial nerve with cell body located in peripheral structure (nasal mucosa). Pass through cribriform plate of ethmoid bone and go on to olfactory bulbs at floor of frontal lobe. Final interpretation is in temporal lobe.	Smell. However, system is more than receptor/interpreter for odors; perception of smell also sensitizes other body systems and responses such as salivation, peristalsis, and even sexual stimulus. Loss of sense of smell is termed *anosmia.*
II Optic		
Sensory	Ganglion cells of retina converge on the optic disc and form optic nerve. Nerve fibers pass to optic chiasm, which is above pituitary gland. Some fibers decussate, others do not. The two tracts then go to the lateral geniculate body near the thalamus and then on to the end station for interpretation in the occipital lobe.	Vision.
III Oculomotor		
Motor	Originates in midbrain and emerges from brain stem at upper pons.	Extraocular movement of eyes.
	Motor fibers to superior, medial, inferior recti, and inferior oblique for eye movement; levator muscle of the eyelid.	Raise eyelid.
Parasympathetic	Parasympathetic fibers to ciliary muscles and iris of eye.	Constrict pupil; changes shape of lens.
IV Trochlear		
Motor	Comes from lower midbrain area to innervate superior oblique eye muscle.	Allows eye to move down and inward.
V Trigeminal		
Sensory	Originates in fourth ventricle and emerges at lateral parts of pons. Has three branches to face: ophthalmic, maxillary, and mandibular.	*Ophthalmic branch:* Sensation to cornea, ciliary body, iris, lacrimal gland, conjunctiva, nasal mucosal membranes, eyelids, eyebrows, forehead, and nose. *Maxillary branch:* Sensation to skin of cheek, lower lid, side of nose and upper jaw, teeth, mucosa of mouth, sphenopolative-pterygoid region, and maxillary sinus. *Mandibular branch:* Sensation to skin of lower lip, chin, ear, mucous membrane, teeth of lower jaw and tongue.

From Rudy E: *Advanced neurological and neurosurgical nursing,* St. Louis, 1984, Mosby.

Continued

Table 19-2 Cranial nerves—cont'd

Cranial nerve	Origin and course	Function
V Trigeminal—cont'd		
Motor	Goes to temporalis, masseter, pterygoid gland, anterior part of digastric muscles (all for mastication), and the tensor tympani and tensor veli palatini muscles (clench jaws).	Muscles of chewing and mastication and opening jaw.
VI Abducens		
Motor	Arises from a nucleus in pons to innervate lateral rectus eye muscle.	Allows eye to move outward.
VII Facial		
Sensory	Lower portion of pons goes to anterior two thirds of tongue and soft palate.	Taste anterior two thirds of tongue. Sensation to soft palate.
Motor	Pons to muscles of forehead, eyelids, cheeks, lips, ear, nose, and neck.	Movement of facial muscles to produce facial expressions, close eyes.
Parasympathetic	Pons to salivary gland and lacrimal glands.	Secretory for salivation and tears.
VIII Acoustic		
Sensory	*Cochlear division:* Originates in spinal ganglia of the cochlea, with peripheral fibers to the organ of Corti in the internal ear. Goes to pons, and impulses transmitted to the temporal lobe.	Hearing.
	Vestibular division: Originates in otolith organs of the semicircular canals in the inner ear and in the vestibular ganglion. Terminates in pons, with some fibers continuing to cerebellum. Only cranial nerve originating wholly within a bone, petrous portion of temporal bone.	Equilibrium.
IX Glossopharyngeal		
Sensory	Posterior one third of tongue for taste sensation and sensations from soft palate, tonsils, and opening to mouth in back of oral pharynx (fauces). Fibers go to medulla and then to the temporal lobe for taste and sensory cortex for other sensations.	Taste in posterior one third of tongue. Sensation in back of throat; stimulation elicits a gag reflex.
Motor	Medulla to constrictor muscles of pharynx and stylopharyngeal muscles.	Voluntary muscles for swallowing and phonation.
Parasympathetic	Medulla to parotid salivary gland via otic ganglia.	Secretory, salivary glands. Carotid reflex.

From Rudy E: *Advanced neurological and neurosurgical nursing,* St. Louis, 1984, Mosby.

Table 19-2 Cranial nerves—cont'd

Cranial nerve	Origin and course	Function
X Vagus		
Sensory	Sensory fibers in back of ear and posterior wall of external ear go to medulla oblongata and on to sensory cortex.	Sensation behind ear and part of external ear meatus.
Motor	Fibers go from medulla oblongata through jugular foramen with glossopharyngeal nerve and on to pharynx, larynx, esophagus, bronchi, lungs, heart, stomach, small intestines, liver, pancreas, kidneys.	Voluntary muscles for phonation and swallowing. Involuntary activity of visceral muscles of heart, lungs, and digestive tract.
Parasympathetic	Medulla oblongata to larynx, trachea, lungs, aorta, esophagus, stomach, small intestines, and gallbladder.	Carotid reflex. Autonomic activity of respiratory tract, digestive tract including peristalsis and secretion from organs.
XI Spinal accessory		
Motor	This nerve has two roots, cranial and spinal. Cranial portion arises at several rootlets at side of medulla, runs below vagus, and is joined by spinal portion from motor cells in cervical cord. Some fibers go along with vagus nerve to supply motor impulse to pharynx, larynx, uvula, and palate. Major portion to sternomastoid and trapezius muscles, branches to cervical spinal nerves C2-C4.	Some fibers for swallowing and phonation. Turn head and shrug shoulders.
XII Hypoglossal		
Motor	Arises in medulla oblongata and goes to muscles of tongue.	Movement of tongue necessary for swallowing and phonation.

The return to a familiar world and the home setting may dramatically improve cognition. Old picture albums, newspapers, and favorite television and radio programs can be therapeutic and entertaining. A multidisciplinary team care plan should reflect a cognitive plan of care that becomes increasingly challenging and rewarding.[9]

Medications. Patients may have received anticoagulants, such as heparin or warfarin sodium during their acute illness. Warfarin is a commonly prescribed anticoagulant for patients at discharge. The effects of warfarin are judged by prothrombin time. The prescribed quantity may range from 1 to 2 times the dose given at baseline prothrombin time

based on typical home dosage of 2 mg/day to 10 mg/day PO. Anticoagulation therapy will continue for as long as the patient is considered to be at risk. The nurse may be asked to collect weekly or biweekly blood specimens to determine prothrombin time values and to immediately report any abnormal values or adverse reactions.

Patients and family must be taught the risks of warfarin or antiplatelet (aspirin) therapy. The nurse will routinely assess for bleeding, evidenced by hematuria, hemoptysis, hematemesis, melena, bleeding gums, bruising of skin, or petechiae. Instructions for gentle toothbrushing, care when shaving, and prevention of nicks or skin cuts is emphasized.

Short Portable Mental Status Questionnaire (SPMSQ)

Instructions: Ask questions 1-10 in this list and record all answers. Ask question 4a only if patient does not have a telephone. Record number of errors based on 10 questions.
Allow one more error if subject has had only a grade school education.
Allow one less error if subject has had education beyond high school.

+	–

1. What is the date today?_____
    Month   Day   Year
2. What day of the week is it?_____

3. What is the name of this place?_____

4. What is your telephone number?_____

4a. What is your street address?_____
    (Ask only if patient does not have a telephone)
5. How old are you?

6. When were you born?

7. Who is the President of the United States now?

8. Who was the President just before him?

9. What was your mother's maiden name?

10. Subtract 3 from 20 and keep subtracting 3 from each new number, all the way down.

_____ Total Number of Errors

0–2	Errors	Intact intellectual functioning
3–4	Errors	Mild intellectual impairment
5–7	Errors	Moderate intellectual development
8–10	Errors	Severe intellectual impairment

To be completed by interviewer

Patient's name: _____Date:_____

Sex: 1. Male   Race: 1. White
      2. Female   2. Black
                            3. Other

Years of education:_____   1. Grade school
                                          2. High school
                                          3. Beyond high school

Interviewer's name:_____

Figure 19-1 Short Portable Mental Status Questionnaire (SPMSQ). (From Pfeiffer E: A short portable questionnaire for the assessment of organic brain deficit in elderly patients, *J Am Geriatr Soc* 23(10):433, 1975.)

Mini-Mental State Examination

Maximum
Score   Score

Orientation

Maximum Score	Score	
5	( )	What is the (year) (season) (date) (day) (month)?
5	( )	Where we are: (state) (country) (town) (hospital) (floor)?

Registration

3	( )	Name three objects: 1 second to say each. Ask the patient all three after you have said them. Give 1 point for each correct answer. Then repeat them until he/she learns all three. Count trials and record. Trials

Attention and Calculation

5	( )	Serial 7s. 1 point for each correct. Stop after 5 answers. Alternatively, spell "world" backwards.

Recall

3	( )	Ask for the three objects repeated above. Give 1 point for each correct.

Language

9	( )	Give the name of objects: a pencil and a watch (2 points)

Repeat the following "No ifs, ands, or buts." (1 point)
Follow a three-stage command:
   "Take a paper in your right hand, fold it in half, and put it on the floor." (3 points)
Read and obey the following:
   "Close your eyes" (1 point)
Write a sentence (1 point)
  Copy design (1 point)
  Total score
ASSESS level of consciousness along a continuum_____

                                   Alert Drowsy Stupor Coma

Instructions for Administration of Mini-Mental State Examination

Orientation
(1) Ask for the date. Then ask specifically for parts omitted (e.g., "Can you also tell me what season it is ?"). One point for each correct.
(2) Ask in turn "Can you tell me the name of this hospital?" (e.g., town, country) 1 point for each correct.

Registration
Ask the patient if you may test his/her memory. Then say the names of three unrelated objects clearly and slowly, about 1 second for each. After you have said all three, ask him/her to repeat them. This first repetition determines his/her score (0-3), but keep saying them until he/she can repeat all three, up to six trials. If he/she does not eventually learn all three, recall cannot be meaningfully tested.

Attention and Calculation
Ask the patient to begin with 100 and count backward by 7. Stop after 5 subtractions (93, 86, 79, 72, 65).
Score the total number of correct answers.
If the patient cannot or will not perform this task, ask him/her to spell the word "world" backward. The score is the number of letters in correct order (e.g., dlrow = 5, dlorw = 3).

Recall
Ask the patient if he/she can recall the three words you previously asked him/her to remember. Score 0-3

Figure 19-2 Mini-Mental State Examination. (From Folstein MF and others: Mini-mental state: a practical method for grading the cognitive state of patients for the clinician, *J Psychiatr Res* 12(3):189, 1975.)

Language

Naming: Show the patient a wrist watch and ask him/her what it is. Repeat for pencil.
　Score 0-2.

Repetition: Ask the patient to repeat the sentence after you. Allow only one trial. Score 0 or 1.

Three-stage command: Give the patient a piece of plain blank paper and repeat the command.
　Score 1 point for each part correctly executed.

Reading: On a blank piece of paper print the sentence "Close your eyes" in letters large
　enough for the patient to see clearly. Ask him/her to read it and do what it says. Score 1
　point only if he/she actually closes his/her eyes.

Writing: Give the patient a blank piece of paper and ask him/her to write a sentence for you.
　Do not dictate a sentence; it is to be written spontaneously. It must contain a subject and
　verb and be sensible. Correct grammar and punctuation are not necessary.

Copying: On a clean piece of paper, draw intersecting pentagons, each side about 1 inch and
　ask him/her to copy it exactly as it is. All 10 angles must be present, and 2 must intersect
　to score 1 point. Tremor and rotation are ignored.

Estimate the patient's level of sensorium along a continuum, from alert on the left to coma
　on the right.

Figure 19-2—cont'd For legend see p. 341.

Sensory status. Problems related to hemianopsia, field cuts, impaired depth perception, and unilateral neglect require that the patient be approached in a manner to avoid the "blind spots." Furniture in the home should be arranged appropriately and not moved about. Spatial disorders and impaired vision make it difficult for patients to be independent until they have readjusted to the home environment.

Patients with a parietal lesion of the nondominant side may experience a condition known as "neglect" and totally ignore the opposite side of the body. If asked to draw a picture of a clock, this patient will draw numbers only on one side of the clock's face. The neglected side needs to always be carefully protected. The patient can be reminded of the neglected side with visual attention and range of motion exercises to prevent injury and muscle wasting.

Pain in the affected limb may be one of the first signs of neural recovery. The repetitive exercises and physical therapy help to restore the lost neural circuitry and stimulate the neurons to rewire the damaged brain. Motor recovery follows sensory recovery. The healthy side may be stimulated to communicate with the damaged side. The home care nurse may observe that when the patient moves the unaffected arm, the opposite limb with the deficit also moves, but only slightly. These compensatory reactions should be recorded.

The occupational therapy (OT) and physical therapy (PT) rehabilitation team's contribution is important to help the patient gain confidence and overcome sensory obstacles that interfere with autonomy and independence (see Chapter 17).

Language and communication. Left-sided stroke survivors may have receptive and expressive language deficits that impair meaningful communication. After discharge to home, patients' full awareness of their deficit may cause fear, anger, frustration, despair, hopelessness, and even rebellion as they develop nonverbal or healthy attempts to express themselves and make their needs known. It is therefore important to maintain the same caregivers who, over time, learn the meaning of damaged speech (much as a mother understands her baby's utterances). During this phase it is vital that the home care nurse address the patient in a respectful way and refrain from using slang or babytalk communication.

Communication aids (e.g., Talking Pictures) for patients with communication difficulties following stroke augment and supplement communication and are useful for language therapy. Communication boards (Figure 19-3) may be the only means of communication for some patients after a stroke.

Physical mobility and musculoskeletal function. A rigidly adhered to routine of getting the patient out of bed (OOB), sitting in a specialized chair, and ambulating as soon as possible is vital to

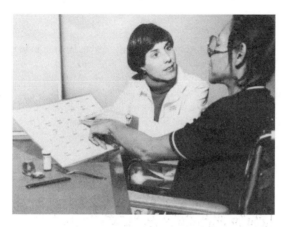

Figure 19-3 Using the Talking Pictures communication board. (Copyright Crestwood Company, Milwaukee, Wisconsin.)

the prevention of long-term complications of immobility and to achieve the expected outcome. Special equipment, the training of caretakers or volunteers, and a schedule for OOB activities are needed. The physical therapist (PT) and occupational therapist (OT) prescribe the type and amount of therapy with range of motion (ROM) exercises that can be passive or active. Exercises performed independently by the patient or by the family should be repeated up to 8 or more times per day. As soon as the patient can ambulate, daily walks with measured distances are incorporated into the daily routine. Walkers and any necessary assistive devices should be in the home and monitored for safety and maintained in good repair. The amount of time OOB and ambulation distance are increased until normal functions are restored. Efforts to eliminate falls and prevent injury are part of the patient and family teaching. The home should be checked for safety hazards at each visit. (Refer to Chapter 17 for more information on patient rehabilitation needs and care.)

Nutrition. A nutritionist should be consulted before discharge to assist in the evaluation of nutritional needs and to develop a home nutrition program. Copies of the diet should be available to everyone participating in the patient's dietary activities.

The nurse will be responsible for the assessment of cranial nerves, particularly the lower cranial nerves IX through XII involved in the gag reflex and voluntary muscles for swallowing. The assess-

ment includes evaluation of the patient's ability to chew, swallow, protect the airway from choking and aspiration, and manage different textures and foods; a recording of weight, intake and output, calorie count; condition of the oral cavity and teeth; and a check to determine if the food that is purchased and prepared is adequate.[7]

Patients on steroids or medications that affect fluids and electrolytes require further evaluation to maintain the integrity of the gastrointestinal tract and also to test for occult bleeding and electrolyte imbalance. For continued healing, patient teaching will focus on the importance of increased metabolic needs during recovery.

The use of supplemental or tube feedings for patients unable to tolerate oral feedings requires additional assessment and teaching to meet the patient's hypermetabolic requirements until adequate oral intake is safe and feasible. Determining when to switch and what to institute is best done in consultation with the nutritionist/speech therapist. Percutaneous endoscopic gastrostomy (PEG) tubes are widely used to provide long-term nourishment and can be easily managed in the home setting. Protocols provided by the physician or home care organization should be maintained until the PEG tube is discontinued.

The problems of dysphagia, dehydration, and malnutrition should be closely monitored during the home visit in conjunction with the neuroassessment to evaluate any relationship between the neurological deficits and these potential complications. Creative methods are needed to promote adequate fluid intake and nutrition for the stroke survivor.

In addition, financial considerations may factor into the family's abilities to provide nutrition for the patient. Social services should be notified along with other community agencies as needed.

Bladder elimination. A bladder training program is best initiated during hospitalization and continued at home. Assess the stroke survivor's ability to eliminate by observing toilet routine, degree of continence, use of bladder aids, urinary and dietary intake and output, activity level, skin integrity surrounding the genitalia, and the patient's ability to verbalize toileting needs and/or problems. (Refer to Chapter 16 for more information on elimination problems.)

Bowel elimination. Bowel incontinence may develop from neurological dysfunction resulting from impaired defecation reflexes and loss of motor control and weakness following a stroke. The home care nurse will assess the following:

- Toilet habits
- Bowel evacuation
- Constipation and diarrhea
- Communication skills to verbalize bowel problems
- Balance and strength
- Dietary fluid and fiber
- Stress and anxiety related to bowel evaluation

Every home care provider is familiar with checking patients for fecal impaction, diarrhea, and skin integrity associated with bowel incontinence and dealing with the patient's embarrassment from loss of bowel control. These same principles are discussed in Chapter 16.

Skin integrity. Thin, dry, flaky skin is vulnerable to prolonged immobility and will quickly break down into pressure ulcers if not well protected. Powders, soaps, and lotions should be used with caution. Mild soap and warm water for remoisturization, gentle toweling to toughen the skin, and meticulous repositioning prevent breakdown. Padding and assistive devices over heels, elbows, and bony prominences are encouraged until the patient is OOB. Strong bleaches and detergents should be avoided in laundering bed linen. Silk sheets are ideal for heavy patients who must be turned frequently. (Refer to Chapter 14 for further guidelines on wound or skin care.)

Stroke prevention. Recovering stroke patients and their families require special teaching to prevent recurrent attacks. The importance of medication compliance, blood pressure control, adherence to diet, smoking cessation, weight control, and other identified controllable risk factors need frequent reinforcement.[1] Teaching the prompt reporting of the earliest warning signs of a "brain attack" for immediate intervention may prevent future death or disability from stroke. The most difficult challenge is motivating the patient to change a lifestyle that precipitated the earlier attack. Wellness promotion and a healthy lifestyle are the most effective therapy we can offer. A stroke risk screening (see Appendix XIX-I) can impact the incidence, morbidity, and mortality of stroke and should be incorporated into the assessment of every homebound elderly patient.[3]

Conclusion

Stroke survivors challenge the home care nurse with many situations during recovery. Patience is needed by everyone during the long period of brain healing and subsiding of the edema. Recovery varies from patient to patient. Compensatory coping skills, a high degree of motivation, compliance to a structured regimen, and family support combine for success in overcoming this devastating insult to the brain.

Patient/family/professional resources for stroke

American Stroke Association
A Division of the American Heart Association
National Center 7272
Greenville Avenue
Dallas, TX 75231-4596
(214) 706-1293

National Stroke Association
9707 East Easter Lane
Englewood, CO 80112
(800) 787-6537

MULTIPLE SCLEROSIS

Multiple sclerosis (MS) is the most common neurological illness affecting young adults.[6] The disease usually begins in young adulthood with a progressive course characterized by disseminated demyelination of nerve fibers of the brain and spinal cord with remissions and exacerbation that continue throughout life. When myelin is destroyed in multiple areas, the ability of the nerves to conduct electrical impulses to and from the brain is disrupted by the scars, or sclerosis. According to the National Multiple Sclerosis Society, approximately 350,000 people in this country have MS, and each may have a different pattern of demyelination. Symptoms depend on which areas of the central nervous system (CNS) have been attacked and the amount and scatter of lesions. It is one of few diseases that affect women more than men and is more common among whites.

The etiology is unknown; however, most theories suggest an immunogenetic-viral cause in which the immune system attacks the body's own myelin.[5] As shown in Table 19-3, symptoms correlate with areas of dysfunction.

Pathophysiology

Multiple plaques in the CNS that consist of demyelinated nerve fibers, sparing of axons, gliosis,

Table 19-3 Clinical manifestations of multiple sclerosis

Area of dysfunction	Symptoms
Cranial nerve dysfunction	Blurred central vision; faded colors; blind spots (optic neuritis)
	Diplopia
	Dysphagia
	Facial weakness, numbness, pain
Motor dysfunction	Weakness
	Paralysis
	Spasticity
	Abnormal gait
Sensory dysfunction	Paresthesias
	Lhermitte's sign (electric shock-like sensation radiating down spine into the extremities)
	Decreased proprioception
	Decreased temperature perception
Cerebellar dysfunction	Dysarthria
	Tremor
	Incoordination
	Ataxia
	Vertigo
Bowel and bladder dysfunction	Fecal urgency, constipation, incontinence
	Urinary frequency, urgency, hesitancy, nocturia, retention, incontinence
Cognitive dysfunction	Decreased short-term memory
	Difficulty learning new information
	Word-finding trouble
	Short attention span
	Decreased concentration
	Mood alterations (depression, euphoria)
Sexual dysfunction	Women: decreased libido, decreased orgasmic ability, decreased genital sensation
	Men: erectile, orgasmic, and ejaculatory dysfunction
Fatigue	Overwhelming weakness not overcome with increased physical effort

From Beare PG, Myers JL: *Adult health nursing,* ed 3, St. Louis, 1998, Mosby.

and inflammatory cells are the principal pathological findings in MS. Plaques range in size from 1 mm to 4 cm and are found scattered throughout the white matter and to a lesser degree in the gray matter. Areas that show a predilection for development of plaques include the optic nerves and chiasm, regions of the brainstem, cerebellum, cerebrum, and cervical spinal cord.[4,5]

Acute complications

Respiratory failure occurs in patients with MS secondary to aspiration, atelectasis, and pneumonia. Sepsis related to urinary tract infections (UTIs) and respiratory infections is not uncommon. Hospitalization is often required during a severe exacerbation for corticosteroid administration, feeding tube placement, insertion of a suprapubic catheter, or for spasticity management. As soon as these problems are under control, the patient is discharged for home care.

Treatment

Patients often experience years of frustration until they are finally diagnosed with MS. It has been called "the great imitator" because it can mimic other diseases. After an unexplained remission, patients often dismiss the early signs of MS and disregard the milder symptoms. Magnetic resonance imaging (MRI) has emerged as an important neurodiagnostic study to offer earlier supportive evidence; however, diagnosis of MS is one of exclusion because there is no single test for absolute confirmation. Clinical diagnosis is made when the patient has neurological dysfunction in more than one area of the nervous system that tends to appear more than once. For some, diagnosis is often a relief when they finally have a name for their illness and can begin treatment. Symptom management (refer to the list in Table 19-3) by a multidisciplinary team is recommended to assist the individual in living a normal life until the onset of an acute attack. Corticosteroids (usually oral prednisone), beginning with a high dose and then tapering, will reduce the inflammatory flare-up. Treatment with plasma exchange, immunosuppressive agents, and other modalities have been studied with the best results attributed to a new drug, Betaseron (interferon beta-1b). It has been shown to decrease the incidence and severity of exacerbations for patients with relapsing-remitting MS and may actually alter the course of the disease.[6] Other medications may be prescribed for relief of symptoms, such as, spasticity (baclofen), urinary retention (bethanechol or oxybutynin), or urinary tract infections (antibiotics).[6]

HOME CARE APPLICATION
Assessment

Homebound patients with MS may be wheelchair-bound, bedridden, or only minimally ambulatory depending on the progression of the disease. A review of the patient's record and a thorough history taken on the initial visit will determine which symptoms are apparent. A complete baseline neuroassessment is needed that will be used for all future comparisons. It is therefore important for the nurse to assess and record findings in a systematic manner. A flow sheet is recommended. Standardized scales may be used, such as the Short Portable Mental Status Questionnaire (SPMSQ) or Mini-Mental State Examination (see Figures 19-1 and 19-2), the Bartherl Index and the Brody Instrumental ADL Scale, the Kurtzke Scale, or the minimal record of disability (MRD). Each patient has unique physiological and psychological requirements that may also include environmental and home modifications.

Home care nursing interventions

Cognition, behavior, and psychosocial. Changes in cognition, short-term memory, mood swings, and depressive states should be evaluated and given consideration in planning home care.

Once family and caregivers understand that changes in behavior are disease related and not purposeful, it is easier for them to accept and live with these changes.

Strategies such as keeping notes, making a list for daily activities and routines, and reducing stressful episodes are helpful. Fatigue, one of the most common problems experienced by individuals with MS, can interfere in coping with cognition and behavior. The National Multiple Sclerosis Society describes fatigue in the following ways: (1) normal, due to overactivity, (2) short-circuiting, in which damaged nerves tire with use, (3) lassitude, which is overpowering exhaustion requiring medication, and (4) fatigue of depression, best managed with psychological counseling and/or medication. Fatigue should be evaluated and considered in the overall management of cognitive/behavioral problems.

Euphoria, or loss of control with laughing or crying, can be addressed by the nurse with suggestions (e.g., when you can't stop laughing, think of the saddest thing in your life or pretend that you are in church). Uncontrollable crying or sadness can be countered by visualizing feelings of joy and happy events. Active listening and help with coping skills in an empathetic manner will help the patient learn to manage unwanted behavior and deal with psychosocial concerns.

Mobility. After the amount and safety of ambulation has been planned, the home care nurse in conjunction with the rehabilitation team can teach or reinforce the following:

- Position changes from a lying or sitting position
- Balance
- Coordination
- Gait
- Toilet, tub, or shower safety
- Strengthening exercises
- Assistive devices that aid in mobility
- Wheelchair/bed/chair transfer techniques
- Application and removal of orthotics, braces, or appliances for improved support for mobility

The home care nurse will need to use motivational strategies to impress upon patients with MS that they cannot give in to their weakness, ataxia, and fatigue because it will only make them more incapacitated. Pride may interfere in the use of assistive devices such as a cane, wheelchair, or visible tools that bring attention to the illness. Some patients use denial to cope with their disease and do not want to be seen as handicapped. After the home care nurse explains that energy conservation is more important than pride and will enable the patient to be more mobile, the patient is usually more receptive. Canes, walkers, and wheelchairs can be personalized with artful decorations, paint, and glitter. Safe footwear (usually leather-soled, flat tie shoes) is recommended. The home care nurse should periodically check all equipment to see that it is still appropriate, fits, and is being used.

Sensory. Lhermitte's phenomenon is a sudden, transient, electric-like shock that spreads down the body when the head is flexed forward and is a characteristic finding in MS. Numbness, tingling, loss of joint sensation, and other sensory losses often accompany demyelination from MS. Intolerance of heat from exercising, an overheated environment, a hot bath/shower, or a swimming pool decreases the efficiency of nerve conduction. Keeping the environmental temperature in the cool range helps to avoid discomfort and associated sensory and motor symptoms.

Pain. Pain and discomfort from musculoskeletal dysfunction may result from compensation to maintain balance, from spasticity, or from nerve damage. Correction of the underlying problem or a rehabilitation program may reduce or eliminate the pain. After a complete pain assessment, the physician, nurse, and rehabilitation team can devise remedies to address the patient's pain and discomfort. For the bedridden patient, gentle massage, a warm bath, good body alignment with pillow support to the back and between the legs, a rigid turning schedule with proper protection of the bony prominences, and frequent ROM exercises to decrease spasticity will ease the pain. These interventions will also aid in the prevention of skin breakdown, deep vein thrombosis (DVT), and pulmonary embolism. See Chapter 24 for further information on pain assessment and management.

Language and communication. Brain lesions that affect speech and swallowing require the nurse to help the patient adapt or seek appropriate communication aids. A speech pathologist referral should be requested to devise a treatment plan to improve speech. Helpful suggestions to the patient include the following:

- Speak slowly.
- Use better breath control.
- Make a tape recording for feedback on tone, pitch, and inflection.
- Use a voice amplifier to generate more volume.

Self-care issues. Enlisting the OT to assess the plan interventions for self-care for ADLs will help the patient gain independence in bathing, toileting, dressing, eating, cooking, cleaning, and living safely in the home. The use of electronic devices may serve not only to decrease energy use, but also to provide more freedom and independence. Depending on the availability of financial resources, there is a wide selection of electronic equipment available. The ability to do housekeeping chores may be minimal or not possible for homebound patients. Every resource should be used to allow for maximal home independence until the needs and interventions change during the terminal phase. See Chapter 2, which identifies key concepts of self-care in the home.

Elimination. Bowel problems of constipation and continence plague many patients with MS because of lesions on nerves that control bowel motility. Recommendations made earlier in the chapter are applicable to patients with MS.

The most common problems affecting the bladder are increased frequency, leakage between voidings, storage, incomplete emptying, and difficulty in urinating. Self-catheterization, the use of prescribed medications, and the prevention of UTIs are all important in helping the patient successfully manage MS in the home. See Chapter 16 for further information on bowel and bladder management in the home.

Sexuality. The nurse may find that no one has discussed sexuality with the patient or that the patient has not asked questions regarding changes in sexuality.[11] The neurological changes may be manifested in the following ways:

Difficulty in achieving or maintaining an erection for males

Decreased libido from fatigue, anxiety, embarrassment

Decreased sensation in the genital area that inhibits arousal for females

Vaginal dryness for females

Interference with coitus by the urinary catheter
Mental, emotional, or psychological concerns

A frank discussion opens the door to dealing with sexual concerns. The home care nurse may suggest that the couple communicate openly and honestly. Professional help may be needed until the problems can be overcome and the patient can relax and enjoy a satisfying sexual relationship with his or her partner. Attention to dress and appearance, good personal hygiene, and relaxation techniques help set the mood for romance and sexual encounters and improve the patient's quality of life.[11]

Conclusion

Primary nursing diagnoses and primary themes of patient education are listed in Boxes 19-3 and 19-4. Because patients with MS live a near-normal life span, they will be faced with a myriad of problems from the remissions and exacerbations that accompany this disease until the nerve fiber degenerates and the symptoms become permanent. Research is promising, but until a prevention or cure is found, nurses will be important in helping the patient attain the best possible quality of life.

Patient/family/professional resources for MS

The National Multiple Sclerosis Society
733 Third Avenue
New York, NY 10017-3288
Phone: (212) 986-3240
FAX: (211) 986-7981

DEMENTIA: ALZHEIMER'S TYPE

Dementia, Alzheimer's type is a progressive degenerative disease of the brain in which cells die and are not replaced. It results in impaired memory, thinking, and behavior and is the most common form of dementing illness according to the national Alzheimer's Association (AA), which has developed the following checklist of 10 common symptoms:

- Recent memory loss
- Difficulty performing familiar tasks
- Problems with language
- Disorientation of time and place
- Poor or decreased judgment
- Problems with abstract thinking
- Misplacing things
- Changes in mood or behavior
- Changes in personality
- Loss of initiative

Incidence

With over 4 million Americans afflicted with Alzheimer's disease, it is considered the fourth leading cause of death among adults in the United States.[10] The AA predicts that by the year 2050 over 14 million Americans will have the disease. People are affected regardless of gender, race, ethnicity, or socioeconomic group. The incidence appears to be higher in women. The symptoms usually begin to appear after age 60 with increasing incidence with aging. By the age of 80, up to 40% of the elderly may be affected. Dementia, with im-

Box 19-3 PRIMARY NURSING DIAGNOSES/PATIENT PROBLEMS

Multiple Sclerosis (MS)
- Impaired memory
- Impaired physical mobility
- Sensory/perceptual alterations
- Pain
- Impaired verbal communication
- Self-care deficits
- Alterations in elimination
- Altered sexuality patterns

Box 19-4 PRIMARY THEMES OF PATIENT EDUCATION

Multiple Sclerosis (MS)
- Information on MS and available resources
- Overcoming physical disadvantages
- Disability prevention/physical fitness
- Coping strategies
- Energy conservation and prevention of fatigue
- Activities of daily living (ADLs)
- Communication
- General self-care strategies

paired intellectual or cognitive function that affects speech, language, memory, and personality is a broad term that often defies diagnosis until autopsy.[10] Terms other than Alzheimer's that nurses may hear associated with dementia include Pick's disease, multiinfarct dementia, organic brain disorder, and organic brain syndrome. In the following sections, dementia, Alzheimer's type will be used to describe the care for patients in the home who suffer from some type of dementia.

Pathophysiology

The cause is unknown; however, there are several theories of causation. The abnormal protein theory suggests that the large concentrations of amyloid-rich plaques, identified on autopsies from patients with Alzheimer's dementia, consist of neurofibrillary tangles most dense in the hippocampus.[4] They are thought to interfere with neural transmission.[4] The brain of patients with the disease becomes atrophic with primary atrophy in the temporoparietal and anterior frontal lobes. The degeneration of neurons in the cerebral cortex allows the ventricles to enlarge, giving a characteristic image on computed tomography (CT) or MRI.

It is believed that Alzheimer's dementia is related to a gene on the X chromosome with autosomal dominant inheritance accounting for a small percentage of the disease. Genetic factors, viral agents, and environmental toxins are also being studied.

Progression

Alzheimer's dementia may progress in stages that last several years before the onset of the next stage. The Global Deteriorating Scale (GDS) developed by Reisberg and others is based on the clinical progression of the disease. For example, in stage I for a period of 1 to 3 years there is memory loss and loss of visuospatial skills (e.g., difficulty finding the way around the house, language changes, and personality changes). Changes begin with minor slipups and slight forgetfulness. For the next 2 to 10 years these same symptoms may get worse with the addition of praxis and acalculia. In stage III intellectual function severely deteriorates; patients are bedridden, mute, incontinent, unable to breathe normally, sleep most of the time, and suffer with rigid limbs or remain in the fetal position. They no longer recognize self or loved ones. A simple way

to remember the stages are four words: forgetful, confused, ambulatory, and dementia[10] (Box 19-5). Certain groups of nerve cells no longer function and are destroyed. Death from aspiration, pneumonia, or infection follows the prolonged bed rest.

Treatment

Because there is no treatment or cure to stop the disease progression, care is supportive and symptomatic with the goals of keeping the patient safe from injury (e.g., falling) and from succumbing to complications of immobility. Management is directed at four areas:

- Behavior
- Cognition
- Slowing the progression of the disease
- Delaying onset of symptoms

The approval of tacrine hydrochloride (Cognex) as a palliative measure during clinical trials was shown to improve scores on the cognitive scale, with a tendency for the effect to plateau, and to delay the disease's effects in mild to moderate Alzheimer's dementia. Side effects include liver toxicity, cholinergic effects with nausea, vomiting, and diarrhea. Other medications that may be prescribed during home care are for sleep disturbance, depression, delusions, constipation, and antibiotics for UTIs or respiratory infections.

HOME CARE APPLICATION
Assessment

Patients with Alzheimer's dementia requiring home care are often in the late stage of the disease and present a challenge to the family and to the home care nurse. When dementia impairs memory and the ability to learn and is associated with behavior that may not be socially acceptable, caregivers may feel stressed and frustrated in their attempts to help.

After completion of a general physical assessment to evaluate vital signs, weight, nutrition, elimination, hydration, and skin, the home care nurse should focus on the following neurologic changes:

- Cognition (Mini-Mental State Examination if appropriate)
- Memory
- Level of consciousness

Box 19-5   SIGNS AND SYMPTOMS OF STAGES OF DEMENTIA

Early Stage (Stage I)

- Memory—forgetfulness, need for notes related to new learning, may appear absentminded
- Disorientation—cannot associate natural cues with time of day, gets easily flustered under stress
- Personality changes—mood swings, changes in affect, may appear depressed, irritable, and develop delusions of persecution, may call 911 to report burglary, may make accusations that people around them are stealing their money and personal items
- Impaired judgment—lack of judgment or unable to make logical decisions (e.g., with finances by taking money out of the bank or giving away personal property), very vulnerable
- Speech and language—inappropriate use of words or unable to name familiar objects
- Concentration—short attention span with impaired ability to concentrate
- Spatial orientation—topographic disorientation
- Activity—may appear careless, nondependable, but otherwise no motor deficits
- Nutrition—within normal limits of premorbid level of nutrition

Late Stage (Stage II)

- Memory—short-term and long-term memory impaired, may or may not recognize significant others
- Orientation—not oriented
- Personality—apathetic and indifferent to surroundings, socially acceptable behaviors impaired, may say things that offend, verbally abusive, very irritable, sundowning syndrome
- Judgment—cannot comprehend and make judgments
- Speech and language—aphasia more apparent
- Concentration—lost

- Spatial orientation—disoriented
- Activity—restless, need supervision for ambulation, unsteady, apraxic, difficulty dressing, wandering becomes a safety hazard, may become combative
- Nutrition—may have higher caloric needs related to agitation and restlessness, too restless to sit still long enough for adequate intake of food and fluids unless supervised

Final Stage (Stage III)

- Memory—lost
- Orientation—lost and impaired, Glasgow Coma Score decreasing
- Personality—intellect so impaired that personality is indefinable, family no longer "knows who this person is"
- Judgment—totally impaired
- Speech and language—may moan and groan to stimuli
- Concentration—totally impaired
- Spatial orientation—totally impaired
- Activity—bedridden, totally dependent, rigid and may assume fetal position, prone to skin breakdown
- Nutrition—difficult to feed, may require tube feeding or PEG tube, weight loss, incontinent of bladder and bowel
- Death—from complications of aspiration, infection, malnutrition, decubitus

The rate of progression from stage to stage varies with the individual and may depend on the quality of care and the prevention of secondary complications. The stages may span a period of 5 to 20 years. Serial electroencephalogram (EEG), CT, and MRI assist the professional caregiver and families to correlate signs and symptoms of the disease with the neurodiagnostic findings and mental status assessments.

- Motor—apraxia with impaired ability to perform purposeful activity, ataxia unless bedridden
- Agitation and paranoia
- Combativeness
- Potential for injury

Nursing interventions

Stimulation to promote brain activity and reduce agitation and boredom are recommended. A calm,

reassuring, and respectful manner is needed to assess and treat the patient (Box 19-6). Verbal communications may fail, but a demonstration using body language can substitute for teaching the patient appropriate activities such as taking medications, eating, or transferring from bed to commode. Distraction can be used to stop unwanted aggressive behavior (Box 19-7).

Simple speech face-to-face, calling the patient's name, and speaking slowly with a single command

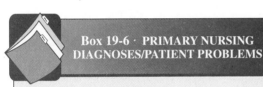

Box 19-6 · PRIMARY NURSING DIAGNOSES/PATIENT PROBLEMS

Alzheimer's Dementia

- Altered thought processes
- Impaired memory
- Impaired communication skills
- High risk for injury
- Alterations in elimination
- Altered nutrition, less than body requirements
- Constipation/diarrhea
- Sleep pattern disturbance
- Impaired mobility
- Caregiver role strain

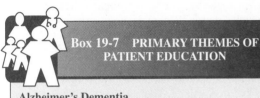

Box 19-7   PRIMARY THEMES OF PATIENT EDUCATION

Alzheimer's Dementia

- Preparation for long-term fatal illness
- Coping skills
- Safety
- Estate planning and/or living will
- General self-care strategies

or statement are more effective than engaging in conversation. Attention span is short, and repetition may be required along with a gentle touch.

Dehydration, malnutrition, and weight loss can be prevented by offering small frequent feedings, providing finger-food snacks, feeding the patient, and making sure dentures fit. A large tray of food may provoke confusion, whereas one choice at a time that is ground or pureed can be eaten quickly.

Supportive care focuses on a planned schedule of ADLs that begins with awakening the patient at the same hour each day, consistent mealtimes and snacks, toileting the patient every 2 hours, and preventing long naps that may lead to nocturnal wakefulness. If the patient is ambulatory and wandering is a problem, find a safe place to walk in a nonstimulating location. Using large muscles for exercise

such as walking is a way to decrease agitation. If agitation is related to the need for bladder or bowel evacuation, offer the patient an opportunity to walk to the bathroom or use a bedside commode.

Medications for sleep are appropriate so that the patient is rested and less agitated during the day and also for the family's benefit so that their sleep is uninterrupted during the night; however, a walk before bedtime, a warm bath, and a back massage help relax the patient and may obviate the need for medications. Psychiatric or geriatric clinical nurse specialists can also evaluate the patient and assist in making additional referrals as necessary.

Elder abuse has been recognized in the older patients whose behavior is unpredictable and stressful to the caregivers. When the family's ability to cope is stretched to the limits and the potential for abuse is suspected, the nurse's role is significant in giving the family "permission" to relinquish care to others. Home care nurses can collect and compile information for community services that offer respite care. The insurance or health care payer may have a program to provide a 1- or 2-week respite program to allow the caregivers a vacation. Moving the patient from the home to a new and strange environment for this short period, although advantageous for the caregiver, may cause the patient to react in negative behavior that could appear as regression. If this happens, families should be warned beforehand and prepared to cope with any temporary regression. The home care nurse can make arrangements with the respite agency for continuation of the plan of care. The nurse is encouraged to continue seeing the patient during respite care for continuity and to forewarn the family of any behavioral or physical changes to expect on their return.

Protective services must be called if the patient shows evidence of any type of abuse (verbal or physical). The home care nurse is responsible for detecting abuse and should develop a "high index of suspicion" and confront the patient with questions about the appearance of bruises, fractures, burns, and pinch marks. Check the wrist and feet for evidence of physical restraints or signs of overmedication for chemical restraints. Signs that the patient has not been properly fed or nourished along with poor personal hygiene are important hallmarks of abuse. Ask the patient about family social interaction versus long periods of sensory deprivation and isolation. Reporting of inadequate funds for medical supplies may reveal that the family is reallocating or diverting the patient's finances. See Chapter 8 and Chapter 23 for further information on abuse and neglect issues.

After the diagnosis and recognition of dementia, families are at risk for a strain on relationships that may be expressed with anger, frustration, and resentment. Because dementia affects its victims as they look forward to and approach their retirement years, couples often feel robbed of a lifetime of working hard for the rewards of retirement. Roles must be reversed, plans for the future scrapped, and finances used for treatment and support rather than the pleasures of retirement. A spouse no longer has the mate to turn to for advice and help. On the contrary, the healthy spouse often feels compelled to conceal the stress and strain of the consequences of the illness from the spouse who is ill. The healthy spouse may try to conceal the illness from friends and relatives and go into isolation. Denial may result in frequent doctor visits to find a physician who disagrees with the diagnosis of dementia. Loss of jobs affects income and available funds for everything except necessary expenses.

Children of affected parents may feel embarrassed and refuse to participate in the care or support of the ill parent, causing further hardship for the patient. Fatigue and caregiver burnout are not uncommon. In order to prevent the depletion of lifetime savings or sale of the family home, a divorce may seem to be the only solution. Some couples have chosen this solution to bypass the regulations for health care coverage and support. Medical care and/or home care may not be prescribed during the early phase when these problems are so troublesome.

As the late stage of the illness is reached by the patient, the care and supervision become more intense. The patient may not be safe left alone. Cigarette or pipe smoking becomes particularly dangerous with patients in bed or falling asleep on a sofa or stuffed chair that could catch fire and cause serious burn wounds to the patient. Simple acts like making a cup of coffee may result in leaving a burner turned on that creates a fire or spilling hot liquid that results in skin burns. Falling in the home when the gait becomes unsteady is problematic because the patient uses poor judgment and no longer understands limitations and safety hazards. The routine of getting up, brushing teeth, dressing, and eating becomes impaired as the disease progresses. It is not only frightening to the patient, who has no understanding of the disease process, but it can also be devastating to the family members who must watch and wait with nothing to offer other than help with basic needs.

Physicians may prescribe medications (e.g., haloperidol, thiothixene, loxapine, or thioridazine) to control some of the symptomatic delusions, hallucinations, agitation, or depression or to help the patient sleep.

Eventually the patient will become completely bedridden and totally dependent. Home care nursing focus is the same as for any bedridden patient with problems of immobility. The family must decide if they can continue home care or if a long-term care facility is in the best interest of the patient. After a family conference, including the physician, caregivers, and social services, the necessary plans for transfer can be completed once the decision is made. Hospice care, long-term skilled care, and even special facilities for patients with Alzheimer's dementia are options for the family to consider. The guilt of "giving up" or abandonment should be dealt with during this period to calm the family's emotions. Financial concerns may complicate the decision after the cost of care is considered.

Conclusion

Degenerative disorders pose hardships for everyone concerned. Until further advances are made in pharmacological therapy to reduce the effects, and until scientific researchers discover the cause of this devastating disease, nurses will play a vital part in helping the patient to function as long as possible until the ravages of the neuronal destruction cause death. The statistics for Alzheimer's dementia in the future are frightening as Americans live longer only to be afflicted with a disease that robs the mind of the ability to think, to learn, to love, and to enjoy the golden years of retirement.

Patient/family/professional resources for Alzheimer's dementia

Alzheimer's Association
919 North Michigan Avenue, Suite 1000
Chicago, IL 60601-5997
Phone: (800) 272-3900

SUMMARY

Three important neurological diseases commonly seen in the home are stroke, multiple sclerosis, and dementia. Care for other neurological illnesses has similarities in case management that can be generalized from this information. Reading this chapter, the home care nurse can see the importance of having a thorough understanding of neuroanatomy and neuroassessment. (For a comprehensive review of neuroscience nursing, the reader is referred to *Neuroscience Nursing,* by Ellen Barker.[2])

The nurse managing patients in the home may need to plan additional time for patients with neurological diseases to allow for a detailed history taking, complete general assessment, and a thorough neuroassessment. Family teaching is more demanding because of a knowledge deficit among the public concerning the cause, treatment, and outcome of neurological disorders. Recovery may not be an option in some cases with the nursing focus on comfort and palliative care until the disease runs its course. Despair has to be countered with hope; helplessness countered with every possible community resource. Support groups, local chapters for stroke, MS, and Alzheimer's dementia, and related groups (e.g., geriatric services) should be made available to the patient and family. Day care, elder care, respite care, and religious organizations can be consulted for possible assistance.

The satisfaction of easing the family's burden of care and the joy of managing patients with neurological dysfunction who can recover in their own environment surrounded by their family is a nursing specialty reserved for the home care nurse.

REFERENCES

1. America's Health Network: AHN chat room: nurses make stroke top priority, http:www.ahn.com; April 8, 1999.
2. Barker E: Cranial surgery. In Barker E, editor: *Neuroscience nursing,* St. Louis, 1994, Mosby.
3. Barker E: Brain attack: a call to action, *RN* 62(5):54, 1999.
4. Bunting L, Fitzsimmons B: Degenerative disorders. In Barker E, editor: *Neuroscience nursing,* St. Louis, 1994, Mosby.
5. Donohoe KM: Autoimmune disorders. In Barker E, editor: *Neuroscience nursing,* St. Louis, 1994, Mosby.
6. Kelly CL, Smeltzer SC: Betaseron: the new MS treatment, *J Neurosci Nurs* 26(1):52, 1994.
7. McLearn S, Green S: Nutritional screening and assessment, *Professional Nurse* 13(6):S9, 1998.
8. National Stroke Association: *Be smart stroke facts,* Englewood, Colo, 1998, The Association.
9. Ronning OM, Guldvog B: Outcome of subacute stroke rehabilitation: a randomized controlled trial, *Stroke* 29(4):779, 1998.
10. Stolley JM: When your patient has Alzheimer's, *Am J Nurs* 94(8):34, 1994.
11. Walters AS, Williamson GM: Sexual satisfaction predicts quality of life: a study of adult amputees, *Sexuality and Disability* 16(2):103, 1998.
12. Whitney F: Stroke. In Barker E, editor: *Neuroscience nursing,* St. Louis, 1994, Mosby.

Appendix XIX-I

Stroke Risk Screening

STROKE RISK SCREENING

Site and address of screening ――――――――――――――――――――――――――――――― Date: ――― / ――― /―――

PART I - DEMOGRAPHICS, AGE AND ETHNICITY

Name: (last) ―――――――――――――――――― (first) ―――――――――――――― (middle initial) ―――――

Gender:___Male ___Female - Highest Level of Education: ____High School or less―――― College ―――― Graduate School

Address: ―――――――――――――――――― (city) ――――――― (state) ――――― (zip) ――――――― (county) ―――――

Phone: Home (_____) _____ Work (____) _____ Date of Birth: ___ /___ /___ Age today____

Do you have a primary health care provider? --- ―― Yes ―― No
Have you seen a health care provider in the past year? --- ―― Yes ―― No
Do you have medical insurance? --- ―― Yes ―― No

Ethnicity/Race: _____ African-American _____ Caucasian_____ Hispanic White _____ Hispanic Non-White
―――――― Asian/Pacific Islander ―――――― American Indian or Alaskan Native―――――― Other or Unknown

PART II - HISTORY FOR KNOWN AND ESTABLISHED HIGH RISK FACTORS FOR STROKE

1. Have you ever been told that you have high blood pressure?... ―― Yes ―― No
2. Do you take medication for high blood pressure?... ―― Yes ―― No
3. Do you have a history of abnormal heart rate or rhythm called atrial fibrillation?...................... ―― ―― No
4. Have you ever been checked for or been told that you have narrowing of the arteries to the brain?... ―― Yes ―― No
5. Have you had a heart attack, heart by-pass surgery, angioplasty, or another disease of the heart?.... ―― Yes ―― No
6. Have you had a previous stroke, mini-stroke, or TIA?.. ―― Yes ―― No
7. Do you have diabetes mellitus (DM), or are you on insulin or medication for high blood sugar?......... ―― Yes ―― No
8. Have you ever smoked cigarettes?.. ―― Yes ―― No
9. Do you currently smoke cigarettes?.. ―― Yes ―― No

PART III - HISTORY FOR SIGNIFICANT BUT SLIGHTLY LOWER RISK FACTORS FOR STROKE

10. Has a family member had a stroke or heart attack when they were less than 45 years of age? .... ―― Yes ―― No
11. Do you consume more than two ounces of alcohol per day on a daily basis? .... ―― Yes ―― No
12. Do you have a cholesterol level greater than 200? .... ―― Yes ―― No

PART IV - HISTORY OF OTHER/UNCOMMON IMPORTANT RISK FACTORS FOR STROKE

13. Do you smoke cigarettes and take birth control pills? .... ―― Yes ―― No
14. Do you have sickle cell anemia? .... ―― Yes ―― No
15. Do you use one or more of the following drugs: cocaine, crack, heroin, amphetamines? .... ―― Yes ―― No
16. Are you overweight or obese? .... ―― Yes ―― No
17. Do you consider your activity level as generally inactive? .... ―― Yes ―― No

PART V - BLOOD PRESSURE AND PULSE

Blood pressure (BP) recorded sitting _____ (Systolic) _____ (Diastolic) _____ Right Arm _____ Left Arm
Radial pulse rate for 60 seconds (beats/minute) _____ Irregular pulse rate? _____ Yes _____ No

PART VI - IDENTIFICATION OF RISK FOR STROKE AND RECOMMENDATION

1. __ **Low Risk for Stroke:**
   Under the age of 55, responded "**No**" to questions 1-17 (self-reported risk factors), and was not identified to have an irregular pulse rate, or a measured systolic BP equal to or greater than 140 or diastolic equal to or greater than 90.
   RECOMMENDATION: Take this completed screening form to your health care provider at your next appointment.

2. __ **Moderate Risk for Stroke:**
   Age equal to or greater than 55 with no self-reported risk factors and no risk factors identified on screening **OR** - Age up to 64 with one self-reported risk factor, or an irregular pulse rate or a measured systolic BP equal to or greater than 140 or a diastolic equal to or greater than 90.
   RECOMMENDATION: Notify your health care provider within a week with the results of your screening and request an appointment for an evaluation and care to prevent a stroke.

3. __ **High Risk for Stroke:**
   Age equal to or greater than 65 with one self-reported risk factor, or an irregular pulse, or a measured systolic BP equal to or greater than 140 or a diastolic BP equal to or greater than 90.
   OR - Any age with **two or more risk factors,** either self-reported and/or identified on measurement of an irregular pulse or systolic BP equal to or greater than 140 or a diastolic equal to or greater than 90.
   RECOMMENDATION: Notify your health care provider TODAY with the results of your screening and request an appointment for evaluation of your risks for stroke and care to prevent a stroke.

4. __ **PRESENTS WITH WARNING SIGNS OF STROKE, OR TIA (MINI-STROKE)**
   RECOMMENDATION: CALL OR HAVE SOMEONE CALL 911 IMMEDIATELY!

PART VII - THE EARLY WARNING SIGNS OF STROKE
* Sudden weakness, numbness, or paralysis of the face, arm or leg on one or both sides of the body

* Sudden blurred vision or blindness in one or both eyes

* Sudden difficulty speaking, slurring of speech or difficulty understanding

* Sudden severe headache with sudden onset that occurs without apparent reason

* Sudden loss of balance, dizziness, or falling without any apparent reason

Call 911 immediately if you experience any of these symptoms.

I have received a screening for the risk of stroke and agree to follow up with the recommendations. I understand this is only a screening. I agree that this data can be entered into a database for research without identifying me by name.
(Signature of Participant) _____ **Signature of Health Care Provider** _____

The **Stroke Risk Screening** was developed in 1999 jointly by the Division on Research Delaware Nurses Association and Ellen Barker, MSN, RN, CNRN, Neuroscience Nursing Consultants, Wilmington, Delaware. Marian P. LaMonte, M.D., M.S.N., Assistant Professor of Neurology and Co-Director of the Maryland Brain Attack Center, University of Maryland Medical Center, Baltimore, Maryland, served as Nurse/Neurologist advisor. There is no Copyright and permission is not needed to duplicate this form. For more information, visit Ms. Barker's website at http://neuronurse.com.

20 THE PATIENT WITH AIDS

Robyn Rice and David J. Ritchie

The term acquired immunodeficiency syndrome (AIDS), a disorder of the immune system, is used to describe only the most severe diseases (e.g., opportunistic infections, neoplasms, wasting, encephalopathy) associated with infection by the human immunodeficiency virus (HIV).[15,17] Two strains of HIV (HIV-1 and HIV-2) cause AIDS, and at least 10 families of HIV-1 exist around the world.[12]

AIDS was initially reported in the United States with an outbreak of 25 cases in 1981.[5] Symptomatology was related to an ineffective immune system. We now know that AIDS predisposes individuals to various intermittent and debilitating diseases. These so-called opportunistic infections are rarely seen in people with intact immune systems. For example, *Pneumocystis carinii* pneumonia (PCP) and Kaposi's sarcoma, hallmark diseases of AIDS, normally do not occur in young and middle-age adults.

At present, a person who is HIV positive and has a CD4$^+$ T cell count of less than 200 mm^3 is considered to have AIDS. In addition, the current Centers for Disease Control and Prevention (CDC) surveillance case definition of AIDS in the United States cites a number of clinical indicator diseases associated with AIDS[6,45] (Box 20-1). Using the CDC case definition for medical management, the lowest, but not necessarily the most recent, documented CD4$^+$ T cell count is used for classification purposes.

HIV infection and AIDS are not synonymous terms; primary HIV infection is followed by AIDS. In addition, HIV infection does not usually imply an immediate diagnosis of AIDS. There seems to be some time lag between initial infection and the full-blown manifestation of AIDS.[15] In a study of HIV infected persons, Pantaleo and others[34] reported that clinical signs and symptoms of AIDS developed after a median time period of 10 years. Although scientists continue to discover new information about AIDS, at present there is no known cure. The course of the disease has a very wasting effect on the body. Acute infection and comorbidities eventually result in the patient's death.[14,18]

The social ramifications of AIDS have been tremendous because AIDS appears to be primarily a sexually transmitted disease.[11] In the United States the homosexual and bisexual population have experienced the majority of reported cases.[11] However, the disease has now moved into the heterosexual population in the United States in increasing numbers.[11]

Sexual taboos, social prejudices regarding how the virus is contracted, and fears of getting the disease have made case reporting and public education very difficult. In many instances an almost universal hysteria and phobia have occurred in communities confronted with issues of caring for and living with persons with AIDS (PWAs). For example, it has been very difficult for parents to get children with AIDS enrolled in school and to keep them there.[29] Although community alliances have improved since the 1980s, historically the homosexual population has had problems getting the public involvement and social networking needed to respond to this epidemic.

An epidemic it is, for surveillance studies indicate that as of 1999 approximately 1 million persons in the United States are infected with HIV-1.[12] CDC statistics indicate that there are approximately

---

Box 20-1   1993 CDC SURVEILLANCE CASE DEFINITION OF AIDS

CD4$^+$ T Cell Categories

Category I: Greater than or equal to 500 cells g/ml
Category II: 200 to 499 cells g/ml
Category III: Less than 200 cells g/ml

Clinical Categories

Category A

Asymptomatic HIV infection (HIV positive with no
 evidence of illness)
Persistent generalized lymphadenopathy (chronically
 swollen glands)
Acute (primary) HIV infection with accompanying
 illness or history of acute HIV infections (HIV
 positive with flulike illness)

Category B

Conditions with symptoms not included in the category C list but that occur in any HIV positive person
and are attributed to HIV infection. Examples of category B illnesses include thrush, early (noninvasive)
cervical cancer, fever, or chronic diarrhea.

Category C

HIV positive persons who have or who have had any
of the following: candidiasis of bronchi, trachea, or

lungs; candidiasis, esophageal; cervical cancer, invasive ('93 revision); coccidioidomycosis, disseminated
or extrapulmonary; cryptococcosis, extrapulmonary;
cryptosporidiosis, chronic intestinal (>1 month duration); cytomegalovirus disease (other than liver, spleen,
or nodes); encephalopathy, HIV related; herpes
simplex: chronic ulcers (>1 month duration), or bronchitis pneumonitis, or esophagitis; histoplasmosis, disseminated or extrapulmonary; isosporiasis, chronic intestinal (>1 month duration); Kaposi's sarcoma;
lymphoma, Burkitt's (or equivalent term); lymphoma,
immunoblastic (or equivalent term); lymphoma,
primary of brain; *Mycobacterium avium* complex, or
M. kansasii, disseminated or extrapulmonary; *Mycobacterium tuberculosis,* pulmonary ('93 revision);
Mycobacterium, other species, any site; *Pneumocystis
carinii* pneumonia; pneumonia, recurrent ('93 revision); progressive multifocal leukoencephalopathy;
Salmonella septicemia, recurrent; toxoplasmosis of
brain; wasting syndrome due to HIV.
  NOTE: The CDC states that HIV-infected persons
should be classified using the lowest accurate, but not
necessarily the most recent, CD4$^+$ count.

Source Centers for Disease Control and Prevention: 1993 Revised classification system for HIV infection and expanded surveillance
case definition for AIDS among adolescents and adults, *MMWR Morb Mortal Wkly Rep* 41 (RR-17):1, 1992.

297,137 persons currently living with AIDS in the
United States.[11,12] Of significance, a substantial
decline of AIDS incidence has continued since first
reported in 1996.[11] This provides evidence of the
widespread beneficial effects of new treatment regimens. Such a decline also highlights the importance of HIV prevention strategies such as promoting knowledge of HIV risk behaviors and ways to
reduce the risk of infection, as well as improvement
in access to care and medical treatment regimens.

   More PWAs will likely be seen in home care
over the next decade because this is probably the
most cost-effective and patient preferred way to
manage a disease that has become more chronic in
nature as related to the impact of new drug therapies on overall patient survival time.

   Typically, PWAs contract infections and recover, only to contract further infections. Therefore most PWAs go about their normal work rou-

tines, receiving only periodic medical attention.
Advanced symptomatology of AIDS requires a
great deal of nursing and personal care that can be
done at home.

   The purpose of this chapter is to give a general
overview of HIV infection and AIDS in order to
assist home care nurses to prepare a plan of care for
adult patients.

PATHOPHYSIOLOGY

T-cell lymphocytes (white blood cells) are responsible for cell-mediated immunity, which involves
graft rejections, antigen-specific responses to intracellular parasites, and the stimulation of B-cells to
make antibodies.[17,23] HIV invades the bloodstream
and preferentially infects T cells. After penetrating
the T cell, HIV uses the enzyme reverse transcrip-
tase to copy its own genetic structure into the
genome of the infected cell.

The mechanism for activation of the immune system with subsequent viral replication of HIV is still under investigation. Although the infected T cell appears to remain dormant, an active battle for control of the host is ongoing. It is known that when stimulated by antigens (e.g., by a common cold), the infected CD4[+] T cell (CD4[+] is the receptor for HIV on the T-cell lymphocyte) can reproduce the virus instead of itself.[14,15,23] The new HIV "buds" out and essentially lyses the infected CD4[+] T cell, spilling into the bloodstream only to infect other CD4[+] T cells. At first, HIV interferes with the function of the CD4[+] T cell. Eventually, CD4[+] T cells die or do not reproduce themselves, whereas B-cell function (humoral immunity) remains intact and is often hyperactive.[18]

Of note, some HIV strains may be more cytotoxic, destroying CD4[+] T cells more rapidly than other strains. Also, evidence suggests that an infected individual usually becomes infected with just one strain of HIV, but soon after infection the virus mutates progressively into many different quasispecies.[14] Once an individual has become infected, superinfection with a strain from another individual does not seem to occur.[14]

Rates of HIV replication may be enhanced by factors such as viral burden, age, gender, coexisting infections, congenital defects, stress, and recreational drug and alcohol use.[15,23] In addition, HIV replication may be minimal if CD4[+] T cells are not stimulated to reproduce.[18]

The role of HIV in the pathogenesis of AIDS remains a subject for discussion. Current thinking suggests that the presence of HIV along with the existence of other infectious agents may be a major factor driving the pathophysiological manifestations of AIDS.[22,30,46]

The pathophysiology of AIDS is of a progressively destructive nature. Serologically, monocyte-macrophage dysfunction, hypergammaglobulinemia, leukopenia, thrombocytopenia, and anemia can occur. Involvement of alveolar macrophages corresponds to the high incidence of pulmonary infections experienced by PWAs.[31] In addition, the virus enters the central nervous system (CNS) via infected macrophages that cross the blood-brain barrier and cause further damage.[25] As a result the loss of functional CD4[+] T cells and the infection of macrophages and monocytes appear to correlate with the clinical course of AIDS.[15,17,23] Death usually results from opportunistic infections or tumors such as *Mycobacterium tuberculosis, Pneumocystis carinii* pneumonia, Kaposi's sarcoma, or lymphomas. Others are noted to die from a progressively disabling neurologic syndrome involving dementia (AIDS dementia complex) or from a progressively disabling wasting syndrome without apparent development of any secondary infections or tumors.[14,45]

HIV PRESENTATION AND CLINICAL COURSE OF AIDS

The typical course of HIV infection involves (1) initial infection with HIV virus associated with flulike symptoms, followed by (2) a period of clinical latency (median, 10 years) during which the individual is usually symptom free, followed by (3) physical manifestations of disease, (4) the development of AIDS-indicator disease(s), and (5) eventual death.[31,34]

Primary infection, also referred to as acute retroviral syndrome, usually develops within 3 to 6 weeks after exposure.[14] Acute retroviral syndrome can produce clinically symptomatic illnesses such as night sweats, the flu, or mononucleosis. At this point the HIV-infected individual may look and feel essentially well. The significance here is that it is during this time period that the individual is at highest risk for transmitting the infection to others.

Although an HIV-infected individual can die from an initial opportunistic infection, it is much more common for a person to suffer episodes of severe illness interspersed with periods of relative wellness. HIV destroys the lymph node architecture and depletes the CD4[+] T-cell population.[14] Eventually, recurring infections and related symptoms of AIDS exhaust the body's reserves and ability to respond to therapy, and death results. It should be noted that, as related to individual HIV virulence and other factors, some individuals may rapidly progress to full-blown AIDS and die quickly.

MECHANISM OF TRANSMISSION

HIV has been isolated from blood, semen, vaginal secretions, saliva, tears, breast milk, cerebrospinal fluid, amniotic fluid, alveolar fluid, urine, and feces.[8,9,11] Blood, semen, vaginal secretions, and breast milk have been implicated in transmission of HIV.[8,9,11] At present, transmission of HIV is believed to occur in three ways[7,8,11]:

1. Through sexual contact
2. Through exposure to infected blood or body fluids
3. From HIV-infected women to their fetus or infant

EPIDEMIOLOGY

Although AIDS has been reported in every state, rates are highest in the more heavily populated states. The AIDS population primarily resides in metropolitan areas, but the epidemic continues to reach smaller communities.

Homosexuals and bisexuals

In the United States, homosexual and bisexual males constitute the largest group of the AIDS population and are at highest risk for HIV infection.[11] This is thought to be related to sexual practices and exposure to large numbers of sexual partners. Anal intercourse and practices such as "fisting" (inserting the hand into the anus) cause repeated tearing of mucous membranes and bleeding. Therefore the "receptive partner" is probably at highest risk for HIV infection, although an open sore or lesion on the penis also provides a route of entry for the virus. The risk of oral exposure to HIV-containing semen is unknown and difficult to evaluate, because most homosexuals practice both oral and anal sex.[16]

Common infections that initially occur in HIV-infected homosexuals and bisexuals include genital and perianal warts, along with a variety of sexually transmitted diseases. Bowel disease is common in this group.

Intravenous drug users and sex workers

Cases of HIV-infected intravenous drug users (IDUs) have been reported in increasing numbers since the late 1980s.[7,11] The mechanism of transmission of HIV in IDUs involves sharing used or "dirty" needles.[38] Practices such as "booting," whereby blood is drawn back into the syringe to extract any remaining drug, allow small amounts of HIV-infected blood to be left in the needle. This blood becomes a source of contamination for further infection. The problem of sharing dirty needles and syringes or "works" is magnified by the existence of "shooting galleries," where IDUs meet to share drugs and works.[16]

Offering commercial sex is another primary mechanism of HIV for IDUs. Considering the pres-

ence of HIV within the U.S. population, sex without protection may be lethal.[39]

Typical infections reported in HIV-infected IDUs included pneumonia, endocarditis with sepsis, tuberculosis, and coinfections with other viruses.[15] Renal disease in HIV-infected IDUs is common.[28] Sexually transmitted diseases among sex workers, especially syphilis, are also common.[39]

Polysubstance abuse among HIV-infected IDUs is common and may complicate treatment. For example, mental illnesses and lifestyles associated with drug use include antisocial personality disorders, depression, isolation, and anxiety.[40]

Women, adolescents, and children

Since the 1990s increasing numbers of women and adolescents are being reported with HIV. Again, this likely reflects modes of transmission into the heterosexual population via intravenous drug use and unprotected sex.

The majority of children with HIV infection are born to African-American and Latino women.[11] Transmission appears to occur in utero or during labor and delivery when the infant is exposed to HIV-infected blood or other infected body fluids. Although rare, transmission through breast-feeding has been reported.[47] From 1996 to date, the number of children (under 13 years of age) who were diagnosed with AIDS has significantly declined, principally reflecting the continued success of efforts to reduce perinatal transmission through promoting voluntary HIV testing and zidovudine therapy for pregnant HIV-infected women and their infants.[11,12]

African-Americans

In the United States, the impact of HIV and AIDS in the African-American community has been devastating. To date, African-Americans make up almost 37% of all AIDS cases reported in the United States.[11,12] Researchers estimate that 240,000 to 325,000 African-Americans—about 1 in 50 African-American men and 1 in 160 African-American women—are infected with HIV.[11,12] Substance abuse is fueling the sexual spread of HIV in the United States, especially in minority communities with high rates of sexually transmitted diseases.[11]

Hemophiliacs

In 1982 the first cases of AIDS among hemophiliacs were reported.[7,12] The mechanism of transmission was exposure to commercially produced factor VIII concentrate. Since March of 1985, mass screening of donated blood and plasma has almost eliminated this route of transmission.[12]

OCCUPATIONAL AND CASUAL TRANSMISSION

The primary route of HIV exposure for health care workers has been by accidental needlesticks.[11] The risk for occupational exposure to HIV is low and estimated to be less than 0.1% for a single mucous membrane exposure (95% confidence interval = 0.006 to 0.05).[21] As of 1999, health care workers represent 5.1% of the total known AIDS population reported to the CDC.[11,12] Nursing ranks highest in the category of jobs at risk for exposure to HIV.[11,12]

Isolated case studies have documented other mechanisms of exposure and subsequent HIV infection of home care workers. For example, one woman who provided home care to a neighbor with AIDS subsequently contracted AIDS.[18] This woman had no known risk factors. The care she provided involved frequent and prolonged contact with the patient's secretions and excretions. The woman did not use gloves and recalled numerous small cuts on her hands and an exacerbation of chronic eczema.

In studies of family members of PWAs, approximately eight cases of casual transmission in the home have been reported since the 1980s.[8,12] Activities examined in these reports included kissing, embracing, and sharing common household items (dishes, linens, and toilet facilities) with the HIV-infected family member. HIV infection apparently occurred following mucocutaneous exposures to blood or other body substances in persons who received care from or provided care to HIV-infected family members residing in the same household.[8,12]

SCREENING

Laboratory tests to detect HIV infection identify serological response to the virus.[17] After initial infection, antibodies usually appear within 3 to 6 weeks. Detection of HIV antibodies indicates that the individual has been exposed to HIV, initiated an immune response, and is infectious.[15,23]

Initial screening for HIV antibodies is done by the enzyme-linked immunosorbent assay (ELISA). Positive results are confirmed by the Western blot test to establish that the antibody in question is HIV specific.

HOME CARE APPLICATION

The goals of home care for PWAs should be directed toward the following:

- Treating disease and ongoing symptoms
- Preventing exacerbations of disease (restoration and maintenance)
- Instructing patients and families regarding self-care management of health care needs at home
- Anticipating and planning for any assistance the patient may require in performing activities of daily living (ADLs)
- Providing for the psychosocial and spiritual needs of the patient and family or caregiver

Developing the plan of care

Initial interview. During the first visit, home care nurses should develop a plan of care based on patient and family needs. An ongoing nutritional and physical assessment and an in-depth interview will provide clues to the appropriate interventions for PWAs (see Chapter 5 for assessment parameters).

When first interviewing the patient and family, ask them what their biggest concerns are and how the home care agency can be of help. Obtaining answers to the questions in Box 20-2 will help in mutually determining the plan of care (see also Box 20-3).

Patient education. Health teaching for patients and their designated caregivers is very important (Box 20-4). Patient education strategies should focus on fostering the patient self-care management and best level of functioning. Disease process, infection control, diet, equipment, medications, procedural care, bowel/bladder management, and tips for home maintenance should be a part of health teaching. Instruct the patient/caregiver to immediately call the physician for severe changes in mental status, temperature, pulse, and respirations or with sudden onset of bleeding, diarrhea, vomiting, pain, seizures, or loss of vision or sensation in a body part.

This patient group can be quite challenging to teach. This may be due to problems with dementia that affect memory and to behavioral problems resulting from possible substance abuse or unusual lifestyle issues. Any difficulties with noncompliance or nonparticipation with the plan of care must

<table>
<tr><td>

Box 20-2   INTERVIEWING PERSONS WITH AIDS AND THEIR FAMILIES FOR ASSESSMENT OF INITIAL NEEDS

What are your living arrangements?

Does your significant other or family know that you have AIDS? (It is not uncommon for patients to request that their mother not be told they have AIDS.)

Are there family members or a lover or a significant other who can assist you with care as needed?

Who cooks and prepares the meals? Would a referral to a registered dietitian be helpful?

What are your finances like in terms of getting needed medical supplies? Would a referral to social services be helpful?

Do you have transportation to the grocery store or physician, and is there someone who can assist with travel as needed?

Do you need help with activities such as grooming, cooking, laundry, and general housekeeping? Would a referral to the home care aide or personal chore worker be helpful?

What do you and your family know about AIDS? Do you have any questions about AIDS or transmission of HIV? How do you think you became infected with HIV? Are you on any medications? Do you know what your CD4$^+$ count is?

What do you know about infection control precautions? For example, how would you or your family care for an accidental cut on your arm or clean up a blood spill?

Are you sexually active? If so, what means are being used to protect your partner?

Are you actively using drugs? Alcohol? (Alcohol and drug abuse can cause serious complications with prescribed therapy and treatment.)

What are your wishes with respect to advance directives? Do you have a living will, durable power of attorney for health care, or health care proxy?

</td></tr>
</table>

Box 20-3   PRIMARY NURSING DIAGNOSES/PATIENT PROBLEMS

- Fatigue
- Pain
- Knowledge deficit; home management of AIDS
- Risk for altered body temperature
- Altered nutrition; less than body requirements
- Impaired memory
- Ineffective family coping
- Risk of impaired skin integrity
- Altered oral mucosa
- Incontinence; functional
- Altered sexuality pattern
- Diarrhea; risk for fluid volume deficit

Box 20-4   PRIMARY THEMES OF PATIENT EDUCATION

- Disease process; when to call the case manager and physician
- Medications
- Procedural care
- Diet
- Infection control
- Home management of AIDS (e.g., infection control, AIDS symptomatology, women's health, procedural care, home safety issues)
- Positive coping skills
- Energy conservation techniques
- Diet
- General self-care strategies

be addressed if treatment is to be effective and safe. (See Chapter 6, which provides guidelines for working with patients who do not participate with the plan of care.)

Chemical dependence and substance abuse. As stated previously, HIV infection is strongly correlated with intravenous drug use, and home care nurses may encounter patients who are experiencing chemical dependance. If possible, refer these patients to a drug treatment program as needed. If working with chemically dependant patients, consider the following suggestions for care:

- Do not bargain.
- Actively address each and every harmful behavior that is observed.
- Speak truthfully and do not preach.

Be aware that active drug usage in the home or abusive or violent patient behaviors should warrant termination of home care services as related to staff safety issues. (See Chapter 8: Legal and Ethical Issues, which discusses the home care nurse's rights.)

Medications. During the initial interview, review all medications with the patient, including purpose, action, dosage, side effects, and methods of administration. Although experimental studies are ongoing, at present no cure for AIDS exists. Antiretroviral therapy, vaccines, and immune therapy are principal areas of drug research.[10,24,26] See Table 20-1 for medications currently being used to treat HIV and associated infections in the home; be aware of the side effects that should immediately be reported to the physician. The goals of drug therapy for PWAs include[32]:

- Decrease HIV RNA levels to less than 5000 copies.
- Maintain or raise $CD4^+$ T cell counts to greater than 500 cells.
- Delay the development of HIV-related symptoms and opportunistic infections.

Infection control. During the first visit, assess the patient and family's knowledge of infection control and the management of AIDS. PWAs may excrete many other infectious agents (e.g., cytomegalovirus) aside from HIV. Infection control precautions and good personal hygiene should be reinforced on each visit. Therefore instruct patients and family members in standard precautions for blood and body fluids as discussed in Chapter 6. *Most important, emphasize that gloves must be worn whenever there is the possibility of contact with the patient's blood, vomitus, urine, feces, or other body substances (e.g., draining wounds).*

Instruct PWAs to avoid cleaning the cat box or bird cage (potential source of infections) unless gloves and a mask are worn. They should not clean the fish tank because it may contain mycobacteria, which can cause acute respiratory disease.[16] Keep pets indoors exclusively so they do not pick up any infections to subsequently transmit. Also, keep pets out of the patient's bed.

When discussing infection control, try to reassure the patient and the family that household transmission of HIV—although possible—is rare. It is important for all household members to follow infection control precautions. However, also make the point that the virus does not just jump off one person and onto another. Reinforce the idea that the

patient is at greatest risk for infection because AIDS destroys the immune system. Therefore PWAs should avoid situations that would expose them to colds or flus. Family members with a cold or flu should wear a mask when providing care. Sick or ill friends should not visit. Pregnant women should avoid caring for relatives with AIDS because of the many possible infections that PWS may have.

Home care nurses should be aware that the most important protective measure against HIV is safe and immediate disposal of needles or sharp objects. Masks should be worn if the patient is coinfected with a contagious respiratory pathogen.

Be aware that there is a significant relationship between HIV infection and tuberculosis (TB).[9,33] In fact, TB is the leading cause of death among PWAs. Therefore all PWAs should be tested for TB and, if infected, should immediately begin therapy to prevent TB disease.[9,12,33]

Physical assessment and nursing care

AIDS is a disease that affects multiple body systems. In treating existing problems and preventing exacerbation of AIDS, it is important for home care nurses to continuously use holistic assessment skills as a basis for practice. Nursing care should focus on symptom control and an understanding of any preexisting health problems, behaviors, or activities that might influence treatment. For example, gay male patients who consume large quantities of alcohol place themselves at risk for developing pancreatitis if they are taking didanosine.[16]

General appearance. Patients typically experience premature aging and graying of hair.[25] Hair loss is common. Loss of facial fat, along with profound weight loss, can give these patients a gaunt appearance. Skin and mucosal membranes are typically pale in color. Problems with fatigue, fever, weight loss, and nausea are common.

Fatigue. A common complaint of most PWAs is fatigue. Low-flow oxygen therapy and frequent rest periods may be helpful. Promote adequate sleep. Keep needed items at the bedside (e.g., iced water, urinal, and a towel to absorb perspiration). Plan and prioritize activities throughout the patient's day. For example, suggest resting after breakfast and before bathing. (See Chapter 11 for energy conservation tips in the home.) Consider a referral to rehabilitation and home care aide services.

Table 20-1 Medications currently used in the treatment of HIV infection and AIDS

Medication	Dose/route	Adverse effects	Major use(s)
Nucleoside reverse transcriptase inhibitors (NRTIs)			
Zidovudine (ZDV)	200 mg PO q8h or 300 mg PO q12	Anemia, leukopenia, myopathy, hepatotoxicity, headache	A component of highly active antiretroviral therapy (HAART)
Didanosine (ddI)	125-200 mg PO bid	Pancreatitis, peripheral neuropathy, insomnia	A component of HAART
Zalcitabine (ddC)	0.75 mg PO tid	Peripheral neuropathy, pancreatitis, oral ulcers	A component of HAART
Stavudine (d4T)	30-40 mg PO bid	Peripheral neuropathy, anemia, hepatotoxicity	A component of HAART
Lamivudine (3-TC)	150 mg PO bid	Peripheral neuropathy, headache, gastrointestinal (GI) disturbances	A component of HAART
ZDV/3-TC (Combivir)	1 (ZDV 300 mg/3-TC 150 mg) PO bid	Anemia, leukopenia, myopathy, hepatotoxicity, headache, peripheral neuropathy, GI disturbances	Combination product for HAART therapy
Abacavir	300 mg PO bid	Hypersensitivity reactions, malaise	A component of HAART
Adefovir	120 mg PO qd × 1 month, then 60 mg PO qd with L-carnitine 500 mg PO qd	Nephrotoxicity, Fanconi's syndrome, decreased serum L-carnitine	A component of HAART (investigational)
Non-nucleoside reverse transcriptase inhibitors (NNRTIs)			
Nevirapine	200 mg PO qd × 14 days, then 200 mg PO bid	Rash, headache, depression	A component of HAART, often as a protease inhibitor substitute
Delavirdine	400 mg PO q8h	Rash, headache, GI disturbances	A component of HAART, often as a protease inhibitor substitute
Efavirenz	600 mg qd	Central nervous system (CNS) disturbances, rash	A component of HAART, often as a protease inhibitor substitute

Continued

Table 20-1 Medications currently used in the treatment of HIV infection and AIDS—cont'd

Medication	Dose/route	Adverse effects	Major use(s)
Protease inhibitors (PIs)			
Saquinavir	1200 mg PO q8h (soft-gel); 600 mg PO q8h (hard-gel)	GI disturbances, lipodystrophy, hypertriglyceridemia, glucose intolerance	A component of HAART
Ritonavir	300 mg PO q12h (day 1), 400 mg PO q12h (days 2 & 3), 500 mg PO q12h day 4, then 600 mg PO q12h thereafter	Paresthesias, GI disturbances, taste perversion, lipodystrophy, hypertriglyceridemia, glucose intolerance	A component of HAART
Indinavir	800 mg PO q8h	Nephrolithiasis, hyperbilirubinemia, lipodystrophy, hypertriglyceridemia, glucose intolerance	A component of HAART
Nelfinavir	750 mg PO q8h or 1250 mg PO q12h	Diarrhea, lipodystrophy, hypertriglyceridemia, glucose intolerance	A component of HAART
Amprenavir	capsules: 1200 mg PO q12h; oral solution: 22.5 mg/kg bid or 17 mg/kg tid (maximum daily dose = 2800 mg)	GI disturbances, rash	A component of HAART
Miscellaneous anti-HIV therapy			
Hydroxyurea	500 mg PO bid	Hematologic disturbances, ulcerated extremities	Adjunctive agent to potentiate didanosine activity
Antifungals			
Amphotericin B (AmB)	0.25-1.5 mg/kg/day IV	Nephrotoxicity, hypokalemia, hypomagnesemia, anemia, fever, chills	Cryptococcosis, candidiasis, histoplasmosis, blastomycosis, coccidiodomycosis
Amphotericin B lipid complex (ABLC)	5 mg/kg IV qd	Nephrotoxicity, hypokalemia, hypomagnesemia, anemia, fever, chills	Alternative therapy in patients intolerant of AmB
Amphotericin B colloidal dispersion (ABCD)	3-4 mg/kg IV qd	Nephrotoxicity, hypoxia, hypokalemia, hypomagnesemia, anemia, fever, chills	Alternative therapy in patients intolerant of AmB

Table 20-1 Medications currently used in the treatment of HIV infection and AIDS—cont'd

Medication	Dose/route	Adverse effects	Major use(s)
Antifungals—cont'd			
Liposomal amphotericin B	3-5 mg/kg IV qd	Nephrotoxicity, hypokalemia, hypomagnesemia, anemia, fever, chills	Alternative therapy in patients intolerant of AmB
Fluconazole	100-800 mg/day IV or PO	GI disturbances, hepatotoxicity	Candidiasis, cryptococcal meningitis
Itraconazole	200-400 mg PO or IV qd	GI disturbances, hepatotoxicity, hypokalemia	Histoplasmosis, aspergillosis, blastomycosis
Ketoconazole	200-400 mg PO qd	GI disturbances, hepatotoxicity, adrenal insufficiency	Candidiasis
Clotrimazole	10 mg troche dissolved in mouth 5 times/day	Mild local burning or irritation	Oral candidiasis
Nystatin	400,000-600,000 units PO suspension swish and swallow qid	GI disturbances	Oral candidiasis
Amphotericin B suspension	100 mg PO suspension swish and swallow qid	GI disturbances, rash	Refractory oral candidiasis
Flucytosine (5-FC)	25-37.5 mg/kg q6h (target serum level range 25-100 mcg/mL)	Leukopenia, anemia, thrombocytopenia, GI disturbances	Cryptococcal meningitis (with AmB)
Antivirals			
Ganciclovir	5 mg/kg IV q12h (treatment)-24h (maintenance) or 300 mg PO bid (prevention)	Leukopenia, anemia, thrombocytopenia	Cytomegalovirus (CMV) treatment and prevention
Foscarnet	60 mg/kg IV q8 (treatment); 90-120 mg/kg IV qd (maintenance)	Nephrotoxicity, electrolytes disturbances, seizures, phlebitis	CMV treatment
Acyclovir	200-800 mg PO 3-5 times/day or 5-10 mg/kg IV q8h (severe disease)	Nephrotoxicity, seizures	Herpes simplex virus (HSV), varicella zoster virus (VZV)
Valacyclovir	1000 mg PO q8h (VZV treatment); 1000 mg PO q12h (HSV treatment); 500 mg PO q12h (HSV recurrences)	Headache, nephrotoxicity, CNS disturbances	HSV, VZV
Famciclovir	500 mg PO q8h (VZV treatment); 125-500 mg PO q12h (HSV recurrences)	Headache, nausea	HSV, VZV

Continued

Table 20-1 Medications currently used in the treatment of HIV infection and AIDS—cont'd

Medication	Dose/route	Adverse effects	Major use(s)
Antivirals—cont'd			
Cidofovir	5 mg/kg IV q week × 2 weeks, then 5 mg/kg IV q 2 weeks	Nephrotoxicity	CMV treatment
Ganciclovir insert	insert q several months	Retinal detachment, visual acuity disturbances	CMV retinitis treatment
Fomivirsen	330 mcg intravitreally q 2 weeks × 2 doses, then q 4 weeks	Uveitis, retinal detachment, visual disturbances	CMV retinitis treatment
Antiprotozoals			
Trimethoprim-sulfamethoxazole (TMP-SMX)	15 mg/kg/day IV or PO (based on TMP); 1 DS tablet PO 3-7 days/week (PCP prophylaxis)	Anemia, leukopenia, thrombocytopenia, rash, nephropathy	*Pneumocystis carinii* pneumonia (PCP) treatment and prevention
Pentamidine	3 mg/kg/day IV (treatment); 300 mg inhaled q month (prophylaxis)	Nephrotoxicity, hypotension, arrhythmias, hypoglycemia or hyperglycemia, hypocalcemia	PCP treatment and prevention
Dapsone	100 mg PO qd (treatment); 100 mg PO qd (prophylaxis)	Hemolytic anemia, rash	PCP prevention and as a component of treatment with trimethoprim
Atovaquone	750 mg PO bid (treatment); 1500 mg PO qd (prophylaxis)	GI disturbances	PCP treatment and prevention
Trimetrexate	45 mg/m^2 IV qd × 21 days (plus leucovorin 20-40 mg/m^2 qd × 24 days	Neutropenia, anemia, thrombocytopenia, hepatotoxicity, fever	PCP salvage treatment
Pyrimethamine	50-100 mg PO qd (treatment); 25-50 mg PO qd (suppressive therapy); 50 mg PO q week (prophylaxis)	Anemia, leukopenia, thrombocytopenia	Toxoplasmosis treatment or PCP prophylaxis
Sulfadiazine	1-1.5 grams PO q6h (plus pyrimethamine and leucovorin)	Anemia, leukopenia, thrombocytopenia, rash, nephropathy	Toxoplasmosis
Paromomycin	500 mg PO qid	GI disturbances	Cryptosporidiosis
Antibacterials			
Clarithromycin	500 mg PO bid	GI and taste disturbances	*Mycobacterium avium* complex (MAC) treatment and prevention

Table 20-1 Medications currently used in the treatment of HIV infection and AIDS—cont'd

Medication	Dose/route	Adverse effects	Major use(s)
Antibacterials—cont'd			
Azithromycin	500 mg PO qd (treatment) or 1200 mg PO q week (prevention)	GI disturbances	MAC treatment and prevention
Rifabutin	300 mg PO qd	Uveitis, neutropenia, body fluid discoloration, GI disturbances	MAC prevention
Growth factors			
Filgrastim (G-CSF)	5-10 mcg/kg subcutaneously or IV qd	Bone pain, fever	For ZDV- or ganciclovir-induced neutropenia
Sargramostin (GM-CSF)	250 mcg/m^2 IV or subcutaneously qd	Bone pain, fever	For ZDV- or ganciclovir-induced neutropenia
Erythropoietin (EPO)	100 units/kg subcutaneously 3 times/week	Hypertension, headache, arthralgia, diarrhea	For ZDV-associated anemia

Risk for altered body temperature. Instruct patients to take their temperature the same time each morning. Research suggests that 99.9° F should be the upper limit of the normal body temperature in healthy adults 40 years of age or younger.[19,27] Apply a sheet or loosely woven blanket to the patient's trunk to promote heat loss. If no skin lesions are present and the patient is ambulatory, immerse the patient in a tub bath with a water temperature at 102.2° F.[19] Avoid tepid sponge baths and alcohol sponging; these cause shivering. Use cooling blankets and ice packs when core temperature is rising uncontrollably to prevent seizures. Instruct the caregiver to call an ambulance if the feverish patient has a convulsion, becomes delirious, or is combative because the patient will require immediate medical attention.

For chronic recurrent night sweats, instruct the patient to take a prescribed antipyretic before going to bed. Keep an extra set of pajamas and bed sheets on hand at night for profuse diaphoresis. Keep a plastic cover on the pillow.

Be aware that the patient is also at risk for dehydration. Increase caloric and fluid intake as needed. See the gastrointestinal section later in this chapter.

Altered nutrition; less than body requirements. Weight loss and many nutrient deficiencies seen in PWAs are a result of the disease. The "wasting" effect of AIDS is related to diarrhea, malabsorption, oral-esophageal problems, fever, and difficulties with swallowing and vomiting. Visually appealing meals, food supplements, and measures to control unpleasant odors may be helpful in promoting appetite.

Malnutrition augments the course of AIDS.[38,44] Therefore a well-balanced diet is important to preserve lean body mass and to provide the body with reserves needed to fight infection. Take a dietary history to identify eating habits. Recommend a diet that provides adequate amounts of all nutrients, taking into account particular symptoms or difficulties the patient may be experiencing with eating. Indulge desires for favorite foods. High-calorie snacks are recommended. Keep easy-to-prepare foods such as frozen dinners on hand. The patient should drink liquids a half an hour before eating instead of with meals in order to preserve appetite.[16]

Difficulties with diet may also be related to the patient's ability to chew, swallow, or digest food. For painful sores in the mouth, instruct the patient to avoid acidic foods (e.g., citrus or pineapple), extremely hot or cold food and beverages, and rough foods (e.g., raw fruits and vegetables). Encourage patients to eat nonabrasive, easy-to-eat foods such as ice cream, pudding, noodle dishes, and soft cheeses. Eating popsicles will numb mouth pain. Instruct the patient to use a straw to make swallowing easier. Consider a referral to the registered dietitian and refer the patient to community resources for support services (e.g., Meals-On-Wheels or community-based HIV/AIDS food outreach programs).[42]

Knowledge deficit; nausea management. Problems with nausea and vomiting are frequently a side effect of the various medications prescribed to treat the symptoms of AIDS. Discontinuation of the offensive medications is one solution. Administration of antiemetics (e.g., Reglan or Compazine) may be useful. Consider the use of cannabinoids such as dronabinol; they may control nausea and stimulate appetite.[36] Nasogastric feedings may be required for patients with severe nausea and vomiting associated with significant weight loss.[44]

Avoid offensive cooking odors by keeping windows open and the home well aerated. Instruct the patient to try cold entrees rather than hot ones because they have less odor and are often better tolerated.[44]

Soft foods, liquid meals, or canned supplements may be tolerated better than solids, depending on the type of infection or gastrointestinal disease.[44] The patient may want to avoid greasy, fatty, or spicy foods because they can aggravate gastrointestinal absorptive disorders.[38]

Head, ears, eyes, nose, and throat. There are many oral opportunistic disorders associated with HIV, including infections, cancers, and other lesions.[41] Examine the lips for vesicles or pustules indicative of herpes simplex virus (HSV). HSV can be treated with intravenous or oral acyclovir.

Oral cavity disease is common, especially oral thrush and hairy leukoplakia. Oral thrush appears as yellowish-white plaques on the mucosa. These can progress into the esophagus, causing a sore throat and difficulty swallowing. Hairy leukoplakia has a white-ribbed or fibrous appearance and is most commonly found along the sides of the tongue. Fungal infections of the mouth can be treated with clotrimazole troches and lozenges, nystatin, or systemic azole antifungals.[30,41]

Altered oral mucous membrane. Erosion of the gingiva, associated with painful and bleeding gums, is common in HIV disease. Therefore good dental hygiene should be recommended as a part of the treatment. Patients should routinely brush the teeth using a soft toothbrush and avoid flossing near the gum line. Dental visits should also be encouraged.

If an infection or lesion is in the mouth, suggest that patients use Toothettes (small sponge-tipped swabs) when brushing their teeth. This may be followed with a half-strength hydrogen peroxide mouthwash. A betadine rinse or antibacterial mouthwash (e.g., chlorhexidine) may be helpful.

Avoid commercial mouthwashes with alcohol or glycerine that dry out the mouth. Suggest commercially prepared artificial saliva for problems with a dry mouth; use lip balms to keep lips moist. Instruct the patient to suck on sugarless hard candies or popsicles for dryness of the mouth.

Acute and painful ulcerations may develop on the soft palate, making eating difficult. Topical applications of viscous lidocaine, triamcinolone acetonide (0.1% in Orabase), or thalidomide may relieve the pain of swallowing. Patients should avoid wearing loose-fitting dentures, which may cause a mouth lesion. Using a straw can help to bypass painful lesions when consuming liquids.

Impaired vision. Cytomegalovirus (CMV) retinopathy is the most frequently occurring eye infection in PWAs and essentially destroys the retina. If the infection reaches the optic nerve, a total loss of vision occurs. CMV retinitis is typically treated with ganciclovir. Because PWAs are prone to eye infections, do not allow them to wear contacts overnight.

What is the patient's ability to perform activities of daily living (ADLs)? Check vision and assist patients to cope with any loss. For example, instruct the patient and family to place items required for ADLs in a familiar spot. Talking clocks and watches are available. Patients may enjoy listening to the radio or audiocassette tapes of books.

Encourage home independence in activities such as feeding. For example, suggest the use of finger foods as snacks and use cups for liquids such as soaps. In addition, describe the location of eating utensils when serving food and identify locations of food on a plate referring to a clock (e.g., the meat is at 6 o'clock and the potatoes are at 2 o'clock).

Review general safety measures for the home. Avoid changing or moving furniture in the home and the use of unsecured area rugs.

Cardiopulmonary. Cardiac disorders are common in HIV-infected patients and may include pericardial effusions, mitral valve regurgitation, and dysrhythmias. Kaposi's sarcoma can invade the heart wall, causing valvular dysfunction. Auscultate for abnormal heart sounds and murmurs, and check the patient's heart rate. Report deviations from baseline status and whenever the patient is symptomatic to the physician.

Pulmonary infections are also common. Approximately 60% of PWAs develop pneumonia.[15] *Pneumocystis carinii* pneumonia (PCP) and TB also occur in this group. Assess the patient for changes in cough, sputum production, and lung sounds; such changes could indicate a new or recurring lung infection. See Chapter 6 for respiratory precautions.

Activity intolerance; ineffective breathing pattern. Instruct patients to notify the physician or home care nurse immediately if they experience excessive coughing, shortness of breath, and changes in color or amount of sputum; these are signs and symptoms of pulmonary infection.

If coughing is an ongoing problem, encourage the patient to take cough medications as scheduled. Cough drops and tea with lemon and honey may be helpful. Warm saline gargles may relieve a sore throat. Hydrate the patient with 2 to 3 L of fluid a day if possible to reduce coughing related to viscous pulmonary secretions.

If dyspnea is an ongoing problem, instruct the patient in energy conservation techniques such as pursed-lip breathing and planned rest periods between activities. Have the patient avoid environmental stressors such as cold air, smoke, and air pollution. As appropriate, instruct patients to increase fluid intake to thin their mucus secretions for easier expectoration. Also, room humidification may be helpful. As ordered, encourage use of prn oxygen to help with dyspnea. A referral to rehabilitation services may be appropriate in order to improve activity tolerance.[35] See Chapter 11 for energy conservation guidelines.

Neurologic. Depending on central nervous system (CNS) involvement, PWAs may experience behavioral changes such as forgetfulness and difficulty with recall. A photophobia may indicate cryp-

tococcal meningitis, which is accompanied by mood swings and headaches. If the spinal cord becomes involved, paralysis may develop. Fluconazole and amphotericin B are being used to treat cryptococcal meningitis.[2,43] The use of fluconazole is promising because this drug does not have the extreme side effects caused by amphotericin B.[2,43]

Impaired memory. Personality changes and a decline in judgment and comprehension can occur and may be followed by blindness and seizures. The patient may realize that mental functioning is deteriorating and become angry or depressed.

AIDS dementia may result with brain infection. As the disease advances, the patient may lose interest in outside activities and become indifferent and withdrawn. These patients sometimes assume an almost fetal position in bed. Provide written schedules for patients with mental status changes and encourage everyone involved in the patient's care to adhere to the schedule as much as possible. Keep calendars with current dates and pictures of loved ones nearby to help the patient orient to reality. Use clocks with AM and PM indicators. Always address the patient by name and maintain face-to-face contact during interactions. Have the patient dress and groom daily; do not permit patients to go unkempt and unbathed.

Be aware that PWAs are at increased risk for falls as the disease progresses. Provide for home safety; include the caregiver in all aspects of health teaching. Maintain good lighting. Eliminate throw rugs to decrease the possibility of falls. Remove all loose wires and electrical cords from high-traffic areas. **Never leave household cleansers or other potential poisons in unmarked containers near medications or food.** Instruct patients/caregivers to keep a list of vital telephone numbers within reach at all times (e.g., physician, hospital, emergency ambulance service, poison control center, suicide/crisis/substance abuse intervention hotline, police, fire department). Discourage guns in the home.

Dark glasses may help if the patient complains of photophobia. Consider a referral to the psychiatric home care nurse for behavioral problems (see Chapters 19 and 22).

Pain. Remember that the patient's self-report of pain is the most reliable indicator of location and intensity. Generally, pain incidence in PWAs increases as the disease progresses.

Medication for pain management depends on patient symptoms and stage of the disease. The AIDS pain experience is much like that of cancer, but the pain tends to be much more dramatically undertreated. Neuropathic pain syndromes are among the most common seen in PWAs.[4] Hydrocodone bitartrate and acetaminophen (Vicodin), oxycodone and acetaminophen (Percocet), and morphine sulfate (Roxanol) are administered for mild, moderate, and severe pain respectively. A continuous infusion of morphine may be required for end-stage disease or for severe, unrelenting pain. Physicians should order "rescue" doses when regularly scheduled doses are insufficient. In addition, consideration for concomitant administration of nonsteroidal antiinflammatory drugs (NSAIDS), even if the pain is severe because of the potential for additive analgesia and opioid sparing. Finally, adjuvant analgesics may be added as needed. See Chapter 24 for further pain assessment and management guidelines. Nursing care should also focus on basic patient comfort measures such as backrubs and an occasional hug.

Integumentary. Depressed cellular immunity is responsible for the majority of the viral and fungal infections common with AIDS patients. Skin disorders increase as the number of CD4[+] T cells declines.[14,15]

Inspect the skin for lesions, rashes, wounds, or signs of inappropriate needle marks. Examine the axillary and inguinal lymph nodes for swelling or tenderness. Report findings to the physician as appropriate.

Risk for impaired skin integrity. Typically, AIDS patients have very dry, scaly skin. This may be related to malabsorption of fatty acids, which causes dryness and premature aging of the skin. Dry skin and problems with immobility and poor nutrition can predispose these patients to pressure sores. If the patient suffers from diarrhea, skin integrity is threatened.

Report reddened areas or signs of skin breakdown to the physician for a wound care protocol. Avoid occlusive dressings because they are contraindicated in immunocompromised patients.

Bath oils, liquid emollient soaps, and moisturizers can be used to alleviate dry skin. Avoid tub baths if skin lesions are present. As appropriate, instruct the family in wound and skin care (see Chapter 14).

Gastrointestinal. Patients with AIDS are at risk for a variety of gastrointestinal infections and disease. Instruct the patient/caregiver to thoroughly scour all fresh vegetables because PWAs are vulnerable to *Salmonella, Shigella,* and other bacteria. Unpasteurized milk products should be avoided, and meats should be thoroughly cooked.

Diarrhea; risk for fluid volume deficit. Cryptosporidiosis and CMV are frequently the cause of diarrhea in PWAs.[15] Ganciclovir may be useful in treating CMV diarrhea.

A low residue, high protein, high calorie diet is recommended. Potassium-rich foods such as bananas, apricots, or baked potatoes (without butter) will help correct the hypokalemia that is often associated with large fluid losses.[38] It may be necessary to restrict dietary fiber and provide nutrient supplements (e.g., Ensure) until diarrhea is resolved.

Instruct the patient to avoid raw vegetables and fresh salads. With acute onset of diarrhea, PWAs may lose gallons of fluid each day and be at risk for dehydration. Limiting caffeine, which stimulates gastrointestinal motility, may also help control diarrhea.

Assess the patient for signs and symptoms of dehydration such as hypotension and poor skin turgor. When appropriate, encourage fluids (2 to 3 L a day) and instruct the caregiver to offer fluids to the patient frequently. For severe dehydration, the patient may require normal saline intravenously. It may be necessary to obtain a blood specimen for laboratory evaluation (e.g., SMA6) of electrolyte status. Kaopectate and Immodium or Lomotil may be useful to treat diarrhea.

Incontinence; functional. Chux, a type of incontinence pad or adult diaper, may be helpful in managing acute episodes of diarrhea. Recommend the use of moisture barrier creams around the anus to prevent excoriation. Instruct the patient/caregiver to cleanse the area with warm, soapy water **and** commercial spray cleansers (e.g., Peri Wash) immediately after episodes of diarrhea; then rinse, pat dry, and apply A and D Ointment or skin barrier cream (gloves should be worn during this procedure). For severe diarrhea, fecal incontinence pouching devices can be worn. Instruct the patient to avoid anal intercourse or oral-anal sexual activities.

Genitourinary. Ask patients if they are having any problems with itching, warts, or sores. Examine areas of concern. HSV often appears around the anus or vulva. These lesions appear as small, red ulcers and are painful. Acyclovir is the treatment of choice for HSV.

Evaluate males for testicular swelling, which could indicate that Kaposi's sarcoma has invaded the inguinal area.[17] A scrotal support or sling may provide comfort.

Ask female patients if they are having any problems with vaginal discomfort or unusual discharge. As appropriate, obtain a specimen for laboratory analysis and institute treatment. *Good personal hygiene should be highly reinforced.*

Altered sexuality pattern; sexual dysfunction. It is advisable to ask the patient about sexual habits. Sexual practice is a very personal and sensitive subject; respect it as such. Encourage safe sex, and discourage multiple sexual partners.[13] Review the proper use of condoms, which have been shown to be helpful in preventing infection (Figures 20-1 and 20-2; Boxes 20-5 and 20-6). Make sure the patient understands that AIDS is most often transmitted during sex. The patient may wish to refrain from sex or explore other methods of expressing affection.

Incontinence; functional. Urinary incontinence related to neurologic impairment or weakness may become a problem for PWAs. Male patients may benefit from an external or condom catheter in controlling incontinence. A urinary incontinence pouching device can be worn by female patients. Avoid indwelling catheters when possible because of the risk of infection in immunosuppressed patients. Problems with urinary retention can be managed by intermittent or straight catheterization (see Chapter 16).

Knowledge deficit; women's health. Women with AIDS may not always continue to menstruate, depending on how the physical and emotional stressors of the disease have affected their hormones. It will be important for women with AIDS to keep track of their menstrual period so they can inform their physician of any missed cycles or change in the frequency, flow, or length of their periods. HIV-infected women should be encouraged to use a reliable method of birth control to avoid becoming pregnant because of the risk of transmission of HIV from mother to child.

Instruct caregivers to always wear gloves when changing a sanitary napkin or tampon for a female patient. Tampons should be changed every 2 to 4 hours and not worn overnight. Follow local health ordinances regarding disposal of infectious waste.

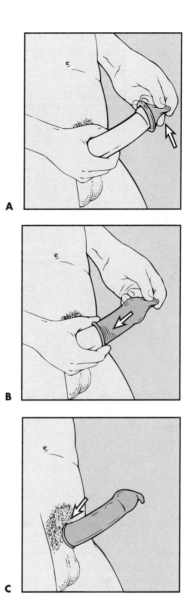

Figure 20-1 Proper placement of the male condom. **A,** The condom is placed over the glans of the erect penis, being careful to squeeze air out of the reservoir. **B** and **C,** The condom is then rolled down the shaft of the penis to the hairline. (From Grimes DE, Grimes RM: *AIDS and HIV infection,* St. Louis, 1994, Mosby.)

Instruct women with AIDS to wear cotton underwear in order to avoid vaginitis. In addition, douching or wearing scented sanitary napkins or tampons

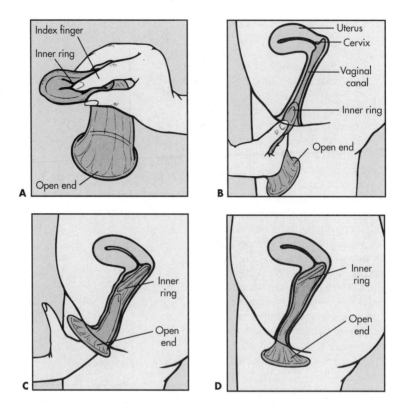

Figure 20-2 Proper placement of the female condom. **A,** Inner ring is squeezed for insertion. **B,** Sheath is inserted similarly to a diaphragm. **C,** Inner ring is pushed up as far as it can go with the index finger. **D,** Proper placement of female condom. (From Grimes DE, Grimes RM: *AIDS and HIV infection,* St. Louis, 1994, Mosby.)

is not recommended because it may promote vaginal infections.

When providing care for PWAs, treatment addresses the symptoms of the disease and the infection itself. (Refer to *HIV/AIDS: A Guide to Nursing Care* by J.H. Flaskrud and P. Ungvarski as an additional resource when caring for PWAs.[16])

Nursing interventions should consider comfort level along with maintenance and restoration of health. Once basic physiological needs are met, it is then possible to address the psychosocial and spiritual needs of PWAs and their families. Therein may lie the greatest challenge for effective intervention.

LIVING AT HOME WITH AIDS

The reality for many PWAs is that they have a horrific disease for which there is no known cure. Psychosocial problems are largely related to loss.[1,3]

Perhaps the best insight into what living with AIDS is like comes from considering what patients have lost as a result of the disease:

- General good health, supplanted by a persistent feeling of malaise and weakness
- Independence and mobility, which may create changes in role and identity
- Attractive appearance or body image, as a result of the many infections and skin disorders, cancers, premature aging, and hair and weight loss related to AIDS
- Appetite and the ability to swallow
- Support systems and networking (possibly family, friends, and lover), as part of the social stigma and fear connected with AIDS
- Financial stability, resulting from job loss and resources drained by medical bills
- The right to a long and happy life

Box 20-5   PATIENT EDUCATION GUIDE: PROPER USE OF THE MALE CONDOM

- Use only condoms (rubbers) that are made out of latex or polyurethane.
- "Natural skin" condoms have pores that are large enough for HIV to penetrate.
- Store condoms in a cool, dry place and protect them from trauma. The friction caused by carrying them in a back pocket, for instance, can wear down the latex.
- Do not use a condom if the expiration date has passed or if the package looks worn or punctured.
- Lubricants used in conjunction with condoms must be water soluble.
  - Oil-based lubricants can weaken latex and increase the risk of tearing or breaking.
  - Non-lubricated, flavored condoms can provide protection during oral intercourse.
- The condom must be placed on the erect penis before any contact is made with the partner's mouth, vagina, or rectum to prevent exposure to preejaculatory secretions that may contain HIV.
- See Figure 20-1 for proper steps in male condom placement.
- Remove the penis and condom from the partner's body immediately after ejaculation and before the erection is lost.
  - Hold the condom at the base of the penis and remove both at the same time.
  - This keeps semen from leaking around the condom as the penis becomes flaccid.
- Remove the condom after use, wrap in tissue, and discard. Do not flush down the toilet, as this can cause plumbing problems.
- Condoms are not reuseable! A new condom must be used for every act of intercourse.

Modified from Lewis SM and others: *Medical-surgical nursing: assessment and management of clinical problems,* ed 5, St. Louis, 2000, Mosby.

Such losses are not easy for the patient and family to accept. AIDS strikes most patients at a very creative and productive time of life. Issues of death and dying are understandably hard for this relatively young population to contemplate, much less accept.

Ineffective family coping

Conflicts among the patient and family or significant others may occur and are exacerbated by the

Box 20-6   PATIENT EDUCATION GUIDE: PROPER USE OF THE FEMALE CONDOM

- Female condoms consist of a polyurethane sheath with two spring form rings.
  - The smaller ring is inserted into the vagina and holds the condom in place internally. This ring can be removed if the condom is to be used for anal intercourse. It **should not be removed** if the condom is to be used for vaginal intercourse.
- The larger ring surrounds the opening to the condom. It functions to keep the condom in place externally while protecting the external genitalia.
- Use only water-soluble lubricants with female condoms.
  - Female condoms come prelubricated and with a tube of additional lubricant.
  - Lubrication is needed to protect the condom from tearing during sexual intercourse and can also decrease the noise that results from friction of the penis against the condom.
- Some men have reported that the female condom feels better than the male condom. Other men like male condoms better. The only way to find out which type of condom works best is to try them both.
- Practice inserting the female condom. The steps for proper insertion are shown in Figure 20-2. Lubrication makes the condom slippery, but do not get discouraged, just keep trying.
- During sexual intercourse, ensure that the penis is inserted into the female condom through the outer ring. It is possible for the penis to miss the opening, thus making contact with the vagina and defeating the purpose of the condom.
- Do not use a male condom at the same time as a female condom.
- After intercourse, remove the condom before standing up.
  - Twist the outer ring to keep the semen inside, gently pull the condom out of the vagina, and discard.
  - Do not flush down the toilet, as this can cause plumbing problems.
- Do not reuse a female condom.

Modified from Lewis SM and others: *Medical-surgical nursing: assessment and management of clinical problems,* ed 5, St. Louis, 2000, Mosby.

exhaustive nature of the disease. If the patient is gay, the family may still be adjusting to that fact, and feelings of guilt or fear of gossip or social prejudice may incline family members to isolate themselves from relatives, neighbors, or friends who could otherwise be a source of comfort and support. Eventually, most PWAs will be unable to live by themselves and alternate living arrangements will have to be made. Therefore home care nurses should assist the patient to identify potential caregivers to assist with everyday care, as well as basic end of life needs.

Considering the losses involved in living with AIDS, the home care nurse should be prepared to witness feelings of anger, guilt, and depression expressed by the patients, families, and significant others.[4,20] Opening lines of communication is the best intervention when providing care for these patients and their families. Listen to patient and family concerns, and provide reassurance and resources as needed. Maintain confidentiality. Find out what the patient's wishes are with respect to aggressive medical therapy should the patient become unable to make decisions. Make sure the patient's wish is communicated to the family because they may have influence in this decision.[37] If appropriate, do not hesitate to suggest pastoral care or hospice as a way of furthering good communication and support and possibly preparation for death.

Caregivers may become overwhelmed with the patient's multiple health care needs. The key to successful caregiving is to encourage caregivers to attend to their own needs, too. As a result, caregiver respite services or alternate living arrangements for the patient may become necessary. A referral to social services is suggested as the patients are often faced with the need to apply for entitlements.

A multidisciplinary team approach is best when providing the many services required by PWAs. Plan visits and coordinate the services of other disciplines on the basis of evolving patient needs and losses during the course of illness. Exploring financial concerns will also give insights into the patient's/caregiver's needs and worries.[3] A community assessment should identify easily accessible grocery stores and transportation for the patient/caregiver. See Chapter 4, which discusses family focused care.

SUMMARY

It is likely that a larger number of PWAs will be cared for outside the hospital in the next decade. As a result, home care organizations will be providing service for great numbers of these patients. In today's society, HIV infection and AIDS are associated with powerful emotional issues and the vast complexities of disease manifestation. Understanding AIDS, its mechanisms of transmission and pathogenesis, along with the psychosocial issues involved with this epidemic equips home care nurses with the scientific knowledge and the sensitivity needed to care for PWAs at home.

HIV has no known cure. However, in this world, all things are possible and our patients' hopes for a better tomorrow should never be discouraged. Key interventions are to provide our patients with information that alleviates symptoms of the disease. Support of the family or caregiver will be an important part of this process. As professionals, it is important to offer ourselves as caring individuals. For PWAs, being home does not necessarily mean being alone . . .

REFERENCES

1. Aranda-Naranjo B: The effect of HIV on the family, *AIDS Patient Care* 7(1):27, 1994.
2. Arndt C and others: Fluconazole penetration into cerebrospinal fluid: implications for treating fungal infections of the central nervous system, *Infect Dis* 157:178, 1987.
3. Baker S: Addressing the needs of people living with aids and their caregivers, *Nurs Clin North Am* 34(1):201, 1999.
4. Breitbart W: Pain management-psychosocial issues in HIV and AIDS, *Am J Hospice Palliat Care* 13(1):20, 1996.
5. Centers for Disease Control and Prevention: Pneumocystis pneumonia—Los Angeles, *MMWR Morb Mortal Wkly Rep* 30:250, 1981.
6. Centers for Disease Control and Prevention: 1993 Revised classification system for HIV infection and expanded surveillance case definition for AIDS among adolescents and adults, *MMWR Morb Mortal Wkly Rep* 41(RR-17):1, 1992.
7. Centers for Disease Control and Prevention: Revised guidelines for the performance of CD4+ T-cell determinations in persons with human immunodeficiency virus (HIV) infection, *MMWR Morb Mortal Wkly Rep* 42(17):280, 1994.
8. Centers for Disease Control and Prevention: Human Immunodeficiency virus transmission in household settings—United States, *MMWR Morb Mortal Wkly Rep* 43(19):347, 1994.
9. Centers for Disease Control and Prevention: Tuberculosis morbidity-United States, 1997, *MMWR Morb Mortal Wkly Rep* 47(13):256, 1998.
10. Centers for Disease Control and Prevention: Report of the NIH panel to define therapy of HIV infection and guidelines for the use of antiretriviral in HIV-infected adults and

adolescents, *MMWR Morb Mortal Wkly Rep* 47(RR-5):1, 1998.

11. Centers for Disease Control and Prevention: HIV/AIDS surveillance report—1999, *MMWR Morb Mortal Wkly Rep* 11(1):1, 1999.
12. Centers for Disease Control and Prevention: Telephone conversation with statistics department in March, 2000.
13. Daigle B and others: *HIV homecare handbook,* Sudbury, Mass, 1999, Jones & Bartlett.
14. Farthing C: Aids—a historical overview. In Friedman-Kien AE, Cockerell C: *Color atlas of aids,* ed 3, 2000, Philadelphia, WB Saunders.
15. Fauci A: Immunopathogenic mechanisms of HIV infection, *Ann Intern Med* 124:654, 1996.
16. Flaskrud JH, Ungvarski P: *HIV/AIDS: a guide to nursing care,* Philadelphia, 1999, WB Saunders.
17. Gold JW: HIV-1 infection, diagnosis and management, *Med Clin North Am* 76(1):1, 1992.
18. Grint P, McEvoy M: Two associated cases of the acquired immunodeficiency syndrome (AIDS), *Communic Dis Rep* 1:42, 1986.
19. Holtzclaw BJ: The febrile response in critical care: state of the art science, *Heart Lung* 21(5):482, 1992.
20. Ingram KM and others: Social support and unsupportive social interactions: their association with depression among people living with HIV, *AIDS Care* 11(3):313, 1999.
21. Ippolito G and others: Italian study group on occupational risk of HIV infection, the risk of occupational human immunodeficiency virus infection in health care workers: Italian multicenter study, *Arch Intern Med* 153:1451, 1993.
22. Lemaitre M and others: Role of mycoplasma infection in the cytopathic effect induced by human immunodeficiency virus type-1 in infected cell lines, *Infect Immun* 60(3):742, 1999.
23. Levy JA: HIV pathogenesis and long-term survival, *AIDS* 7(11):1401, 1993.
24. Lewis SM and others: Medical-surgical nursing: assessment and management of clinical problems, ed 5, St. Louis, 2000, Mosby.
25. Libman H: HIV pathogenesis, natural history and classification of HIV infection, *Prim Care* 19(1):1, 1993.
26. Lundgren JD and others: Comparison of long-term patients with AIDS treated and not treated with zidovudine, *JAMA* 271(14):1088, 1994.
27. Makowiak PA and others: A critical appraisal of 98.6 degrees F, the upper limit of the normal body temperature, and other legacies of Carel Reinhold August Wunderlick, *JAMA* 268(12):1578, 1993.
28. Miller FH and others: Renal manifestations of AIDS, *Radiographics* 13(3):587, 1993.

29. Monmaney T: Kids with AIDS, *Newsweek* 9:51, 1987.
30. Montagnier L, Blanchard A: Mycoplasmas as cofactor in infection due to human immunodeficiency virus, *Clin Infect Dis* 17(Suppl 1):S309, 1992.
31. Nahlen BL and others: HIV wasting syndrome in the United States, *AIDS* 7(2):183, 1993.
32. National Institutes of Health: Report of NIH panel to define principles of therapy of HIV infection, 1997, http://www.hivatis.org/upguidaa.html.
33. Occupational Safety and Health Administration: Tuberculosis. OSHA technical links www.osha-slc.gov/SLTC/tuberculosis/index.html.
34. Pantaleo G and others: The immunopathogenesis of human immunodeficiency virus infection, *N Eng J Med* 328(5):327, 1993.
35. Pfeiffer N: Long-term survival and HIV disease—the role of exercise and $CD4^+$ response in HIV disease, *AIDS Patient Care* 6(5):237, 1992.
36. Plasse TF and others: Recent clinical experience with dronabinol, *Pharmacol Biochem Behav* 40(3):695, 1994.
37. Ragsdale D and others: How HIV+ persons manage everyday life in the hospital and at home, *Qualitative Health Res* 4:411, 1994.
38. Resler S: Nutrition care of the AIDS patients, *J Am Dietetic Assoc* 88(7):828, 1988.
39. Rolfs RT: Risk factors for syphilis: cocaine use and prostitution, *Am J Public Health* 80(7):853, 1990.
40. Ross HE and others: The prevalence of psychiatric disorders in patients with alcohol and other drug problems, *Arch Gen Psychiatry* 45(11):1023, 1988.
41. Sears C: The oral manifestations of AIDS, *AIDS Patient Care* 3(4):8, 1989.
42. Shields MF, Cook A: Food outreach, inc: a community-based nutrition program for people with HIV/AIDS, *Home Health Care Manage Prac* 10(1):62, 1997.
43. Sugar A, Saunders C: Oral fluconazole as suppressive therapy of disseminated cryptococcus in patients with acquired immunodeficiency syndrome, *Am J Med* 85:481, 1988.
44. The Task Force on Nutrition Support in AIDS: Guidelines for nutrition support in AIDS, *AIDS Patient Care* 3(4):32, 1989.
45. Tu XM and others: Survival differences and trends in patients with AIDS in the United States, *J AIDS* 6(10):1150, 1993.
46. Wang RY and others: High frequency of antibodies to mycoplasma penetrans in HIV-infected patients, *Lancet* 340(8831):1312, 1991.
47. Ziegler J and others: Postnatal transmission of AIDS-associated retrovirus from mother to infant, *Lancet* 1:896, 1985.

PART III

SPECIAL CLINICAL AND COMMUNITY ISSUES

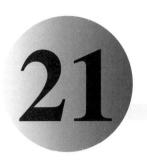

MATERNAL-CHILD NURSING: POSTPARTUM HOME CARE

Annette M. Lynch, Roberta A. Kordish, and Lenore R. Williams

After birth moved from home to hospital almost a century ago, the hospital length of stay (LOS) steadily declined until 1996. The Newborn and Mothers' Protection Act of 1996 was enacted in response to consumer demand, professional medical organizations, media attention, and heavy lobbying efforts for improvements in maternal-child care. This law mandated insurers to reimburse a minimum length of stay of 48 hours following a vaginal birth and 96 hours following a cesarean birth.

However, current health care coverage may compromise the ability of providers to meet health care needs of mothers, infants, and new families after birth. These needs have been documented in medical, nursing, and sociological research and continue to exist regardless of LOS. Mothers need to recover physically and emotionally. Infants need to make a successful transition to extrauterine existence. Families need to reorganize as they incorporate the infant into the family unit.

Such needs of childbearing families can be met through implementation of a comprehensive postpartum home care program. Such a program is essential to ensure desired clinical outcomes of modern maternity care. The purpose of this chapter is to describe key concepts and practice issues of postpartum home care.

HISTORICAL PERSPECTIVES

In 1890, 25% of births occurred in a hospital setting; Sloan Memorial Hospital in New York City reported an average LOS of 17.4 days.[48] By 1968, 99.5% of all births occurred in the hospital,

and the average LOS was 4 to 5 days.[13] From 1970 until 1996, the LOS continued to decline because of consumer choice for more homelike, family-centered experiences and payer demand for less costly care (Figure 21-1). The current LOS for all births in the United States is 2.2 days. The LOS for vaginal births averages 1.8 days. For cesarean births, the average LOS is 3.5 days.[20,55,56]

Research has described postpartum home care programs beginning with the Bradford experiment in 1959 in England and spanning the United States and Canada for over 35 years.* In these studies, a shortened hospital stay was combined with follow-up care at home to ensure safe recovery of mothers and infants and to address health care needs of the entire family. Each study demonstrated that a well-planned program resulted in successfully met goals. Even with federally mandated reimbursement for LOS, lawmakers in several states realized that the time in the hospital was insufficient for needs of the mother, infant, and family to be met and enacted legislation for follow-up care.[18]

Common elements of successful short-stay maternity programs included (1) guidelines for discharge, (2) preparation of qualified visiting nurses, (3) antepartal contact with the childbearing family, (4) multidisciplinary collaborative program design, (5) timely visits matched with the develop-

---

*References 6, 10, 13-19, 26, 28, 30, 32, 33, 34, 36, 38, 44, 53, 54, 58, 59, 62.

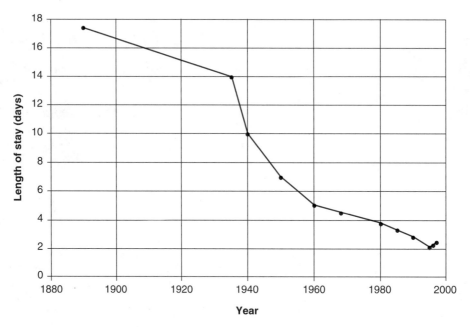

Figure 21-1 Historical changes in maternal length of stay.

mental crisis in families, (6) planned mechanisms for referrals when medical or support services were indicated, (7) caregiver accessibility, (8) outcome measurement, and (9) demonstrated cost-effectiveness.

PHILOSOPHY OF CARE

Today the goals of care for childbearing families are a healthy pregnancy, a healthy infant, and parents who are prepared for and confident in their new roles. To achieve these goals, current standards of care advocate early and regular prenatal care and birth in a hospital or birthing center. However, there is no standard that recognizes the needs of mothers, infants, and families following hospitalization. The Association of Women's Health, Obstetric and Neonatal Nurses (AWHONN) published a position statement[8] and guidelines for perinatal home care.[7,9] In addition, both the American Nurses Association (ANA)[5] and the March of Dimes[42] developed similar documents. These publications advocate skilled postpartum home care as an equally *necessary* component in meeting national health care goals for childbearing families.

Postpartum nursing has always made a valuable contribution to the recovery of mothers and infants from childbirth and to the successful launching of new families. Regardless of the environment, such nursing care continues to be necessary to achieve the following goals:

- Monitor and ensure the physical and emotional well-being of family members.
- Identify developing complications early, preventing exacerbations and costly rehospitalizations.
- Bridge the care gap between discharge and ambulatory follow-up for mothers and infants with their primary care providers.*

SCOPE OF SERVICES

Differences exist between home care for patients with medically diagnosed conditions and home care for postpartum families. Of note, childbirth is a healthy event. Although services to treat an illness or injury are not indicated, birth does involve a recovery period that must be monitored

---

*Primary care providers exist for both mother and infant. They can include an obstetrician, a certified nurse midwife (CNM), a family practitioner, a pediatrician, and/or a pediatric nurse practitioner.

and a developmental crisis that the new family must resolve to maintain health. A program approach to postpartum home care recognizes these differences and structures services to match this unique population.

A comprehensive and cost-effective skilled postpartum home care program is a hybrid of traditional inpatient postpartum care and traditional home care. It is based on the understanding that when mothers and infants are discharged in 48 hours after vaginal birth or 96 hours after cesarean birth, only initial stabilization has occurred. Health promotion activities have just been initiated, and few learning needs have been identified or met. The intent of such a program is to begin where hospital or birthing center care has ended, neither duplicating nor omitting any essential elements. These postpartum home care services span the time from late pregnancy to follow-up after birth.

Whereas each mother and infant is the focus of a different primary care provider, only the home care nurse has a whole family perspective. The home care nurse is aware of family dynamics, can assess the health care needs of each family member, and facilitates the initial stages of family reintegration (see Chapter 4).

The postpartum home care program includes the following services:

- Case management from discharge to ambulatory care followed by an experienced registered nurse
- Prenatal and/or previsit contact with the referred family
- Coordination of care with primary care providers, hospital or birthing center nurses, and community agencies[3]
- Visits made 24 to 72 hours following discharge
- Skilled nursing assessment and intervention for mothers, infants, and families
- Use of a risk management documentation tool
- Postvisit telephone call(s)
- Availability of a 24-hour help line
- Continuous measurement of quality variables such as health status, complications, readmission rates, patient satisfaction, and cost-effectiveness

In addition to the role preparation for the home care nurse outlined in Chapter 3, qualifications for a registered nurse providing skilled postpartum

---

Box 21-1 PRACTITIONER COMPETENCIES FOR POSTPARTUM HOME CARE

Didactic Content

- Physiology of lactation
- Postpartum involution
- Postpartum missing pieces
- Postpartum timetable
- Postpartum depression
- Physiological transition of infant to extrauterine existence
- Infant nutrition and feeding
- Infant growth and development
- Infant behavior
- Infant/parent cue/response pattern
- Infant hyperbilirubinemia
- Infant metabolic screening
- Family theory
- Family developmental tasks
- Communication theory
- Teaching/learning theory
- Crisis theory and intervention

Clinical Skills

- Physical assessment of the postpartum woman
- Psychosocial assessment of the postpartum woman
- Physical assessment of the infant
- Feeding assessment of the infant
- Specimen collection—maternal (venipuncture or finger stick, urine and stool, vaginal culture, wound culture)
- Specimen collection—infant (heel stick, urine)

---

home care include a minimum of 1 year maternal-infant care experience with the theoretical and clinical competencies to assess and care for mothers, infants, and families at home[7,9] (Box 21-1).

HOME CARE APPLICATION
Prenatal contact

Case management begins with preparation of patients at 34 to 36 weeks' gestation. Although a home care agency may not always have access to a patient before delivery, some hospitals or managed care organizations may provide a vehicle for prenatal contact with the client. The home care nurse can contact the patient by phone, in person, or via written communication. The objectives of this contact are as follows:

- Explain the purpose, content, and length of the home visit.
- Facilitate the coordination of care with primary care providers, hospital/birth center nurses, insurers, and community agencies.
- Obtain baseline data on the mother and family (health status during pregnancy, preparation for the infant, availability of help at home following hospital discharge, infant feeding method, and pediatric provider).
- Provide anticipatory guidance for identified needs, especially for patients who plan to breast-feed or those who have yet to select a pediatric provider.
- Determine address and telephone number of family location following hospital discharge.

The nurse gives the patient instructions on how the agency is to be notified of the patient's delivery. Documentation of this contact is kept with the patient's chart.

Referral process

The home care nurse can be likened to the "next shift." Although some home care agencies have their own coordinators to obtain discharge data, the health care system of the future dictates efficiency. An expedient method for the transfer of information is for the inpatient nurse to "give report" to the home care nurse. This allows the home care nurse to continue or modify the nursing plan of care already established. Since visits should be scheduled within 72 hours of discharge, it is best to obtain the referral information and medical orders for care on the day of discharge. Figure 21-2 shows an example of a comprehensive referral form.

Scheduling visits

The home care nurse determines when the visit should be made based on prenatal contact, referral information, and any specific physician order(s). For example, an infant of 37 weeks' gestation who is having feeding difficulty, an inexperienced breast-feeding mother, or a multipara who was discharged on a regimen of methylergonovine maleate would all warrant visits earlier in the 72-hour time frame.

Mothers should be contacted within 24 hours of discharge to determine recovery status, schedule the visit, verify location, and provide the 24-hour help line number. Considerations for scheduling visits include a mutually convenient time and the presence of support persons. Home care for the postpartum family necessitates use of equipment unique to this population (Box 21-2).

Maternal assessment

The nurse determines the mother's progress toward the goal of physical and psychological recovery from childbirth and instructs the mother in self-monitoring techniques. The three major assessment categories are physical, activities of daily living, and psychological. In order to establish a comfort level, it is more appropriate to assess the mother's psychological status and to review activities of daily living before doing the physical examination. However, in this section, physical assessment of the mother will be addressed first. Abnormal findings are always reported to the primary care provider.

Physical assessment. Suggest an area of privacy before initiating the physical assessment of the mother. The mother needs to assume a supine position on a mattress or sofa. A waterbed is not ideal because of instability. Sensitive issues such as contraception and domestic violence may be addressed more appropriately at this time.

Vital signs. Although the mother's temperature may be elevated during the first 24 hours after delivery and again when the milk comes in, the upper limit of normal elevation is 100.4° F (38° C). Tachycardia (greater than 100 beats per minute) may indicate a potential for infection, hemorrhage, vaginal hematoma, or other types of cardiovascular compromise. At the time of the home visit, the mother should be normotensive. Elevation may indicate postpartum pregnancy–induced hypertension (PIH). Hypotension may indicate excessive bleeding.

Breasts. Identify whether the mother is breast- or bottle-feeding. Inspect and palpate breasts for size, tension, color, heat, and discharge. If the bottle-feeding mother is engorged, assess her understanding of using ice packs, analgesics, a breast binder, or a tight bra for comfort. Current obstetric guidelines do not recommend antilactogenic medications.[23,24,39] If the mother is breast-feeding, assess tenderness, nodularity, and milk production. Inspect the nipples for integrity and erectility. If

✖ Hollister.

Postpartum Family Referral Form
Hollister Maternal/Newborn Record System
To order call: **1.800.323.4060**   Re-order No. 5841

Date of
Birth __MO__ / __DAY__ / __YR__   Home Phone _____   Visit Address (if different) _____
Marital Status S M W D Sep   Contact Phone _____
Special Cultural/Religious/Language Considerations ☐ None   Identify_____

	OBSTETRICIAN	PEDIATRICIAN	HOSPITAL	INSURANCE
NAME	_____	_____	_____	Company _____
ADDRESS	_____	_____	_____	Phone _____
	_____	_____	_____	Holder _____
TELEPHONE	_____	_____	_____	Policy No. _____

Maternal Information
EDD_____   Record No. _____
G____T____P____A____L____
Medication Allergy   ☐ None   Identify _____
Significant Health History   ☐ None   Identify _____

Birth Data
Date ____ / ____ / ____   Time _____
Type ☐ Spontaneous Vaginal ☐ Forceps ☐ Vacuum
     ☐ Cesarean
Episiotomy   ☐ No ☐ Yes ☐ Midline ☐ RML ☐ LML
              ☐ Extension _____
Laceration   ☐ No ☐ Yes ☐ Perineal _____
              ☐ Periurethral ☐ Vaginal
Anesthesia   ☐ None ☐ Local ☐ Epidural ☐ Spinal ☐ General
Complications ☐ None
    Identify _____

Discharge Data
Date ____ / ____ / ____   Time _____
Temp _____ Pulse _____ Resp _____ BP _____ / _____
Emotional Status ☐ Happy ☐ Ambivalent ☐ Anxious
                  ☐ Depressed ☐ Angry ☐ Other _____

Level of Maternal/Infant Attachment (Key on reverse side)
☐ 0   ☐ 1   ☐ 2   ☐ 3   ☐ 4

Level of Paternal/Infant Attachment (Key on reverse side)
☐ 0   ☐ 1   ☐ 2   ☐ 3   ☐ 4   ☐ Father Not Involved

Support Person(s) ☐ None   ☐ Father of Baby
    Other_____

Significant Lab Data   ☐ None
    Blood Type/RH _____
    Hgb/Hct _____
    Other _____

Medications/Treatments   ☐ None
    Identify _____
Abnormal Findings/Special Needs ☐ None
    Identify _____
Referrals/Follow Up Appointments ☐ None
    Identify _____

Newborn Information
Name _____   Record No. _____
☐ Male ☐ Female   Apgar ____ 1 min ____ 5 min ____ 10 min
Birth Weight _____   Discharge Weight _____
Length _____   Head/Chest Circumference ____ / ____
Gestational Age Exam ____ wks ☐ SGA ☐ AGA ☐ LGA
☐ Preterm ☐ Term ☐ Postterm
Circumcision ☐ No ☐ Yes ☐ Problems _____

Discharge Data
Date ____ / ____ / ____   Time _____
Temp _____ Pulse _____ Resp _____
Feeding   ☐ Breast   ☐ Formula Type _____
  Problems ☐ None   ☐ Positioning   ☐ Latch
           ☐ Suck   ☐ Sleepy   ☐ Mucousy
           ☐ Other
Jaundice   ☐ None
           ☐ Head (3mg/dl)
           ☐ Head & Chest (6mg/dl)
           ☐ Head & Entire Chest (9mg/dl)
           ☐ Head, Chest & Abdomen to Umbilicus (12 mg/dl)
           ☐ Head, Chest & Entire Abdomen (15 mg/dl)
           ☐ Head, Chest, Abdomen, Legs, & Feet (18 mg/dl)
Significant Lab Data   ☐ None
    Blood Type/RH_____ Coombs ☐ Neg ☐ Pos

Test	Date	Time	Results
Bilirubin	_____	_____	_____
	_____	_____	_____
	_____	_____	_____

Metabolic Screen ☐ Done ☐ Initial Needed ☐ Repeat Needed
                  ☐ Kit/Card Given
Medications/Treatment   ☐ None
    Identify_____
Abnormal Findings/Special Needs ☐ None
    Identify_____
Referrals/Follow up Appointments ☐ None
    Identify_____

COMMENTS _____
_____
_____
_____
_____

Signature _____   Date_____

Hollister Incorporated, 2000 Hollister Drive, Libertyville, Illinois 60048

Postpartum Family Referral Form #5841 998

Figure 21-2 Postpartum family referral form. (Reprinted with permission of Professional Nurse Associates, Inc., Cleveland, Ohio.)
Continued

Maternal / Paternal Attachment Key

0	=	No visual contact No verbal response, demanding or rejecting tone No attempt to touch infant, rough handling
1	=	Occasional glances Single words, no inflection Minimal touch, holding baby away from body
2	=	Looks at infant at intervals Short phrases, average tone Holds infant, explores with finger tips
3	=	Seeks en face with infant, smiles at infant Long phrases, soft, soothing tone Comments on infant appearance Enfolds infant, explores with hands
4	=	Maintains en face with infant Speaks in rhythmic pattern, loving tone Uses infant name or "pet" name Enfolds infant, cuddles, strokes, rocks

Hollister Incorporated, 2000 Hollister Drive, Libertyville, Illinois 60048

POSTPARTUM FAMILY REFERRAL FORM #5841 998

Figure 21-2—cont'd For legend see p. 383.

Box 21-2   EQUIPMENT FOR POSTPARTUM HOME CARE

- Record system (Hollister Postpartum Home Care Record System)
- Foamed alcohol surgical hand scrub
- Gloves
- Thermometer and probe covers
- Sphygmomanometer, regular and large cuffs
- Stethoscope
- Penlight
- Infant scale
- Tape measure
- Cord clamp remover
- Lactation devices (lactaids, shells)
- Specimen collection supplies (metabolic screening cards; urine specimen containers; laboratory kit with alcohol swabs, lancets, spring-loaded automatic puncture device, microtainers, capillary tubes, clay, tourniquet, Vacutainer system, gauze sponges, adhesive bandages; specimen labels; specimen bags; sharps container; Clinistix; Dextrostix; culture tubes)
- Educational materials
- Community resources information

---

nipple integrity is altered, determine the use and effectiveness of any topical agent. Advise cleansing the nipples with water only as soap may dry the nipple tissues. A well-fitting, supportive bra may be worn for comfort. An ill-fitting or underwire bra may cause plugged ducts and ultimately mastitis in the breast-feeding mother.[47] This is an ideal time to teach or reinforce the mother in the technique of breast self-examination (BSE). Inform the breast-feeding mother about changes in breast configuration and in the timing of BSE during lactation.

Abdominal musculature. Following birth, the mother's abdomen is usually soft, distended, and a cause for potential body image alteration. Pregnancy can distend the abdomen and cause an actual separation of the two rectus abdominis muscles (diastasis recti). To assess this phenomenon, have the mother assume a supine position (head flat or elevated with a low pillow, knees bent, feet flat on surface). Instruct the mother to attempt a chin-to-chest maneuver, as if doing a modified sit-up. Measure the width and length of any separation in centimeters. Have the mother palpate the diastasis

recti to understand the reason for her figure changes and enable her to self-monitor resolution. Instructions in exercise progression can be suggested at this time. If a cesarean or bilateral partial salpingectomy (BPS) (tubal ligation) incision is present, assess the mother's abdomen for presence of sutures/staples/steri-strips, approximation, redness, swelling, and discharge. Physician orders and agency policy should govern the nurse's removing sutures or staples.

Reproductive tract. The puerperium is the period of time from the end of the third stage of labor until the pelvic organs have returned to normal.[23,39] Usually by 6 weeks post partum, the uterus returns to its prepregnant state by the process known as involution. During involution the actual number of uterine cells does not change, but each cell decreases in size by approximately 90%.

Approximately 12 hours after delivery, the uterine fundus can be palpated 1 cm above the umbilicus. The fundus descends about 1 to 2 cm every 24 hours. The uterus should not be palable after the ninth postpartum day.[39] Uterine discharge (lochia) is made up of blood and debris from the necrosis of the decidua (uterine lining). Lochia progression is described in Table 21-1. Lochia should always have a fleshy smell. A strong odor resembling spoiled meat could signify infection.

Progression of uterine involution is measured by the location and consistency of the uterine fundus. When assessing the fundus, first instruct the mother to empty her bladder. The stretched uterine ligaments allow the uterus to move easily in the abdominal cavity. A full bladder can displace the uterus to the right or left of midline. Begin by assessing the perineal pad for the color and amount of lochia, while noting the lochia odor. With the mother in a recumbent position place one hand immediately above the symphysis pubis, and the other on top of the fundus. The fundus should feel firm. If the fundus is relaxed, gently massage it until firm. Assess lochia by noting the type and number of perineal pads and the percentage of pad saturation. Instruct the mother how to monitor normal uterine involution by palpating her fundus, identifying normal involution progression, and recognizing appropriate lochial flow. Fundal height and lochia can vary slightly due to multiparity, infant size, cesarean birth, or the presence of fibroids. Delayed uterine involution or a persistent relaxed

Table 21-1 Lochia progression[23,24,39]

Stage	Time postpartum	Characteristics
Rubra	Delivery-3 days	Red, possibly small clots
Serosa	4-10 days	Brownish to pink, serosanguineous
Alba	11-21 days	Yellowish to white

uterus is abnormal. Significant uterine tenderness or foul-smelling lochia may indicate the presence of endometritis.[23]

Assess the perineum by having the mother assume a side-lying position with the top leg flexed over the bottom leg. Use a penlight to illuminate the area. Lifting the buttock to visualize the perineum and anal area, note the condition of the perineal body, any laceration/episiotomy (REEDA scale[21]), and the presence/condition of hemorrhoids. Question the mother about perineal hygiene and the use and effectiveness of sitz baths and topical agents.

Elimination pattern. Immediately after delivery, there may be swelling or bruising near the urethra. The bladder has increased capacity following delivery, but the sensation to urinate may not be present due to the use of conduction anesthesia. The pregnancy-induced ureteral dilatation persists for 2 to 4 weeks after birth. In addition, the body must rapidly rid itself of 2000 to 3000 ml of extracellular fluid that accumulates in normal pregnancy. The newly delivered mother experiences diuresis and diaphoresis to accomplish this task. A history of pregnancy-induced hypertension complicates this resolution because of the presence of edema.[39] The bladder should not be palpated above the symphysis pubis. Identify presence of urinary symptoms such as urgency, frequency, dysuria, burning, incontinence, or tenderness. Because any of these signs and symptoms may indicate a urinary tract infection, be prepared to obtain a clean catch urine specimen.

Birth causes decreased intraabdominal pressure. Hormonal alterations may cause decreased intestinal peristalsis. Fear of defecation because of the presence of hemorrhoids and/or laceration/episiotomy may also delay return to normal bowel habits. Assess bowel elimination pattern, and identify the use and effectiveness of stool softeners or laxatives. Be aware that nutritional and fluid deficiencies will impact bowel function.

Lower extremities. Following the delivery of the placenta, there is an increase in clotting factors. This can be exacerbated if the mother has a cesarean delivery, pregnancy-induced hypertension, obesity, or a history of vascular disorders or thromboembolytic disease.[39] Ambulation is recommended to avoid venous stasis. Assess the mother's legs for heat, swelling, redness, or pain. Pain in the calf on dorsiflexion is known as a positive Homans' sign and may indicate thrombophlebitis. To elicit this response, with the leg extended, gently hold the knee flat and dorsiflex the foot. Note the presence of any edema. Measure the extent by depressing the leg surface. Residual edema may not be resolved, especially if the mother has had a prolonged induction of labor or pregnancy-induced hypertension. Pitting edema of 2+ or more is significant.

Pain. Many mothers experience altered comfort in the postpartum period. Common sites of pain include head, breast, uterus, abdomen, back, perineum, hemorrhoid, and leg. Determine the intensity, duration, and cause of the pain. Identify use of analgesics and their effectiveness. Persistent or intractable pain is abnormal.

Instruct the mother in reportable danger signs. A handout that instructs when to call her provider may be offered.

Activities of daily living. Returning to the realities of household management and infant care may preclude adequate nutrition. If the mother's nutritional needs are not met, recovery may be delayed, and lactation may be inhibited. Decreased appetite may also signify postpartum depression.[11,12,23] Obtain a 24-hour diet history (including fluids), assess for nutritional adequacy, and counsel on apparent deficits. Identify intake of iron and vitamin supplements. Most practitioners recommend that lactating mothers continue to take prenatal vitamins.

Fatigue is common. Sleep was interrupted in the last trimester of pregnancy, labor caused energy expenditure, and infant caretaking activities prevent optimal sleep. Identify day and night periods of uninterrupted sleep. Determine maternal activities, including infant care, household management, and exercise. The activities of daily living should be correlated with physical and psychological findings in order to determine their appropriateness. Help the family prioritize and reorganize activities to facilitate the mother's recovery.

Psychological assessment

General comments. Use principles of therapeutic communication such as active listening, maintaining eye contact, reflecting, clarifying, empathizing, encouraging, and the use of touch to elicit information. Ask open-ended questions such as "What has bringing this baby home been like?" to obtain information about feelings, body image, and self-concept.

Integrating the birth experience. The term *missing pieces* refers to a woman's inability to recall her birth events clearly.[1] The labor and birth experience must be resolved before the woman can take on her new role as a mother. Allow the mother time to reflect and determine if missing pieces exist. Reports from the referring institution or information from a support person can clarify details so the mother has a total picture of the birth experience.

Postpartum timetable. Following birth, the mother must progress through tasks of maternal psychological adaptation (Table 21-2). Although Rubin's classic stages[49] of "taking in," "taking hold," and "letting go" have been artificially accelerated by the advent of shortened hospital stays and may seem blended in contemporary American women,[43] identification of the mother's place on this timetable allows for effective intervention in meeting her needs.

Postpartum depression. The initial exhilaration of delivery is often changed by the time the nurse sees the family in the home. A fluctuation in hormones, fatigue, and feelings of unmet self-expectations and societal expectations may precipitate negative feelings during the postpartum period (Table 21-3). Beck[11,12] offers a checklist to facilitate identification of postpartum depression and mood disorders. Address any negative feelings

Table 21-2 Maternal psychological adaptation

Phase postpartum	Maternal characteristics
Taking in (1-2 days)	Passive, dependent, concerned with own needs; verbalizes delivery experience
Taking hold (3-10 days)	Strives for independence; strong anxiety element; maximal stage of learning readiness; mood swings may occur
Letting go (10 days - 6 weeks)	Achieves interdependence; realistic regarding role transition; accepts baby as a separate person; new norms established for self

Modified from Rubin R: Puerperal change, *Nurs Outlook* 9:753, 1961.

Table 21-3 Postpartum depression[11,12,61]

Type	Characteristics	Incidence
Blues	Benign, brief, occurring 2-10 days after birth	80%
Atypical	More disabling, physical and psychological symptoms, longer-lasting	10%
Psychosis	Incapacitating, may be long-term, risks of suicide and infanticide	0.5%-3.0%

or anxiety the mother expresses. Acknowledging that many new mothers feel down (blues) but are not emotionally incapacitated (atypical depression or psychosis) gives families guidelines to do self-monitoring.

Sexuality. Partners can resume intercourse when lochia has ceased, the perineum is healed, and contraceptive issues are addressed.[3] Inform the couple that the breasts of a nursing mother may leak during orgasm and that vaginal dryness can cause discomfort. Fatigue in one or both partners can interfere with sexual expression. Lack of desire in one or both partners can adversely affect the couple's sexual relationship at a time when mutual support is vital. Partners need to be informed that conception is possible prior to the return of menses. Address family planning preferences. If contraception is desired, suggest options. Over-the-counter measures (e.g., foam and condoms) can be used prior to the woman's visit to her health care provider for the postpartum checkup. Although some low-dose oral contraceptives are safe to take during breast-feeding,[23,39] they are transmitted in breast milk. Long-acting hormonal contraceptives such as Depo-Provera or Norplant are not usually recommended for the first 6 weeks during which a mother is breast-feeding. Because the inner pelvic structure changes following birth, a diaphragm must be refitted. Uterine healing and cervical closure occurs over a 4-week period, precluding placement of an intrauterine contraceptive device (IUD) before this time. Due to irregularities incurred in the menstrual cycle during lactation, natural family planning may not be effective.

Infant assessment

Assess the newborn infant's progress in achieving the goal of healthy adaptation to extrauterine life. The three major assessment categories are physical, nutritional, and behavioral. The presence of parents and other family members allows the nurse to demonstrate infant capabilities and caregiving techniques. Safety of the infant is paramount. Never leave the infant unattended. Perform the assessment on a bed, sofa, table with padding, crib, or changing table. To prevent heat loss, undress the infant only for weighing and measuring. Other assessments may be performed with the infant partially clothed. Abnormal findings are always reported to the primary care provider.

In several states, newborn metabolic screening must be repeated if the infant is not at least 48 hours of age at the initial screen. The tests generally include phenylketonuria (PKU), hypothyroidism, and galactosemia. Included in some screening programs are congenital adrenal hypoplasia, homocystinuria, maple syrup urine disease, sickle cell disease and other hemoglobinopathies, tyrosinemia, histidinemia, and various other screening tests.[39,60] Follow the directives of individual state statutes.

Physical assessment

Descriptive data. Weigh the infant and measure the length from head to heel. Weight loss of greater than 10% of birth weight is reportable. Head circumference (normal range, 33 to 35 cm) may be slightly altered from birth, and molding may initially decrease head circumference. Chest circumference (normal range, 30.5 to 33 cm) should be 2 to 3 cm less than head circumference.

Vital signs. Axillary temperature should register 36.4° to 37.2° C (97.5° to 99° F). Crying or excessive environmental heat will elevate temperature; exposure or environmental cooling may produce hypothermia.

Assess apical pulse (normal range, 120 to 160 beats per minute) by auscultation in the fourth to fifth intercostal space, medial to the left midclavicular line. This is the point of maximum intensity (PMI). Displacement of the PMI may indicate cardiac malposition, pneumothorax, or diaphragmatic hernia. Crying can increase the rate to 180 beats per minute; sleep can decrease the rate to 100 beats per minute. Assessing specific components of heart sounds is difficult because of the rapid pulse and respiratory rate. The first (S_1) and second (S_2) should be clear, with the S_2 being somewhat higher in pitch and sharper. Although murmurs may be heard because of incomplete transition from fetal to newborn circulation, they may also indicate major cardiac anomalies and should always be reported. Although irregular rhythm is possible in infants, it is also a potential sign of distress or major abnormality and should always be reported.

Respirations (normal range, 30 to 60 breaths per minute) are irregular and abdominal, with periodic apnea of up to 15 seconds. Breath sounds should be equal and bilateral. Grunting, nasal flaring, and substernal retracting are abnormal findings indicative of respiratory distress.[60] Auscultation of respiratory sounds and cardiac status are best done when the infant is quiet and should be counted for 60 seconds.

Head. The oval contour of the infant's head is usually apparent by the second day of life. Palpate the infant's skull to determine the presence and condition of the **fontanels** and **sutures.** The normal anterior and posterior fontanels feel firm, flat, and are easily demarcated against the skull bones. Depressed fontanels indicate dehydration. A bulging fontanel signifies increased intracranial pressure caused by crying, coughing, or a pathological occlusion of the flow of cerebrospinal fluid. Residual molding, caput succedaneum, cephalhematoma, or overriding sutures may be present after delivery. Caput succedaneum is identified as a soft swelling caused by fluid in the subcutaneous tissue of the scalp and is not limited by suture lines. A cephalhematoma is identified as firm swelling that does not cross suture lines. If a vacuum extractor was used during delivery, there may be an area resembling caput succedaneum but appearing slightly cyanotic. Abnormal findings include fused sutures and the presence of a snapping sensation along the lambdoid suture.

The eyelids may be swollen as a result of the use of prophylactic eye treatment at delivery. Normal **eyes** are symmetrical with pink conjunctiva and white sclera. There may be a subconjunctival hemorrhage caused by capillary rupture at the time of delivery. Pupils should be equal and reactive to light. Infants are able to fixate on an object held 8 to 10 inches away from the eyes and follow the object to midline. The iris is usually slate grey or dark blue in light-skinned infants and brown in dark-skinned infants.

Normal **ear** position aligns the top third of the pinna with the outer canthus of the eye. Pinnae are flexible with cartilage present. The infant in the alert or light sleep state exhibits the startle reflex when a loud noise is apparent. Some states require parents and hospital staff to complete a screening tool that identifies hearing deficit risk factors.

Infants are obligatory **nose** breathers and are unable to breathe if the nares are occluded. Hold one hand over the infant's mouth and one nostril while noting air passage through the open canal, and then repeat on the other side. This is an opportune time for the nurse to instruct the family on nasal suctioning with a bulb syringe.

Assess the **mouth** for a high-arched, intact palate and the uvula at midline. Assess tongue mobility. A shortened frenulum may cause immobility and impair breast-feeding. Check for the sucking, rooting, and gag reflexes. Mucous membranes should be pink. Thrush (a white, patchy coating on the tongue or buccal membranes) is an abnormal condition requiring treatment. If a mother has vaginal moniliasis at the time of birth, transmission to the infant's oral mucosa is almost ensured.

Thrush interferes with infant feeding, may cause candidal diaper dermatitis, and can be transmitted to the nipples and breasts of the nursing mother. [60]

Neck. The infant's neck is usually short, thick, and surrounded by skin folds. There is complete range of motion. Identify movement, shape, and the ability of the infant to exhibit some degree of head control. Palpate clavicles for the presence of crepitus, which indicates fracture. This may or may not be accompanied by brachial plexus palsy. [60]

Chest. The chest appears almost circular with symmetrical expansion. The xiphoid process is prominent. Due to the influence of maternal hormones, breasts of infants of either sex may be enlarged and exude a milky white discharge ("witches' milk") around the third day of life.

Cardiovascular. In addition to heart sounds (see the section on vital signs), assess brachial and femoral pulses for strength and equality. Color changes in the skin may indicate cardiac compromise (see the section on skin).

Abdomen. The abdomen is almost cylindrical in nature. Bowel sounds are audible with a stethoscope. The liver can be palpated approximately 1 to 3 cm below the right costal margin. A liver that is larger may indicate hepatomegaly, especially in the presence of jaundice. Occasionally the tip of the spleen can be palpated approximately 1 cm below the right costal margin, and a skilled practitioner can palpate the kidneys soon after birth. Abdominal masses are abnormal.

The **umbilical cord** is white, gelatinous, and moist at birth. The cord may still be clamped from birth. Inspect the cord for drying and if not moist, remove the clamp. Instruct in cord care and placement of the infant's diaper below the level of the cord to promote continued drying and prevent infection. Tub baths are not recommended until the cord stump falls off, usually 7 to 14 days after birth. Although some serosanguineous drainage may occur, there should be no active bleeding. The presence of erythema, purulent drainage, and foul odor indicate an infection.

Genitalia. The **female** infant at term may exhibit swelling of the clitoris and labia majora, especially with a breech presentation. A hymenal tag may be present at the posterior end of the vagina, gradually disappearing by a few weeks of age. Due to the influence of maternal hormones, vaginal discharge is usually white, mucous, and may be blood tinged

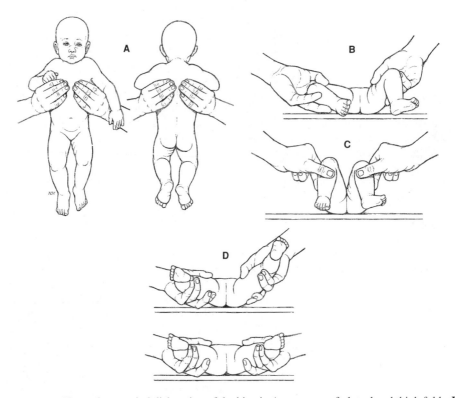

Figure 21-3 Signs of congenital dislocation of the hip. **A,** Asymmetry of gluteal and thigh folds. **B,** Limited hip abduction with flexion. **C,** Apparent shortening of femur, indicated by knee height when knees are flexed. **D,** Ortolani click (under 4 weeks of age). (Modified from Wong DL and others: *Whaley and Wong's nursing care of infants and children,* ed 6, St. Louis, 1999, Mosby.)

(pseudomenstruation). Explain to parents that this is normal and usually disappears by 4 weeks of age.

Inspect the **male** infant for urethral opening *at the tip of the penis.* The uncircumcised male has a foreskin covering the glans. Forcibly retracting the foreskin is not necessary for hygiene and may cause adhesions. Smegma, a thick white substance, may be present. If the infant is circumcised, a yellow exudate may be present on the glans. This granulation is part of the normal healing process and should never be removed. Petrolatum may be applied to prevent adherence of the circumcised penis to the diaper. Bleeding or swelling is abnormal. If a Hollister Plastibell is used for circumcision, the residual plastic ring usually falls off in 5 to 8 days. No petrolatum should be used with the Plastibell because it may cause deterioration of the plastic.

The scrotum in the term male infant is usually large and pendulous, with greater edema in the breech infant. Testes are normally palpated in the scrotal sac. Undescended testes in the inguinal canal, inguinal hernia, scrotal masses, or hydrocele are abnormal.

Skeletal. Place the infant on the abdomen. Inspect the back for any curves, masses, or openings along the spinal column. Any degree of spina bifida or pilonidal cyst or sinus is abnormal. Extend the legs to examine for symmetry and equality of gluteal and thigh folds. Inspect the anus at this time for fissures or fistulas.

Examine the extremities with the infant in a supine position. Asymmetry, limited range of motion, malformations, polydactyly, and syndactyly are abnormal. Check for congenital dislocation of the hip by techniques shown in Figure 21-3. The

Table 21-4 Infant stool patterns[39,60]

Type	Characteristics	Time frame
Meconium	Thick, tarry, dark green	Birth - 2 days
Transitional	Loose, green-brown to yellow-brown, seedy	2-5 days
Breast-fed	Mushy, golden yellow, often after each feeding, odor similar to sour milk	posttransitional
Formula-fed	Firm, pasty, yellow-brown, strong odor	posttransitional

Table 21-5 Selected infant reflexes[39,60]

Reflex	Assessment technique	Expected response
Moro's	Stimulate by sudden noise, movement, or change in position/equilibrium.	Extends and abducts all extremities; forms *C* shape with thumbs and forefingers; adducts, then flexes extremities
Palmar grasp	Place finger in palms.	Grasps examiner's finger
Babinski's	Stroke outer sole of foot upward from the heel across the ball of the foot.	Hyperextends toes; dorsiflexes great toe; fans toes outward

test for Ortolani's sign should be reserved for experienced practitioners.

Elimination. Infants void 3 to 4 times per day in the first few days of life. By the end of the first week, the infant who is adequately hydrated will void 6 to 10 times per day. Urine is almost colorless, although there may be some orange-red uric acid crystals present. Stool frequency can vary widely from one per feeding to one every few days[39] (Table 21-4).

Neuromuscular. The term infant is in a flexed posture and exhibits neither hypotonia nor hypertonia. Occasionally the infant may demonstrate trembling activity. Several reflexes are present at birth and are bilaterally equal, indicating central nervous system integrity (Table 21-5). Diminished or unequal responses are abnormal. Expect the infant's cry to be strong and lusty. Cries that are high pitched, shrill, weak, groaning, absent, or exceeding 4 hours per day are abnormal.

Skin. The skin is smooth and pink. By the second day there may be some dry and peeling areas, especially in the postmature infant. Acrocyanosis or transient mottling may occur when the infant becomes chilled. Pallor or generalized cyanosis may indicate cardiovascular compromise

and is considered abnormal. Normal variations include telangiectatic nevi, mongolian spots (especially seen in infants of African, Asian, and Hispanic descent), milia, miliaria, erythema toxicum, and birthmarks. Petechiae or ecchymoses may be present if birth was traumatic. A scalp lesion may result if an internal electrode was used for fetal monitoring.

Jaundice. Jaundice is one of the most common conditions present in infants, with incidence of 50% to 80% reported.* Physiological jaundice is caused by an accumulation of bilirubin, a product of red blood cell (RBC) breakdown. A high volume of fetal RBCs is needed to circulate oxygen in utero. At birth, natural destruction of excess RBCs occurs. The infant's immature liver is unable to remove the bilirubin as rapidly as the demand is made. This physiological process is compared with other types of jaundice in Table 21-6. Physiological jaundice can be exacerbated by ethnic predisposition (Asians, Native Americans, Eskimos), maternal medical complications (diabetes or infection), birth injury, prematurity, or hypoxia. Assess the

---

*References 2, 31, 40, 41, 51, 52.

Table 21-6 Types and characteristics of neonatal jaundice*

Type	Etiology (incidence)	Onset	Progression	Prevention/treatment
Physiological jaundice	RBC hemolysis and immature liver function (5%-80% of all infants)	After 24 hours, usually second or third day	Peaks third to fifth day, declines fifth to seventh day	Sufficient caloric/fluid intake, resulting in increased stooling. Possible phototherapy.
Breast-feeding–associated jaundice	Decreased caloric and fluid intake associated with insufficient milk production in early breast-feeding (10%-25% of breast-fed infants)	Usually second to third day	Peaks second to fourth day	Early initiation of breast-feeding. Breast-feeding 8-12 times per 24 hours. Temporary formula supplement may be required if infant exhibits significant dehydration, poor feeding behavior, lethargy, and infrequent stooling. Possible phototherapy.
Breast milk jaundice	Beta-glucuronidase in some mothers' milk, inhibiting conjugation and fecal excretion of bilirubin (1%-4% of breast-fed infants)	After 7 days	Peaks 10-15 days	Diagnosis may be confirmed by temporary cessation (24-48 hours) of breast-feeding with formula replacement. Monitor levels. Requires no intervention in most cases.
Pathological jaundice	Excessive RBC hemolysis caused by RH/ABO maternal-fetal incompatibility	Within first 24 hours	Variable	Requires medical management. Treatment related to cause. May include phototherapy and/or exchange transfusion.
	Deficient carrier protein or binding sites caused by prematurity, sepsis, hypoxia, or certain drugs	After first week of life		
	Liver/metabolic disease or malformation	Within first 24 hours		

*References 2, 31, 40, 41, 51, 52.

jaundice level by visual inspection. Jaundice appears in a cephalocaudal progression and usually resolves in the opposite direction. Use the "rules of three"[50] to estimate the approximate serum bilirubin level as follows:

- Head (3 mg/dl)
- Head and upper chest (6 mg/dl)

- Head and entire chest (9 mg/dl)
- Head, chest, and abdomen to umbilicus (12 mg/dl)
- Head, chest, and entire abdomen (15 mg/dl)
- Head, chest, abdomen, legs, and feet (18 mg/dl)

Lowdermilk and others[39] also refer to a zone determination for visual estimation of bilirubin levels.

A serum bilirubin level verifies the estimated level of significant jaundice. Because unconjugated bilirubin is extremely toxic to neurons, an infant with severe jaundice is at risk of developing kernicterus, or bilirubin encephalopathy, from the deposit of unconjugated bilirubin in the brain cells. The level of serum bilirubin required to cause brain damage is unknown.[42,60] It is imperative that the nurse assess not only the degree of jaundice, but also hydration and behavior.

Draw a blood specimen to determine serum bilirubin level by heel stick per agency protocol and medical order. Warm the heel prior to site preparation. Puncture the outer aspect of the heel no deeper than 2.4 mm to avoid osteochondritis.[60] Use of a spring-loaded automatic puncture device permits optimal depth of puncture to reach the vascular bed and provides a safer, more uniform option (Figure 21-4). A free flow of blood is necessary. Squeezing the heel or scraping it on the collection tube may cause excessive hemolysis, giving a false high bilirubin level. Apply pressure to the site with gauze until bleeding has stopped, and then apply an adhesive bandage. Use universal precautions when obtaining and transporting specimens (see Chapter 6). Protect the specimen from light during transport to prevent bilirubin breakdown (which could result in a false low reading).

Nutrition assessment. In the first few days of life, the infant may lose up to 10% of birth weight.[39] Therefore an infant nutritional assessment is an important aspect of home visits.

Breast-feeding. Due to its immunologic, nutritional, and psychological advantages, breast milk is the optimal food for infants. There are three stages of milk production in the lactating mother: colostrum (thick, yellow), transitional milk (2 to 4 days after birth), and mature milk (approximately 2 weeks post partum). Mature breast milk has a high fluid component, resembles skim milk, and provides 20 calories/ounce. Although breast-feeding is more economical than bottle-feeding, it does require adequate nutrition, hydration, and rest for the mother.

Breast-feeding is a learned behavior. To promote an adequate milk supply, the breast-feeding infant should feed on demand, 8 to 12 times per day during the first few weeks of life. Encourage the mother to alternate the breast she offers first and to offer both breasts at each feeding without time re-

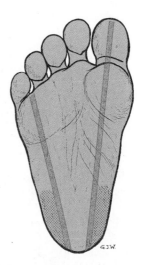

Figure 21-4 Puncture sites (stippled area) on sole of infant's heel. (From Wong DL and others: *Whaley and Wong's nursing care of infants and children,* ed 6, 1999, St. Louis, Mosby.)

striction to stimulate milk production.[37,39,47] Alternate feeding positions (cradle, side-lying, football) to prevent nipple trauma. Position the infant "tummy-to-tummy." Ensure the infant's mouth is wide open with tongue down. Check that the mother's nipple and as much of the areola as possible is grasped before latch and sucking begin. Improper latch may cause painful, cracked, and bleeding nipples (see the section on maternal assessment). Assess for nutritive sucking (characterized by coordinated suck-swallow and audible swallowing). Discourage use of supplemental bottle feedings and pacifiers in the first 2 weeks to prevent nipple confusion and refusal of the breast. Parents can gauge adequate nutrition and hydration by infant satisfaction between feedings and 6 to 8 wet diapers per day after the first week of life. Assure parents that it takes 2 to 3 weeks for breast-feeding to be established. Weight gain of at least 0.6 ounce/day in the first 6 months of life is appropriate for the infant who is breast-fed.[47]

Bottle-feeding. Bottle-fed infants are fed with a commercially prepared formula, usually recommended by the primary care provider. These formulas are available in ready-to-feed, concentrate, and powder. Assess the parents' knowledge of formula preparation and storage. Instruct parents to

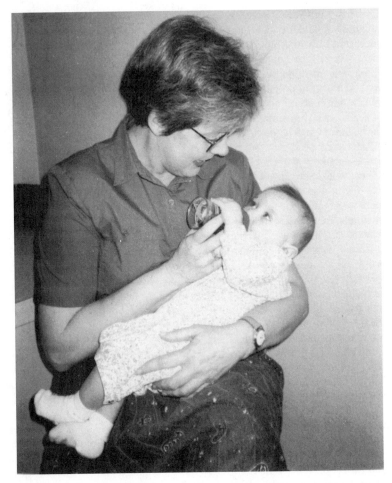

Figure 21-5 Parent-child interaction may be observed during feeding time. (Photo courtesy Robyn Rice.)

feed the infant cradled in the en face position and never to prop bottles (Figure 21-5). Infants need about 2 hours of sucking time each day.[60] Allowing the infant approximately 20 minutes to take a feeding every 3 to 4 hours will ensure sucking needs are met. Calculate the nutritional needs for each infant, based on 50 calories/pound/day and 20 calories/ounce of formula. Infants who receive formula gain 1 ounce/day in the first 6 months.[60] Instructing families about infant nutritional needs can prevent underfeeding or overfeeding. An infant who is overfed can be irritable, may frequently regurgitate, and exceeds recommended weight gain.

Suggest burping the infant at the middle and end of each feeding. The infant who cries prior to being fed or feeds too rapidly may need to be burped prior to feeding and more frequently to prevent gastric distention, excessive gas, and regurgitation.

Whether the infant is breast- or bottle-feeding, the nurse should observe and assess the following:

- Method of feeding
- Frequency of feeding
- Length of time or amount at each feeding
- Feeding reflexes (root, suck, swallow, gag)
- Environment during feeding

- Infant and maternal cue-response patterns before, during, and after feeding
- Amount, frequency, and character of regurgitation
- Type and pattern of use of a pacifier

Behavioral assessment. Assess the infant's sleep/activity pattern for the preceding 24 hours by identifying the amount of time in the sleep, awake-alert, and awake-crying states. Often parental expectations do not coincide with the reality of an infant who is "always crying." Although the duration of crying is highly variable, 1 to 4 hours per day is considered normal. Infants under 3 months of age may have paroxysmal abdominal pain (colic), a condition manifested by long periods of intense crying, drawing the legs up to the abdomen, and inability to be comforted.[60]

Consolability is the ability of the infant to self-quiet or be quieted with assistance. The level of consolability can be measured after an infant has been crying for at least 15 seconds. The infant who is difficult to console may evoke intense feelings of helplessness in parents. Wood and others[61] report that women who suffer from postpartum depression often perceive their infants as demanding and difficult and in turn see themselves as inept at child care. Identifying individual differences in consolability will help parents cope with infant crying. Does the infant continue to cry regardless of consoling maneuvers such as movement, enfolding, sounds, or sucking? Does the infant respond to minimal consoling maneuvers by caregivers? Does the infant make an effort to self-console by sucking on fist, fingers, or tongue?

Family assessment

Incorporation of a new family member is a developmental crisis, the resolution of which is facilitated by the presence of supportive others. The nurse is part of this support network. Identify family members living in the home, others whom the family can mobilize for support (parents, grandparents, neighbor, friend), and family dynamics (see Chapter 4).

Family-infant interaction. Most parents develop an expectation of their infant during pregnancy. When the reality of their infant's gender, appearance, and/or temperament does not correlate with this "fantasy" infant, bonding may be delayed

and interaction compromised. Assess both expectations and current perceptions of parents about their infant.

Communication, a reciprocal process involving a sender and a receiver, is an integral part of parent-infant interaction. Assess the parents' awareness of, interpretation of, and response to infant cue patterns. Determine the level of both verbal and tactile response to infant cues. Some factors influencing diminished parental response may include lack of knowledge, anxiety, or cultural variations. Absence of or negative parental response (demonstrated by neglecting, scolding, shaking, or striking the infant) necessitates referral to social services.

Response patterns may also be influenced by parental attitudes toward discipline and spoiling. Attitudes may be shaped by the parents' own childhood experiences, experience with other children, or by extended family participation in care. A belief that infants require discipline may predict abusive behavior. Assess discipline by observing interactions with other children in the home and/or through questions such as the following:

- Are you concerned about spoiling your infant?
- When and how do you think you will start disciplining your infant?
- What do you remember about your parents disciplining you?

Assure parents that the newborn infant cannot be "spoiled" by responding to cues.

Caution parents to avoid shaking an infant as a method to awake the infant or in attempts to quiet the infant when they experience frustration. "Shaken baby syndrome" can cause severe brain trauma or death.[60]

Knowledge of infant capabilities. Knowledge of physical, sensory, and behavioral capabilities of the infant enhances family interaction and parental development. Physical capabilities include reflexes and developmental milestones of the first month of life. Informing parents that infants interact with all senses helps them understand the need for appropriate sensory stimulation. Identify behavioral capabilities by assessing the infant's response to and interaction with the environment.

Infant care abilities of the family. Assess family members' ability to bathe, diaper, clothe, and feed the infant; to provide appropriate skin, cord, and circumcision care; and to offer sensory stimulation. In addition, determine the family awareness of health promotion and illness prevention activities. Increased infant irritability, lethargy, hypothermia, or hyperthermia, signs of dehydration, recurrent and/or forceful vomiting, diarrhea, and poor feeding are signs of illness that require medical evaluation. Make certain family members are aware of appropriate thermometer use. This is an opportune time to discuss the importance of ongoing well-child care, especially the schedule of immunizations.

Instruct the family in reportable danger signs. A handout that instructs when to call the infant's provider may be appropriate.

Adjustment to parental roles. A change in factors such as division of labor, financial status, and communication between partners can add stress to the lives of new parents. Help identify strengths and potential problems and support parents in developing effective coping mechanisms. Families experiencing financial difficulties may be eligible for federal programs (such as the Special Supplemental Nutrition Program for Women, Infants, and Children [WIC]) or for state/county programs (such as family assistance, housing assistance, or utilities financing). Be aware of available programs and refer families where appropriate. Discuss plans for the mother's return to work, including options for child care.

Injury prevention. Determine if any environmental hazards exist in the home. Accidents are the highest cause of death for children under 2 years of age. In addition to safety of the crib, car seat, infant equipment, and age-appropriate toys, it is important that the nurse counsel the family on carrying the baby, risk for choking, and sleep positioning. Stress the effects of secondhand smoke. If a family has a pet, acknowledge it may require special attention at this time. Check the home for adequate heat, refrigeration, and water and for the presence of environmental hazards. Advise a mother never to feed or sleep with her infant on a water bed because of the danger of suffocation.

Family violence. Nearly 4 million women in the United States were physically hurt by their partners in 1994.[27] Violence is not limited by socioeconomic status or race. The addition of a new family member may exacerbate an existing abuse cycle.[4,27,29] Assess for adult domestic violence, es-

pecially toward the woman, through such questions as the following:

- Are you in a safe relationship?
- Do arguments ever involve slapping, pushing, shoving, or threats with a weapon?

There may be signs of abuse detected during the maternal physical assessment. Several sources identify how to monitor these injuries.[4,27,29] Be aware of community resources and refer to domestic violence hot lines or shelters where appropriate. Laws on mandatory reporting of domestic violence vary from state to state.[29] A business card format with hot line/shelter phone numbers and a safety plan for escape (Box 21-3) is a safe, convenient way to relay this information.

Adjustment of siblings. Parents bringing home a second or subsequent child may have concerns about the impact the new infant will have on the

---

Box 21-3   SAFETY PLAN FOR VICTIM SURVIVORS OF DOMESTIC VIOLENCE

Have the following items hidden in one central place:

- Credit cards and cash
- Extra keys for car and house
- A small bag with extra clothing for you and children
- These important documents:
  - Bank accounts
  - Insurance policies
  - Health insurance cards and medications
  - Deed or lease for house or apartment
  - Marriage license
  - His date of birth
  - Social security numbers (his, yours, and children's), green card or work permit
  - Birth certificates (yours and children's)
  - List of important phone numbers (family, friends)
  - Court papers or orders
  - Driver's license or photo identification
  - Sentimental valuables
  - Children's school records

Modified from Ohio Department of Human Services, Domestic Violence Network: *ACOG Educational Bulletin No. 257,* December 1999.

family constellation. Determine reactions of the sibling(s) through observation and interview. Identify developmental stages of older children that could positively or negatively influence their adjustment. Encourage parental reinforcement of positive behaviors and appropriate limit setting when indicated.

A family copes through identifying their needs, seeking information, reorganizing their lifestyle, mobilizing their resources, and adapting to the changes in their lives. Most families exhibit strength and growth potential with the addition of a new family member. When ineffective coping exists, facilitate appropriate intervention and counseling.

Box 21-4 PRIMARY NURSING DIAGNOSES/PATIENT PROBLEMS

Maternal

- Pain, related to episiotomy/perineal laceration, cesarean incision, breast engorgement, backache, uterine cramping
- Altered nutrition: less than body requirements
- Constipation
- Risk for infection (cesarean/BPS incision, urinary tract, episiotomy, uterine, breast)
- Risk for injury (elevated blood pressure, anemia, postpartum hemorrhage, postpartum PIH, thrombophlebitis, domestic violence)
- Ineffective individual coping
- Altered sexuality patterns
- Anxiety
- Risk for caregiver role strain
- Fatigue
- Hyperthermia

Infant

- Ineffective breast-feeding
- Altered nutrition: less than body requirements
- Risk for injury (hyperbilirubinemia, heart murmur, anemia)
- Risk for infection (cord, eye, circumcision)
- Risk for altered body temperature
- Effective breast-feeding

Family

- Knowledge deficit (infant care, feeding, growth and development)
- Family coping: potential for growth

Planning and intervention

Postpartum home care programs usually include one visit. Based on maternal and infant nursing diagnoses,[58,59] patient teaching is a major intervention. (Boxes 21-4 and 21-5). Mothers have difficulty learning and retaining in the first 2 days post partum.[16,25,49] Learning occurs in incremental steps. Reinforce teaching with written materials. Select brochures or pamphlets that are culturally sensitive, appropriate to language and reading level, and specific to the needs identified. Pay careful attention to brochures written by product manufacturers. Although educational, they are also marketing tools. In addition, brief written recommendations for self and infant care ("nursing prescriptions") can help the mother recall key interventions to meet identified needs.

Families may have ongoing needs for support and/or social services beyond the scope of the postpartum home visit. In these circumstances, do not hesitate to refer to appropriate organizations or agencies (e.g., support groups for parenting or postpartum depression, La Leche League, county health departments, extended visiting programs).

Box 21-5 PRIMARY THEMES OF PATIENT/FAMILY EDUCATION

- Maternal pain management
- Maternal nutrition
- Signs and symptoms of postpartum complications
- Modification of activities of daily living to promote rest and recovery from childbirth
- Health maintenance
- Infant care
- Infant feeding (general)
- Breast-feeding
- Normal infant growth and development
- Signs and symptoms of infant illness
- Family planning
- Community resources: socioeconomic, breast-feeding support, domestic violence, postpartum depression, infant cardiopulmonary resuscitation (CPR) classes
- Identification and management of emergencies
- General self-care strategies

Evaluation

Evaluation is the final step of the nursing process. In a postpartum home care program, this can be done by a follow-up phone call 7 to 10 days after the final visit. Individual needs may require calls being made sooner or more frequently. During the phone call, ask questions to determine physical and emotional status of the mother. Areas for maternal assessment include breasts, nutrition, elimination, lochia, incision/laceration, sleep/activity pattern, and emotional needs. Areas for infant assessment include feeding, elimination, condition of cord and circumcision, and sleep/activity pattern. Assess family support and adjustment. If problems identified during the visit have not been resolved or new problems are detected, suggest additional interventions or make referrals. Ascertain that the mother and infant are scheduled to receive follow-up care via primary care providers. Terminate the relationship and document findings.

SUMMARY AND IMPLICATIONS FOR THE FUTURE

The Newborn and Mothers' Protection Act of 1996 mandates reimbursement for a minimum length of stay but fails the public in that it does not address continuing health care needs of the new mother and child. The majority of mothers and newborns will have a healthy recovery after birth. However, no one can predict which infant will have feeding problems or become septic or which mother will develop infection or postpartum depression. It is up to home care nurses to meet the needs of mothers, infants, and families, maintaining professional standards of practice while containing costs. This challenge presents an opportunity for home care nurses to expand health promotion activities of the fourth trimester.

Some insurers provide follow-up care to mothers and newborns as part of their benefits structure. Although the visit may be designated as "supportive/educative" in nature, nurses doing the visits must be competent in assessment skills should any needs be identified.

The Prenatal and Infancy Home Visitation by Nurses Program studied by Olds and others[45] in multiple sites during the past 20 years demonstrated one way to prevent low birth weight, child abuse and neglect, and recidivism for pregnant adolescents. The findings indicate that the func-

tional and economic benefits of the program are greatest for families at risk. What happens when public funding is nonexistent? How does this impact the 40-year-old primigravida who has limited support but does not fit the "qualifications" for families at risk? Nurses must be willing to challenge the status quo to meet the health care needs of families in the twenty-first century.[22]

In 1999 the Ohio Department of Health created a state-funded initiative, Welcome Home, for registered nurse visits to all primigravidas and adolescent mothers within 2 weeks of hospital discharge. Preliminary findings are positive, and the program has received additional public and private funding.

An objective of the Healthy People 2000 Initiative was to increase to at least 75% the proportion of mothers who breast-feed their infants in the early postpartum period and to at least 50% the proportion who continue breast-feeding until their babies are 5 to 6 months old. In a report recently released[57] the 1997 figures indicate those numbers are 62% and 26%, respectively, for all women, with significantly reduced numbers for low-income and minority mothers. Studies indicate that regardless of length of stay, the two most common reasons that women cited for discontinuing breast-feeding were the perception that the infant was not getting enough milk and the mother's need to return to work or school.[46] Professional support and education for mothers and infants at home contribute to successful breast-feeding.[35] If there is a hope to reach the benchmark established by the Healthy People initiative, funding must be allocated for home visits or other measures that provide lactation support.

Postpartum home care is a natural progression in the redesign of maternity care. There is a national standard of care that all women receive prenatal care in order to facilitate health promotion activities and identify complications. The majority of women do have a healthy pregnancy and birth. That same concept should be applied to the postpartum recovery period, which extends beyond a 48- or 96-hour length of hospital stay. Comprehensive evaluation by a professional registered nurse during this time would manage postpartum recovery and associated risks, as well as meet educational needs.

Home care nurses need to be proactive in establishing postpartum home care as an integral component of maternity care. Doing so would ensure the safety and well-being of mothers, infants, and families, and in the long run, promote a healthier society.

REFERENCES

1. Affonso D: Assessment of maternal postpartum adaptation, *Public Health Nurs* 4(1):9, 1987.
2. American Academy of Pediatrics: Practice guideline: Management of hyperbilirubinemia in the healthy term newborn, *Pediatrics* [online] 94(4), 1994. Available at: http://www.aap.org/policy/hyperb.htm.
3. American Academy of Pediatrics, American College of Obstetricians and Gynecologists: *Guidelines for perinatal care,* ed 4, Elk Grove, Ill, 1997, American Academy of Pediatrics.
4. American College of Obstetricians and Gynecologists: *Domestic violence,* ACOG Technical Bulletin No 257, Washington, DC, 1999, The College.
5. American Nurses Association: *Position statement on home care for mother, infant and family following birth,* Washington, DC, 1995, The Association.
6. Arnold L, Bakewell-Sachs S: Models of perinatal home follow-up, *J Perinat Neonatal Nurs* 5(1):18, 1991.
7. Association of Women's Health, Obstetric, and Neonatal Nurses (AWHONN): *Didactic content and clinical skills verification for professional nurse providers of perinatal home care,* Washington, DC, 1994, The Association.
8. Association of Women's Health, Obstetric, and Neonatal Nurses (AWHONN): Position statement: issues: shortened maternity and newborn hospital stays, *Voice* 2(5):20, 1994.
9. Association of Women's Health, Obstetric, and Neonatal Nurses (AWHONN): *Standards and guidelines for professional nursing practice in the care of women and newborns,* ed 5, Washington, DC, 1998, The Association.
10. Avery M: An early discharge program: implementation and evaluation, *J Obstet Gynecol Neonatal Nurs* 11(4):233, 1982.
11. Beck CT: A checklist to identify women at risk for developing postpartum depression, *J Obstet Gynecol Neonatal Nurs* 27(1):39, 1998.
12. Beck CT: Postpartum depression: stopping the thief that steals motherhood, *AWHONN Lifelines* 3(4):41, 1999.
13. Bennett MD: Influence of health insurance on patterns of care: maternity hospitalization, *Inquiry* 12:59, March 1975.
14. Bennett RL, Tandy LJ: Postpartum home visits: extending the continuum of care from hospital to home, *Home Healthc Nurse* 16:294, 1998.
15. Britton JR and others: Early perinatal hospital discharge and parenting during infancy, *Pediatrics* 104(5, pt 1):1070, 1999.
16. Brooten D and others: A randomized trial of early hospital discharge and home follow-up of women having cesarean birth, *Obstet Gynecol* 84(5):832, 1994.
17. Brown SG, Johnson BT: Enhancing early discharge with home follow-up: a pilot project, *J Obstet Gynecol Neonatal Nurs* 27(1):33, 1998.
18. Carpenter JA: Shortening the short stay, *AWHONN Lifelines* 2(1):28, 1998.

19. Carty E, Bradley C: A randomized, controlled evaluation of early postpartum hospital discharge, *Birth* 17(4):199, 1990.
20. Centers for Disease Control and Prevention/National Center for Health Statistics: National hospital discharge survey: annual summary, 1996, DHHS Publication No (PHS) 99-1711, Series 13, No 140, Washington, DC, 1999, US Government Printing Office.
21. Cohen S and others: *Maternal, neonatal and women's health nursing,* Springhouse, Pa, 1991, Springhouse Publishing.
22. Cox RP: Family health care delivery for the 21st century, *J Obstet Gynecol Neonatal Nurs* 26(1):109, 1997.
23. Cunningham F and others: *Williams obstetrics,* ed 20, Norwalk, Conn, 1997, Appleton & Lange.
24. DeCherney A, Pernoll M, editors: *Current obstetric and gynecologic diagnosis and treatment,* ed 8, Norwalk, Conn, 1994, Appleton & Lange.
25. Eidelman A and others: Cognitive deficits in women after childbirth, *Obstet Gynecol* 81(5, pt 1):764, 1993.
26. Evans C: Description of a home follow-up program for childbearing families, *J Obstet Gynecol Neonatal Nurs* 20(2):113, 1991.
27. Fishwick NJ: Assessment of women for partner abuse, *J Obstet Gynecol Neonatal Nurs* 27(6):661, 1998.
28. Gagnon AJ and others: A randomized trial of a program of early postpartum discharge with nurse visitation, *Am J Obstet Gynecol* 176(1, pt 1):205, 1997.
29. Gantt L, Bickford A: Screening for domestic violence, *AWHONN Lifelines* 3(2):36, 1999.
30. Gillerman H, Beckham M: The postpartum early discharge dilemma: an innovative solution, *J Perinat Neonatal Nurs* 5(1):9, 1991.
31. Grupp-Phelan J and others: Early newborn hospital discharge and readmission for mild and severe jaundice, *Arch Pediatr Adolesc Med* 153(12):1283, 1999.
32. Haupt BJ: Deliveries in short stay hospitals: United States, 1980, *NCHS Advancedata 83* 12:1, October 8, 1982.
33. Hellman I and others: Early hospital discharge in obstetrics, *Lancet* 1:227, 1962.
34. Jansen P: Early postpartum discharge, *Am J Nurs* 85(5): 547, 1985.
35. Johnson TS and others: A home visit program for breastfeeding education and support, *J Obstet Gynecol Neonatal Nurs* 28(5):480, 1999.
36. Kotagal UR and others: Safety of early discharge for Medicaid newborns, *JAMA* 282(12):1150, 1999.
37. Lawrence RA, Lawrence RM: *Breastfeeding: a guide for the medical profession,* ed 5, St. Louis, 1999, Mosby.
38. Lemmer C: Early discharge: outcomes of primiparas and their infants, *J Obstet Gynecol Neonatal Nurs* 16(4):230, 1987.
39. Lowdermilk DL and others: *Maternity and Women's Health Care,* ed 6, St. Louis, 1997, Mosby.
40. Maisels MJ: Clinical rounds in the well-baby nursery: treating jaundiced newborns, *Pediatr Ann* 24(10):547, 1995.
41. Maisels MJ, Kring E: Length of stay, jaundice and hospital readmission, *Pediatrics* 101(6):995, 1998.
42. March of Dimes: *Early hospital discharge for mothers and infants,* White Plains, NY, 1996, March of Dimes.
43. Martell LK: Is Rubin's "taking in" and "taking hold" a useful paradigm? *Health Care Women Int* 17(1):1, 1996.

44. Norr K, Nacion K: Outcomes of postpartum early discharge 1960-1986: a comparative review, *Birth* 14(3):135, 1987.

45. Olds DL and others: Prenatal and infancy home visitation by nurses: recent findings, *The Future of Children: Home Visiting: Recent Program Evaluations* 9(1):44, 1999.

46. Quinn AO and others: Breastfeeding incidence after early discharge and factors influencing breastfeeding cessation, *J Obstet Gynecol Neonatal Nurs* 26(10):289, 1997.

47. Riordan J, Auerbach K: *Breastfeeding and human lactation,* ed 2, Boston, 1999, Jones & Bartlett.

48. Ropp A, Thorn K: Historical perspectives. In *Short stay postpartum programs.* Presented at a course conducted by the Nurses' Association of the American College of Obstetricians and Gynecologists, Pittsburgh, June 1986.

49. Rubin R: Puerperal change, *Nurs Outlook* 9:753, 1961.

50. Scanlon J: *A system of newborn physical examination,* Baltimore, 1979, University Park Press.

51. Schwoebel A, Sakraida S: Hyperbilirubinemia: new approaches to an old problem, *J Perinat Neonatal Nurs* 11(3):78, 1997.

52. Seidel H and others: *Primary care of the newborn,* St. Louis, 1993, Mosby.

53. Temkin E: Driving through: postpartum care during World War II, *Am J Public Health* 89(4):587, 1999.

54. Theobald G: Home on the second day: the Bradford experiment: the combined maternity scheme, *Br Med J* 2:1364, 1959.

55. U.S. Department of Health and Human Services: *Health United States and prevention profile,* DHHS Pub No. 90-1232, Hyattsville, Md, 1990, The Department.

56. U.S. Department of Health and Human Services: *Health United States 1993,* DHHS Pub No. 93-1232, Hyattsville, Md, 1994, The Department.

57. U.S. Department of Health and Human Services: *Healthy People 2000 review: 1998-99,* DHHS Pub No. (PHS) 99-1256, Hyattsville, Md, 1999, The Department.

58. Williams L, Cooper M: Nurse-managed postpartum home care, *J Obstet Gynecol Neonatal Nurs* 22(1):25, 1993.

59. Williams L, Cooper M: A new paradigm for postpartum care, *J Obstet Gynecol Neonatal Nurs* 25(9):745, 1996.

60. Wong DL and others: *Whaley and Wong's nursing care of infants and children,* ed 6, St. Louis, 1999, Mosby.

61. Wood AF and others: The downward spiral of postpartum depression, *MCN Am J Matern Child Nurs* 22(6):308, 1997.

62. Yanover M and others: Perinatal care of low risk mothers and infants: early discharge with home care, *N Engl J Med* 294(13):702, 1976.

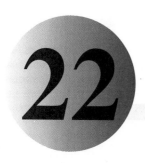

THE MENTAL HEALTH PATIENT

Patricia E. Freed

Today many individuals with chronic and acute mental illness are receiving health care in the community. Many of these individuals and their families are attempting to manage complex recovery protocols, while dealing with diminished coping abilities, financial strains created by illness, loss of significant social support, and often additional physical health problems. Medicare now reimburses for psychiatric home nursing care for patients who have a primary diagnosis of mental illness and whose care is supervised by a psychiatrist or physician. Patients must be homebound and require intermittent skilled nursing care.

Patients other than those with chronic mental illness can also benefit from the services of a psychiatric home care nurse (PHCN). Among them would be patients in crisis, those with a history of not following their treatment plan, those who require frequent hospitalization, the dually diagnosed (e.g., psychiatric illness and substance dependence), those whose symptoms contribute to isolation and decreased function, those with both mental and physical illnesses, and those who neglect to care for themselves.[29] In addition, psychiatric home care nurses could provide consultation and support to families with parenting dilemmas such as are faced when children and adolescents have developmental difficulties and delays, chemical dependence, behavioral problems, or other mental health issues.[24] The services the PHCN can provide the following:

- Assessment and evaluation of mental status
- Assessment and monitoring of medication effectiveness and side effects
- Administration of medications and management of compliance
- Assessment of family and community support systems and their effectiveness
- Basic education concerning the diagnosis of mental illness and its treatment
- Personal and family counseling
- Crisis intervention
- Social skills training
- Individual and family psychotherapy
- Assistance with developing problem-solving and daily living skills and coping strategies
- Basic health promotion (e.g., stress management, teaching principles of exercise, nutrition, sleep, safe sex, oral health, and stressing the avoidance or limited use of drugs, tobacco, and alcohol)
- Assistance and support to families and caregiver
- Referrals to community resources to maintain home independence
- Encouragement to follow-up with physician and clinic appointments in order to prevent rehospitalization
- Referrals to social service, dietitian, or occupational or physical therapy as indicated for multidisciplinary collaboration
- Supervises assistance of home care assistant
- Evaluation of the plan of care

These services are provided by the PHCN to stabilize and maintain the individual in the community.[14] The care plan, mutually established with the patient and family/caregivers empowers patients to develop their resources and take responsibility for their own life situations.

401

Ideally, home care agencies employ a certified psychiatric nurse who is experienced in working with individuals with mental illness and disorders.[28] For resources on mental illness, see Box 22-1. Home care agencies are recognizing that PHCNs can make additional contributions to the agency, including staff consultation, role modeling, prediction of nursing outcome, effective group skills, and psychoeducational and community health education and support services. However, *all home care nurses may be required to attend to the complex needs of patients experiencing mental health problems and of their families.*

All home care nurses may encounter patients with mental illness, often because many individuals have both physical and mental illnesses. For example, a newly diagnosed diabetic patient may also have an acute depressive disorder. Both physical and psychological needs should be addressed, even when the primary referral is for diabetic teaching and management. This is related to the fact that people, not body parts, experience healing. Of interest, in one study it was noted that home care nurses failed to recognize

depression in half of their homebound clients and did not plan care accordingly.[9] The purpose of this chapter is to review the two most common mental disorders treated in the home, depression (acute and chronic) and schizophrenia, and to provide information to assist home care nurses with the plan of care for these patients and their families. For consistency purposes the term home care nurse is used throughout this chapter. However, it is emphasized that patients whose primary problem is that of mental illness should receive care from a PHCN. See Chapter 19, which discusses clinical guidelines for patients who experience dementia.

PHILOSOPHY OF MENTAL HEALTH HOME CARE SERVICES

The purpose of psychiatric home care is to provide continuous and comprehensive treatment that addresses a broad range of issues, including medication and treatment, housing, education, psychosocial skills training, health promotion, and work rehabilitation. Nursing activities include home visits to provide individual and family-focused therapies that are carried out in the patient's home or residential treatment setting. See Box 22-2 for a list of possible nursing diagnoses that the home care nurse might identify.

After a nurse-patient relationship is established, work can begin toward mutual exploration of problems and maladaptive behaviors. The ability of patients to participate in such exploration may depend on the effectiveness of the medication in

---

Box 22-1   INTERNET RESOURCES FOR PATIENTS AND FAMILIES

National Alliance for the Mentally Ill

http://www.nami.org/

Informational site for patients, families, and health care workers. Sections on research, medication, diagnosis, and policy. Also suggestions about how advocates may get involved and how those with mental illness might help others.

Self-Help Sourcebook

http://www.mentalhelp.net/selfhelp/

Tons of links to support groups of all kinds. Search under a heading or by the name of the group. Information and articles about forming your own on-line support group.

Schizophrenia

http://www.mentalwellness.com

Covers lots of financial issues, how to find a support group, and a section called "Behind the Mask," in which individuals with mental illness have their achievements and contributions highlighted.

Box 22-2   PRIMARY NURSING DIAGNOSES/PATIENT PROBLEMS

- Social isolation
- Suicidal thoughts
- Medication compliance
- Nutrition, hydration, weight loss, weight gain
- Loss of interest, lack of enjoyment in usual interests
- Altered sleep patterns
- Diminished physical activity, fatigue
- Irritability, anxiety
- Feelings of guilt, worthlessness
- Poor concentration, indecisiveness

lifting the patient's mood and providing the energy level necessary to participate actively in problem solving. Because depressed patients tend to make progress slowly, any progress—however slow and tenuous—is significant. Problems such as anxiety, powerlessness, suspicion, low self-esteem, anger, negative thinking, impulse control, or egocentricity can be addressed and dealt with until success is achieved in some area. Success with one area can serve to increase self-esteem and enhance the possibility of success in other areas.

Home visits

The importance of the nurse-patient relationship has been well documented, and it is seen as the heart or essences of psychiatric nursing.[31] Relationships with the patient and family must be intentionally fostered, carefully maintained and gently terminated. Mentally ill patients often do not request home care services, and sometimes they refuse to allow nurses to enter their homes. Because they are often ambivalent about receiving home care services, the establishment of a nurse-patient relationship must begin immediately. Without such a relationship, future visits may not be allowed and the many needs of these patients will not be met.[33] Sound communication and interpersonal skills are required to establish trust and rapport. It is important for home care nurses to maintain a professional demeanor yet convey empathy and demonstrate an understanding of the patient's feelings in order to help patients and their families feel accepted and understood. The more accurately home care nurses reflect patient and family feelings, the more helpful the interactions.

Issues related to stigma, drug use, the possibility of abuse, and the potential for suicide must be addressed by all home care nurses caring for patients with mental illness. Much ignorance and misconceptions exist in regard to mental illness, resulting in fear and negative attitudes. Such stigma may prevent individuals from seeking or accepting treatment, may create feelings of isolation and victimization, and may pose barriers to hope and a positive future.[12,27] See Box 22-3 for a few tips on how to help patients and their families cope with mental illness.

Smoking, alcohol, and substance abuse must also be considered. Even small amounts of alcohol or other drugs may be dangerous for individuals

---

> **Box 22-3   LIVING WITH MENTAL ILLNESS**
>
> Identify your own feelings about having a mental illness.
> Find friends who accept you and support you as you are.
> Accept that you or your family member has an illness for which there is no blame.
> Know your rights. Workplace and housing discrimination are illegal!
> Decide what you *are* going to tell people and what you are *not* going to tell people.
> Join an advocacy group.
> Be alert and be involved at the legislative level.
> Educate others and encourage them to find out more about mental illness.

---

with mental illnesses, so no recreational use is appropriate. Home care nurses quickly recognize alcohol intoxication and substance abuse when it is associated with aggressive behavior but often overlook other behaviors such as self-neglect, burns, falls or other accidents that many indicate drug use.[23] Smoking is addicting and leads to many serious health problems such as cancer, bronchitis, and an increased risk of heart disease.[2] Nicotine in cigarettes increases the levels of dopamine in the brain, interfering with the effectiveness of many medications that the patient may be taking.[8] Pharmacological treatment (nicotine patches) and smoking cessation programs are available resources. It is believed that smoking may be a means by which the patient self-medicates negative symptoms. Varying smoking activity (e.g., increasing, stopping, and restarting) may contribute to the development of psychotic symptoms.[16] It is important to support efforts to stop or reduce smoking for general health reasons, but carefully monitor symptoms so that medication dosages can be adjusted as necessary. While assuming a relaxed and nonthreatening approach, home care nurses should ask patients about their use of tobacco, drugs, and alcohol and get a list of all of the prescription and over-the-counter medications used. Nurses should remind patients and their families that chemical dependence is a disease for which treatment is available. In fact, such treatment has been shown to decrease psychiatric symptoms, increase sobriety, and result in less frequent hospitalization.[21] Some general guidelines for talking with patients about alcohol and drug use appear in Box 22-4.

Individuals with mental illness may also be the victims of abuse. The home care nurse should be alert for any type of abuse in the home.[17] Mandatory abuse reporting laws cover children, the dependent elderly, and those whose physical or mental conditions impair their judgment or reason. Laws vary from state to state as to where reports are sent, but most social workers keep up-to-date with this information and can be consulted as needed.

All patients with a psychiatric diagnosis may entertain suicide or death thoughts and these should be assessed each visit. Predicting suicide is not always possible, but studies indicate that depression predicts suicide thoughts.[40] Males, those with a history of suicide attempts, those who abuse alcohol and/or drugs, and those recently discharged from a psychiatric hospital are at increased risk for suicide.[30] Home care nurses should be alerted to the fact that when antidepressant medications reduce apathy and fatigue, the patient may suddenly have more energy to complete a suicide plan.[11] The fear that bringing up the subject of suicide instills the idea of self-harm is unfounded. Offering patients an opportunity to discuss the subject openly and honestly may reduce tension and convey concern. Direct and indirect questions are used to make an assessment of suicide potential. The following questions are helpful:

Box 22-4   GUIDELINES FOR TALKING ABOUT ALCOHOL AND DRUG USE

Avoid stigmatizing words (e.g., alcoholic or drug addict).

Focus on the effects of alcohol and/or drugs.

Consider the individual's ability to understand.

Don't have a discussion while the person is using drugs or alcohol.

Avoid confrontation. Speak from your concern.

Encourage the individual to strive toward sobriety and/or decreased use.

Explore the relationship of drug and/or alcohol use to symptom management.

Promote problem-solving and decision making about drug and/or alcohol use.

- Are you thinking about killing yourself right now?
- Do you have a plan?
- Do you have access to the things you need to carry out your plan?
- Do you trust yourself to keep your thoughts and feelings under control?

If the patient answers yes to the first question, it is imperative to continue. Having a plan is much more serious than simply having thoughts of suicide. If the plan is vague and there is no convenient way to carry it out, the threat is probably not immediate. However, if the plan is in place, the necessary means are available, and the patient feels out of control, then danger is imminent and further steps must be taken to protect the patient. Evaluation of the plan includes considering its lethality (How deadly is the method?), its specificity (How detailed and elaborate is the plan?), and provision for rescue (How likely is it that the patient can carry it out?). These additional considerations help the home care nurse plan appropriate interventions.

Some indirect behavioral cues that may indicate that the patient is thinking about suicide require further investigation and include:

- Verbal remarks or comments about committing the act
- Giving away personal items, especially those that have been cherished for the patient's entire life
- Hallucinations
- Marked restlessness, anxiety, or agitation
- Delusions about severity of real or imagined physical illness, such as cancer
- Sudden calm or happiness in a previously depressed individual
- Purchasing a gun, going on spending sprees, or stockpiling pills

Life stressors such as a loss, stressful event, sudden change in life situation, or change in health or financial status may also precipitate suicidal behavior. Intervening in suicidal thoughts requires careful decision making and judgment on the part of the home care nurse and is usually made in collaboration with the attending psychiatrist or physician. Often, admission to a psychiatric in-patient setting is in the best interest of the patient who requires careful monitoring and safety precautions.[20]

Collaboration with family members to keep a patient safe may be an appropriate course of action if the family has been supportive in the past and can provide responsible supervision.[18,19] Removing a lethal amount of drugs from the home or preventing access to a firearm might be another intervention (a 1-week supply of medication is usually not a lethal amount). Additional interventions include:

- Making a no-suicide, no-harm contract
- Providing a crisis or hot-line number
- Referring the patient to support groups
- Return visits and telephone checks
- Counseling or problem-solving sessions

Home care for suicidal patients should focus on relieving stress, improving support, and lessening the individual's vulnerabilities.

Working with families

A collaborative arrangement with family members respects the needs of the family unit while focusing on the needs of the identified patient. Generally family members want to be involved in care and report greater satisfaction with service when they are included.[43] Family members struggle to understand the patient, find ways to influence the illness, and help the patient with the mental illness progress.[36] Understanding the concerns of families can help the home care nurse interact with families in more effective ways.

Families and friends of individuals with mental illnesses may feel angry or guilty that they cannot help the individual. It is very frustrating when the individual doesn't respond to repeated encouragement, doesn't return phone calls, and may not even get out of bed. Depression is particularly pervasive, and it is difficult to be around someone who is depressed for long periods without feeling a bit depressed yourself.

The behaviors of individuals with schizophrenia are difficult to understand. Families need support and outlets to maintain their own well-being. The home care nurse should remind family members that they cannot change the other person whose behavior is the result of an illness and that their continued attempts at interaction and encouragement do have a positive effect over the long term. Nurses should remind families that they must take care of themselves by developing other outlets, activities,

hobbies, and outside interests. Children of depressed parents should be reassured that the illness is not their fault and encouraged to express their feelings. Family members should be provided with informational resources and community support services. They should be introduced to the National Alliance for the Mentally Ill, an organization for patients, family, and professional caregivers whose mission is to support, educate, and advocate for those with mental illness. See Chapter 4 for more information about family care.

HOME CARE APPLICATIONS FOR DEPRESSION

Depression is a mental disorder that nurses will encounter frequently in home care. Depression is categorized, according to the *Diagnostic and Statistical Manual of the American Psychiatric Association* (DSM IV), as one of the major depressive disorders, a disturbance of mood not caused by any other physical or mental disorder.[1] Typical patients referred to a home care agency have recently been hospitalized with either some manifestation of depression or, less commonly, a bipolar disorder.

Etiology and pathophysiology

The etiology of depression is presently unknown. There are psychoanalytic, cognitive, biochemical, genetic, and sociocultural theories of depression; however, at present there is no overriding evidence to support any one theory. Depression occurs at all ages. It occurs more frequently in women than in men and in persons who live alone. The elderly are particularly at risk for depression secondary to medical conditions and the side effects of many commonly prescribed medications.[7,37]

Nursing assessment of depression

According to the DSM IV, a major depressive episode includes five or more of the following symptoms having been present during the same 2-week period.[1] A depressive episode represents a change from the person's previous functioning with symptoms that include:

- Depressed mood most of the day, nearly every day
- Diminished interest or pleasure in activities
- Significant weight loss when not dieting or weight gain

- Insomnia or hypersomnia nearly every day
- Psychomotor agitation or retardation nearly every day
- Fatigue or loss of energy nearly every day
- Feelings of worthlessness or excessive or inappropriate guilt nearly every day
- Diminished ability to think or concentrate or indecisiveness nearly every day
- Recurrent thoughts of death, recurrent suicidal ideation without a specific plan, or a suicide attempt or a specific plan for committing suicide

Presenting symptoms may endure for a few weeks or for long periods of time and may be intense or mild. They may be confined to a one-episode experience or occur over and over during the life of the patient.

Physical appearance provides significant information in determining the presence of depression or mania. Personal hygiene, nonverbal behaviors, and indicators of general health and nutrition should be assessed. Specific symptoms and behaviors appear in Box 22-5.

A complete physical assessment and history is taken during the initial home visit. This should include information regarding previous episodes of depression or other mental illness. A depression assessment scale may be used for this evaluation. For the geriatric patient, the Yesavage Geriatric Depression Scale (Figure 22-1) may be useful. It can be administered quickly and involves only "yes" and "no" answers, which are easier for elderly patients to follow. Because the depressed individual may exhibit signs of paranoia or cognitive impairment, the Folstein Mini-Mental State Assessment Tool is frequently useful for determining the presence of dementia[15] (see Figure 19-2). A sample patient care plan for depression is presented in Table 22-1.

Treatment modalities for depression

There are many different treatment modalities available for depression. Most commonly, antidepressant medications are prescribed for patients over 60 years of age. Electroconvulsive therapy (ECT) treatment is effective in about 80% of the cases. For some patients nonpharmacological treatments such cognitive therapy may be effective, and for others, medications can be very effective. However, patient stress and lifestyle choices con-

---

Box 22-5   BEHAVIORAL SIGNS OF DEPRESSION

Sadness, crying, discouragement, or brooding
Anxiety, panic attacks, irritability, or paranoia
Talking of feeling sad, blue, or depressed; that nothing is fun, or down in the dumps
Withdrawal from usual activities
Inability to express pleasure and loss of interest in sex
Feelings of worthlessness
Unreasonable fears
Self-reproach for minor failings
Critical attitude toward self and others
Increased or decreased body movements
Pacing, wringing hands, or pulling or rubbing hair, body, or clothing
Sleep disturbances
Weight and appetite changes
Fatigue
Preoccupation with physical health or somatic complaints
Difficulty concentrating, thinking, or making decisions
Thoughts of death and/or suicide, suicide attempts, or suicide

Modified from Buckwater KC, Stolley J: Managing mentally ill elders at home, *Geriatric Nurse* May/June 1991.[4]

---

tinue throughout life and the best treatment outcomes are those associated with combinations of antidepressants and counseling or psychotherapy. A wide variety of psychotherapeutic approaches assist the depressed patient toward recovery.

Brief psychotherapy based on Caplan's crisis intervention is an approach that is used to help home care patients effectively manage personal stressors and everyday problems, which can be overwhelming.[5] Using this approach the home care nurse determines the patient's perception of the event and helps the patient make a realistic appraisal of its impact, while exploring and strengthening coping mechanism and support systems.

Reminiscence, or life history review, is another strategy that works well in elderly patients whose depressive symptoms follow the loss of a spouse or significant other.[35] Using this approach the patient's grief is explored and support groups are encouraged.

Choose the best answer for how you felt over the past week

1. Are you basically satisfied with your life?	yes/**no**
2. Have you dropped many of your activities and interests?	**yes**/no
3. Do you feel that your life is empty?	**yes**/no
4. Do you often get bored?	**yes**/no
5. Are you hopeful about the future?	yes/**no**
6. Are you bothered by thoughts you can't get out of your head?	**yes**/no
7. Are you good in spirits most of the time?	yes/**no**
8. Are you afraid that something bad is going to happen to you?	**yes**/no
9. Do you feel happy most of the time?	yes/**no**
10. Do you often feel helpless?	**yes**/no
11. Do you often get restless and fidgety?	**yes**/no
12. Do you prefer to stay at home, rather than going out and doing new things?	**yes**/no
13. Do you frequently worry about the future?	**yes**/no
14. Do you feel you have more problems with memory than most?	**yes**/no
15. Do you think it is wonderful to be alive now?	yes/**no**
16. Do you often feel downhearted and blue?	**yes**/no
17. Do you feel pretty worthless the way you are now?	**yes**/no
18. Do you worry a lot about the past?	**yes**/no
19. Do you find life very exciting?	yes/**no**
20. Is it hard for you to get started on new projects?	**yes**/no
21. Do you feel full of energy?	yes/**no**
22. Do you feel that your situation is hopeless?	**yes**/no
23. Do you think that most people are better off than you are?	**yes**/no
24. Do you frequently get upset over little things?	**yes**/no
25. Do you frequently feel like crying?	**yes**/no
26. Do you have trouble concentrating?	**yes**/no
27. Do you enjoy getting up in the morning?	yes/**no**
28. Do you prefer to avoid social gatherings?	**yes**/no
29. Is it easy for you to make decisions?	yes/**no**
30. Is your mind as clear as it used to be?	yes/**no**

Scoring instructions: Score bold answers as 1 point
Rating: 0-9 = normal; 10-19 = mild depressive; 20-30 = severe depressive

Figure 22-1 The Yesavage Geriatric Depression Scale. (From Brink TL and others: Screening tests for geriatric depression, *Clin Gerontol* 1:37, 1982.)

The Internet also offers opportunities for support to homebound patients and may even be less anxiety provoking than attending a group meeting. Support groups have been found to decrease depressive symptoms and improve mood.[22] Both the Internet and support groups help the patient to learn how to effectively manage his or her health problems and concerns. Educational issues that should be addressed appear in Box 22-6.

Medication response

Home care nurses must carefully monitor the effectiveness and side effects of any antidepressant or other medication the patient is receiving. Determining whether patients are taking their medication is essential. If a significant other is present and willing to assume the responsibility for medication compliance, the problem may be solved. However, patients often live alone and are potentially unreliable, forgetful, or easily confused by the medication regimen set up for them. If this is the case, home care nurses must find an alternative way to help these patients comply with their medication schedule. Methods of promoting compliance include making out a plan in graphic form, filling small envelopes with the appropriate medication for each time period and clearly marking the envelope with the date and time of day the medication is to be taken, or suggesting that patients obtain a commercially produced medication box with compartments. Local pharmacies often

Table 22-1 Care plan: depression

Nursing problem	Interventions	Expected outcomes
Date: Alteration in mental status related to depressed feelings, loneliness, preoccupation with physical problems, or poor body image	Assess mental status for increased depression: Downhearted feelings Tearfulness Insomnia Altered eating patterns Anxiety Loss of interest Irritability Difficulty making decisions Lack of enjoyment in usual interests Suicidal ideations Counsel patient in ways to increase activities, ways to deal with health losses, ways to decrease social isolation, ways to assert self effectively, and ways to become less sensitive to the remarks of others Instruct patient in actions and side effects of medications Assess effectiveness and side effects of medications	By _____ (date) patient will: Verbalize that depression has lifted Have no more than two signs and symptoms of depression Identify ways to deal more effectively with social isolation Begin to use identified patterns of dealing with social isolation Acknowledge sad feelings and begin to deal with them positively Make a contract not to harm self and contact MD/RN when having these feelings Verbalize knowledge of actions and side effects of medications Take medication as scheduled Verbalize knowledge of self-care activities to handle common drug side effects (e.g., dry mouth, constipation, postural hypotension)

Box 22-6   PRIMARY THEMES OF PATIENT EDUCATION: DEPRESSION

- Medication effects and side effects; reasons for taking medications
- Missed-dose management of medication
- Information about electroconvulsive therapy
- Information about mental illness; when to call the doctor
- Coping strategies
- Grief resolution
- Suicide prevention
- Community resources
- Basic health promotion
- Social skills
- Self-care management

deliver such boxes or medication packs to the patient's home. Without medication compliance, mental health patients will almost invariably deteriorate and require rehospitalization. Because some medications take weeks before reaching peak activity levels, it is extremely important for home care nurses to monitor medication effectiveness by assessing for changes in behavior and symptomatology. In addition, patient blood levels should be monitored and the patient should be observed for possible side effects and interactions of all medications being administered.[38]

Depressed patients often discontinue medication because of the many side effects they experience. They may not believe the drug is effective, or they may believe they are cured and no longer need the medication. When patients are informed of the slow onset of therapeutic response from many drugs and given information about coping with side effects, they are much more likely to accept the prescribed regimen and follow instructions. These instructions often require frequent repetition because many patients have difficulty concentrating or may have memory problems that make learning difficult or impossible.

Home care nurses should also teach patients to manage those times when a medication dose is forgotten or when they are unable to take their medication at the regularly scheduled time. The following are general instructions for missed-dose management[44]:

- Take the missed dose as soon as possible.
- If the missed dose is remembered when the next regularly scheduled dose is due, take only the regularly scheduled dose.
- Take any remaining doses for the day as prescribed.
- Do not take double doses.

Patients must be made aware of the reasons they are taking each medication, the effects and side effects of each medication, and the consequences if the regimen is not followed. Teaching patients to associate medication times with routine daily activities (e.g., mealtimes, early morning awakening, or bedtime) can make medication taking as routine as other habits of daily life.

Patients and their families may also need information and support regarding ECT. Patients may have received a series of ECT in the hospital or may be continuing treatment on an outpatient basis. One of the primary problems of ECT is temporary loss of memory. Patients may not remember having been instructed that memory loss is usually only temporary. These patients may be very bewildered and frightened by the memory loss and need to be reminded repeatedly that it is usually of a temporary nature. Families should be instructed that after ECT, the patient is often lethargic and will require transportation to and from the treatment setting.

HOME CARE APPLICATIONS FOR SCHIZOPHRENIA

The typical patient with schizophrenia who is seen by home care nurses lives alone in a subsidized apartment or lives with an aging parent in the family home. Frequently these patients have social workers assigned to them through the department of mental health for case management. If a case worker is assigned, the home care nurse should establish contact and strive to develop a collaborative relationship. In this way conflicts and duplication of services can be prevented. Collaborative care means partnerships with patients and families and among all health care providers (e.g., medical, psychiatric, and behavioral health providers) who may be involved with the patient. Such multidisciplinary collaboration helps individuals with mental illnesses to continue to live in the community and enjoy a satisfactory quality of life. See Chapter 9 for case management strategies.

Etiology and pathophysiology

Schizophrenia is the most common and disabling of the mental disorders. It is thought to stem from some malfunction of the brain and is classified as a thought disorder in the DSM IV.[1] It might best be thought of as a group of psychotic disorders characterized by disturbances in thought, perception, affect, behavior, and communication that last longer than 6 months. There is no known prevention.

The etiology of schizophrenia is unknown. Various theories have been presented to explain the disorder. Excessive activity of neurotransmitters in the brain, particularly dopamine, have been investigated, but other neurotransmitters may play a role.[39] Structural and functional abnormalities identified by brain-image techniques have also been explored.[26] Genetics plays a role in the disorder, and family history is the only known risk factor. The disorder is found in all races and is more common in men than in women. Psychological and social factors, such as disturbed family and interpersonal relationships, may also contribute to its development.

There are no laboratory tests that provide a definitive diagnosis, and no single feature is present in all types of schizophrenia. The clinician's diagnostic judgment is based on presenting clinical features, developmental background, genetic or family history, current stress factors, premorbid functioning, and patient response to therapy. Schizophrenia usually has an onset before the age of 45, with continuous presence of symptoms for 6 months or longer, resulting in deterioration in functioning in self-care, work, and social relations. Although 25% of this population recover spontaneously, there is no cure for schizophrenia. The majority of such patients become chronically ill with symptoms that usually last throughout the life span.

Nursing assessment

Schizophrenia effects people in several ways. Like other chronic medical illnesses, it can be in remission or treatment may have effectively controlled many of the symptoms by balancing neurochemical activity in the brain. There are five subtypes of this disorder: catatonic, paranoid, disorganized, un-differentiated, and residual.

The clinical features of schizophrenic disorders include:

- Presence of psychotic features (e.g., hallucinations or delusions) during the active phase
- Characteristic symptoms effecting thought, perception, affect, and integrity
- Deterioration from a previous level of function (e.g., work, interpersonal, social, or self-care)
- Onset before age 45 (usually adolescence or early adulthood)
- Duration of at least 6 months

Thought, affect, perception, volition and integrity disturbances also occur. Both content and form of thought may be disturbed. Delusions and false beliefs despite contrary reality, may be multiple, bizarre, grandiose, fragmented, or persecutory. The origin of thoughts may be attributed to others, or they may be disowned. Events, objects, and other people may have particular and unusual significance in patient delusions of reference. The patient may be preoccupied with egocentric ideas and fantasies and withdraw from reality.

Inappropriate emotional expressions may occur or the patient may display a flat and blunted expression. Of importance, many of the drugs used to treat schizophrenia mimic the symptomology. Perceptual distortions commonly include auditory hallucinations, which are voices perceived as external to the patient. These voices are often familiar and may make insulting comments. Tactile hallucinations also occur, usually associated with a tingling or burning sensation. Other types of sensory hallucinations may occur, but their association with medical illness should be evaluated. Body boundary disturbances also occur, and it may be difficult for the patient to accurately differentiate between self and others.

Frequently there are disturbances in the patient's sense of self and motivation. These disturbances may grossly impair functioning and self-care activities and make it difficult for the patient to have the feelings of uniqueness, individuality, and self-integrity that others normally experience. The home care nurse may also recognize the disorder through patient behaviors such as withdrawal; aloofness; apathy; ambivalence; suspiciousness;

immature or impulsive emotional reactions; and episodes of destructiveness, which often create family conflicts and general family attitudes, that make it difficult for the family to form relationships and to utilize resources in the community.[34]

Treatment modalities in schizophrenia

Treatment consists of administering antipsychotic medications, which act on chemicals in the brain (blocks the excess release of neurotransmitters) to reduce schizophrenic symptoms. However, about 5% to 20% of patients with schizophrenia do not respond to medication. Many of these individuals spend their lives in and out of hospitals, suffer uncontrolled symptoms, are often homeless, and sometimes are permanently institutionalized.

Medication response

Assessment of the effectiveness and side effects of drugs is particularly important for patients with schizophrenia, who sometimes forget or disregard appointments with their physicians. It is also important for home care nurses to explore medication compliance. Positive patient attitudes toward medication have been found to be related to satisfaction with interpersonal relationships and social activities.[42] Problems may arise when the patient is taking other drugs with antipsychotic medications (Table 22-2). Home care nurses may be the only link these patients have with their physician for months at a time. They must make appropriate assessments to evaluate medication response and engage in patient and family education (Box 22-7).

One of the most frequent reasons for seeing schizophrenic patients in the home is to administer injections of fluphenazine decanoate (Prolixin) or haloperidol decanoate (Haldol) on an intermittent schedule, usually every 4 to 6 weeks. The rationale for these visits may be that these patients are non-compliant in going to the mental health center for regular injections or that they have no one who can or will assume the responsibility for getting them to the center.

Although injections are the primary purpose for home visits, nurses must assess the effectiveness and side effects of the medications that the patient is taking, making certain that no problems are emerging and that the medication dosages remain adequate to control symptoms. Frequently the home care nurse is the only health care provider

Table 22-2 Drug interactions with antipsychotic medications

Antacids	Can inhibit the absorption of the phenothiazine neuroleptics, reducing their effectiveness.
Anticholinergic drugs	Can intensify the anticholinergic effects of neuroleptic drugs, causing more dry mouth, blurred vision, constipation, and ejaculatory problems.
Anticoagulants	Can become more active when taken with phenothiazines, increasing the risk of bleeding. When given with aloperidol, anticoagulants may be less effective.
Antidepressants	In the tricyclic family (e.g., imipramine [Tofranil] and nortriptyline [Pamelor]; can raise neuroleptic blood levels, increasing the likelihood of adverse effects.
Antihypertensives	Become more potent when taken with neuroleptics. Propranolol (Inderal) and other beta blockers may exacerbate neuroleptics' cardiotoxic effects.
Bromocriptine (Parlodel)	May need to be given in larger doses to control parkinsonism-like symptoms when the patient is taking antipsychotics. By raising dopamine levels in the brain, bromocriptine, like other antiparkinsonian agents, can intensify the symptoms of schizophrenia.
Caffeine	Counteracting antipsychotic effect.
Carbamazepine (Tegretol)	Can lower neuroleptic blood levels, reducing the effectiveness of the drug.
Corticosteroids	Are more efficiently absorbed when taken with neuroleptics, making them more potent.
Digoxin (Lanoxin)	Is more likely to reach toxic levels when taken with antipsychotic agents.
Levodopa (Larodopa)	Is less effective when taken with neuroleptics, which also are less effective. Methyldopa (Aldomet), when taken with haloperidol, may cause dementia.
Morphine and other narcotic analgesics	Can make patients taking neuroleptics more drowsy and increase the risk of respiratory side effects (e.g., bronchospasm, laryngeal edema, and suppression of the gag and cough reflexes).
Quinidine (Duraquin)	Affects the myocardium more powerfully when taken with neuroleptics, increasing the risk of hypotension, bradycardia, and heart block.

Modified from Vallone DC, Stephanos MJ: Minimizing adverse drug reactions, *RN* p. 36, 1990.[41]

who sees the patient on a regular basis. Therefore it is imperative that the nurse be aware of neurological impairments that are common to antipsychotic drugs, such as extrapyramidal symptoms (EPS), tardive dyskinesia, and neuroleptic malignant syndrome.

Managing extrapyramidal symptoms. The home care nurse must be able to recognize EPS because these symptoms must be reported to the physician as soon as they occur. If the symptoms appear minor, some physicians will choose not to treat EPS, whereas others may lower the dose at the first sign of EPS. Some physicians may add an anti-EPS agent, such as benzotropine (Cogentin), to the medication regimen when EPS appears. As discussed next, EPS is usually not difficult to assess and fairly easy to treat.

Dystonic reactions are involuntary, spastic muscle movements. They may consist of sustained or intermittent muscle spasms that produce abnormal postures and contortions of the eyes, face, neck, or throat. Slower dystonic movements and postures occur when the trunk or extremities are involved. An oculogyric crisis, when the eyes roll back and up, can be a serious problem. Further developments can include life-threatening events when the tongue, neck, or pharyngeal areas become distorted, blocking the airway. The physician must be notified, and an anti-EPS agent must be given at the first sign of acute dyskinesia. Dystonic reactions usually occur a few minutes or several hours after the first dose of an antipsychotic drug.

Parkinsonism (drug-induced) reactions consist of symptoms identical to idiopathic Parkinson's disease: rigidity, postural abnormalities, slowed movements, blunted spontaneity, and tremor (especially of the hands and fingers). "Pill rolling" movements of the fingers and "cogwheel" rigidity of the arms are rather easily assessed. These symptoms occur early in treatment, usually within the first week or before the second month of beginning the antipsychotic medication. They are usually controlled by antiparkinsonian agents, such as trihexyphenidyl, amantadine, or benztropine.

Akinesia consists of a fixed and flat facial expression, a dulled speech, an apathetic manner, and lethargy or excessive sleeping. It can be confused with psychosis, organic brain syndrome, or depression. It is reversed by lowering the dose of the antipsychotic and adding anticholinergics.

Akathisia is restlessness and motor agitation. Shuffling, tapping, shifting of weight from foot to foot, or rocking may be part of the agitated clinical picture. A more severe manifestation might be running or pacing constantly or being unable to stand or sit for any length of time. It may be difficult to differentiate from signs of anxiety. Often patients can state that the movements are related to their medication. A single dose of an antipsychotic can trigger this EPS. Sometimes self-destructive behaviors such as suicide or homicide may result from severe akathisia. Confusing these behaviors with anxiety and increasing the dosage of antipsy-

chotic medication, or giving antianxiety medication, only worsens the problem. Anticholinergics can be given routinely or as needed to effectively control such problems.

Tardive dyskinesia, considered an irreversible form of EPS, should be prevented by identifying it as early as possible.[13] Chewing movements, licking and smacking of the lips, sucking, repetitive protrusion of the tongue or tongue movements within the oral cavity, tongue tremor or wormlike myokynic (twitching) movements on the tongue surface, grotesque grimaces, and facial spasms constitute tardive dyskinesia. Early signs after initiating neuroleptic drug therapy consist of facial tics, ill-defined oral or ocular movements, chewing, rocking, or swaying. Frequently, tardive (meaning late or delayed) dyskinesia appears late in treatment, often after 3 to 6 months of taking antipsychotic medications. These chronic, involuntary movements may also be observed in the extremities and trunk, with restless, agitated movement of the hands, feet, fingers, and toes. The physician must be informed as early as possible of such developments so that the offending neuroleptic drug can be discontinued while the condition is still reversible.

The most serious form of EPS is neuroleptic malignant syndrome (NMS). Approximately 1% of all patients treated with neuroleptic medications develop NMS. It has a 15% to 30% mortality rate. NMS has been described as an exaggerated form of neuroleptic-induced parkinsonism. Hyperthermia (a sudden and rapidly rising temperature) is the main signal indicating NMS, along with central nervous system symptoms such as confusion, seizures, and autonomic instability (widely fluctuating blood pressure, tachycardia, and diaphoresis). Creatine phosphokinase (CPK) is elevated. Diffuse tremor, dystonic posturing, drooling, and changes in mental status that may lead to stupor or coma may also be present. Rapid and severe muscle rigidity with difficulty moving or breathing is the final indicator of this potentially fatal syndrome. NMS often goes unrecognized by health care professionals in the community.[6] Treatment consists of immediate discontinuance of the antipsychotic medication and appropriate support of cardiovascular, respiratory, and renal functions. Home care nurses should notify the physician as soon as these indications are noted and make arrangements for closer medical supervision.

Table 22-3 Signs of relapse

Personal appearance and hygiene	Personal care, grooming, and hygiene deteriorate. Patient may lose or gain weight.
Thinking	Negative thoughts, preoccupation with death, difficulty concentrating, distraction, and auditory negative hallucinations may occur.
Interpersonal relationships	Withdrawal and avoidance of others occurs. Patient may quit taking medication, though not all relapse is a result of medication discontinuance.

Home care nursing of schizophrenic patients includes attending to their physical and psychosocial health care needs. This may require monitoring vital signs, weight, and blood sugar levels for diabetic patients; urine screening; venipuncture for any needed blood specimens; assessment and instruction concerning any bowel problems; and behavioral counseling as needed. Schizophrenia is characterized by relapse and remission. Early intervention in relapse may prevent serious disruption. Individualized triggers that would not seem catastrophic to others contribute to relapse.[34] Over time the patient may be better able to recognize signs of relapse and develop a self-monitoring proactive response.[3] Signs of a relapse may also be detected by the home care nurse (Table 22-3). Home care nurses should be aware that adequate patient sleep, nutrition, and exercise may provide a buffer against such relapses.[34]

Working with detached or withdrawn patients

Nursing care of patients with schizophrenia involves establishing an emotional bond with patients who are frequently detached, withdrawn, or hallucinating. Communication is often difficult, and patience on the part of the home care nurse is essential. Patients frequently view efforts to establish a relationship with them as attempts to deprive them of the protective facade they have built around themselves. Home care nurses must allow patients time to become familiar with them and to test their reliability while never personalizing such behaviors. Home care agencies should take this into account and consistently send the same nurse to the same patient as often as possible.

When assisting patients who remain detached to establishing relationships, home care nurses should identify the behaviors used to avoid relating and help the patients to relinquish such behaviors by helping them to see that there is no need for avoidance. Home care nurses also must identify and rely on healthy aspects of behavior presented by patients. Nurses can discover clues about what raises anxiety levels by carefully observing patients' behaviors and noting what is being discussed when avoidance begins. In this way home care nurses can then help patients to overcome anxiety and develop some success in relating to others. No one approach works for all patients, so home care nurses must be resourceful and willing to attempt innovations when original strategies fail. The belief that all patients are potentially reachable is an essential attitude for all nurses who care for the mentally ill.

Working with elusive patients

Patients who do not keep appointments, either by running away when they know their nurse is coming or by refusing to answer the door, pose another problem for home care nurses. Later the patient may or may not offer an excuse such as, "I forgot," "I had to go to my doctor," or "I didn't hear your knock." The nurse should wait for a few minutes and then leave the patient a note clearly stating when the visit was scheduled to occur, when the next visit will be, and that the patient is expected to be present and available at that time. Patients often test their nurses to see if they mean what they say and will care enough to come back. If the behavior persists, family or friends may have to intervene and assist in making sure that patients are available for visits. Home care agencies can seldom afford to allow their nurses to go repeatedly to homes only to find no one at home or no one to answer the door. Home care nurses must confront patients who miss visits about their behavior, conveying an attitude of concern and interest in understanding what actually happened. Home care nurses should express their worry and annoyance at being "stood up," presenting their own reality to the patients. Let the patient know that the behavior has affected someone else. A written contract should be established when these behaviors interfere with the provision of care. Failure to abide by the agreement results in notification of the attending psychiatrist and probable termination of services by the home care agency.

Working with suspicious/hostile patients

Suspicious patients present special problems to home care nurses because they frequently do not allow the nurses into their homes or to give them injections or make assessments. They also are very difficult to engage in any kind of problem-solving activities. Their suspicion is grounded in a persistent tendency to mistrust or doubt the sincerity or honesty of others. They are unable to consider any viewpoint valid except their own. They cannot admit that they might ever be wrong about anything. Home care nurses must approach suspicious patients with a goal of helping them learn to trust. They must very carefully define their own role in working with these individuals, because such patients tend to misinterpret words and behaviors. Home care nurses must also be very honest and extremely consistent to build trust. It is important for home care nurses to realize that any trust that does develop is fragile and can be destroyed by even a casual remark or action. Suspicious patients tend to avoid interpersonal relationships because they cannot believe another person could ever be reliable. Sometimes patients become angry, hostile, or aggressive with the home care nurse, or this may be problem behavior that occurs toward family members. Aggression may be used to intimidate or control another person or situation, or it may represent a loss of self-control, because the patient is feeling powerless and frightened.[32] Such behaviors may be difficult to differentiate when the home care nurse is unfamiliar with the patient. However, the family usually knows the patient quite well and can be helpful to clarify and differentiate patient expressions of anger. Using anger to intimidate is not appropriate, and the goal of care is to defuse it while teaching the patient more appropriate ways of getting his or her needs met. If an individual is losing control, emotional and physical distance might be more appropriate, and the issue can be discussed when the patient is calmer. In any event, the home care nurse must consider personal safety and use sound judgment about entering or staying in a home where safety may be jeopardized. A sample patient care plan for the suspicious or paranoid patient is presented in Table 22-4.

Social skills training

Schizophrenia is associated with severe and persistent disability. The home care goal is to ensure

Table 22-4 Care plan: suspicious or paranoid patient

Nursing problem	Intervention	Expected outcomes
Alteration in mental status related to suspicion and fear of interpersonal relationships	Assess mental status for signs of paranoia, violence, physical assault of others, or verbal abuse of others Counsel patient on working through fears of relating to other people and on developing an increased ability to trust other people Be honest; keep promises; do not argue or disagree; do not whisper or talk with others if the patient cannot hear what you are saying Keep the patient informed of any changes in care; give concise explanations; use a simple and matter-of-fact approach	By _____ (date) patient will: Have no episodes of violent or verbally abusive behavior Verbalize or admit to having suspicions fears of relating to other people Verbalize feelings of anxiety, inadequacy, and helplessness Verbalize learning of the ability to clarify doubts, suspicions, and possible misinterpretations of other people's motives Identify coping behaviors that have been effective in the past Express thoughts and feelings related to real life events and concerns

that physical, emotional, social, and problem-solving skills needed to live, learn, and independently work in the community have been provided. Although newer antipsychotic medication may be addressing negative symptoms (e.g., amotivation, social withdrawal, apathy, slovenliness, and anhedonia), drugs do not teach life and coping skills.[25] Most schizophrenic patients need to learn or relearn social and personal skills to survive in the community.[10] By knowing the patient within the context of his or her home environment, nurses can help patients and families select realistic health goals and develop improved social skills that are necessary for self-care.

SUMMARY

Schizophrenia and depression are two of the many mental health disorders that a nurse encounters in the home setting. No two patients will manifest identical symptoms. As inpatient hospitalization stays are reduced (e.g., because of DRG criteria; insurance limitations; or reduced federal, state, and local funding), more and more mentally ill persons are discharged to their homes in states of disequilibrium and instability. Providing home care to individuals with mental illness and their families is a greatly needed service. Many gaps exist in the current psychiatric health care system, and patients and their families can be confused, overwhelmed, or frustrated when trying to negotiate needed care and support. The psychiatric home care nurse is certainly an advocate to the patient and family and provides care that bridges traditional inpatient psychiatric services into the community. Moreover, all home care nurses may have contact with such patients and their families because home care is a very open system. Delivering services characterized by mutual trust, respect, and accountability while holistically addressing the health care needs of the individual and family is a very rewarding experience.

REFERENCES

1. American Psychiatric Association: *Diagnostic and statistical manual of mental disorders,* ed 4, Washington, DC, 1994, The Association.
2. Anonymous: Nicotine addiction, *U.S. Department of Health & Human Services Publications,* National Institutes of Health, 1998.
3. Baker C: The development of the self-care ability to detect early signs of relapse among individuals who have schizophrenia, *Arch Psychiatr Nurs* 9(5):261, 1995.
4. Buckwalter KC, Stolley J: Managing mentally ill elders at home, *Geriatr Nurs,* p. 136, 1991.
5. Caplan G: *Principles of preventive psychiatry,* New York, 1964, Basic Books.
6. Cardy S and others: Neuroleptic malignant syndrome: an assessment of registered psychiatric nurses' knowledge, *Aust NZJ Ment Health Nurs* 6(4):156, 1997.
7. Cosgray RE, Hanna V: Physiological causes of depression in the elderly, *Perspect Psychiatr Care* 29(1):26, 1993.
8. Dalack GW and others: Nicotine dependence in schizophrenia: clinical phenomena and laboratory findings, *Am J Psychiatry* 155(11):1490, 1999.
9. Dalton JR, Busch KD: Depression: the missing diagnoses in the elderly, *Home Healthcare Nurse* 13(5):31, 1995.
10. Daniels L, Roll D: Group treatment of social impairment in people with mental illness, *Psychiatr Rehab J* 21(3):273, 1998.
11. D'Arrigo T: Depression and recovery in home care patients, *Caring,* p. 42, June 1994.
12. DeNiro DA: Perceived alienation in individuals with residual-type schizophrenia, *Issues Ment Health Nurs* 16(3):185, 1995.
13. Dillon NB: Screening system for tardive dyskinesia: development and implementation, *J Psychosoc Nurs* 30(10):3, 1992.
14. Felten BS: The geropsychiatric clinical nurse specialist in home care, *Home Healthcare Nurse* 5(9):635, 1997.
15. Folstein MF: "Mini-Mental State": a practical method for grading the cognitive state of patients for the clinician, *J Psychiatric Res* 12:189, 1975.
16. Foulds J: The relationship between tobacco use and mental disorders, *Curr Opin Psychiatry* 12(3):303, 1998.
17. Freed P, Drake VK: Mandatory reporting of abuse: practical, moral, and legal issues for psychiatric home health nurses, *Issues Ment Health Nurs* 20(4):433, 1999.
18. Freed PE, Rudolph S: Protecting partial-hospitalization patients from suicide, *Perspect Psychiatr Care* 34(2):14, 1998.
19. Goldacre M and others: Suicide after discharge from psychiatric inpatient care, *Lancet* 342:744, 1993.
20. Goldblatt MJ: Hospitalization of the suicidal patient, *Death Stud* 18:453, 1994.
21. Havassy BE, Arns PG: Relationship of cocaine and other substance dependence to well-being of high-risk psychiatric patients, *Psychiatr Serv* 49(7):935, 1998.
22. Hays JC and others: Social correlates of the dimensions of depression in the elderly, *J Gerontol B Psychol Sci Soc Sci* 53(B):31, 1998.
23. Herring R, Thom B: The role of home caregivers: findings from a study of alcohol and older people, *Health Care Later Life* 3(3):199, 1998.
24. Iglesias GH: Role evolution of the mental health clinical nurse specialist in home care, *Clin Nurse Spec* 12(1):38, 1998.
25. Keltner NL: Risperidone: the search for a better antipsychotic, *Perspect Psychiatr Care* 31(1):30, 1995.
26. Keltner NL: Pathoanatomy of schizophrenia, *Perspect Psychiatr Care* 32(2):32, 1996.
27. Kirkpatrick H and others: Hope and schizophrenia: clinicians identify hope-instilling strategies, *J Psychosoc Nurs* 33(6):15, 1995.

28. Kozlak J, Thobaben M: Treating the elderly mentally ill at home, *Perspect Psychiatr Care* 28(2):31, 1992.
29. Lapierre ED, Soileau JC: In-home behavioral health services: establishing a program, *Caring* 14(7):7, 1995.
30. Litman RE: Predicting and preventing hospital and clinic suicides, *Suicide Life Threat Behav* 21:56, 1991.
31. McElroy E: Uncovering clinical knowledge in expert psychiatric nursing practice (Doctoral dissertation, University of Alabama at Birmingham), *Dissertation Abstracts International,* 52(03),1355B, 1995.
32. Missouri Department of Mental Health: *Basic family guide to schizophrenia,* Jefferson City, Mo, 1991, Division of Comprehensive Psychiatric Services and the Office of Public Affairs.
33. Murphy MF, Moller MD: Relapse management in neurobiological disorders: the Moller-Murphy symptoms management assessment tool, *Arch Psychiatric Nurs* 7(4):226, 1993.
34. Palmer-Erbs VK, Anthon WA: Incorporating psychiatric rehabilitation principles into mental health nursing, *J Psychosoc Nurs* 33(3):36, 1995.
35. Rife JC: Clinical comments: use of life review techniques to assist older workers in coping with job loss and depression, *Clin Gerontol* 20(1):75, 1998.
36. Rose LE: Gaining control: family members relate to persons with severe mental illness, *Res Nurs Health* 21(4):363, 1998.
37. Shua-Haim JR and others: Depression in the elderly, *Hosp Med* 33(7):44, 1997.
38. Smith M, Buckwalter KC: Medication management, antidepressant drugs and the elderly: an overview, *J Psychosoc Nurs Ment Health Serv* 30(10):30, 1992.
39. Spitzer VM: Biological aspects of schizophrenia, *JAPNA* 1(6):204, 1995.
40. Uncapher H and others: Suicidal thoughts in male nursing home residents, *Ann Long Term Care* 6(10):301, 1998.
41. Vallone DC, Stephanos MJ: Minimizing adverse drug reactions, *RN* p. 36, 1990.
42. Van Dongen CJ: Attitudes toward medications among persons with severe mental illness, *J Psychosoc Nurs* 35(3):21, 1997.
43. Whelton C: Involving families in psychosocial rehabilitation, *Psychiatr Rehab J* 20(3):57, 1997.
44. Zind R and others: Educating patients about missed medication doses, *J Psychosoc Nurs Ment Health Serv* 30(7):10, 1992.

23

THE ELDERLY PATIENT

Gail F. Wilkerson

The provision of quality care for older adults is challenging our society. The increasing number of older adults requiring diverse health care services necessitates the development of cost-effective, quality care.[31] More and more older adults are deciding to live at home even though many of them have chronic health problems that require assistance. Four out of 10 persons 65 years of age or older require assistance, and the need for home care assistance increases with age.[22]

The high cost of health care and a desire for independence are two primary factors that influence the older adult's decision to remain at home as long as possible. In addition, the demands for home health care are growing in response to the diagnostic-related groups (DRGs) and managed care groups, which encourage shorter hospital stays and provide limited reimbursement for acute care services.

The purpose of this chapter is to provide information that will assist home care nurses in developing a plan of care for older adults. Included in the chapter are a profile of the elderly population, a review of the normal physiology of aging, a description of the characteristics of elderly patients receiving home health care services, and an examination of patient care issues relevant to the needs of older adults.

DEMOGRAPHICS
Age

Persons 65 years of age or older represent 12.7% of the U.S. population.[14] The number of older adults has increased by 10% since 1990, compared to an increase of 8% in the under-65 population. The most rapid increase can be expected between the years 2010 and 2030, when the baby boom generation reaches age 65.[12] By the year 2000 approximately 13% of the population will be 65 years of age or older; this percentage may climb to 20% by 2030.[14]

In addition, during the twentieth century the average life span for Americans rose from 47 years to 76 years.[14] In other words, a child born in 1997 can expect to live 76.5 years, about 29 years longer than a child born in 1900.[8,14]

Living arrangements

The majority (67%) of noninstitutionalized older persons live with family members[14]; only 31% live alone. The percentage of older persons living in nursing homes dramatically increases with age. At present approximately 5% of persons 65 years of age or older, 6% of persons from 75 to 84 years of age, and 20% of persons 85 years of age or older are living in nursing homes.[14]

The elderly population is less likely to change residence than other age groups. Twenty-eight percent of older persons live in inner cities, whereas 49% live in suburbs.[14]

Income

The median income of older persons is $18,166 for men and $10,504 for women. Approximately 14% of family households with a person 65 years of age or older have incomes of less than $15,000; 63% of these households have incomes of $25,000 or more. The incomes of 10.5% of the elderly population are at or below the poverty level.[14]

Housing

Seventy-nine percent of the elderly population own their own homes, and 21% are renters.[14] The housing of elderly Americans is generally older and less adequate than that of younger age groups, and structural problems are common.[3]

Employment

Employment status does not often change for individuals after the age of 65. Twelve percent of older Americans (3.6 million) are in the labor force; this constitutes 2.8% of the U.S. labor force.[14]

Education

The length of formal education of the older adult population is increasing; between 1970 and 1998 the percentage who completed high school rose from 28% to 67%. The percentage varies with race and ethnic origin: 69% of whites, 43% of African-Americans, and 30% of Hispanics.[14]

PHYSIOLOGY OF AGING

Many physiological functions decline at a rate of approximately 1% per year after age 30.[2] A decline in any one major organ system such as the cardiovascular, respiratory, or genitourinary system is not always significant. It is the gradual deterioration of several organ systems that typically affects the functional ability of the older individual.

Goldstein[19] defines aging as "a progressive unfavorable loss of adaptation and a decreasing expectation of life with the passage of time that is expressed in measurement as decreased viability and increased vulnerability to the normal forces of mortality." Age-related functional loss follows several patterns. A function can be totally lost, as is the female reproductive ability, or a function can be retained with an altered level, as occurs with musculoskeletal disease or kidney changes. As age-related changes occur, some people develop chronic problems and therefore become more vulnerable to illness.

For home care nurses to accurately assess an older person, it is important that they have a clear understanding of how the human body ages.

Cardiovascular

With age the heart loses elasticity; therefore decreased contractility and cardiac output occur in response to increased metabolic demands.[43] Increased systolic and diastolic blood pressure result from increased peripheral resistance and pulse pressure. These changes in cardiac output and peripheral resistance cause a decrease in organ perfusion. By age 80 renal blood flow is reduced by half and cerebral blood flow by 20%.[2] Electrical changes produce a decrease in the heart rate and an increase in premature beats. The heart rate during rest changes little with age. Pedal pulses may be weaker as a result of arteriosclerotic changes. Lower extremities may be cool to the touch and appear mottled on inspection.

Respiratory

A decrease in pulmonary blood flow and diffusion is found in older adults. Respiratory accessory muscles undergo degeneration that results in decreased muscle strength. The maximum breathing capacity, vital capacity, residual volume, and functional capacity all diminish with age.[2] Airway closure occurs at higher tidal volumes in an older adult. Ventilation is less than adequate in dependent lung regions where perfusion is greatest. As a result, a decrease in PaO_2, the amount of oxygen in the blood, would be associated with a significant decrease in oxygen delivery in someone over age 60.[34] Respiratory disorders such as chronic obstructive pulmonary disease (COPD) or emphysema put an elderly patient at greater risk for hypoxemia than a younger patient (see Chapter 11).

Integumentary

The amount of subcutaneous adipose tissue decreases with age, resulting in poor thermal insulation. Extremities are cooler, and perspiration decreases. There is less fat distributed on the extremities and more on the trunk. Epidermal sweat glands and hair follicles atrophy, pigmentation increases unevenly, and the supporting collagen and elastin degenerate. These changes cause discolored, thin, dry, and wrinkled skin.[48] Senile purpura and senile keratosis are common. Such changes in the integument, along with poor peripheral circulation, predispose the elderly population to tissue breakdown and the formation of dermal wounds (see Chapter 14).

Hair color may be dull gray, white, yellow, or yellow-green. Hair distribution thins on the scalp, axillae, pubic area, and all extremities. Nail growth slows with age; nails become hard, thick, and brittle and are difficult to keep groomed. Insufficient calcium may make fingernails and toenails turn yellow. Older adults often need to be referred to a podiatrist because they are unable to reach their feet, see their feet, or manipulate clippers to cut the nails.

Genitourinary

The glomerular filtration rate (GFR) and kidney mass decrease with age. By age 80 the GFR declines by 50%, and creatinine clearance declines by 33% compared with age 50.[24] Men may have increased micturition as a result of prostatic enlargement. Women have a decrease in perineal tone and therefore may have urgency and stress incontinence (see Chapter 16).

Reproductive

In older males testosterone production decreases, the phases of intercourse are slower, and there is a lengthened refractory time. No changes are seen in libido and sexual satisfaction. Testes decrease in size, sperm count decreases, and seminal fluid has a diminished viscosity.

Female estrogen production decreases with menopause, and breast tissue diminishes. The uterus decreases in size, and mucous secretions cease. Uterine prolapse may occur as a result of muscle weakness.

Gastrointestinal

Chewing may be impaired due to partial or total loss of teeth, malocclusion, or ill-fitting dentures.[21] Swallowing may be more difficult due to diminished salivary secretions.[16] A decrease in esophageal peristalsis may cause an increased incidence of hiatal hernia with gaseous distension. Digestive enzyme production is decreased, and fat absorption is delayed, affecting the absorption rate of fat-soluble vitamins A, D, E, and K. Intestinal peristalsis is reduced, causing a decrease in motility and, as a result, constipation. Gastric emptying is markedly slower in older persons. Some studies report that transit time for a liquid meal in elderly persons is more than double that in young adults.[42]

Musculoskeletal

Muscle strength and function decrease with loss of muscle mass. Bone structure is more porous but maintains normal demineralization. Connective tissue increases in density and contains less water as a person becomes older. Joints are less mobile, and tightening and fixation occur.[17,20] Physical activity will delay loss of function. Posture changes with age, and kyphosis is often seen. Normal height decreases 1 to 3 inches from that in young adulthood.

Neurological

The majority of the elderly population have normal cognitive function in learning, memory, and abstract thinking.[20] A common concern of the aged is forgetfulness, which becomes a problem when it interferes with the performance of activities of daily living.[33] It has been found that an elderly person may take longer to learn and remember new information but is capable of doing so.[1,20]

Slowing is one of the most significant nervous system changes.[23] This affects learning new information, motor tasks, and reaction to multiple stimuli. Activities that show a functional decline include getting up from a chair, writing rapidly, and buttoning or zipping clothing.[23]

Proprioception is less efficient with age. As a result the elderly person often demonstrates a gait change, such as a Parkinson-like gait. Gait changes, combined with reduced position sense, complicate the older person's ability to maintain balance.

Sleep patterns

With age there may be a decrease in the total hours slept. This is caused by an increase in the number of nocturnal awakenings and an overall decrease in sleep efficiency. Sleep becomes fragmented as brief or complete awakenings occur, causing the older person to spend more time in bed awake. Frequent complaints of the older person are insomnia and disrupted sleep.

Sensory

All senses gradually decline with age. Sight, hearing, taste, tactile sensitivity, and perception of vibration all diminish because of anatomical changes.

As the eye ages, structural and functional changes take place. The eyelids atrophy and become wrinkled. The lenses lose elasticity and frequently become opaque and cloudy, causing cataracts and a sensitivity to glare.[4] Changes in the iris and pupil slow down the ability to adapt to darkness. Sclerosis of the iris causes the pupils to become smaller, which limits the amount of light reaching the retina.[2] Many older adults find it difficult to drive at night because of a visual inability to adapt to darkness and bright lights. A decrease in lacrimation (tearing) causes many older people to complain of dry eyes.

The four most common diseases that affect vision are cataracts (opacity of lens), macular degeneration (retina), glaucoma (increased intraocular pressure), and diabetic retinopathy.[2] Conditions that should be reported to the physician are blurred vision, double vision, changes in pupil color, a film over the eye that does not go away with blinking, and frequent changes in the prescription for corrective lenses.

Hearing and vestibular function normally decrease with age. Significant hearing impairments are found in 90% of nursing home residents and 30% of the ambulatory noninstitutionalized elderly population.[2]

Gustatory sensation has a diminished acuity because the tongue papillae and taste buds decrease in number with aging. These changes can result in a change in taste and loss of appetite, which may lead to inadequate nutrition.

Tactile sensitivity for touch and pain decreases with age, and the ability to detect vibration is reduced, especially in the feet. These changes are thought to be a result of slowed peripheral nerve conduction and central conduction of peripheral impulses associated with aging.

Understanding the normal aging process and how it may interfere with activities of daily living will improve home care nurses' abilities to identify significant changes in the condition of their patients. Knowledgeable nurses will readily recognize changes in the patient's status that should be communicated to the physician and incorporated into the plan of care.

THE ELDERLY HOME CARE PATIENT

To develop a realistic and meaningful plan of care, home care nurses should be familiar with the health characteristics of elderly patients admitted to home care services.

Van Ort and Woodthi[52] studied 66 elderly patients admitted to home care to determine the home care patient/caregiver characteristics and to iden-

tify the nursing needs of these patients. In their study 70% of the home care patients were women from 70 to 89 years of age, 50% of whom were married. A majority (80%) of the patients were living with a caregiver; only a small number (14%) were living alone. Patients received home care an average of 19 days, having approximately three health-related visits a week.

This study also identified the most frequent medical and nursing diagnoses for elderly home health patients; 75% of the primary medical diagnoses fell into four categories: orthopedic, cardiovascular, diabetes, and pulmonary-related. This corresponds with Fowles's list of the most common ailments found in the noninstitutionalized elderly population.[14] See Box 23-5, which lists nursing diagnoses related to the geriatric client.[26]

This study is significant because it reflects the health care problems found most frequently among the elderly—problems related to dementia, nutrition, immobility, polypharmacy, and safety. These problems represent the patient care issues that home care nurses should consider in designing and implementing plans of care that promote symptom management and enhance patients' return to optimal health.[52]

PATIENT CARE ISSUES IN THE HOME SETTING
Dementia

As many as 10% to 15% of persons over the age of 65 may have cognitive impairment.[2,6] Once a dementia is recognized, the cause or type should be determined. Dementia is a clinical syndrome characterized by a decline from a previous level of intellectual function.[51] It has many different causes. True cognitive impairment or dementia takes place when there is deterioration in at least three of the following: cognition, memory, language, recognition, visual spatial skills, and personality.[2,28] Some illnesses that cause dementia can be stopped or reversed, but the illnesses most frequently associated with dementia are not reversible.[51]

Four common treatable causes of dementia in the elderly are (1) drugs, (2) hypothyroidism and other metabolic conditions, (3) destructive or mass lesions of the central nervous system, and (4) depression.[25,30] The most common untreatable type is dementia of the Alzheimer's type (DAT), which is present in 65% to 75% of the patients seen in dementia clinics.[51] A diagnosis of DAT is based on four criteria[3]: (1) global cognitive dysfunction that interferes with daily activities, (2) gradual onset, with symptoms lasting for 6 months or longer, (3) progressive deterioration over time, and (4) lack of strong evidence for another illness causing the dementia.

Nurses caring for elderly patients need to recognize the difference between dementia and delirium, both of which occur frequently in the elderly. Delirium is characterized by a sudden change in the level of consciousness and is therefore a cognitive change. It is usually associated with an acute illness. Fever, hypoxemia, and other metabolic dysfunctions associated with acute illness can affect consciousness or mental state, thereby producing delirium.

Frequently dementia and depression are both present in elderly people at the same time.[35] It is difficult to distinguish between depressed elderly individuals and those with a true dementia, but there are some differences. Depressed patients are dysphoric, with mild or no cognitive impairment.[44] The onset of depression is often abrupt, and the patients frequently have a history of affective problems. Patients with dementia are less aware of cognitive problems, have a more gradual onset of symptoms, and have serious deficits in memory, thinking, judgment, and problem-solving abilities.[54] Such deficits eventually lead to these patients being totally dependent on others for care.[13]

The care of a patient with an illness causing dementia is complex and requires a multidisciplinary approach that considers the needs of both the family and the patient. Few people with chronic illnesses such as Alzheimer's disease receive in-home nursing care.[10] Therefore home care nurses assist these patients intermittently when acute health problems occur (Box 23-1). (For further information about Alzheimer's disease and depression refer to Chapters 19 and 22.)

Nutrition

Because aging is associated with a decline in body function, nutrition is also affected. People age at different rates and to different extents, but the effects on body functions appear similar. The ability to digest food and use nutrients depends on the range of age-related changes in the body. Morley and Silver[38] list five factors that affect the nutritional status of the older adult: (1) social factors, (2) psychological factors, (3) physical factors, (4) anorexia of aging, and (5) disease.

Social factors that affect eating behaviors include poverty, problems with food shopping and preparation, and lack of socialization at mealtime. It sometimes is assumed that the reason older adults eat inadequately is lack of knowledge about nutrition, but often the reason is poverty. Older persons may skip meals, eat pet food, and exist on snack foods because they have limited financial resources. Lack of transportation and physical impairment may also interfere with their ability to buy and prepare food. Because 30% of the elderly population live alone, there is often a decreased interest in preparing nutritious meals. Socialization at meals enhances the intake of a well-balanced diet.[42]

Bereavement and depression are psychological factors that may affect nutrition in the elderly person. It is estimated that one third of people over age 60 have a depressed mood.[15] When people are sad, blue, or depressed, they often lose interest in eating and may lose weight without trying. Decreased appetite is a very common symptom of depression.[47]

Physical conditions that affect eating behavior are immobility, inability to feed oneself, and diffi-

---

Box 23-1   DEVELOPING A PLAN OF CARE FOR THE DEMENTIA PATIENT/CAREGIVER AT HOME

- Provide ongoing education about the disease process.
- Identify effective techniques that assist patients/caregivers with day-to-day tasks.
- Assist patients and families with behavioral management strategies that facilitate appropriate behavior.
- Locate community resources that assist with respite care and long-term care decisions, especially for the patient living alone.
- Provide ongoing emotional support for patients/caregivers.
- Identify safety issues, such as environmental modifications.
- Assume a case management role as the patient advocate.

culty chewing. It has been found that nutritional intake is related to dentition and self-perceived chewing problems.[45] Persons who believe they have a chewing problem will eat less and therefore have a decreased intake of protein and calories and an increased carbohydrate intake.[21] Some carbohydrates are softer and more tolerable than proteins.

Factors that contribute to anorexia or weight loss with aging are decreased basal metabolic rate, hunger, and feeding drive. Not only do older people have a decreased metabolic rate, but also they become physically less active. Deterioration of taste, smell, and visual acuity may cause older adults to lose pleasure in eating. There is a natural decline in gastric secretions with age, and as a result digestion is less efficient. A change in gastric hormones affects the drive to eat.[33,42] The gastrointestinal tract sends messages to the central nervous system that cause a feeling of fullness when food passes through the intestines.

The most extreme changes in nutritional status in older adults are caused by diseases. For example, with dementia, memory deficits affect the amount of food eaten, and therefore weight loss is common.[11] Patients with dementia are at increased risk for malnutrition because of indifference (they do not care about eating), memory loss (they cannot remember if they have eaten), and impaired judgment (they do not recognize the need to eat). Many elderly patients are dependent on others for providing adequate nutrition, and their needs are not always met.

Meeting the nutritional needs of the elderly is complicated by individual differences in aging and by the roles played by social, psychological, and physical factors in each patient's lifestyle. A thorough assessment of a patient's food intake is necessary to determine caloric and nutritional status. This assessment should include medical, social, nursing, and dietary histories and a physical examination. Home care nurses should be aware of normal aging changes that may mask themselves as a nutrient deficiency. Patients are at nutritional risk when they have three or more of the warning signs listed in Box 23-2.[37]

Immobility

Impaired physical mobility is a state in which the individual experiences a limitation of the ability for

---

Box 23-2	WARNING SIGNS OF POOR NUTRITIONAL HEALTH

- Disease
- Eating poorly
- Tooth loss/mouth pain
- Economic hardship
- Reduced social contact
- Multiple medicines
- Involuntary weight loss/gain
- Assistance needed in self-care
- Age above 80 years

---

independent physical movement.[26] Most diseases and rehabilitative states involve some degree of immobility. Approximately 30% of those 85 years of age or older have extreme limitations in the activities of daily living.[29] These limitations are of major significance to the health care system.

Alteration in mobility may be short-lived or chronic. A patient who is hospitalized because of an acute medical problem is at risk for developing a chronic problem as a result of the hazards of immobility. Observable signs and symptoms of immobility are associated with many different acute health conditions (see Chapter 17).

The hazards of immobility affect all people with impaired physical mobility, but older adults are at increased risk. Age and disease affect functional reserves, and more energy is needed to maintain functional status as capabilities and resources decline.[4] Many organ systems are affected by decreased mobility.[32] These systems and the effects of immobility are listed in Table 23-1. The hazards of immobility make it important for home care nurses to maximize mobility within the limits of the patient's condition.

Mobility is potentially the most important factor in assessing the independence of the elderly and their needs for health care.[4] Restricted ability to move affects the performance of all other tasks. The ultimate nursing goals are maintenance of mobility and prevention of impairment.[7]

When selecting interventions for a patient who has limited mobility, the nurse needs to consider three things: (1) the condition that caused the disability, (2) the medical restrictions on activity, and

Table 23-1 Hazards of immobility

Body system	Hazard
Skin	Skin breakdown
Musculoskeletal	Muscle weakness
	Increased immobilization
	Backache
	Joint stiffness
	Disuse osteoporosis
Cardiovascular	Increased workload of heart
	Orthostatic hypotension
	Thrombus formation
	Peripheral edema
Respiratory	Decreased chest expansion
	Stasis of secretions
	Pneumonia
	Carbon dioxide narcosis
	Respiratory acidosis
Renal	Difficult urination
	Urinary stasis
	Renal calculi
Gastrointestinal	Constipation
	Fecal impaction
Psychological	Depression
	Boredom

(3) the individual's abilities and limitations.[44] Risk factors also should be taken into consideration when instituting a plan of care. Risk factors associated with immobility in the elderly population include contractures, severe dementia, poor vision, hip or leg fractures, and environmental safety hazards.[37,49]

Polypharmacy in a shoe box

Of all prescription drugs ordered, 25% are for the elderly.[11] Because many elderly people have at least one chronic health condition, they are more likely than other age groups to be taking multiple medications. This makes them highly susceptible to adverse drug reactions caused by multiple drug use, which is the most common reason for such reactions. Adults over the age of 65 are twice as likely as other age groups to have an abnormal response to medication.[36]

The problem of adverse reactions is often compounded by improper management and administration of medications at home. Self-medication errors and subsequent adverse reactions may be related to

(1) methods of storage or organization in which both current and out-of-date medications are stockpiled in shoe boxes, bowls, paper bags, or dresser drawers, (2) impaired visual acuity and memory associated with aging, (3) a knowledge deficit regarding the action of medication and need for adherence to medication, (4) multiple physicians ordering multiple medications, and (5) lack of financial resources to purchase medications.

Numerous age-related physiological changes affect the absorption, distribution, and metabolism of medications. These changes may alter the reaction to medication and influence the type and dosage of medication prescribed by physicians.

A decline in gastric acid secretions and motility affects the rate at which drugs are absorbed.[27] Medications that rely on acid in the stomach for dissolving often do not produce the expected therapeutic response in older adults.

Distribution to tissues is less effective because of changes in cardiac output that affect circulation. An increase in body fat compared with total body mass causes drugs to build up in the adipose tissue. Therefore drugs are active longer as a result of slower distribution throughout the body.[36]

Metabolism, detoxification, and excretion of medications are altered by age-related changes in the kidney and liver. Decreased glomerular filtration rate, tubular reabsorption, and cardiac function lead to a less efficient kidney. Medications are not filtered as rapidly and are present in the body longer. The time it takes for drugs to be excreted is almost doubled with advanced age.[36] Decreases in the size and function of the liver alter the enzyme system. The detoxification of drugs declines, causing medications to remain in the bloodstream longer.

To avoid adverse reactions and yet achieve therapeutic levels, elderly patients usually require lower doses of medication. Since no two individuals are alike, drug response will vary. All home care nurses should keep current on the use and side effects of medications. There are many risks associated with drug therapy in older adults, and the benefit from drug therapy should outweigh any problems a drug may induce.

The initial home care visit should include a thorough nursing assessment of drug use in the elderly patient. (See the home care application section later in this chapter.) From this assessment the nurse can develop a plan of care that promotes safety and prevents noncompliance in medication use. This plan should include ongoing patient education and assessment of medication administration, tolerance, and effectiveness.

Safety

Risk for injury is a nursing diagnosis that should routinely be considered with an elderly individual requiring home care assistance. This is defined as "interactive conditions between individual and environment which impose a risk to the defensive and adaptive resources of the individual."[26]

The elderly are more susceptible to accidents, falls, and elder abuse as their capabilities diminish.[39,41] Internal and external factors work together to influence this susceptibility. Among these are biological factors such as sensory dysfunction, physiological factors such as immobility, and increased demands on caregivers related to growing older.[50] Deficits of sight, hearing, equilibrium, and reaction time[10] (all of which predispose older adults to accidents) may be a result of aging, disease, or a side effect of medication. Specific accidents common among the elderly are related to fire, carbon monoxide poisoning (from a faulty heating system), medication reactions, drowning, and auto use.[12] The elderly have a high rate of hospital admission and death as a result of trauma.[12] Prevention of accidents can be enhanced by a comprehensive assessment of the home situation. Escher and others[12] describe a mnemonic, ACCIDENTS, to help home care nurses assess the older adult's risk for an accident in the home (Box 23-3). This assessment may lead to interventions that range from simple oral or written reminders to suggestions for changing a person's lifestyle. The family and/or caregiver should be included in the plan of care to prevent accidents in the home.

Falls are the leading cause of death from injury in persons older than 65.[44] Although the majority of falls do not cause sufficient injury to require medical attention, serious injury from falls is significant. Approximately 250,000 hip fractures per year occur among persons 65 years of age or older, with an annual cost of $7 billion.[25] The people who fall most often are those who have multiple medical impairments or functional disabilities. These individuals

---

> **Box 23-3 ASSESSMENT OF POTENTIAL RISKS FOR ACCIDENTS IN THE HOME**
>
> **Accidents**
> A = Activities of daily living (level of function)
> C = Cognition, emotional state (memory, depression)
> C = Clinical findings (health history)
> I = Incontinence
> D = Drugs (complete inventory)
> E = Eyes, ears, environment (sensory deficits)
> N = Neurologic deficits (gait, balance)
> T = Travel history (driving ability)
> S = Social history (alcohol, drug)

From Escher JE and others: Typical geriatric accidents and how to prevent them, *Geriatrics* 44:54, 1989. Reprinted with permission.

---

should be identified in the plan of care as being at risk for falls.[7,29] The risk of falling is greater among older adults who have decreased abilities and are taking a number of medications. Other factors that may indicate a risk of falling are confusion, corrective lenses, nocturia with urgency, weakened or impaired gait, the use of assistive devices, and a history of falls.[7,34] The patient who uses furniture or railings for support, has poor balance, or requires assistance when rising from a chair is assessed by the nurse as having impaired gait. By thoroughly and accurately assessing the patient's status on the initial home visit and pursuing the appropriate safety measures, home care nurses can identify characteristics and physiological changes that place a patient at risk of falling and implement measures to prevent falls.[7] The mnemonic ACCIDENTS may assist home care nurses in assessing functional ability and safety in the home.

Elder abuse represents a shocking and still largely hidden phenomenon affecting hundreds of thousands of our nation's most helpless and vulnerable citizens.[5,15] It crosses all classes of society and occurs in large urban areas and small towns.[36] Estimates suggest that between 500,000 and 2.5 million elderly people in the United States are victims of abuse, neglect, exploitation, or abandonment each year.[31] Because the abused elderly are reluctant to admit that their children, their loved ones, or those entrusted with their care have mistreated them, only one out of every six cases is ever reported.[31] Home care nurses who are knowledgeable about signs and symptoms of elder abuse can assist in providing a safe, clean environment and protection from those who are not genuinely concerned about the health and best interests of the older adult.[33]

Neglect is a situation in which a caregiver intentionally or unintentionally fails to some degree in providing care for an individual. Signs that could be suggestive of neglect are alterations in nutrition evidenced by weight loss or dehydration, impaired skin integrity evidenced by pressure sores, or alterations in elimination evidenced by a decrease in bowel movements. Neglected patients may appear dirty and ill clothed, with hair and nails that show no signs of personal grooming. Their environment may display features such as poor ventilation or heating, bug-infested or filthy surroundings, and isolation from the rest of the household (Box 23-4). Careful evaluation is needed when neglect is suspected. It is important for the nurse to remember that every caregiving situation is different and to consider the intent of the caregiver. In assessing older adults, it is also important to differentiate the effects of age-related changes or disease from the effects of neglect. Even conscientious caregivers can experience great difficulty with the nutrition, skin care, and elimination needs of the impaired older adult.

Characteristics of those susceptible to abuse include the following: over the age of 65, living with a spouse or another person, poor health, and significant dependence on caregivers for basic needs, love, and social interaction. This dependency may lead to abuse or neglect when caregivers lack the resources to meet the demands made on them.[5,9] Potential abusers may be members of families that have high levels of stress (e.g., alcoholism, marital problems, financial difficulties)[15] or a pattern of violence within the family,[40] pathologic individuals who inflict harm for unknown reasons, or individuals who are unable to meet the physical and emotional needs of an elderly patient.

The presenting symptoms of abused individuals often fall into two categories: physical and behavioral. Physical abuse may result in unex-

---

Box 23-4   CLINICAL INDICATORS OF ABUSE AND NEGLECT

- Poor hygiene
- Decubiti
- Dehydration
- Poor skin integrity
- Fecal impaction
- Contractures
- Malnutrition
- Urine burns/excoriation
- Witnessed beatings
- Emotional abuse (verbal assaults, threats of violence, or harassment)
- Inappropriate touching or fondling
- Unexplained or questionable bruises or burns
- Financial exploitation
- Signs of unnecessary confinement; victim is tied to the bed or locked in a room
- Failure to seek medical care for the patient
- Self-neglect; elderly who live alone may fail to provide for themselves and meet basic needs; this is a reportable form of elder abuse in most states

---

plained fractures of the skull, nose, or facial structures. Other physical signs of abuse include abrasions, bleeding, bone fractures, bruises, burns, and drug toxicity. Because physical evidence of abuse does not always exist, home care nurses also need to be sensitive to behavioral signs that may indicate abuse. Behavioral signs of abuse include cowering and guarded, indifferent, or passive behavior.

The health condition and home environment of geriatric patients should be assessed by home care nurses in determining the potential for injury. Accidents, falls, and mistreatment are only a few of the many outcomes that may result from the physical decline that accompanies increasing age.

HOME CARE APPLICATION

When assessing the geriatric patient, attention should be directed toward the following goals of home care[1]:

- Treating the symptoms of disease
- Maintaining functional ability
- Preventing impairment of physical ability

- Providing patient and family instruction regarding care management in the home
- Identifying or anticipating assistance the patient and family may require in performing activities of daily living (ADLs)
- Identifying physical and environmental safety issues
- Providing for the psychosocial and cultural needs of the patient and family
- Locating community resources to meet short-term and long-term needs of the patient and family

During the first visit, home care nurses should develop a plan of care based on the special needs of the elderly patient and family as related to health problems (Boxes 23-5 and 23-6). Because many different nonfatal, chronic health conditions interfere with the independent functioning of older adults, home care nurses must consider many factors when evaluating the elderly patient in the home. The assessment should be structured to identify patient problems and the appropriate interventions to be initiated. When planning care for these patients, there may be a need for multidisciplinary referrals and various state and community resources.

When first interviewing the patient and/or family, consider issues and questions that influence the plan of care (for example, the patient's primary concerns, health history, recent life changes, daily activities, cognitive patterns, and support systems).[46]

Primary concerns

Determine the reasons the patient/caregiver sought home care. Ask why the patient requires skilled nursing care. Investigate the patient's stated problems. The information may be obtained from the patient or the family by asking the following specific questions:

What changes in health status have taken place?
When did these changes begin?
How have they affected lifestyle?
How can the home care agency be of help?

The patient's and family's perceptions of changes will help focus the assessment.

Health history

Patterns of recurrent injury or illness disclose situations involving physical or psychological abuse, financial limitations, and the effectiveness of past treatment. Questions to ask include the following:

When and where did the patient last receive health care?
What was the outcome?
How often has the patient been hospitalized and for what reasons?
For what reason was the patient referred to home care services?

Medication use

Patients should be asked to *show* the home care nurse all medications they have in the home, in-

---

Box 23-5   PRIMARY NURSING DIAGNOSES/PATIENT PROBLEMS

- Knowledge deficit
- Altered thought processes
- Impaired physical mobility
- Activity intolerance
- Impaired skin integrity
- Altered comfort
- Self-care deficit
- Ineffective respiratory function
- Potential for nonparticipation with the therapeutic regimen

---

Box 23-6   PRIMARY THEMES OF PATIENT EDUCATION

- The normal physiology of aging
- Medications: purpose, action, dosage, side effects, and methods of administration
- Safety issues: recognition and treatment
- Dementia: recognition and treatment
- Hazards of immobility and treatment (skin care, exercise programs, proper body positioning, range of motion exercises, pressure reduction/relief devices, bowel and bladder management)
- Diet: food selection, dentition, appetite, weight
- General self-care strategies

cluding over-the-counter medications. Asking the patient how, when, and why each drug is taken is very important. This information should be checked against prescription bottles and physician orders. The following questions may assist home care nurses in reviewing patients' medication history, their habits, and their knowledge:

History:

What medicines are you taking? Please show them to me.

How long have you been taking each medication?

How and when do you take your medication?

Do you ever forget to take your medicines? If you do forget them, what do you do?

Where do you purchase medications? Is cost a problem?

How often are your medicines reviewed by your physician?

Have you ever had an unpleasant reaction to medication?

Storage:

What medications do you have at home that you are not currently using?

Where do you keep medications?

How long do you keep a medication before discarding it?

Problems:

Do you have any problems taking medications such as tablets, eyedrops, or insulin? Be specific in your assessment here; for example, ask the patient to read the medication labels to you or to demonstrate how he or she administers the insulin.

A thorough medication history may prevent adverse reactions to medications. If the history reveals problems with reading medication labels or remembering when to take medications, systems such as the following may be helpful:

- Medication placed into envelopes marked in large black letters that are easily read
- Pills placed in an egg carton or plastic organizer
- Prefilled insulin syringes stored in the refrigerator
- Cross-off-the-pill chart, devised by home care nurses, on which patients "X" out time and dosage box or square after the medication is taken
- A talking medication dispenser (there are several brands now out on the market)

- Medication boxes or "punch cards" dispensed by the pharmacist
- Use of a magnifying glass to read labels
- Color coding the tops of medication bottles for easy reference
- Assistance of caregivers to administer and monitor the patient's medication regimen

Patient education in regard to purpose, side effects, route of administration, and *when* to take the medication, should be a routine component of the plan of care. Medications should be reviewed on *every visit* with emphasis on both compliance and patient response.

At times the home care nurse may do a pill count to verify medication compliance for patients with memory or sensory impairments. Pill counts should be conducted with the patient or family member.

Recent life changes

Older adults experience many losses and significant changes. These may include the death of a spouse, the loss of close friends, a decrease in financial resources, or separation from family.

Physical problems such as weight loss or malnutrition may be a result of serious life changes. As indicated earlier, a person who is sad, blue, or depressed may lose interest in eating, preparing meals, or socializing. Often a referral to the registered dietitian, mental health nurse, or social worker is helpful to resolve some of these problems.

Activities of daily living

Activities of daily living are ambulating, bathing, dressing, toileting, and eating. The level of function in these areas indicates the amount of assistance needed in the home. Referrals are made for assistance according to the needs of each individual patient. The home care aide can assist the patient with personal care such as bathing and grooming. Rehabilitation services can assist the elderly patient in improving mobility and independence by providing a therapeutic exercise regimen that increases strength and endurance along with patient education regarding use of assistive devices for safe ambulation and transfer activities.

Cognitive patterns

Assessment of cognition includes a review of recent stressful life changes and current medication routine. Focus on a patient's reasoning ability, memory, behavior, mood, and activities to determine intellectual function. Changes in cognitive ability should be investigated when they interfere with a patient's functional capacity and safety in the home.

Support systems

The last step in doing a thorough assessment of an elderly patient is an evaluation of available support systems. Answers to the following questions will influence the plan of care:

- What are the patient's living arrangements?
- Are there family members or a significant other who can assist the patient as needed?
- Who cooks and prepares the meals?
- What is the home environment like? (Consider safety issues such as handrails, steps, lighting, rugs, and clutter.)
- Is there evidence of patient abuse or neglect?
- How does the patient travel and get around in the community?

Investigating the patient's support system will guide the selection of interventions. Intraagency referrals and external referrals to other health care professionals are made according to the individual needs of the patient.

If patient abuse, neglect, or inadequate living arrangements are believed to exist, home care nurses must share their concerns with their managers and the patient's physician. Issues of neglect should also be addressed with the family. All states now require the reporting of suspect or observed elder abuse and/or neglect; social services can direct the nurse to the appropriate state agency for assistance and provide the hot line phone number. When initiating a hot line call for suspected or observed abuse or neglect, the home care nurse should report the following:

- The name, age, and address of the victim
- The nature and extent of the victim's condition
- Any other relevant information

Plans should be made to revisit to assess patient safety in the home.

SUMMARY

As a result of a gradual decline of physiological function, older adults may experience deterioration of several organ systems that affect functional ability. Common health concerns or problems among the elderly include knowledge deficits, impaired mobility, impaired skin integrity, altered comfort, and self-care deficits.

Nursing care of older adults requires special skill and sensitivity. The goal of a successful plan of care for older adults is to maintain their maximum potential. Regardless of the specific disease process or treatment that serves as the basis for the home care referral, decisions for nursing intervention must be based on the unique behavior of the individual. A comprehensive assessment by the home care nurse is the key to developing an effective plan of care. This is facilitated by having knowledge about the physiology of aging, the specific issues relevant to the elderly population, and resources available for care. This not only will promote symptom management but will enhance the older adult's return to optimal health and an independent lifestyle at home.

REFERENCES

1. Backman K: Models for the self-care of home-dwelling elderly, *J Adv Nursing* 30(3):564, 1999.
2. Berman R and others: Physiology of aging. I. Normal changes, *Patient Care* 1:20, 1988.
3. Braun K, Rose C: Geriatric patient outcomes and costs in three settings: nursing home, foster family, and own home, *J Am Geriatr Soc* 35:387, 1987.
4. Brown MD: Functional assessment of the elderly, *J Gerontol Nurs* 14:13, 1988.
5. Comijs HC: Elder abuse in the community: prevalence and consequences, *J Am Geriatr Soc* 46(7):885, 1999.
6. Consensus Conference: Differential diagnosis of dementing diseases, *JAMA* 258:3411, 1987.
7. Cuming RG: Home visits by an occupational therapist for assessment and modification of environmental hazards: a randomized trial of falls prevention, *J Am Geriatr Soc* 47(12):1397, 1999.
8. Darney AJ: *Life expectancy at birth and age 65: statistical record of older Americans,* Detroit, 1998, Gale Research.
9. Davis D: Elderly abuse: a national disease, *Caring* 1:5, 1986.
10. Edwards D: Home-based multidisciplinary diagnosis and treatment of inner-city elders with dementia, *Gerontologist* 39(4):483, 1999.
11. Eliopoulous C: *Gerontologic nursing,* ed 3, Philadelphia, 1992, JB Lippincott.
12. Escher JE and others: Typical geriatric accidents and how to prevent them, *Geriatrics* 44:54, 1989.
13. Fairburn CG, Hope RA: Changes in eating in dementia, *Neurobiol Aging* 9:28, 1988.

14. Fowles D: *A profile of older Americans,* Washington, DC, 1998, Program Resources Department, American Association of Retired Persons and Administration on Aging, US Department of Health and Human Services.

15. Fulmer T, Street S: Abuse of the elderly: screening and detection, *J Emerg Nurs* 10:131, 1984.

16. Geokas MC and others: The aging gastrointestinal tract, liver and pancreas, *Clin Geriatr Med* 1:177, 1985.

17. Gianturco D, Busse E: Psychiatric problems encountered during a long-term study of normal aging volunteers. In Isaacs A, Post F, editors: *Studies of geriatric psychiatry,* New York, 1978, John Wiley & Sons.

18. Golden AG: Inappropriate medication prescribing in homebound older adults, *J Am Geriatr Soc* 47(8):948, 1999.

19. Goldstein S: The biology of aging, *N Engl J Med* 285:1120, 1971.

20. Gordon GS, Genant HK: The aging skeleton, *Clin Geriatr Med* 1:95, 1985.

21. Gordon SR and others: Relationship in very elderly veterans of nutritional status, self-perceived chewing ability, dental status and social isolation, *J Am Geriatr Soc* 33:334, 1985.

22. Johnson K: Exploring home health care opportunities as a result of the prospective payment system, *Caring* 4:54, 1985.

23. Katzman R, Terry R: *The neurology of aging,* Philadelphia, 1984, FA Davis.

24. Kaysen GA, Meyers BD: The aging kidney, *Clin Geriatr Med* 1:207, 1985.

25. Kelsey JL, Hoffman S: Risk factors for hip fracture, *N Engl J Med* 316:404, 1987.

26. Kim MJ and others: *Pocket guide to nursing diagnoses,* ed 4, St. Louis, 1991, Mosby.

27. Lamy PP: Adverse drug effects, *Clin Geriatr Med* 6:293, 1990.

28. Larsen EB and others: Dementia in elderly outpatients: a prospective study, *Ann Intern Med* 100:417, 1984.

29. Larsen EB and others: Evaluation and care of elderly patients with dementia, *J Gen Intern Med* 1:116, 1986.

30. Lauder, W: A survey of self-neglect in patients living in the community, *J Clin Nurs* 8(1):95, 1999.

31. Lowenstein S, Schrier R: Social and political aspects of aging. In Schrier R, editor: *Clinical internal medicine in the aged,* Philadelphia, 1982, WB Saunders.

32. Lund C, Sheafor M: Is your patient about to fall? *J Geriatr Nurs* 11:37, 1985.

33. Lynch SH: Elder abuse: what to look for, how to intervene, *Am J Nurs* 1:26, 1997.

34. Mahler PA and others: The aging lung, *Clin Geriatr Med* 2:215, 1986.

35. Marsden CD, Harrison MJG: Outcome of investigations in patients with presenile dementia, *Br Med J* 2:249, 1972.

36. Meiner S: Polypharmacy in the elderly: early intervention can prevent complications, *Adv Nurse Pract* 5(7):28, 1997.

37. Miceli DG: Evaluating the older patient's ability to function, *J Am Acad Nurs Pract* 5:167, 1993.

38. Morley JE, Silver AJ: Anorexia in the elderly, *Neurobiol Aging* 9:9, 1988.

39. Morse JM and others: Characteristics of the fall prone patient, *Gerontologist* 27:516, 1987.

40. Patwell T: Familial abuse of the elderly: a look at caregiver potential and prevention, *Home Health Care Nurs* 4:10, 1985.

41. Pillemer K, Finkelhor D: The prevalence of elder abuse: a random sample survey, *Gerontologist* 28:51, 1988.

42. Posner BM and others: Nutrition and health risks in the elderly: the nutrition screening initiative, *Am J Public Health* 83:944, 1993.

43. Rehman Hu: Age and the cardiovascular system, *Hosp Med* 60(9):645, 1999.

44. Reifer BV and others: Coexistence of cognitive impairment and depression in geriatric outpatients, *Am J Psychiatr* 139:623, 1982.

45. Roe DA: Geriatric nutrition, *Clin Geriatr Med* 6:319, 1990.

46. Santo-Noval DA: Seven keys to assessing the elderly, *Nursing* 8:60, 1988.

47. Selikson S and others: Risk factors associated with immobility, *J Am Geriatr Soc* 36:707, 1988.

48. Shenefelt PD, Fenske NA: Aging and the skin: recognizing and managing common disorders, *Geriatrics* 45:57, 1990.

49. Tinetti ME and others: Risk factors for falls among the elderly persons living in the community, *N Engl J Med* 319:1701, 1980.

50. Tinetti ME and others: Fall index for elderly patients based on number of chronic disabilities, *Am J Med* 80:429, 1986.

51. US Department of Health and Human Services: Quick reference guide for clinicians: early identification of Alzheimer's disease and related dementias, *J Am Acad Nurse Pract* 9(2):85, 1997.

52. Van Ort S, Woodthi A: Home health care providing a missing link, *J Geriatr Nurs* 15:4, 1989.

53. Yurick AG and others: *The aged person and the nursing process,* ed 3, Norwalk, Conn, 1989, Appleton & Lange.

54. Zung WW: Depression in the normal aged, *Psychosomatics* 8:287, 1967.

THE HOSPICE AND PALLIATIVE CARE PATIENT

Gail Nichols and Robyn Rice

You matter because you are you.
You matter to the last moment of your life,
and we will do all we can
not only to help you die peacefully,
but to live until you die.
—Cicely Saunders[11]

HISTORY AND DEVELOPMENT OF HOSPICE

The origin of the word *hospice* dates back to the Middle Ages, when the expression was used to describe a shelter or haven for the weary traveler.[4,11] From that beginning, the term has come to be associated with support and care. In hospice, dying is looked on as a normal part of living. Consequently hospice programs assist patients and families to prepare for death in a positive manner. Hospice primarily reflects comfort and caring interventions. It embraces the philosophy that quality of life is much more important than quantity and emphasizes caring rather than curing.[36]

The modern hospice concept began in 1967 with the founding of St. Christopher's Hospice in southern London by Dame Cicely Saunders, a nurse, physician, and social worker.[3,4,11] She believed that cancer pain could be better controlled by administering regular doses of pain medicine rather than giving the medicine on an as-needed basis. She also stressed the importance of listening to patients, really hearing and paying attention to what they have to say. Sometimes just the listening itself can produce a dramatic decrease in patients' pain.[38]

Contemporary hospice care began in the United States and Canada with groups in Connecticut, New York, and Montreal. Today approximately 3100 programs exist in the United States.[34] Most people want to remain at home in the end stages of illness, and their wish is usually supported by the family.[4,32,33] The home is viewed as a familiar, comfortable, and realistic place for patient care. More than 90% of hospice care hours are provided in patients' homes.[34] Inpatient services are used when problems arise that cannot be handled at home.[4,32,33]

Hospice programs are frequently a division of home care services. This is particularly true for Medicare-certified hospice programs. Ideally a specially trained hospice nurse provides and coordinates care for terminally ill patients. However, all home care nurses may come into contact with hospice patients. As a future trend, hospice patients may be more likely seen in palliative care programs that provide a continuum of care beginning at diagnosis and continuing through the end stages of terminal illness.

The purpose of this chapter is to review the hospice philosophy and to provide guidelines for the care of terminally ill patients. This information will help all home care staff gain insights into caring for these patients and their families.

Hospice concept and care

Hospice is a philosophy of care and a program of services for people in the end stages of a terminal illness. Hospice treatment is palliative rather than curative. By treating pain and other symptoms, it attempts to give the patient the best quality of life possible in the time remaining. It focuses on the patient, not the disease, and treats the patient and family as a single unit of care. Treatment is delivered by a multidisciplinary team under the direction of a physician. Treatment is holistic, addressing not only the physical needs of the patient and his or her family, but also their psychological, social, and spiritual needs. Although most hospice care is provided in the home, it can also be provided in the nursing home setting. Respite care is provided for tired caregivers, continuous care in the home or nursing home if needed during a crisis. Inpatient care is available as needed for pain and symptom control.[35]

THE MEDICARE HOSPICE BENEFIT

Hospice care is reimbursed under Medicare Part A. Hospice coverage can be 100% for persons with Medicare or Medicaid; private insurance plans have varying degrees of coverage. For terminally ill patients, hospice benefits have advantages not available with standard Medicare coverage (Table 24-1).[33] In addition to the benefits listed in Table 24-1, the Medicare hospice benefit also covers physician and nursing services, medical social services, spiritual counseling, dietary counseling, physical and occupational therapy, speech therapy, trained volunteers, and bereavement services.[35]

Patients must meet certain criteria to qualify for hospice benefits. They must be certified by their attending physician and by the hospice medical director to have a life expectancy of 6 months or less if the terminal illness runs its expected course. They must sign a consent choosing hospice care for their terminal illness instead of standard Medicare A benefits, and they must receive care from a Medicare-certified hospice program.[35]

Patients who choose hospice care under the Medicare hospice benefit receive noncurative medical care and support services for their terminal illness. Treatment for the terminal illness that is not for symptom management or pain control will not be covered by the Medicare hospice benefit, which covers only palliative care that focuses on comfort, relief from pain, and quality of life in the end stages of terminal illness. Standard Medicare benefits are relinquished only for treatment of the terminal illness and may continue to be used for the treatment of health problems unrelated to the terminal illness.[35]

ADMISSION TO A HOSPICE PROGRAM

Admission into a hospice program follows certain guidelines. After a physician has stated on a medical assessment form the opinion that the illness is terminal, an evaluation of the patient's physical and psychological problems must be documented by a nurse or social worker. If the patient meets agency admissions criteria, the patient is notified and necessary consent forms are signed.

An important criterion for admission to a hospice program is that the patient and family should be able to discuss the patient's diagnosis and prognosis openly.[13] Otherwise intervention by the hospice team will be less effective. Open dis-

Table 24-1 Comparison of standard Medicare and hospice benefits

Standard Medicare benefits	Medicare hospice benefits
Patient must be homebound to qualify for home care	Homebound status not required
Prescription drugs not covered	Drugs related to terminal illness fully covered
No custodial home care allowed	Custodial home care may be provided by homemakers and home health aides
Medical equipment and supplies: pays 80% of allowed charge after deductible	Medical equipment and supplies fully covered if related to terminal illness
No respite care allowed	Inpatient respite care allowed for limited days during each benefit period
No more than 8 hours of home care a day allowed	Continuous care available, up to 24 hours a day if needed
Inpatient hospital care is subject to a deductible and co-payment after 60 days per benefit period	Short-term inpatient care fully covered, no deductible or co-payment ever required

From Nassif JZ: *The home health care solution,* New York, 1985, Perennial Library.

cussion of death and dying does not mean that all hope has been removed; rather, it reduces the stress that is involved when caregivers and patients have to watch what they say to one another. At the time of assessment and after admission to the hospice program, home care nurses should answer patients' questions honestly. However, it is not necessary to force a discussion of topics about which no one is ready to speak. In time, patients will usually tell the nurse what they want to know and are ready to hear. Many patients would like to plan their own funeral services but find this a difficult topic of discussion. Sometimes anxiety can be relieved if patients update their wills or make amends with an estranged friend or relative. Facilitating these kinds of discussions can assist both patient and family in realizing that death is actually going to occur.[3,4] Consequently admission into a hospice program can help terminally ill patients and their families say their last good-byes.

PATIENT PROFILES

In 1995, 60% of hospice patients had cancer; 6%, heart-related diagnoses; 4%, acquired immunodeficiency syndrome (AIDS); 1%, renal diagnoses; 2%, Alzheimer's disease; and 27%, "other."[34] Other patients may have terminal lung conditions such as end-stage chronic obstructive pulmonary disease (COPD), neurological conditions such as amyotrophic lateral sclerosis or end-stage dementia, end-stage liver diseases such as cirrhosis, or the patient may be terminally ill as a result of stroke or coma. In 1995 approximately 73% of hospice patients were 65 or older, 17% were between 50 and 64, 9% were between 18 and 49, and 1% were 17 or younger.[34]

THE HOSPICE TEAM: A MULTIDISCIPLINARY APPROACH

The hospice multidisciplinary team is responsible for development and implementation of the plan of care for the hospice patient. Team meetings discuss patient and family needs at all levels—physical, psychological, emotional, social, and spiritual— and develop an individualized plan to respond to those needs. Members of the hospice team must understand the special needs of patients and families dealing with a terminal illness and be able to respond with sensitivity and caring to them. Each member of the hospice team has a special role.

Physicians

Physicians are an important part of the hospice team, responsible for directing the clinical aspects of patient care, the development of the care plan, and the ongoing review of patient care. Many hospices have a medical director, who collaborates with the hospice staff as needed regarding special patient-related problems and may serve as a liaison between the hospice, the community, and other physicians.[22]

The hospice nurse

The hospice nurse assesses patient and family needs on an ongoing basis and coordinates the varied components of hospice services necessary to meet those needs. The nurse must therefore be adept at communication, not only with patient and family but with other members of the hospice team as well.

Hospice nurses must also demonstrate expertise in clinical assessment, pain control, and symptom management. They must be able to modify the plan of care as the disease progresses, communicate patient and family needs to other members of the hospice team, and make referrals as indicated.[22] Perhaps the most difficult task for the hospice nurse is changing the focus of practice from curative to palliative. For example, nursing interventions for managing a bowel obstruction comfortably for the hospice patient at home will be very different from the curative interventions required by the nonhospice patient.

The nurse is also responsible for teaching the patient and family about the disease process, death, and dying and how the family can meet the changing needs of their loved one as illness progresses (Figure 24-1).

Home care aide

Home care aides are responsible for personal care such as nail, mouth, skin, and hair care, linen changes, and bathing. They also report any changes in condition to the patient's nurse and attend team meetings in order to communicate regularly with the other members of the team. Because home care aides often spend a great deal of time in the patient's home and provide direct, hands-on, personal care, they often develop a very special and intimate bond with the patient and family. The aide can therefore often provide information to the mul-

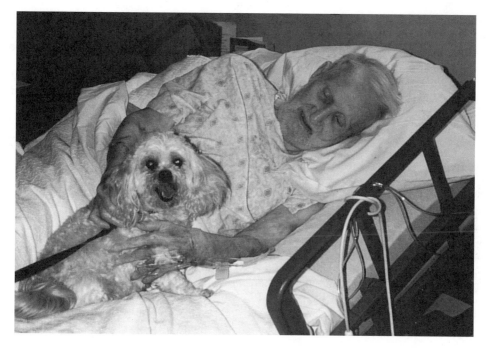

Figure 24-1 Adult hospice caring. (Courtesy St. Anthony's Hospital, Alton, Ill.)

tidisciplinary team that is integral to the plan of care.[22,30]

Social worker

The hospice social worker is also an integral part of the hospice team. The social worker assesses the psychosocial needs of the patient and family and works with the multidisciplinary team to develop a plan of care to meet those needs. Social workers can often clarify family dynamics and assist the team in developing a strategy for working with a particular family. The hospice social worker will also assess the patient and family's support systems and identify community resources to assist them.

Central to the hospice social worker's task is providing counseling and support to the patient and family. The social worker can often assist the patient and family with techniques for stress reduction and nonpharmacological methods of pain and symptom management such as guided imagery, relaxation exercises, and breathing techniques. In addition, the hospice social worker may also counsel the family on financial issues, advance directives, and funeral planning.[10,22,30]

Chaplain

The hospice chaplain is a key component of the hospice multidisciplinary team, providing nondenominational spiritual support for the patient, the family, and the interdisciplinary team. The chaplain may facilitate the patient and family's search for meaning in their experience and assist them in resolving for themselves the end-of-life issues they may face. The chaplain also provides support to the multidisciplinary team members as they also search for meaning in their experiences caring for patients and families.[10,22,30]

Physical, occupational, and speech therapists

The role of the physical therapist in hospice is to enhance function as it relates to quality of life, comfort, and safety for the terminally ill patient. This may mean teaching a hospice patient how to use a cane or a walker, or it may involve teaching a family member how to transfer a patient from bed to chair.[10,22,30] The occupational therapist may contribute expertise on adaptive techniques or assistive devices that would aid the patient in activities of daily living.[10,22,30] The speech/language pathologist may assist the patient with speech or swallowing problems, working with the patient and family to improve communication or instructing the patient and family in certain swallowing techniques.[4,10,11]

Volunteer

Throughout the patient's time at home a very important part of the hospice team—the volunteer—can make a caregiver's life less stressful.[15,36] Each volunteer, working without compensation, tries to do what will help the family the most. This may include shopping for the family (or staying with the patient while the family shops), feeding the patient, or doing laundry. It is up to those involved to decide what is most helpful. If possible, it is best to introduce the volunteer early, before the family has a real need. In the beginning the volunteer can do small chores; then if the time comes when the family has a crisis, they will be less likely to feel shy about asking their volunteer for help.

Dietitian

A dietitian will often act as consultant to the hospice team on nutritional issues and may make patient visits as needed to assess and counsel regarding diet modifications and nutritional supplements or to provide recommendations regarding enteral or parenteral nutrition.[10,22,30]

Bereavement counselor

Bereavement care begins at the start of hospice care, initially addressing anticipatory grief of the family and assessing the family for special bereavement concerns. The bereavement counselor is a part of the multidisciplinary team and along with the other members of the hospice team will develop an individualized bereavement plan of care for the family. The bereavement counselor also orchestrates bereavement follow-up after the loved one's death, including visits, mailings, and phone calls for 1 year following the patient's death.

Caring for the hospice team

Burnout among hospice team members happens but does not have to become an insurmountable problem.[3,15] Difficult circumstances or highly emotional family situations can be stressful for team members. Although in some instances a hospice patient may revoke his or her hospice benefit or be discharged if the patient's condition has stabilized or actually improved, most hospice cases will end in death. The work can be very intense, and there is much interpersonal giving. Regular support sessions or staff conferences help to alleviate work-related stress. Talking with other members of the hospice team and getting feedback (and perhaps a hug) can do a lot to raise lagging spirits. It cannot be overemphasized that team members, like the caregivers, must first take care of themselves.[15]

HOME CARE APPLICATION
Hospice goals of care and fundamentals of patient education

Goals to strive for under the hospice philosophy include general support and palliative measures. The focus of care is pain control, a peaceful death, assistance for the caregiver, and an understanding of the meaning of life.[4,25] These goals are incorporated into the plan of care (Boxes 24-1 and 24-2). Providing care and comfort can include everything from complex pain and symptom management to simple acts such as smoothing sheets, rubbing backs, and drying bottoms. Wrinkled sheets, aching backs, and wet bedclothes become major worries when a person is ill, and counseling will not be effective until these problems are handled.

Competent counseling helps both patients and families see death as inevitable and as a positive event. Looking at life and death in this manner strips away feelings of isolation and makes it easier to view death as a natural part of life. Discussing the patient's terminal condition openly and hon-

Box 24-1   PRIMARY NURSING DIAGNOSES/PATIENT PROBLEMS

- Alteration in comfort: pain
- Alteration in nutrition: less than required
- Knowledge deficit regarding disease process, dying process, diet, medications, hospice services
- Self-care deficit
- Grieving (anticipatory/patient and family)
- Alteration in elimination: bowel and/or bladder
- Alteration in coping: individual, family
- Alteration in skin integrity

estly is the best way to help patients and families cope. It is not a question of taking hope away but instead one of redirecting the patient's goals toward immediate needs such as pain control.[5] This search for meaning in life can provide insightful answers and an acceptance of what has happened and what will happen.[38]

The home environment

Home situations range from calm and well organized to hectic and chaotic. When hospice nurses arrive at the home for the first time, they assess the immediate needs and priorities of the patient and family. This may involve setting up a medication schedule or giving instruction on positioning and transfers. Nurses should try to do what is most helpful for patients/caregivers. The nurse must include the patient and family in establishing the plan of care. Trying to impose the nurse's priorities on the family can lead to frustration for everyone (see Chapters 2 and 4).[5]

Pain management

Although current methods of pain management can effectively treat up to 95% of patients with cancer-associated pain, pain in general and cancer pain in particular is frequently undertreated in the United States.[37,39,41] Approximately 75% of patients with advanced cancer have pain. Of these, 40% to 50%

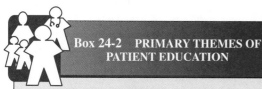

Box 24-2 PRIMARY THEMES OF PATIENT EDUCATION

- Signs and symptoms of dying; when to call the case manager and physician
- Comfort measures: mouth care, skin care, positioning
- Medications: purpose, action, dosage, side effects, route
- Equipment use
- Symptom management: nausea, vomiting, bowels, pain
- Emotional support for caregivers
- Hospice team services
- Concept of palliative care
- Bereavement services
- General self-care strategies

report moderate to severe pain, and 25% to 30% report severe pain.[39,41]

Barriers to pain management. Barriers to effective pain management can be found in the misconceptions of patients and health care professionals regarding pain and pain medications, particularly the opioids. Many patients and health care professionals alike fear addiction and tolerance to analgesics. Physicians may be concerned about the regulatory aspect of prescribing opioids, and both nurses and physicians unfamiliar with chronic pain may not understand the differing physiological response to opioids of patients with chronic as opposed to acute pain. In addition, our health care system does not reward effective pain management or value it as a priority in health care.[8,37,39,41]

Fear of addiction in patients and their families should be addressed, explaining that when opioids are taken for pain, they meet a real and physical need that is very different from the psychological need or dependence of the addict. Tolerance of opioids may develop with long-term use but need not be feared because, unlike most other drugs, opioids have no upper limit or ceiling dose. Because opioids are increased in carefully titrated dosages, the body is able to adapt to and tolerate these increases.[8,37,41]

Dimensions of pain. There are four dimensions of human experience that make up the total pain profile of the patient. These areas are the physical dimension of pain, the psychological or emotional dimension, the spiritual, and the sociological dimension.[13] Physical pain includes other symptoms, such as constipation, nausea, and functional debility. It may also include noncancer pain such as that of joint pain in the patient with arthritis or anginal pain in a patient with a cardiac pathological condition. It may also be related to treatment and the side effects of treatment, as in the case of chemotherapy or radiation therapy. Physical causes of pain must be carefully assessed by the nurse in order to manage pain effectively.

Psychological pain includes the many fears and concerns a person may feel on facing a terminal illness. Fear of pain, of dying, and loss of control over one's life can lead to feelings of helplessness and depression. These fears and concerns must be addressed by the hospice team as emotional pain.[13] Active listening and the emotional support of the hospice team can be key in helping the patient and family work through these painful feelings.

Spiritual pain is highly individual. Feelings of guilt and fear of the unknown as one faces death can lead a person to question the meaning of his or her life. The skilled listening and services of a non-denominational chaplain can help a patient to define areas of spiritual distress and work through them, weaving a meaningful pattern from the fabric of the patient's life.[13]

Sociological pain may include financial concerns, changing roles in the family, loss of a job, changes in relationships, and the inability to continue with former roles in the community. Pain and illness often isolate people in their own homes. The hospice social worker can help the patient and family to identify their support systems in the community, and the volunteer can provide company and support for them. The family may opt to place a hospital bed in the living room so that a bedbound patient will not be alone in a bedroom, but rather in the center of family life.[13]

Types of pain. Cancer pain may be described as visceral, somatic, or neuropathic. Visceral pain is usually associated with abdominal symptoms and is described as deep, dull, aching or as a feeling of fullness or pressure.[8,37] Visceral pain generally responds well to opioid treatment.[37,41]

Somatic pain refers to soft tissue and bone pain. It may be described as aching, throbbing, or stabbing. Opioids and nonsteroidal antiinflammatory drugs (NSAIDs) are often effective in the treatment of somatic pain.[8,37] In neuropathic pain, nerve tissue has been damaged, often as a result of infiltration or compression of nerves by a tumor mass. The resulting pain may be described by the patient as burning, tingling, lancinating, or as shooting into a body area such as the arm or leg.[37] Neuropathic pain can be very challenging to treat successfully because it does not respond as well as visceral and somatic pain to opioids. Neuropathic pain may be treated with adjuvant medications such as tricyclic antidepressants, opioid and nonopioid analgesics, anticonvulsants, steroids, and local anesthetics.[37,41]

Cancer pain can also be described in terms of duration. Most cancer patients describe a chronic, persistent, baseline level of pain, as well as intermittent episodes of breakthrough pain.[42] Chronic, persistent pain should be treated with around-the-clock analgesics such as a slow-release, long-acting morphine or oxycodone, which can be given orally or rectally every 12 hours and provide 24-hour coverage. Some medications, such as Kadian, will last 24 hours and need to be given only once a day. In addition, an immediate-release, short-acting morphine or oxycodone should be prescribed to treat breakthrough pain.

Pain assessment. Careful initial and ongoing assessment of the patient's pain is fundamental to effective management. All factors, including physical, social, spiritual, and psychological, must be assessed and addressed by the hospice team to ensure appropriate pain management. Different types of physical pain must be identified so that the appropriate treatment modalities can be incorporated into the plan of care. Treatment for arthritic pain, for example, will differ from treatment for cancer pain, and treatment for both cancer and arthritic pain may be needed in some patients. A sore mouth and constipation may also be factors contributing to the patient's pain and should be addressed in the plan of care.

Patients with chronic pain will adapt to this pain in time, such that the signs associated with the autonomic nervous system and acute pain, such as anxiety, diaphoresis, rapid pulse, and elevated blood pressure are not seen.[37] Patients may not look as though they are having pain, though in fact their pain may be severe. Patients also learn to mask their pain from others and develop coping mechanisms such as distraction (e.g., watching television), sleeping, pacing, and so on. For these reasons, it is of paramount importance to trust the patient's perception of his or her own pain and to develop the plan of care according to the patient's described need (Box 24-3).[41]

Pain assessment should include a thorough history, and an accurate description of the patient's pain must be obtained (Box 24-4).[41] A pain intensity scale should be used at every visit for clarity and continuity of pain assessment. (Ask the patient to rate his or her pain on a scale of 1 [no pain] to 10 [extreme pain].) For patients who are nonverbal or confused, obtaining an adequate pain assessment can be difficult. The nurse will have to be guided by nonverbal behavioral cues from the patient, such as grimacing, protective or guarding movements, or moaning.

Box 24-3   CLINICAL APPROACH TO PAIN ASSESSMENT AND MANAGEMENT

A   Ask about pain regularly.
    Assess pain systematically.
B   Believe the patient and family in their reports of pain and what relieves it.
C   Choose pain control options appropriate for the patient, family, and setting.
D   Deliver interventions in a timely, logical, and coordinated fashion.
E   Empower patients and their families.
    Enable them to control their course to the greatest extent possible.

From US Department of Health and Human Services, Public Health Service, Agency for Health Care Policy and Research: *Management of cancer pain.* Clinical practice guideline No 9, Pub No 94-1592, March 1994, Rockville, Md.

Box 24-4   GUIDE FOR PAIN ASSESSMENT

1. Location (anatomical site)
2. Description (aching, sharp, knifelike)
3. Intensity (mild, moderate, severe)
4. Duration (constant, intermittent)
5. Exacerbating factors (What makes it worse?)
6. Response to pain (crying, immobility, withdrawal)
7. Current relief measures (What helps? What makes it better?)
8. Acceptable level of pain relief

Pharmacological pain interventions. The World Health Organization (WHO) uses the following approach to drug therapy in cancer pain[41]:

1. By the mouth
2. By the clock
3. By the ladder
4. For the individual
5. With attention to detail

There are many effective interventions for pain control. Pharmacological approaches include nonopioid analgesics, primarily NSAIDs, opioid analgesics, and adjuvant medications.

The WHO analgesic ladder (Figure 24-2) recommends nonopioids for mild pain, with adjuvants as needed; opioids for mild to moderate pain, along with a nonopioid and/or adjuvants as needed; and for moderate to severe pain, opioids are given in increasing doses and in conjunction with a nonopioid medication and/or adjuvant medications as needed.[8,41] If these methods are ineffective, more invasive measures may be used, such as nerve blocks, palliative radiation, and subcutaneous, intravenous, epidural, or intrathecal analgesics.

Nonsteroidal antiinflammatory drugs. Nonsteroidal antiinflammatory drugs, including acetaminophen, are used for mild to moderate soft tissue, bone, and visceral pain. They can be especially effective in the treatment of pain associated with metastasis to the bone and in pain associated with inflammation.[37] Side effects such as gastrointestinal (GI) bleeding should be kept in mind when administering NSAIDs. In addition, NSAIDs are subject to a "ceiling effect," a dosage at which the drugs will no longer provide pain relief and become toxic above recommended dosages (see Appendix XXIV-I for dosing information for acetaminophen and NSAIDs).[37]

Opioids. Opioid-NSAID combinations are often used for mild to moderate pain. Patients with metastatic disease are generally on these medications for only a short time, however, before requiring a switch to a stronger pure opioid agonist.[8] These compound analgesics work best for acute pain of limited duration.[8] It should also be noted that there is no strategy for breakthrough pain for patients taking these short-acting analgesics. In addition, they are subject to the ceiling effect and toxicity level of the particular NSAID used in the opioid-NSAID combination.

For moderate to severe pain, strong opioid analgesics are generally used. These are the pure agonist opioids that act on the central nervous system to block pain and include morphine, hydromorphone, oxycodone, and fentanyl. The advantages of the agonist opioids is that they have no ceiling effect; therefore dosages can be titrated upward to effectively control pain. Meperidine, although it is an agonist opioid, should never be used for chronic pain, because toxic metabolites accumulate with repeated use and may cause central nervous system toxicity producing tremors, confusion, and seizures

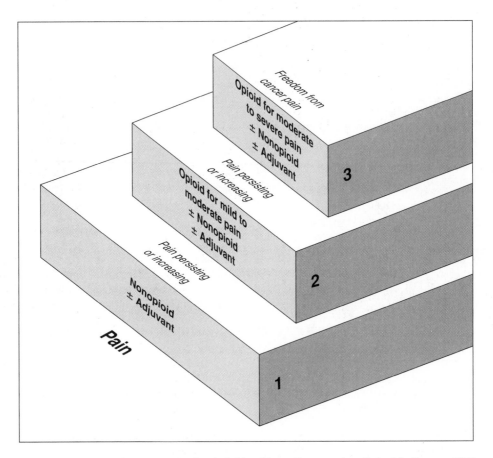

Figure 24-2 The WHO three-step analgesic ladder. (From *Cancer pain relief,* ed 2, Geneva, 1996, World Health Organization.)

(see Appendix XXIV-II for typical starting doses of opioids and equianalgesic opioid doses).[41]

Adjuvants. Adjuvant medications enhance the analgesic effects of morphine and other analgesics. They are often used to treat specific types of pain such as bone pain or neuropathic pain. The most commonly used adjuvants are anxiolytics, corticosteroids, antidepressants, anticonvulsants, and local anesthetics (see Appendix XXIV-III).

Route. Noninvasive analgesic approaches are preferable to invasive palliative approaches.[41] Oral administration is preferred because it is convenient for the patient and family and is usually cost-effective.[2,41] If patients cannot take oral preparations, transdermal or rectal routes should be offered.

Immediate-release opioids can be given rectally but need to be given every 2 to 4 hours. This schedule may be exhausting for caregivers.[41] Long-acting opioids can be administered rectally every 12 hours with blood levels and analgesic effects similar to those seen with oral administration.[8] Administering long-acting opioids rectally makes pain control considerably more manageable for caregivers. Some patients and caregivers, however, may prefer not to administer rectal medications, and this route is contraindicated for patients who have diarrhea, anal/rectal lesions, or mucositis. In these cases, transdermal or parenteral medications are recommended.

Fentanyl is generally given by transdermal route and can be convenient but more costly. This route is not suitable for rapid dose titration but is very effective for stable pain. The transdermal route also allows caregivers to be relieved of a potentially demanding medication schedule because the patch is changed every 72 hours.[12,17]

Parenteral, epidural, and intrathecal routes are generally the last route chosen. Continuous infusions of narcotics can provide excellent pain relief. However, caregivers must be able to manage the equipment, and home care nurses need to be available 24 hours a day for teaching, support, and problems. Both intravenous and subcutaneous routes are acceptable. Often a combination of routes is used to treat pain. The intramuscular route is avoided because of unreliable absorption, pain, and inconvenience to both patients/caregivers.[41]

Radiation therapy may be used for control of cancer pain, primarily for bone metastasis. Localized radiation therapy can provide enough pain relief to substantially (although often temporarily) improve the patient's quality of life.[3,41] Nerve blocks may be used to control localized pain when other, less-invasive pain measures fail.

Opioid side effects. Opioids can cause drowsiness for the first 48 to 72 hours after initial administration or increase in dosage. In addition, a patient may sleep more after beginning opioid therapy because of previous sleep deprivation related to unrelieved pain. Instructing the family in the reasons for drowsiness and its temporary nature will help relieve any anxiety this drowsiness might otherwise provoke. Patients can also use central nervous system stimulants such as caffeine or dextroamphetamine to decrease sedation.[41]

Nausea is another common side effect of opioids. It will generally subside after the first 48 to 72 hours. An antiemetic will help the patient remain comfortable in the meantime.

Constipation always occurs with the administration of opioids. A laxative should be started at the same time as an opioid, and with each increase of the opioid, the laxative should also be increased.

Nonpharmacologic interventions. In conjunction with medication, physical and psychosocial therapies can be used in the management of pain.[36] Physical modalities such as the application of cold or heat, massage, and instruction on repositioning can provide comfort to the patient suffering from muscle aches, pain, and stiffness. Psychosocial therapies, such as focused breathing exercises, re-

laxation techniques, therapeutic touch, meditation, distraction, music therapy and visualization can help relax tense muscles and reduce stress (see Chapter 27).[13,21,41]

Symptom management

Anorexia. Anorexia is common among terminally ill patients. Delayed digestion, a constant feeling similar to seasickness, and decreased or increased olfactory and gustatory sensations all contribute to this symptom. A new narcotic regimen can influence appetite, as can hypercalcemia, copious sputum, uncontrolled pain, or medication taken for problems other than pain. Nausea and vomiting can have a multitude of causes.[15] In addition, a cancer patient may suffer profound weight loss despite a reasonable food intake because of tumor demands. "A tumor approximately 2% of body weight can use over 40% of a person's daily caloric intake."[24] Metabolic rate often increases in cancer patients because of tumor metabolism of glucose and possibly as a result of tumor hormones such as cachectin.[24] Nutritional support becomes very challenging in these patients.

For nausea and vomiting, antiemetics may be given as needed but are probably more effective if administered on a regular schedule. Delayed digestion can be helped by small, frequent meals that are easy to digest. Good oral hygiene can help with intake.[23] Accommodating patients' food desires can be important. Even if a meal of hot, spicy food seems out of line, if patients ask for it, it may be just right for them that day.[32] Many cancer patients cannot tolerate meat, and some cannot bear the taste of anything sweet. Frequently, nutritious meals must be abandoned. Liquid supplements can add vitamins and calories and are easy to consume. Giving patients very small mouthfuls of food and pureeing the food will make eating easier and reduce the energy required for chewing. Small plates of food are also more appetizing and less overwhelming. Encouraging fluid intake by offering frequent sips of liquids will do much to maintain comfort.[15,23] Medications such as steroids, megestrol acetate, and metoclopramide can enhance appetite and intake.[41]

For the most part, caregivers should approach meals in a matter-of-fact way, serving food and removing the leftovers without comment. Too much urging to eat on the part of caregivers can soon make mealtime a battleground where no one wins.[18,23]

Weakness. Decreased food and fluid intake, decreased activity, fever, and shortness of breath all contribute to a lack of energy and drive. As a result, strength and vitality decline. Sometimes a mild exercise program can be physically and psychologically beneficial. Energy conservation techniques can help patients perform activities more efficiently. A referral to rehabilitation services may prove helpful. Providing instruction on cane, walker, or wheelchair use may improve mobility and patient outlook. Being able to move from bedroom to kitchen or even outdoors can lift spirits immeasurably. Adding rails to the bathtub or toilet or raising the height of the toilet in small increments to facilitate use can contribute to feelings of well-being and accomplishment.

Many patients say they have no drive to do anything and no ability to concentrate on a task. Instead, they spend hours each day thinking about the past and future. Some lament the fact that now that they have time to read or do needlework, they no longer have any desire to do these things. One patient remarked, "I never got to see the redwoods. How I wish I could see them." He was strong enough to take the trip, and his family urged him, "We'll take you." But he said, "No, it's really not that important." What he may have meant was that the thought of the trip was too overwhelming, and it was easier to sit in his chair and imagine.[23]

Constipation. A problem frequently encountered in the terminally ill patient is constipation. An assessment of bowel function should be done on the initial visit and a bowel program established. Sometimes the problem is not actually constipation but is instead related to a poor intake and/or narcotic use. It is important to know the patient's past bowel habits. Many older people believe that a daily bowel movement is essential for good health and may have used laxatives for many years to produce this result. In contrast, other patients may have had a bowel movement only every 3 or 4 days. Even with decreased food and fluids, decreased activity, and the addition of pain medication to the patient's regimen, the goal still should be to have a bowel movement at least every 3 days.[26] If this does not occur, the patient should be checked for a fecal impaction. If present, enemas should be used to remove or soften the impaction.

If enemas are unsuccessful, the impaction should be removed manually.

The proper and consistent use of stool softeners, laxatives, suppositories, and/or enemas should then be instituted to try to prevent recurring impactions and to promote more regular bowel movements.[26,29,41] A suppository followed if necessary by an enema will usually produce the desired results.[7] One teaspoon of lactulose 3 times a day will help prevent a high impaction. Patients may have difficulty increasing fiber and fluids in their diet. Liquid supplements that include fiber in their ingredients may prove helpful. In some patients the problem is diarrhea, not constipation. This can often be controlled with medication and a change in diet.[23,32]

Edema. Another common problem is edema, usually occurring in the lower extremities. Edema can be due to a simple cause such as immobility or to more complex causes such as blockage by a tumor, cardiovascular conditions, or liver disease. Treatment may involve the administration of diuretics or digitalis preparations, elevation of the affected part above the level of the heart, the application of elastic hose, or the removal of restricting garments.

Urinary problems. Both urinary incontinence and retention can be controlled with the insertion of a Foley catheter.[4,23,32] However, the families of many patients with incontinence prefer to forgo the indwelling catheter and use pads, diapers, or an external catheter (see Chapter 16).

Dyspnea. Dyspnea can result from a patient's weakened condition or may be due to an actual lung pathologic condition. Morphine is considered the basis of treatment for dyspnea for patients with both cancer and end-stage chronic lung disease.[19] Studies by Bruera and others on cancer patients showed significant improvement in dyspnea without any change in respiratory rate, respiratory results, or changes in carbon dioxide (CO_2) or partial pressure of carbon dioxide ($Paco_2$) levels.[19] Nebulized morphine has been found effective in the control of dyspnea for patients with chronic lung disease and is easy for the family to administer at home.[8,19] Anxiolytics, anticholinergics, corticosteroids, bronchodilators, and diuretics can also be useful in the relief of dyspnea, depending on the cause.[24]

Oxygen therapy is rarely helpful in end-stage dyspnea because few patients are breathless due to hypoxia.[24] In these patients blood gas levels will be normal. The exception to this would be the patient with COPD, who is hypoxic and can benefit from oxygen therapy. Oxygen should be administered by nasal cannula if at all possible, because this makes eating and talking easier for the patient. Oxygen may be administered for psychological effect if a patient feels it increases the level of comfort.[19,24] Many lung cancer and terminal COPD patients continue to smoke and must be warned about combining oxygen and cigarettes. Occasionally there is a singed nose or mustache when patients "forget" that they must turn off the oxygen before smoking, but usually patients and families are overly cautious. Patients who continue to smoke may say that smoking is the only pleasure left in their lives (see Chapter 11).

Nonpharmacological interventions for dyspnea include physical measures such as the use of fans, breathing exercises, a humidifier, and positioning with the head of the bed up—usually at a 45-degree angle. Psychosocial measures include relaxation therapy, active listening, emotional support and reassurance, music, guided imagery, and healing touch, as described in Chapter 27.[19,24] In cases of severe dyspnea, the patient should not be left alone. If the patient remains very distressed, despite all interventions, it may be necessary to give morphine and an anxiolytic in high enough doses to relieve distress, even if this causes drowsiness or sedation.[24]

Skin problems. Dry and/or itchy skin can be another persistent problem. This may be due to poor diet, decreased fluids, medications, the disease process itself, or just the patient's natural propensity for dry and flaky skin. Increasing fluids, using oils in the bathwater, reducing the number of baths, and applying moisturizing lotions are helpful interventions. Fingernails should be kept short and without rough edges. Patients say that itching is more uncomfortable than pain, and an amazing amount of damage can be done when a patient begins scratching. Oral medications can be beneficial in the control of itching.[29]

The more immobile, lethargic, incontinent, and anorexic the patient, the higher the risk for pressure ulcers. Regular repositioning of a bedfast patient is essential to prevent skin breakdown.[23] Sometimes terminally ill patients have particular positions they prefer, and families are reluctant to move the person out of that position. Caregivers need to know that even a few minutes off a preferred side or back can reduce the likelihood of developing pressure areas (see Chapter 14). An alternating pressure pad may also be helpful in preventing skin breakdown.

Insomnia. Insomnia is a problem that often requires attention in the terminally ill patient. The causes are many and varied. For example, some patients begin sleeping more and more during the day and thus have difficulty sleeping at night. These patients are more relaxed during daytime hours and find that sleep comes easily. They are reassured by the daylight and by their awareness that people are moving around and checking on them. In contrast, the nighttime is quiet. Patients may fear that if they call for help they will not be heard, or they may fear the darkness, perhaps even associating it with death. Consequently sleep patterns may become reversed and be exhausting for the family. Caregivers find themselves being up both day and night. Solutions include using sleeping medications to try to restore the normal sleep pattern and counseling patients in an effort to relieve some of their fears of dying. In addition, daytime naps by caregivers when patients are sleeping may help reduce fatigue.

Sometimes patients have a problem simply with going to bed too early. It is not unusual for patients to complain of waking up at 2:00 AM and then admit that they go to bed at 6:00 PM. They often go to bed early out of boredom or just as a way to make the time pass. Patients should be encouraged to try to alter their sleep time, or they must learn to lie quietly at 2:00 AM so that the rest of the family can sleep.

If the patient is depressed, a sedative antidepressant such as amitriptyline may be prescribed. Otherwise a short-acting hypnotic may be more appropriate. If anxiety is a problem, an anxiolytic may provide relief.[24]

Dry mouth and dysphagia. Dry mouth may be caused by decreased fluid intake or medications. Saliva substitutes can help ease dry mouth and improve the health of mouth tissue. If patients are able to increase fluids, this is the most helpful course. Sometimes hard candies and chewing gum can be of temporary benefit. Perhaps a medication that is drying to the mouth can be discontinued.

Dysphagia can be frightening for both patients and caregivers. Causes include candidiasis, dry mouth and throat, weakness, and the disease process itself. Esophageal candidiasis can be present even without evidence or oral thrush and causes painful and difficult swallowing. A systemic antifungal can be used for esophageal candidiasis.[24] If the patient has oral thrush as well, an oral swish-and-swallow antifungal solution may provide relief. Small sips from medicine cups can be used to allow easier swallowing. Straws are not always helpful because patients may have trouble drawing up the liquid and have difficulty stopping the flow once it is started. Offering fluids by eyedropper or syringe can make it possible for patients who have difficulty swallowing to take in at least small amounts. These devices can make it easier to control the amount of fluid being administered. Popsicles, ice chips, sherbet, soft foods, or thick liquids may be tolerated better than plain water or other thin liquids. Nevertheless, it is imperative that patients be aware that fluids are being administered. To prevent choking, caregivers must watch patients swallow before giving the next sip. The lips may also be dry and parched when the mouth is dry. Frequent application of petroleum jelly to the lips provides some comfort.[18,23]

Coughing. Another problem frequently encountered is coughing. Sometimes the cough sounds productive, but the patient is too weak to bring up the sputum. The administration of expectorants, bronchodilators, and perhaps percussion or postural drainage can assist in the expectoration of the mucus. Cough suppressants may prescribed to suppress a dry cough that is exhausting or keeping the patient awake at night.[42] If sputum shows infection, patients may be treated with antibiotics, especially if the infection is interfering with their comfort. Caregivers are encouraged to keep track of sputum's color, consistency, and amount and to report these characteristics to the home care nurse. Some patients produce abnormal amounts of mucus not related to a cough or sputum. These patients will be constantly expectorating saliva because they feel their mouths being flooded with this fluid. Keeping an emesis basin or two at hand and emptying the basin frequently will promote comfort.[23]

Confusion. Confusion is one of the hardest symptoms for families to handle. Family members may find themselves in a constant state of stress because of the patient's unpredictable behavior.

Reorienting patients is sometimes impossible. Even when approached gently and matter-of-factly, confused patients may become very angry when told they are in one place while they insist they are in another. Patients can also exhibit extraordinary strength. It is not unusual for patients considered bedridden to suddenly get up and walk. For example, one patient (a very large man) had been able to be transferred only by a Hoyer lift. One night he got out of bed without anyone's knowledge, walked to his favorite recliner, sat down, and slept. He was not able to get up from that recliner except by the Hoyer lift and in fact never walked again.

In some circumstances, behaviors can be controlled with tranquilizers. Sometimes, however, caregivers feel so much stress from the unpredictability of patients' conduct that they become exhausted and are fearful of sleeping at night lest patients harm themselves. In these cases the family may feel better with extra help during the nighttime hours, either from hospice staff, a volunteer, or by rotating family members. Sometimes the patient may have to be placed in a nursing home for respite or an extended stay.[4]

UNDERSTANDING EMOTIONAL REACTIONS TO DEATH

Having touched first on the most frequently seen physical problems does not mean the psychological problems are less important. Both patients and families may exhibit Kubler-Ross's stages of death and dying, which are denial, anger, bargaining, depression, and acceptance.[14,25,29,40] These stages in death and dying do not represent an orderly progression toward acceptance of death but may occur in any order and combination, and some stages may not be experienced at all. The person's reaction to death and dying will be highly individual.

Denial

Some patients will deny to the end that their disease is really terminal, and families may have to help them with their denial. Poor relationships among family members are usually not improved or resolved when someone is terminally ill. In fact, it is more likely that relationships will deteriorate even further as family members try to fix the blame for an intolerable situation. On occasion, rifts are healed as family members try to make amends for past disputes, but often long-standing feuds continue and counseling will be needed before and after the patient dies.[40] Hospice care can help the family work together, getting family members to talk and opening up lines of communication between parents and children. Emotional support from the team helps the family to cope.[11] A cooperative effort seems to decrease turmoil. Families find that having an outside person such as the hospice nurse who can be called on for advice and counsel makes them feel more confident in their care and more able to share in caregiving chores.

It is also important to explore patients' needs for spiritual guidance. Hospice nurses should encourage visits by the patient's own minister or by the chaplain who is part of the hospice team. Whatever the patient's faith, the nurse must support that faith if it seems helpful and meaningful to the patient.[36] Volunteers can be enlisted to read spiritual writings aloud if the patient so desires. Team members need not worry about saying the "wrong thing" about religion but instead should show care and concern and the ability to listen.[27] Organizing patients' care can provide caregivers with common goals. Hospice personnel can promote stability and give direction or guidance by acting as moderators or supervisors. The disorganization so often seen during the first few visits decreases as family members begin to make lists and diaries and take turns with different chores. If one caregiver is repelled by mucus and another by stool, they may soon learn to laugh at this, and one may take over the area repulsive to the other. Often by the time patients are close to dying, family members who at first were arguing over whether the patient needed one blanket or three are able to gather around the bedside hugging and holding one another.

Providing the encouragement that families may need involves the whole hospice team. Whether the family requests minimal or maximal assistance in the home depends on the family's support systems and personal life experiences. For example, a man in his 80s who has not had much experience with tasks such as changing diapers and cleaning up emesis may feel overwhelmed by these chores. Women without the experience of raising children may feel the same way. Some caregivers feel very insecure but ask for direction and then do what needs to be done. Others take one look at the situa-

tion and call for the home care nurse or aide to remedy it. Frequently all a family needs is for someone to simply listen.[11]

One of the barriers to good communication between patients and caregivers is the mutual use of certain defenses and reactions.[14] Denial of the disease and especially its terminality is common among both patients and their loved ones. Often it is patients who are more realistic about the future, probably because they are the only ones who actually know the extent of their own pain, weakness, or anorexia. There is nothing wrong with hope, but unrealistic hope can be destructive and stand in the way of patient comfort.

Anger

Anger by either the patient or caregivers can also prevent honesty and forthrightness among those involved in the care. Sometimes patients are the angry ones, distressed because they are sick instead of someone else. Caregivers may feel the same way. Family members or patients may be angry with the physicians, hospital, or others in the health care field about procedures done or not done. One source of irritation may be the person's decision about treatment. Terminally ill persons may have decided from the start that they do not want chemotherapy or radiation. Patients who have seen someone with a severe adverse reaction to such therapies may feel that they do not want to take that chance themselves. Caregivers may not agree with the decision and may bring the subject up now and then, in subtle and hurtful ways. Other sources of irritation and anger may be expressed among caregivers who do not get along or when caregivers want patients to do tasks that they do not want to do. For example, caregivers may show their displeasure when patients do not eat, leading patients to exercise control by not eating. Situations can become quite tense and may require counseling.

Families can be just as angry when a patient does not die as when he or she does. In some cases caregivers will take the physician's prognosis very literally, almost counting down the days. If the time passes and the patient does not die, both the patient and family may become confused. "What is going on?" they demand. In other words, they may be asking if the physician was wrong, if maybe the patient is actually getting better. This is the time to reemphasize taking each day as it comes, that life is uncertain and that, at best, predictions are guesses. Usually as emotional responses subside and more rational thinking takes over, patients and their families are able to proceed with more stability and in a more realistic fashion.

Bargaining

Bargaining seems to take several different forms. It may be overt, as when a patient says, "I just have to make it until my first great-grandchild is born," or patients may simply think, "After my sister comes to visit me, then I will be ready." At times the family will urge the patient to hold on. ("We have had this trip planned a long time, and we know John will take good care of you while we are gone.") Amazingly the patient often will stay strong enough to make it to and through the event but may deteriorate quickly afterward. If the patient's and family's attachment to a date or event are the same, everyone seems to work toward that goal. However, anger or silence can result if the patient is not interested in reaching the milestone that the family wants. Communication may be impaired, with the goal becoming more important than the patient. Recognizing that bargaining is taking place can lead to resolution.

Depression

Depression is also a barrier to communication. If the patient/caregiver is depressed, withdrawal leads to silence or to negative talk that can be difficult for everyone. Soon the nondepressed people will start to avoid the depressed one to protect their own outlook. Counseling and the use of antidepressants can be helpful. Certainly there is reason for terminally ill patients to be depressed and for those who love them to feel sad also. True clinical depression is rare, but if the depression seems unreasonably deep or long or suicide is mentioned, home care nurses should be concerned and take appropriate action.[14] Alerting the physician and discussing the patient's feelings with the patient and the family are ways to offer support. A referral to the psychiatric home care nurse may be helpful because suicides occasionally do occur (see Chapter 22).[14]

Acceptance

Some patients may never accept the fact that they are going to die, especially if deterioration is rapid.

Patients may be fearful and anxious regarding what will happen to them or to their family after they die. Encouraging patients to talk about their fears, grief, and concerns may resolve feelings of anger and depression as the end nears. If medication for anxiety and depression is considered, benzodiazepines (Xanax and Valium) are helpful and do not significantly interfere with the patient's level of consciousness. With such interventions, most hospice patients approach their last hours in a calm and peaceful manner surrounded by their loved ones and frequently their nurse.

CAREGIVERS' CONCERNS AND BEREAVEMENT SUPPORT

In hospice, the primary caregiver for the patient is generally a family member or members. Taking care of a dying person is often stressful, exhausting, and traumatic for caregivers. Caregivers frequently lack confidence, saying, "I am not a nurse (i.e., social worker) so I am probably doing everything wrong." It is important to reassure them that if they go by their instincts, they will usually do the right thing. Caregivers are actually more experienced than they realize with tasks such as feeding or bathing. Telling caregivers that knowing the patient gives them an advantage may boost self-confidence. Instilling confidence in caregivers is important so that they feel they are doing a competent job and later feel that they did all they could to make the dying person's last days or weeks comfortable.

"What should I expect—I mean in regard to dying?" is a question often asked by caregivers. Many caregivers fear that the death will be sudden or agonizing because of things they have seen in movies and on television. To learn that patients' conditions usually worsen gradually until they are finally bedridden and that their death will be expected and peaceful relieves caregivers from a lot of anxiety. Another frequent query is, "What will we do when the pain gets excruciating?" Reassuring families that there is usually a medication with a dosage and frequency to take care of problems with patient pain is comforting. "I felt so bad last night when I lost my temper" is another often-heard statement. For some reason, caregivers feel that they should be able to have unending patience with their sick loved ones. However, it is not unusual for patients to awaken their caregivers and then forget what they wanted the caregiver to do. After several nights of this occurring numerous times, tempers get short. In other instances, patients may insist on a treat such as strawberry shortcake at 3:00 AM. When their caregiver finally gets the treat all prepared, the patient may decide that it does not look as good as was imagined and refuse to eat it. The caregiver feels exasperated and then guilty for any outburst. It is important to reassure caregivers that they cannot be expected to be calm every moment. Stress and fatigue make these predicaments look much more serious than they are. They should apologize, explain the reason for the outburst, and then move on.

"How can I get more rest?" is another question commonly asked. Sleeping when the patient sleeps, enlisting the help of friends and neighbors, letting the housework go, and relying more on volunteers are all possible solutions. Caregiving is a full-time job, and even though there may be several people involved, usually there is one main caregiver who accepts responsibility for the majority of the patient's care. If phone calls are interrupting rest periods, caregivers must firmly state that this is rest time, especially if the call will raise the caregiver's anxiety level. If the caregiver is unable to pleasantly ask the person to call back, it might be helpful to have a volunteer stay by the phone during the rest period so that the caregiver can at least relax. Finally, a concern that caregivers often raise is, "I want to go out, but I am afraid to leave the house for fear something will happen while I am gone." Of course this is a worry; however, cabin fever can be depressing. Enlisting the help of a friend, relative, or volunteer to stay with the patient while the caregiver shops, has lunch, or gets a haircut will give a surprising lift to the spirits.

Caregivers often need as much tender loving care as patients. One of the kindest questions a hospice nurse can ask of the caregiver is, "How are you doing?" Caregivers often feel that all the emphasis is on the patient, and this simple question lets them know that they, too, are valuable and appreciated. They must be reassured that they are doing the best they can for the patient and that is all anyone can do.

The time of death and after

During the active dying process, families are instructed to call the hospice nurse. As the patient gets close to dying, some caregivers will ask the nurse or other hospice team member to visit; others want private time with their loved one. Most families appreciate support during this time and also at the time of death.

At this time patients need to feel that they are not alone. Family members should be reassured that holding the dying person's hand and providing small comforts and caring words are meaningful and natural and will be remembered in a positive way. Also families need to know that hearing is the last sense to leave the patient and that they should not speak at the bedside as though the patient has already died. Often families provide strength and encouragement to patients as they are dying. Touching the person who has just died is encouraging and confirms the reality of the situation. It is important to reassure family members that not being able to close the dead person's eyes or mouth is not unusual. Just after the patient dies, the nurse calls the physician, the funeral home, and others who need to be contacted so that the family is free of these concerns. The nurse bathes the patient and stays in the home until the body is removed. Medication is disposed of and equipment is organized for pickup. Saying, "He certainly died peacefully," or relating a touching moment can be comforting to the family. The nurse should use the word *died* rather than a euphemism and should be kind and caring but not overly sentimental. If the home care nurse shares a few tears with the family, this is nothing to be embarrassed about. The nurse should offer to call the minister, priest, rabbi, or other spiritual counselor. The nurse should stay with the family until they seem calm and arrangements have been made. The family is told that the hospice team will stay in touch and is informed that sadness, anger, guilt, and depression are all normal responses. The grieving process may take a long time, and its length will vary for each individual. Family members may need to be told that there is no feeling that they "should" or "should not" have after a certain number of months have passed.

As part of the bereavement follow-up, a letter of condolence is sent from the agency.[16,38] Phone calls may be made to the family members to check on how they are doing and to inquire whether they need assistance of any sort or have any questions that need answering. Formal follow-up by phone or letter is made at 1 month, 3 months, 6 months, and 1 year.[3,16] Home visits may be made at those intervals. In addition, invitations to a monthly bereavement group typically are sent during that period. If more intensive counseling is needed, that also is provided. The monthly bereavement meetings may be a mixture of serious and frivolous topics. There is always the opportunity to "vent your spleen," but there are also meetings that are purely social and fun.[16] Most hospice programs also sponsor a yearly memorial service to honor and remember those who have died during the year. This is beneficial for families and staff.

PEDIATRIC HOSPICE

Pediatric hospice care may be provided by a home care team specifically trained for and dedicated to pediatric hospice care, or it may be provided as part of a primarily adult hospice program. Although the hospice concept remains the same for both adult and pediatric hospice, the needs of the pediatric patient and family are very specialized.

Psychosocial aspects of care

The psychosocial needs of the pediatric hospice patient and family are often complex. The terminally ill child's understanding of illness and death will vary according to developmental level, and the hospice nurse will need to choose a teaching method that will be appropriate to the child's level of understanding.[31]

Preschoolers and older children may feel that the illness is their fault or that treatments are a punishment for wrong behavior. They will need an opportunity to verbalize these feelings, and they will need reassurance that their illness is not the result of having done something wrong.[31] For school-age children, maintaining their social contacts may be very important. The hospice team can facilitate the child's participation in school activities by controlling pain and other symptoms, allowing the child to be active as long as possible. After the child's death, hospice can provide support to the child's friends by

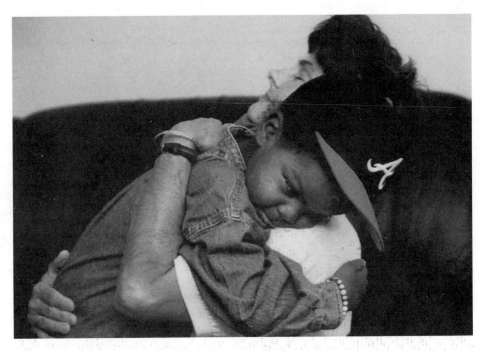

Figure 24-3 Comforting the child. (Courtesy BJC Hospice Services, St. Louis, Mo.)

organizing a school activity in the child's memory, such as making a memory quilt or a memory book.

In addition, the hospice team must often address the needs of siblings. Siblings need to be given simple, age-appropriate information about what is happening to their terminally ill brother or sister. They need the opportunity to talk about their feelings and concerns and to ask questions. They will need to spend time with their dying brother or sister and be involved with their care in whatever small ways possible.[31] The hospice team can assist the family by facilitating their communication and educating the parents on the special needs of their children during the illness and death of a family member (Figure 24-3).

Parents also need special support as they struggle to accept the terminal diagnosis of their child and to learn to care for their child at home as the illness progresses. Parents need to be reassured that they are doing a good job. They also need to be encouraged to spend time with all of their children and to maintain as much normal activity at home as possible.[31]

Pain management

Pain management can be challenging in the pediatric patient. Very young children may not have the verbal skills to describe their pain adequately. Older children may be reluctant to talk about their pain or symptoms. Depending on the developmental age of the child, reactions to pain will vary (Box 24-5).[6] Assessment by the nurse requires close ob-servation of behavioral cues. Irritability, withdrawn behavior, or anger may indicate pain in a child who is usually happy and outgoing. A thorough analgesic history and, in children receiving opioids, an assessment of family attitudes toward opioids will also be necessary (Box 24-6). Determining the location of pain can be accomplished by asking the child to point to where it hurts, on themselves, on a doll, or on an outline drawing of a body.[1] Older children may be able to respond to numbered pain intensity scales (Figure 24-4).[6]

The WHO analgesic ladder is used in pediatric hospice patients as it is in adults. The primary difference is that dosages are adjusted by weight in the pediatric patient.[1] Nonsteroidal antiinflammatory drugs can be used for children with mild pain (Appendix XXIV-I). The drug choice for children with mild to moderate pain is codeine. For severe pain, a strong opioid such as morphine is required (Appendix XXIV-II).[1,9,43] The preferred route is oral, as it is in adults. Nonpharmacological interventions for pain can be very effective in children, and the type of intervention will vary with developmental age (Box 24-7).[6]

Pediatric bereavement issues

Bereavement assessment and planning begins on admission with all hospice patients, but in pediatric hospice it takes on special significance in terms of the special needs of parents and siblings. For parents, losing a child is not considered natural. Most people do not expect to outlive their

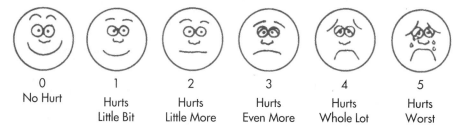

0	1	2	3	4	5
No Hurt	Hurts Little Bit	Hurts Little More	Hurts Even More	Hurts Whole Lot	Hurts Worst

Figure 24-4 FACES Pain Rating Scale. Instructions: Explain to child that each face is for a person who feels happy because there is no pain (hurt) or sad because there is some or a lot of pain. FACE 0 is very happy because there is no hurt. FACE 1 hurts just a little bit. FACE 2 hurts a little more. FACE 3 hurts even more. FACE 4 hurts a whole lot, but FACE 5 hurts as much as you can imagine, although you don't have to be crying to feel this bad. Ask child to choose face that best describes own pain. Record the number under chosen face on pain assessment record. (From Wong DL and others: *Essentials of pediatric nursing,* ed 6, St. Louis, 2001, Mosby.)

Box 24-5	INFANT, TODDLER, PRESCHOOLER, SCHOOL-AGER, AND ADOLESCENT REACTIONS TO PAIN

Infants

Cannot verbally communicate pain
• Sensations are generalized
• Infants *do* feel pain

Age 2 to 7 Years (Pre-operational Thought)

Relates to pain primarily as physical, concrete experience
• Thinks in terms of magical disappearance of pain
• May view pain as punishment for wrongdoing
• Tends to hold someone accountable for own pain and may strike out at that person

Age 7 to 10+ Years (Concrete Operational Thought)

Relates to pain physically (i.e., headache, stomachache)
• Able to perceive psychological pain, such as someone dying
• Fears bodily harm and annihilation (body destruction and death)
• May view pain as punishment for wrongdoing

Age 13 Years and Older (Formal Operational Thought)

Able to give reasons for pain (i.e., fell and hit nerve)
• Perceives different kinds of psychological pain
• Despite mature understanding of pain, has limited life experiences to cope with pain as adult might cope
• Fears losing control during painful experience

From Rice R: *Manual of pediatric and postpartum home care procedures,* St. Louis, 1999, Mosby.

Box 24-6	QUESTIONS TO ASK IN ASSESSING ADEQUACY OF PHARMACOLOGICAL INTERVENTIONS FOR PAIN CONTROL

• Have the child and parent(s) been asked about their previous experiences with pain and their preferences for use of analgesics?
• Does the child or parent(s) have reservations about the use of opioids for pain treatment?
• Is the child being adequately assessed at appropriate intervals?
• Are analgesics ordered for prevention/relief of pain?
• Is the analgesic strong enough for the pain expected or the pain being experienced?
• Is the timing of drug administration appropriate for the pain expected or the pain being experienced?
• Is the route of administration appropriate for the child?
• Is the child adequately monitored for the occurrence of side effects?
• Are side effects appropriately managed?
• Has the analgesic regimen provided adequate comfort and satisfaction from the perspective of the child and/or parents?

From Rice R: *Manual of pediatric and postpartum home care procedures,* St. Louis, 1999, Mosby.

children. Feelings of guilt and/or failure may complicate the parents' grief.[31] Hospices often follow the surviving parents and family in bereavement for longer than the usual 1 year because of the long and often complicated grief the parents and family experience.

SUMMARY

Working with patients who are dying provides many insights into living and the wonders of life. It is essential that those working in hospice look at their own lives and at their own feelings about death before they try to help others. Although very few people want to die tomorrow, for the hospice patient, the family at home, and the hospice team, living each day to its fullest makes death less frightening.

Care and comfort for terminally ill patients are very important. Therefore home care nursing interventions are primarily palliative and supportive with a very holistic focus of care. To die peacefully at home in a familiar spot with those they love gathered around is the way many would prefer their lives to end. With hospice care, that wish is within the patient's and family's reach. For in moments of darkness and despair to touch and be touched signifies our very real and human need for one another.

Box 24-7 NONPHARMACOLOGICAL INTERVENTIONS FOR PAIN APPROPRIATE TO THE CHILD'S DEVELOPMENTAL AGE: REACTIONS/INTERVENTIONS

Infant Reactions to Pain

- Cannot verbally communicate
- Sensations are generalized
- Behaviors:
    - Facial grimacing
    - Pain cry
    - Sweaty
    - Eats less
    - Lethargic
    - Arches back
    - Tense
    - Rocks self to sleep
    - Regression
    - Decreased alert time
    - Unable to suck when agitated

Infant interventions

- Swaddling
- Music
- Pacifier
- Rock from head to toe
- Holding
- Touch

Toddler Reactions to Pain

- No understanding where pain begins or ends
- Cannot explain pain
- Pain as punishment
- Egocentric
- Verbalize pain with words like "owie"
- Common reactions:
    - Regression
    - Hiccough
    - Withdrawal
    - Abnormal postures
    - Resistant
    - Intense, continuous crying
    - Rub, pull painful area
    - Increased frustration
    - Nightmares
    - Grinding teeth
    - Aggressive behavior
    - Won't move

Toddler interventions

- Primarily similar to infant interventions:
    - Blowing bubbles
    - Fantasy storytelling (let child choose the story)
    - Peek-a-boo

Preschool Reactions to Pain

- View as a punishment
- Blame parents for pain
- May beg for forgiveness and/or help
- Common reactions:
    - Deny pain
    - Resist efforts to comfort
    - Regression
    - Irritable
    - Refuses food or drink
    - Repetitive verbalizations
    - Can describe pain
    - Short attention span

Preschool interventions

- Blowing bubbles
- Party blowers
- Feathers
- Pop-up books (let child choose)
- Fantasy storytelling (let child choose story)
- Security object
- Music (let child choose)

School-Age Reactions to Pain

- Can understand cause of pain
- Can describe pain—but might not share
- Behavior consistent with pain experience
- Common reactions:
    - Withdrawal
    - Decreased appetite
    - Sleep disturbances
    - Easily frustrated

School-age interventions

- Mutually determine ways to provide comfort
- Request medication
- Electronic games
- Pop-up books (let child choose)
- Participation in procedure
- Guided imagery
- Breathing techniques
- Massage

Adolescent Reactions to Pain

- Capable of abstract thinking
- Can communicate pain experiences
- Fear of internal and external pain
- Fear of body mutilation
- Loss of control
- Common reactions:
    - Inability to sleep
    - Lack of appetite
    - Withdraw
    - Irritable
    - Angry
    - Frustrated
    - Requests medication

Adolescent interventions

- Note—hard to distract
- Music
- Comedy tapes
- Guided imagery
- Relaxation
- Massage
- TV
- Electronic games

From Rice R: *Manual of pediatric and postpartum home care procedures,* St. Louis, 1999, Mosby.

REFERENCES

1. Amenta M, Sumner L: Terminally ill children in hospice care, *Home Healthc Nurse,* 12(4) 1994.
2. American Pain Society: *Principles of analgesic use in the treatment of acute pain and cancer pain,* Skokie, Ill, 1992, American Pain Society.
3. Baer K: Dying with dignity: a guide to hospice care, *Harvard Health Letter,* special suppl, April 1993.
4. Beresford L: *The hospice handbook: a complete guide,* Boston, 1993, Little, Brown.
5. Buncher P: Hospice nursing: daily challenges, daily rewards, *Caring,* p 67, November 1993.
6. Byrne C: Pediatric hospice care. In Rice R, editor: *Manual of pediatric and postpartum home care procedures,* St. Louis, 1999, Mosby.
7. Colburn L: Preventing pressure ulcers, *Nursing 90* 12:63, 1990.
8. Coluzzi P: Pain management: pharmacologic approaches. In Coluzzi P and others, editors: *Syllabus 2: comprehensive pain management in terminal illness—care beyond cure: physician education in end-of-life care,* Sacramento, Calif, 1996, California State Hospice Association.
9. Corr C, Corr D: Pediatric hospice care, *Pediatrics* 76(5): 1985.
10. Craig D, McDonough P: Multidimensional interdisciplinary model. In Coluzzi P and others, editors: *Syllabus 2: comprehensive pain management in terminal illness—care beyond cure: physician education in end-of-life care,* Sacramento, Calif, 1996, California State Hospice Association.
11. Cundiff D: *Euthanasia is not the answer: a hospice physician's view,* Totowa, NJ, 1992, Humana Press.
12. Doyle D and others, editors: *Oxford textbook of palliative medicine,* Oxford, 1993, Oxford University Press.
13. El-Kurd M and others: Bio-psychosocial/spiritual approaches to pain management. In Coluzzi P and others, editors: *Syllabus 2: comprehensive pain management in terminal illness—care beyond cure: physician education in end-of-life care,* Sacramento, Calif, 1996, California State Hospice Association.
14. Ferszt G, Barg FK: Psychosocial support. In Baird SB: *A cancer source-book for nurses,* Atlanta, 1991, The American Cancer Society.
15. Gentile M, Fello M: Hospice care for the 1990's, *J Home Health Care Pract* 3:1, 1990.
16. Gianino PM: Providing hospice bereavement follow-up services: practicing the art of doing more with less, *J Home Health Care Pract* 3:1, 1990.
17. Groff M: Barriers to effective pain management. In Coluzzi P and others, editors: *Syllabus 2: comprehensive pain management in terminal illness care—beyond cure: physician education in end-of-life care,* Sacramento, Calif, 1996, California State Hospice Association.
18. Holdeen CM: *Nutrition and hydration in the terminally ill patient: the nurse's role in helping patients and families,*
19. Hospice Nurses Association: *Hospice and palliative care clinical practice protocol: dyspnea,* Pittsburgh, Fall 1996.
20. Hospice Nurses Association: *Hospice and palliative care clinical practice protocol: terminal restlessness,* Pittsburgh, 1997.
21. Hover-Kramer S, editor; Mentgen J and others, contributing editors: *Healing touch: a resource for health care professionals,* 1996, Delmar Publishers.
22. Johanson G, Johanson I: The core team. In Sheehan D, Forman W, editors: *Hospice and palliative care,* Sudbury, Mass, 1996, Jones & Bartlett Publishers.
23. Kaiser C: *Home hospice: a caregivers guide,* Wilton, Conn, 1990, Home Health Care.
24. Kaye P: *Symptom control in hospice and palliative care,* Essex, Conn, 1990, Hospice Education Institute.
25. Kubler-Ross E: *On death and dying,* New York, 1972, Macmillan.
26. Levy MH: Pharmacologic management of cancer pain. Lecture at Cancer Pain Symposium, Augusta, Me, June 24, 1994.
27. Lutheran Medical Center: *Hospice,* St. Louis, 1986, National Medical Enterprises.
28. McCaffery M, Portenoy R: In McCaffery M, Pasero C: *Pain clinical manual,* ed 2, St. Louis, 1999, Mosby.
29. McPherson ML: Pharmacologic management of pain and symptoms in terminally ill cancer patients, *J Home Health Care Pract* 3:1, 1990.
30. Marelli T: *Hospice and pallitive care handbook: quality, compliance and reimbursement,* St. Louis, 1999, Mosby.
31. Minter B and others: Care of the terminally ill child. In Hockenberry-Eaton M, editors: *Essentials of pediatric oncology nursing,* Glenview, Ill, 1998, Association of Pediatric Oncology Nurses.
32. Murkland S: Nutritional management of the home hospice patient, *J Home Health Care Pract* 3:1, 1990.
33. Nassif JZ: *The home health care solution,* New York, 1985, Perennial Library.
34. National Hospice Organization: *Hospice fact sheet,* Spring 1999, http:/www.nho.org/facts.
35. National Hospice Organization: *Medicare hospice benefit,* Spring 1999, http:/www.nho.org/facts.
36. Pierce JL: Spiritual care: the soul of hospice, *J Home Health Care Pract* 3:1, 1990.
37. Sheehan D, Forman W: Pain management in cancer. In Sheehan D, Forman W, editors: *Hospice and palliative care,* Sudbury, Mass, 1996, Jones & Bartlett Publishers.
38. Storey P: Goals of hospice care, *Tex Med* 86:50, 1990.
39. Storey P: *Primer of palliative care,* 1996, American Academy of Hospice and Palliative Medicine.
40. Ufema J: Insights on death and dying, *Nursing 90* 12:22, 1990.
41. US Department of Health and Human Services, Agency for Health Care Policy and Research: *Management of cancer pain,* Rockville, Md, 1994, Health Care Financing Administration.
42. West TS: *Hospice medicine: distressing symptoms,* Essex, Conn, 1987, Hospice Education Institute.
43. World Health Organization in collaboration with the International Association for the Study of Pain: *Cancer pain relief and palliative care in children,* Geneva, 1998.

Dosing Data for Acetaminophen (APAP) and NSAIDs

Drug	Usual dose for adults and children ≥50 kg body weight	Usual dose for children[1] and adults[2] <50 kg body weight
Acetaminophen and over-the-counter NSAIDs (oral)		
Acetaminophen[3]	650 mg q4h	10-15 mg/kg q4h
	975 mg q6h	15-20 mg/kg q4h (rectal)
Aspirin[4]	650 mg q4h	10-15 mg/kg q4h
	975 mg q6h	15-20 mg/kg q4h (rectal)
Ibuprofen (Motrin, others)	400-600 mg q6h	10 mg/kg q6-8h
Prescription NSAIDs (oral)		
Carprofen (Rimadyl)	100 mg tid	
Choline magnesium trisalicylate[6] (Trilisate)	1000-1500 mg tid	25 mg/kg tid
Choline salicylate (Arthropan)[6]	870 mg q3-4h	
Diflunisal (Dolobid)[7]	500 mg q12h	
Etodolac (Lodine)	200-400 mg q6-8h	
Fenoprofen calcium (Nalfon)	300-600 mg q6h	
Ketoprofen (Orudis)	25-60 mg q6-8h	
Ketorolac tromethamine[8] (Toradol)	10 mg q4-6h to a maximum of 40 mg/day	
Magnesium salicylate (Doan's, Magan, Mobidin, others)	650 mg q4h	
Meclofenamate sodium (Meclomen)[9]	50-100 mg q6h	
Mefenamic acid (Ponstel)	250 mg q6h	
Naproxen (Naprosyn)	250-275 mg q6-8h	5 mg/kg q8h
Naproxen sodium (Anaprox)	275 mg q6-8h	
Sodium salicylate (Generic)	325-650 mg q3-4h	
NSAIDs (parenteral)		
Ketorolac tromethamine[8,10] (Toradol)	60 mg initially, then 30 mg q6h IM dose not to exceed 5 days	

[1]Only drugs that are FDA approved as an analgesic for use in children are included.

[2]Acetaminophen and NSAID dosages for adults weighing less than 50 kg should be adjusted for weight.

[3]Antiplatelet activities of the other NSAIDs.

[4]The standard against which other NSAIDs are compared. May inhibit platelet aggregation for >1 week and may cause bleeding. Aspirin is contraindicated in children with fever or other viral disease because of its association with Reye's syndrome.

[5]Not FDA approved for use in children as an over-the-counter drug; has FDA approval for use in children as a prescription drug for fever. However, clinicians have experience in prescribing ibuprofen for pain in children.

[6]May have minimal antiplatelet activity.

[7]Administration with antacids may decrease absorption.

[8]For short-term use only.

[9]Coombs-positive autoimmune hemolytic anemia has been associated with prolonged use.

[10]Has the same GI toxicities as oral NSAIDs.

Codes: q = every, h = hour, tid = 3 times a day, IM = intramuscular.

Note: Only the above NSAIDs have FDA approval for use as simple analgesics, but clinical experience has been gained with other drugs as well.

Modified from the Agency for Health Care Policy and Research: *Hypermedia assistant for cancer pain management,* http://www.star.washington.edu/TALARIA/talariahome.html, table 9, 1998.

Appendix XXIV-II

Dose Equivalents for Opioid Analgesics in Opioid-Naive Children and Adults ≥50 kg Body Weight[1]

Drug	Approximate equianalgesic dose		Usual starting dose for moderate-to-severe pain	
	Oral	Parenteral	Oral	Parenteral
Opioid agonist[2]				
Morphine[3]	30 mg q3-4h (repeat around-the-clock dosing) 60 mg q3-4h (single dose or intermittent dosing)	10 mg q3-4h	30 mg q3-4h	10 mg q3-4h
Morphine, controlled-release[3,4] (MS Contin, Oramorph)	90-120 mg q12h	N/A	90-120 mg q12h	N/A
Hydromorphone[3] (Dilaudid)	7.5 mg q3-4h	1.5 mg q3-4h	6 mg q3-4h	1.5 mg q3-4h
Levorphanol (Levo-Dromoran)	4 mg q6-8h	2 mg q6-8h	4 mg q6-8h	2 mg q6-8h
Meperidine (Demerol)	300 mg q2-3h	100 mg q3h	N/R	100 mg q3h
Methadone (Dolophine, others)	20 mg q6-8h	10 mg q6-8h	20 mg q6-8h	10 mg q6-8h
Oxymorphone[3] (Numorphan)	N/A	1 mg q3-4h	N/A	1 mg q3-4h
Combination opioid/NSAID preparations[5]				
Codeine[6] (with aspirin or acetaminophen)	180-200 mg q3-4h	130 mg q3-4h	60 mg q3-4h	60 mg q2h (IM/SC)
Hydrocodone (in Lorcet, Lortab, Vicodin, others)	30 mg q3-4h	N/A	10 mg q3-4h	N/A
Oxycodone (Roxicodone, also in Percocet, Percodan, Tylox, others)	30 mg q3-4h	N/A	10 mg q3-4h	N/A

[1]Caution: Recommended doses do not apply for adult clients with body weight less than 50 kg.

[2]Caution: Recommended doses do not apply to clients with renal or hepatic insufficiency or other conditions affecting drug metabolism and kinetics.

[3]Caution: For morphine, hydromorphone, and oxymorphone, rectal administration is an alternate route for clients unable to take oral medications. Equianalgesic doses may differ from oral and parenteral doses because of pharmacokinetic differences.

[4]Transdermal fentanyl (Duragesic) is an alternative option. Transdermal fentanyl dosage is not calculated as equianalgesic to a single morphine dosage. See the package insert for dosing calculations. Doses above 25 micro g/h should not be used in opioid-naive clients.

[5]Caution: Doses of aspirin and acetaminophen in combination opioid/NSAID preparations must also be adjusted to the client's body weight. Aspirin is contraindicated in children in the presence of fever or other viral disease because of its association with Reye's syndrome.

[6]Caution: Codeine doses above 65 mg often are not appropriate because of diminishing incremental analgesia with increasing doses and continually increasing nausea, constipation, and other side effects.

Codes: q = every, N/A = not available, N/R = not recommended, IM = intramuscular, SC = subcutaneous.

Note: Published tables vary in the suggested doses that are equianalgesic to morphine. Clinical response is the criterion that must be applied for each client; titration to clinical responses is necessary. Because there is not complete cross-tolerance among these drugs, it is usually necessary to use a lower than equianalgesic dose when changing drugs and to retitrate to response.

Modified from the Agency for Health Care Policy and Research: *Hypermedia assistant for cancer pain management,* http://www.star.washington.edu/TALARIA/talariahome.html, table 11, 1998.

Commonly Used Adjuvant Analgesics

Appendix XXIV-III Commonly Used Adjuvant Analgesics

Drug class	Indications	Preferred drugs/routes	Usual starting dose (mg/day)	Usual effective dose range (mg/day)	Dosing schedule	Comments
Alpha$_2$-adrenergic agonist	Multipurpose for chronic pain	Clonidine Transdermal (Catapres)	0.1	?	qd	Doses may be increased by 0.1 mg/day q3-5 days.
		PO	0.1	?	qd	
	Acute nociceptive pain or chronic neuropathic pain	Epidural	25 µg/h	Same	q1h	Added to local anesthetics, clonidine prolongs anesthesia for surgery; combined with epidural opioids, it reduces the oioid dose required. Onset of side effects and analgesia within 30-60 min. Epidural superior to IV.
Anticonvulsants	Multipurpose for chronic pain	Tizandidine PO (Zanaflex)	6	bid		
	First line for paroxysmal (sudden onset) or "shooting" neuropathic pain; second line for nonparoxysmal	Carbamazepine (Tegretol) PO	200	600-1200	q6-8h	
		Clonazepam (Klonopin) PO	0.5	0.5-3	q8h	
		Divalproex sodium (Depakote) PO	500	1500-3000	q8h	
		Phenytoin (Dilantin) PO	300	300	hs	Loading doses may be used (e.g., 500 mg × 2).
		IV	500-1000	?	?	IV dose used for rapidly escalating neuropathic pain.
		Valproate sodium (Depacon) IV	max 20 mg/kg over 5 min	?	?	IV dose used for rapidly escalating neuropathic pain; followed by PO doses.
	Multipurpose for all types of neuropathic pain	Gabapentin (Neurontin) PO	100-300	300-3600	q8h	May increase dose daily.

	Drug	Dose (mg)	Dose (mg)	Frequency	Comment
Antidepressants					
Tricyclics					
Multipurpose for chronic pain; effective for both continuous and "shooting" neuropathic pain, but generally used as second-line agents for paroxysmal (sudden onset) pain	Amitriptyline (Elavil) PO	10-25	50-150	hs	Traditionally amitriptyline was first line. Because of side effects and recent evidence of comparable analgesia, desipramine is preferred for many patients, especially elderly. Less hypotension with nortriptyline. Evaluate and titrate upward q3-5 days. Some patients may prefer divided doses (e.g., q8h).
	Clomipramine (Anafranil) PO	10-25	50-150	hs	
	Desipramine (Norpramin) PO	10-25	50-150	hs	
	Doxepin (Sinequan) PO	10-25	50-150	hs	
	Imipramine (Tofranil) PO	10-25	50-150	hs	
	Nortriptyline (Aventyl, Pamelor) PO	10-25	50-150	hs	
"Newer"					
Same as above	Fluoxetine (Prozac) PO	10-20	20-40	qd	Fewer side effects than tricyclics; less evidence of effectiveness.
	Paroxetine (Paxil) PO	20	20-40	qd	
	Sertraline (Zoloft) PO	50	150-200	qd	
Corticosteroids					
Multipurpose analgesics	Dexamethasone (Decadron) PO	Low-dose regimen: 1-2 mg	Same	qd or bid	May also improve appetite, nausea, and malaise. In patients with advanced medical illness, long-term treatment with low doses is generally well tolerated; used when pain persists after optimal opioid dosing. High doses used for acute episode of severe pain unresponsive to opioids. Risk of serious toxicity increases with dose, duration of therapy, and coadministration of a NSAID.
		High-dose regimen: 100 mg then 96 mg in 4 divided doses	Same	qid	
GABAergic					
"Shooting" neuropathic pain	Baclofen (Lioresal) PO	15	30-200	q8h	
Local anesthetics					
Neuropathic pain of any type	Mexiletine (Mexitil) PO	150	900-1200	q8h	Mexiletine is safer than tocainide and should be tried first. Plasma concentrations should be followed to reduce risk of toxicity.
	Tocainide (Tonocard) PO	400	1200-1600	q8h	
	Lidocaine IV	Brief infusion: 2-5 mg/kg over 20-30 min.	—	—	Analgesia occurs within 15-30 min. May be appropriate for procedural pain or rapidly escalating neuropathic pain.

Continued

From McCaffery M, Pasero C: *Pain: clinical manual*, St. Louis, 1999, Mosby.
?, unknown, unclear; *h*, hour; *hs*, bedtime; *IU*, international units; *q*, every; *qd*, every day.

Appendix XXIV-III Commonly Used Adjuvant Analgesics—cont'd

Drug class	Indications	Preferred drugs/routes	Usual starting dose (mg/day)	Usual effective dose range (mg/day)	Dosing schedule	Comments
		SC, IV	Continuous infusion 2.5 mg/kg/h	Same	—	Used in combination products for headache.
Psychostimulants, oral	Multipurpose for acute or chronic pain; neuropathic or nociceptive; conventionally used to reverse somnolence caused by opioids	Caffeine PO	50-150/dose of opioid or NSAID	?	?	
		Dextroamphetamine (Dexedrine) PO	2.5 after breakfast	10-30	2/day	Administer after breakfast and/or lunch. Avoid evening doses.
		Methylphenidate (Ritalin) PO	2.5 after breakfast	10-30	2/day	Administer after breakfast and/or lunch. Avoid evening doses.
Miscellaneous	Various neuropathic pains; bone pain; osteoarthritis?	Calcitonin Subcutaneous, IV Nasal spray (Miacalcin)	25 IU 200 IU	100-200 IU 200-400 IU	qd qd	
Neuroleptics	Pain associated with anxiety, restlessness, or nausea; multi-purpose analgesic.	Methotrimeprazine (Levoprome) IV, SC	20	80	q6h	Side effects usually limit use to bedridden patients with advanced cancer. 10-20 mg approximately equal to 10 mg morphine. May administer by continuous infusion.
	Trigeminal neuralgia; refractory, paroxysmal (sudden onset) or "shooting" neuropathic pain	Pimozide (Orap) PO	2	4-12	q8h	Neuroleptic drug with side effects typical of this class (e.g., sedation).

From McCaffery M, Pasero C: *Pain: clinical manual*, St. Louis, 1999, Mosby.
?, unknown, unclear; *h*, hour; *hs*, bedtime; *IU*, international units; *q*, every; *qd*, every day.

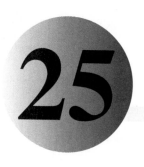

25 MANAGING ENVIRONMENTAL THREATS IN THE HOME

Robyn Rice

The word *home* usually evokes images of comfort, security, and safety. For nurses who make home visits, the word home also represents an environment for caring.[10] Unfortunately, the home environment is not always a safe place. Like a hidden enemy, the home may harbor a number of toxic substances that can pose serious health problems for those who live in it.[4,6,28]

The concept of a healthy environment as important to the health and well-being of the patient is not new to nursing. However, it does have special relevance for today's home care nurses who have contact with patients in their homes. As this paper will describe, toxins in the home not only adversely affect the health of the "patient" but also predispose the entire household to allergies and diseases that are costly to society. By virtue of where they work, home care nurses are in a unique position to identify risk and provide information in order to assist their patients to have toxic-free home environments. Such interventions promote comfort and quality of life and are a key to good health. Moreover, the potential cost-savings to both public and private health care organizations resulting from the improved health of their clientele is an important consequence of "environmental care."[12,23]

The purpose of this chapter is to enhance the home care nurse's awareness of environmental threats in the home. Contextual issues influencing the quality of the home environment are discussed. Recommendations to promote toxic-free home environments are presented. Health care policy issues influencing the delivery of environmental care in the home are considered. Finally, recommendations to improve the health of the home environment are made.

ENVIRONMENTAL THREATS IN THE HOME: PROBLEM IDENTIFICATION

This section highlights common environmental toxins found in the home including lead, volatile organic compounds, radon, fine particulate matter and biological contaminants, pesticides, and electric and magnetic fields.

Lead exposure

Lead is a heavy metal that may cause toxic effects related to exposure. It is considered the most common and socially devastating environmental disease for children.[27] Lead may cause acute toxicity (plumbism) resulting in peripheral neuropathy, anemia, encephalopathy, coma, and even death.[36] Children and adults primarily absorb lead through the gastrointestinal tract and lungs. Common sources of lead found in the home include lead-based paint and lead-contaminated house dust. The route of exposure is usually by direct ingestion of paint chips or inhalation of lead-contaminated house dust, which is thought to originate from the disintegration of lead-based paint and from lead-contaminated soil tracked into the house.[22,38] Action steps for lead screening and intervention are recommended by the Centers for Disease Control and Prevention (CDC).[9]

Volatile organic compounds

Exposure to volatile organic compounds (VOCs) can occur through the ingestion, dermal, and inhalation pathways. As VOCs disintegrate or are heated, they often emit toxic gas. This is referred to as *off-gassing*. Such substances may be found in paints (including household and craft paints, as well as felt-tip pens), beauty products, dry-cleaning fluids, pressed wood, household cleansers, and gasoline, as well other organic chemical compounds.[7]

The adverse health effects resulting from exposure to VOCs are still under investigation. Of concern, VOCs appear to pass from mother to child during pregnancy. Such exposure has been shown to cause birth defects, small for gestational age or low birth weight, and neurological deficits in children.

Contamination of ground water, a primary source of the household drinking water used in the United States, with VOCs is an increasingly common problem. Benzene and other organic chemicals including trichloroethylene, 1,1-dichloroethylene, by-products of chlorine disinfection, carbon tetrachloride, bromodichloromethane, mercury, and halogenic acids have been found in contaminated household water.[4] Dermal exposures of contaminated waters through household activities such as showering, washing dishes, and other forms of dermal contact may be of greater concern than previously thought. A risk assessment of groundwater used for household purposes is advised. Discontinuing both ingestion of and dermal contact with contaminated household water is recommended.[1,31]

Carbon monoxide poisoning, produced from the combustion of organic compounds, is one of the most common causes of accidental death in humans. It is an odorless, tasteless gas that gives no warning of its presence. Kerosene space heaters without proper chimneys, poorly constructed wood stoves, and malfunctioning gas or oil furnaces may emit carbon monoxide and other VOCs such as nitrous oxide, which is a known lung toxin.[18] Proper instillation and maintenance of such equipment, as well as proper ventilation in the home, is a key intervention to prevent poisoning from VOCs.

Radon

Radon is a radioactive gas present in land formations throughout the United States. It is colorless, odorless, and releases harmful alpha particles as it decays to short-lived radionuclide compounds. Lung cancer is the principle disease associated with radon exposure.[3] The Environmental Protection Agency (EPA) has estimated that between 5000 and 20,000 people in the United States die each year from lung cancer caused by indoor radon exposure.[15] Exposure occurs by inhalation. Of note, cigarette smoking is believed to act synergistically with radon exposure, potentiating the risk for cancer.

Soil is the main source of household radon. Radon gas usually enters the home through the foundation.[13] This process results from negative pressure in the home, relative to the soil. Negative pressure can be caused by home ventilation or by warm air rising from the fireplaces or other heat sources.

The EPA recommends that all people in the United States who have basement, first-floor, or second-floor living quarters test their homes for radon.[15] An inexpensive kit may be purchased for this purpose. The primary method of control of radon levels is to increase ventilation within the home.

Fine particulate matter and biological contaminants

Fine particulate matter and biological contaminants in the home are attributed to cigarette smoking, cooking food, burning candles, pet hair, animal dander, asbestos, feces and debris from dust mites and cockroaches, house dust, mold and bacteria, and indoor plant pollens. The method of exposure to fine particulate matter primarily occurs through inhalation. Diseases associated with exposure to fine particulate matter include increased susceptibility to allergies, asthma, respiratory distress, bronchoaveolar pathologies including pulmonary fibrosis, and lung cancer. Children are particularly susceptible to adverse effects.[21,35]

Tobacco smoke contains a wide range of toxic vapors and particles that when inhaled are injurious to the smoker (active smoking) and to those around him or her (passive smoking). The harmful effects of passive smoking are of concern to families who may be chronically exposed to passive smoking. For example, research indicates that there is an increased risk of cardiovascular and lung diseases among people living with spouses who smoke, which is due to the exposure to tobacco smoke in the home.[35] Passive smoking during pregnancy can cause health problems for the mother and fetus alike.[35] In addition, exposure to passive smoking during childhood may predispose the individual to asthma and other pulmonary pathologies in both childhood and adulthood.[28] Identification and elimination of all forms of indoor air pollution is a key intervention for reducing household exposure to these toxins.

Pesticides

Common pesticides and herbicides kept around the home are a source of potentially harmful toxins. Young children are particularly vulnerable to these agents because of their tendency to swallow or drink anything liquid.[37] In addition, after application, pesticides may accumulate on toys and residential "play" surfaces, predisposing children to enhanced exposure through dermal contact. Another important pathway of exposure to pesticides in the home occurs through inhalation.[5,17]

Exposure to pesticides can cause neurological deficits, cancer, and death.[5,32] Proper application of these agents, as well as correct storage, is a key intervention to reducing hazardous exposure. In addition, *Home Safe Home* by D. Dadd describes numerous methods for alternative, natural pesticide control.[11]

Electric and magnetic fields

Electric and magnetic fields are present whenever electrical conduction occurs. Adverse health effects attributable to exposure to electric and magnetic fields are a matter of controversy. However, research suggests an increased risk of cancer with exposure.[26,33] In addition, *chronic* exposure to electric and magnetic fields may impair the immune system and delay wound healing. For example, Colorado ranchers report higher incidences of chronic wounds in cattle that range under their fields.[12] Avoidance and use of alternative energy sources may be helpful. However, no special mode of prevention has been recommended by the CDC.

CONTEXTUAL ISSUES

When identifying environmental threats, contextual issues influencing pollution in the home must be considered. Environmental toxins must be identified within the context of the home milieu. This involves an awareness that toxins are fomented by (1) the design, construction, and upkeep of the home; (2) community issues affecting the health of the home; and (3) family habits and self-care practices influencing the quality of the home environment.

Geological and housing characteristics

Characteristics of the home may influence the nature of environmental threats. For example, Moriske and others found higher indoor air pollution (especially concentrations of carbon monoxide, sedimented dust, and heavy metals) in homes with coal-burning furnaces and open fireplaces than in homes with central heating.[29] Also, research links the presence of mold or mildew growth, water damage, basement water, or presence of damp spots in the home to increased incidence of childhood asthma.[28]

The age and physical condition of the home can also be important factors in an environmental risk assessment. For example, lead from pre-1950's house paint is thought to be the most important source of lead poisoning in children in the United States.[6,9] Since lead dust may be transported from the work environment to the home, the location, age, and physical condition of the home; school; and/or workplace should be taken into consideration when potential sources of lead are identified. In addition, home remodeling projects may result in exposure to lead dust from old painted surfaces.[13]

The presence of radon in the home is also influenced by geological and housing characteristics. For example, the presence of a crawlspace or a concrete slab associated with a basement has been shown to increase radon concentrations in the home.[25] Houses built on a hilly terrain appear more contaminated than those set on even ground.[24] Also, radon levels are lower in houses where central heating (mainly by oil and gas) is used and during summer months when homes are opened up to outside ventilation.[12,24]

In terms of home construction, bedrooms located over garages predispose the family to exposures to carbon monoxide and other VOC fumes. Hence, the bedroom is the obvious room in the house for aggressive environmental controls because of the amount of time family members spend there sleeping.

The impact of the community

Research indicates that African-Americans, Hispanics, and those living in inner-city communities may be at increased risk for exposure to home environmental toxins.[22] In a study with equal numbers of black and white children, blood lead levels were higher in black children.[22] The CDC reported that poor and minority populations, particularly blacks, living in urban areas experience a disproportionate prevalence of asthma and an increase in morbidity and mortality as compared with whites.[6] *These findings suggest that the issue may not be so much a matter of race, rather than minorities may live in communities with a higher incidence of toxic landfills and in poorer, rental housing, which is prone to have lead-based paint and other environmental toxins.*[2]

People living in rural, isolated areas may also experience exposure to environmental threats. For example, Alaska has the highest age-adjusted death rate from unintentional carbon monoxide poisoning in the United States.[18] The problem is related to emissions from water heaters with frozen pipes or incorrectly installed venting systems. Also, rural Alaskan homes are often small (less than 1000 square feet) and tightly sealed to conserve heat.[18] Both of these factors increase the risk of indoor carbon monoxide exposure.

The home's residents

Personal habits and occupations of the home's residents can influence the household's exposure to environmental threats. For example, homes that are not kept clean become a breeding ground for mold, bacteria, dust mites, and cockroaches.[30] Parents who smoke are more likely to have children who experience allergies and respiratory disease.[20,34,35] Pets in the home, especially in the bed with sleeping family members, predispose individuals to allergies and respiratory disease.[34] Also, occupation may influence environmental threats in the home. For example, children of construction workers may be at risk for excessive lead exposure as lead-laden dust is brought into the home on the clothes and shoes of the parent.[38]

ANALYSIS OF THE PROBLEM: HOME CARE NURSING PERSPECTIVES

When deciding on an action plan to reduce environmental threats in the home, certain issues must be considered. Home care nurses should certainly be able to recognize those clients at greatest risk for exposure to toxins. In addition, health care policy issues influencing the public's access to environmental care should be considered. Last, conceptual approaches useful when working with the home-

bound public should also be identified. Such an analysis takes a sharp lens and is paramount to developing innovative change in home care.

Identifying vulnerable populations

Poor access to medical care, unemployment, illiteracy, a lack of education, and residence in older housing are factors that predispose minorities to exposure to environmental threats.[21,22,31] In addition, the growing number of immigrants settling in cities can contribute to crowded and unsafe living conditions.[21] This also places immigrant populations at risk for environmental threats in the home and becomes a public health issue.

In that home care nurses working for Medicare-certified agencies and health maintenance organizations (HMOs) primarily make visits to the elderly, the impact of environmental threats on the health of the older adult is also important to consider. Home health care nurses primarily see elderly patients experiencing a number of chronic disorders including respiratory disease. No study has been found that document the specific impact of environmental care on the health of the home-bound elderly, but Leung and others demonstrated that patients *are* likely to implement environmental recommendations for care after participation in a home health environmental promotional program.[23] Further research is clearly needed in this area.

Pediatric and maternal-child home care nurses should be aware that children are probably more susceptible to home environmental threats than any other population. There are numerous reason for this. Children, by body weight, are smaller than adults and require far less exposure to toxic substances in order to manifest adverse health affects. Children play on floors, surfaces, and places in the home contaminated with environmental toxins. Hence, children are more likely to come into direct contact with toxic substances than adults.[19,32] Also, mouthing behaviors that are common in small children are an important mechanism of exposure to toxins.[22]

Health care policy issues

Recommendations from *Healthy People 2000* call for health promotional activities as a means to decrease morbidity and mortality in the United States.[14] However, from practice perspectives, health care in the United States is primarily delivered on a "fix it" basis. For example, those nurses who work in Medicare-certified home agencies, by virtue of the regulations for reimbursement of services, are not allowed to do a routine environmental risk assessment in the home. Rather, interventions primarily focus on treatments and physical care. Likewise, HMOs send home care nurses out to do physical, but not environmental, care. Postpartum home care nurses teach breast-feeding techniques but rarely discuss toxins in the environment that affect the health of the baby and family. Yet, as this chapter has shown, adverse health effects from environmental toxins affects everyone at a great cost to society.

Virtually all home care nurses provide patient education in order to assist the patient to take care of his or her self at home. It seems logical that environmental care would be a part of health teaching. However, *what* home care nurses teach is very much regulated by health care policy.

Health care policy in the United States primarily has evolved from a bio-medical model. It reflects a philosophy of "take this pill and you will feel better." This approach is not congruent with the realities of today's health care economics. *Smart* health care economics appreciates preventative approaches to care, recognizing the potential savings in the long run from a healthier population that requires less "fix it" medical care. Obviously there is a call for change in how health care is viewed in the United States. It requires that the home care nurse, multidisciplinary team, physician, and health care organization view "patient" and family or caregiver as partners in health rather than objects of care. Consequences of such "partnerships" imply an active patient and family role in care.

Research issues

There is still much debate as to how pollution causes illness. Some researchers argue that significant effects are seen only at so-called "toxic" levels. Others argue that there are many people who are adversely affected even if pollutant levels are well below toxic standards.[12] Consider for a moment sudden infant death syndrome (SIDS). It primarily occurs to infants between 1 and 3 months of age.[8] The cause of SIDS is unknown. Consider for a moment that newborn exposure to toxins in the environment may be a causative factor of SIDS. In terms of the impact of the environment on the health of the public, it is clear that there is much that is not known. Of importance, more research must be done in order to find better answers and solutions to problems with pollution in the home.

Improved self-care as a consequence of environmental caring

Self-care may be thought of as those activities with which each individual is personally involved in order to live productively in his or her environment (see Chapter 2). It reflects a great deal of interaction between members of the household and the nurse as a means to promote independent living and quality of life. Such interactions recognize the existence of a multicultural world where every individual is unique and has a right to determine his or her best level of health. Hence, home care nurses recognize the importance of working *with* families in a culturally sensitive manner in order to foster healthy client behaviors.[23]

Environmental care is a natural antecedent to self-care. Both concepts reflect the patient's right to know and to choose what best balances him or her. Home care nurses can provide environmental care by offering information, promoting decision making, competence, and judgment as a means of assisting the public to attain healthy environments. The author suggests that, in terms of cost benefits to society, the real value of environmental care has yet to be fully appreciated.

RECOMMENDATIONS

Research that validates home environmental care as a positive health outcome is recommended. Nursing interventions to promote a toxin-free home environment include a holistic approach that considers the impact of the environment on the patient and/or family. In addition to basic living conditions and characteristics of the home, contextual factors such as community, household self-care practices, and household member occupation(s) should become a part of a home risk assessment. In addition, public and private agencies that provide home care services are encouraged to adopt the following policies:

1. As part of admission to home care services every patient will assist in developing and maintaining an environmentally safe home environment.

2. Home care nursing and social services staff will receive an in-service and orientation regarding environmental care in the home. The content of the in-service will include identifying potential toxins in the home, contextual influences of environmental pollution, vulnerable populations, concepts of promoting self-care in the home, and interventions to promote a toxin-free home environment.

3. All patients receiving a home visit will also receive an environmental risk assessment as part of the basic admission assessment. With the patient's and/or family's permission, the home care nurse will do a walk through of the home and identify sources of environmental toxins (Box 25-1). After the risk assessment is completed, recommendations to improve the home environment will be reviewed with members of the household; instructional learning materials will be given out. See Appendix XXV-I: Making Your Home Toxin Free.

4. A follow-up telephone visit will be done by the nurse to answer questions, identify the patient's and/or family's level of participation with recommendations, and assess any further needs for environmental care.

5. As part of admission standards, health care organizations reserve the right to terminate services to "unsafe" homes as defined by the environmental standard of care.

Box 25-1 SOURCES OF POTENTIAL TOXINS IN THE HOME
• Moisture
• Pressed wood furniture
• Humidifier
• Moth repellants
• Dry-cleaned goods
• House dust mites
• Personal care products
• Air freshener
• Stored fuels
• Car exhaust
• Paint supplies
• Paneling
• Woodstove
• Tobacco smoke
• Carpets
• Pressed wood subflooring
• Drapes
• Fireplace
• Household chemicals
• Asbestos floor tiles
• Pressed wood cabinets
• Unvented gas stove
• Asbestos pipe wrap
• Radon
• Unvented clothes dryer
• Pesticides
• Stored hobby products
• Lead-based paints
• Dust mites
• Cockroaches
• Pets
• Flowering plants
• Contaminated drinking water

SUMMARY

Although it is considered a haven by most, the home can harbor unseen environmental toxins that pose devastating and costly health problems for the public. Public and private health care organizations should support environmental care as a means to promote quality of life and reduce unnecessary and preventable costs of care. Nurses who make home visits are able to provide recommendations to alleviate such problems in a culturally sensitive and caring manner. Hence, through environmental caring, home care nurses have many opportunities to foster the health of the public in meaningful and innovative ways.

REFERENCES

1. Beavers J and others: Exposure in a household using gasoline contaminated water, *J Occup Environ Med* 38(1):35, 1996.
2. Berry M, Bove F: Birth weight reduction associated with residences near a hazardous waste landfill, *Environ Health Perspect* 105(8):856, 1997.
3. Boice J: Radon, your home or mine, *Radiat Res* 147(2):135, 1997.
4. Bove F and others: Public drinking water contamination and birth outcomes, *Am J Epidemiol* 141(9):850, 1995.
5. Centers for Disease Control and Prevention (CDC): Epidemiologic notes and reports fatalities resulting from sulfuryl fluoride exposure after home fumigation—Virginia, *MMWR Morb Mortal Wkly Rep* 36(36):602, 1987.
6. Centers for Disease Control and Prevention (CDC): Asthma—United States, 1982-1992, *MMWR Morb Mortal Wkly Rep* 43:952, 1995.

7. Centers for Disease Control and Prevention (CDC): Update: mercury poisoning associated with beauty cream, *MMWR Morb Mortal Wkly Rep* 45(29):533, 1996.

8. Centers for Disease Control and Prevention (CDC): Sudden infant death syndrome—United States, 1983-1994, *MMWR Morb Mortal Wkly Rep* 45(40):859, 1996.

9. Centers for Disease Control and Prevention (CDC): Screening young children for lead poisoning: guidance for state and local public health officials (draft), Atlanta, 1997, The Centers.

10. Chopoorian T: Reconceptualizing the environment. In Moccia P: *New approaches to theory development,* New York, 1986, National League for Nursing Press.

11. Dadd D: *Home safe home,* New York, 1997, Penguin Putnam.

12. Delgado A: Interview with Mr. Delgado, CEO of Delgado Ecological Services, Inc. regarding environmental toxins in the home, April 17, 1998.

13. Demers K: Overview of radon, lead, and asbestos exposure, *Am Fam Physician* 44(Suppl 5):51S, 1991.

14. Department of Health and Human Services: *Healthy people 2000.* Washington, DC, 1987, The Department.

15. Environmental Protection Agency (EPA): EPA and surgeon general call for radon home testing (press release), Washington, DC: 1988, The Agency.

16. Environmental Protection Agency (EPA): *The inside story—a guide to indoor air quality,* EPA 402-K-93-0013, Washington, DC, 1995, Office of Air and Radiation.

17. Gurunathan S and others: Accumulation of chlorpyrifos on residential surfaces and toys accessible to children, *Environ Health Perspect* 106(1):9, 1998.

18. Howell J and others: Carbon monoxide hazards in rural Alaskan homes, *Alaska Med* 39(1):8, 1997.

19. Huss K: Controlling allergies by assessing risk in the home, *Pediatr Nurs* 22(5):432, 1996.

20. Jedrychowski W, Flak E: Maternal smoking during pregnancy and postnatal exposure to environmental tobacco smoke as predisposition factors to acute respiratory infections, *Environ Health Perspec* 105(3):302, 1997.

21. Kuster P: Reducing risk of house dust mite and cockroach allergen exposure in inner-city children with asthma, *Pediatr Nurs* 22(4):297, 1996.

22. Lanphear B, Roghmann K: Pathways of lead exposure in urban children, *Environ Res* 74(1):67, 1997.

23. Leung R and others: Behavioral changes following participation in a home health promotional program in King County, Washington, *Environ Health Perspect* 105(10):1132, 1997.

24. Levesque B and others: Radon in residences: influences of geological and housing characteristics, *Health Physics* 72(6):907, 1997.

25. Little D: Children and environmental toxins, *Prim Care* 22(1):69, 1995.

26. McCann J and others: Testing electromagnetic fields for potential carcinogenic activity, *Environ Health Perspect* 105(1):81, 1997.

27. Mahon I: Caregivers knowledge and perceptions of preventing childhood lead poisoning, *Public Health Nurs* 14(3):169, 1997.

28. Maier W and others: Indoor risk factors for asthma and wheezing among seattle school children, *Environ Health Perspect* 105(2):208, 1997.

29. Moriske H and others: Indoor air pollution by different heating systems: coal burning, open fireplace, and central heating, *Toxicol Lett* 88(1-3):349, 1996.

30. Mudd K: Indoor environmental allergy: a guide to environmental controls, *Pediatr Nurs* 21(6):534, 1995.

31. Ott W, Roberts J: Everyday exposure to toxic pollutants, *Sci Am* p. 86, February 1998.

32. Pogoda J, Preston-Martin S: Household pesticides and risk of pediatric brain tumors, *Environ Health Perspect* 105(11):1214, 1997.

33. Sagan L: Epidemiologic and laboratories studies of power frequency electric and magnetic fields, *JAMA* 268:625, 1992.

34. Schmidt C: The abc's of protecting kids, *Environ Health Perspect* 105(7):702, 1997.

35. Shaham J and others: The consequences of passive smoking: an overview, *Public Health Nurs* 20:15, 1992.

36. Silbergeld E: Preventing lead poisoning in children, *Annu Rev Public Health* 18(1):187, 1997.

37. Simko L: Water fluoridation: time to reexamine the issue, *Pediatr Nurs* 23(2):155, 1997.

38. Whelan E and others: Elevated blood lead levels in children of construction workers, *Am J Public Health* 87(8):1352, 1997.

Appendix XXV-I

Making Your Home Toxin Free

Patient's Name:

Date:

Reducing Exposure to Particulates and Biological Contaminants
- Install and use exhaust fans that are vented to the outdoors in kitchens and bathrooms, and vent clothes dryers outdoors.
- Ventilate the attic and crawl spaces to prevent moisture build-up.
- Thoroughly clean and dry water-damaged carpets and building materials (within 24 hours if possible) or consider removal and replacement with tile or hardwood flooring.
- Keep the house clean; vacuum and dust weekly. If a vacuum is not available, dust and sweep daily. House dust mites, pollens, animal dander, and other allergy-causing agents can be reduced, although not eliminated, through regular cleaning.
- Don't smoke, especially in the presence of children.
- If you must have pets in the home, don't sleep with them.
- Consider using miniblinds in the bedroom instead of drapes.
- Heat dry pillow on "high" three times a week to reduce growth of bacteria and molds.
- Have your well water tested for biological contaminants.

Reducing Exposure to Volatile Organic Compounds
- Take special precautions when operating fuel-burning unvented space heaters.
- Install exhaust fans over gas cooking stoves and ranges; keep burners properly adjusted.
- Keep woodstove emissions to a minimum; choose properly sized new stoves that are certified as meeting EPA emission standards.
- Do not idle the car in the garage.
- Have central air handling systems, including furnaces, flues, and chimneys inspected and cleaned annually (replace air filters annually); open and ventilate the home the first day the furnace or air conditioner is turned on.
- To reduce exposure to household chemicals, follow label instructions carefully. Throw away partially full containers of old or unneeded chemicals safely. Buy limited quantities of paints, paint strippers, and kerosene for space heaters or gasoline for lawn mowers; buy only as much as you need right away. Keep exposure to methylene chloride and benzene to a minimum because both are used in household products and are known carcinogens. Keep exposure to perchlorethylene "perc" emissions from newly dry-cleaned materials to a minimum because this chemical has been shown to cause cancer in animals. Avoid using pressed-wood products in the home because they emit formaldehyde, a known carcinogenic agent. Run water through the faucet a few minutes before using it.
- Have well water tested for the presence of toxic chemicals.

Reducing Exposure to Radon
- Test your home for radon.
- Fix your home if your radon level is 4 picocuries per liter or higher; contact your state radon office.

Reducing Exposure to Pesticides
- Use sparingly, according to manufacturer's instructions; consider natural and non-chemical methods of pest control where possible.
- Store in sealed glass jars, preferably in a shed away from the home.

Data from Environmental Protection Agency (EPA): *The inside story—a guide to indoor air quality,* Washington, DC, 1995, The Agency.

- Wear a mask and gloves when spraying with pesticides; keep out of reach of children.
- Make sure you provide plenty of fresh air when using these products; ventilate the area well after pesticide use.
- Mix or dilute outdoors.
- Dispose of pesticides according to the directions on the label or public health directives.
- Take pets or plants outdoors when applying pesticides.
- Store clothes with moth repellents in separately ventilated areas, if possible.
- Keep indoor spaces clean, dry, and well ventilated to avoid pest and odor problems.

Reducing Exposure to Lead

- Keep areas where children play as dust-free and clean as possible.
- Leave lead-based paint undisturbed if it is in good condition; do not sand or burn off paint that may contain lead.
- Do not bring lead dust into the home. If your work or hobby involves lead, change clothes and use doormats before entering your home.
- Vacuum the inside of your car weekly.
- Run cool water through a faucet for a few minutes before using it for eating or cooking purposes; do not use hot faucet water for cooking purposes.
- Have your children tested for lead poisoning; contact your local public health department for screening guidelines. Eat a balanced diet, rich in calcium and iron.

Telephone Numbers for Federal Information Services

- Environmental Protection Agency (EPA), Washington, DC (202) 260-7751
- Indoor Air Quality Information Clearing House, Washington, DC (800) 438-4318
- National Radon Hotline, Washington, DC (800) SOS-RADON
- National Lead Information Center, Washington, DC (800) LEAD-FYI

COMMENTS:

Nurse's Signature and Title:

PART
IV FUTURE TRENDS

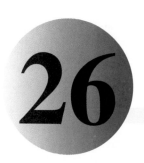

26

FROM TELEHEALTH TO TELECARE: IMPLICATIONS FOR CLINICAL PRACTICE

Robyn Rice

Yes someday nurses will be in space. That will be your future. The age of technology. And, it will be up to you and others like you to figure out how to be a nurse in that time and place.
—Martha Rogers to Robyn Rice, October 1986.[29]

Today's age of technology promises innovations in health care with few boundaries. It also reflects a political climate for cost-effective and quality care. Consequently, health care is moving out of more expensive systems such as the hospital and into alternate settings such as home care.[5,36,38] By the year 2000 it has been estimated that 85% of all health care will be delivered either in the home or in an outpatient setting.[38] This trend is likely to continue to define the health care market because today's baby boomers become tomorrow's consumer-conscious, elder boomers.[36,38] Of consequence, home care nurses are learning to manage issues involving travel and the home milieu and to employ new thinking in practice including self-care theory. They are also being prompted by home care organizations to increase their use of telecommunications as a means to reduce travel time and overall administrative costs of care.[5,36] Consequently, home care nurses will very likely have to learn how to care for their patients using telehealth interventions. Telehealth is broadly defined here as using telecommunications in order to provide patient care. As this chapter indicates, an understanding as to how this transitions into caring, telecare, is yet to be fully understood.

The purpose of this chapter is to describe the impact of telehealth in home care. Critical issues will be examined, a brief review of relevant research will be given, and implications for telecar-

ing will be discussed. Although there are many forms of telecommunications emerging in home care today, this chapter centers on use of the telephone in nursing practice as this is fundamental to understanding future implications of telehealth and telecare.

HISTORICAL PERSPECTIVES

The emphasis on the use of telecommunications in home care largely reflects a push in the health care industry to control overall costs of care. This is probably most true for the Medicare-certified homebound population whose coverage is largely subsidized by the Health Care and Financing Administration (HCFA).[32] At present, reimbursement is retrospective and done on a pay per visit basis. This means that as long as the regulations are followed, the home care agency can bill HCFA for as many home visits as they make. This is changing. Congress has mandated prospective pay for per-episode of patient care for Medicare-certified home care agencies.[32,38] In addition, agencies are expected to demonstrate outcome-based goals of care.[32] Under a per-episode payment, home care agencies will face strong federal pressure to limit costs of health care services.[32,38] Although capitation rates will be set for a per-episode of care, HCFA is essentially leaving it up to home care agencies as to how these monies will be utilized to care for patients. In order to control costs of health care services, managed care organizations (HMOs) are also moving to capitation strategies for home care services. Outcomes of such policies will likely include a reduction of the number of actual visits the patient receives (because fewer and shorter home visits per patient translate into more total visits across greater numbers of patients) with home care market growth in alternative forms of cost-effective care such as telehealth services. Hence, capitation policies will likely prompt increased use of telecommunications such as telephone visits to control costs of care.

Home care nurses have always used the telephone to contact patients and other service providers on behalf of patients. Telephone use has traditionally been an "as needed" addendum to making the actual home visit. However, with the onset of capitation in home care, nurses will likely be required to use the telephone with the *intentionality* to care for the patient. For many home care nurses, *deliberately* assisting patients to achieve outcomes of care via the telephone will be a new perspective on what constitutes care and likely reflects fundamental elements of telecaring.[6,13]

TELEHEALTH AND THE DISCIPLINE OF NURSING

Margaret Neuman, Martha Rogers, and Jean Watson (distinguished nurse theorists, philosophers, and scientists) provide insights on the human experience of life and death that have great relevance for nursing.[24,30,39] Although their approaches differ, these nurses cogitate qualities in the working relationship between nurse and patient that potentiate well-being and best levels of health.[24,34] Key qualities of such a relationship include personal contact and communication. The work of these three nurses has also influenced the author to posit her own clinical nursing theory called *Dynamic Self-Determination for Self-Care* that additionally emphasizes patient choice as key to successful working relationships in home care (see Chapter 2). Hence, the spectre of telecommunications in health care poses numerous questions for nursing. Will telecommunications change the nurse-patient working relationship? How will telecommunications affect the patient? How will it effect the discipline of nursing in terms of clinical practice, education, and research? Should the nursing profession embrace telecommunications as a means for knowing and caring? There are no easy answers to these questions. One thing is true. Technology will not go away and in certain respects could potentially replace the need for the physical presence of the registered nurse. Nursing,

if it is to grow (and survive) as a discipline, must learn workable approaches to telecommunications that enhance nurses' abilities to transcend limitations imposed by equipment, yet, enable them to continue to interact with patients in caring ways. This implies not only an understanding of the use of technology (as equipment) itself but also an awareness of the advantages and disadvantages of the use of electronic mediums in patient care.[6,7,36] This moves nursing practice from a telehealth (disease management) focus to a person (caring) focus. Moreover, a sensitivity to the influence of telecommunications on diverse cultures will be key to nurses forming long-distance relational narratives with patients (and key to successful caring).[12] How such relationships will be expressed remains to be seen. However, nurses should recognize that telecommunications has the ability to empower patients to actively understand, participate in, and influence their health.[7] Such transitions may well represent the demise of the traditional nurse-patient-physician relationship based on the sole authority of the physician.[6,7,24] Rather, the choices, preferences, and self-determination of the patient for self-care will likely play an increased role at every level of health care decision making.[28,31,39]

Appropriate use of telecommunications can forward the discipline of nursing. Such technology can enable nurses to develop global networks for clinical practice, education, and research and to journey where we have yet to imagine. However, in this process, it is important that nursing does not allow technology to objectify the patient as one more piece of equipment, for "pieces" do not experience health.[24,28,30,39] It is also important that nursing does not allow technology to define the discipline but rather come to strong professional resolutions as how to best *use* applications of telecommunications for caring.[24,28,30,39]

IMPLEMENTATION OF TELEHEALTH IN HOME CARE

The literature is replete with descriptions of potential use of telecommunications in home care.[5,38] Such technologies include the following[5,6,16,17]:

- Internet services that offers several distinct features including E-mail; file transfer protocol, which enables computer communication of sounds, pictures (e.g., patient x-rays), and even movies; and the World Wide Web, whereby people can access not just text but virtual reality by using a mouse to point at "hyperlinks" that allow the user to jump through documents quickly. Health care organizations can also use the Internet to promote their services directly to the homebound public. For example, hospice patients may be interested in DeathNet, which serves as a funeral website in which the individual can even listen to and choose musical selections when planning his or her funeral. Most important, the Internet promises to make practically all the information known to everyone on earth available to everyone.

- Telemonitoring devices such as video cameras that can be used for assessment, diagnosis, and health teaching and diagnostic devices that monitor things such as vital signs and electrocardiogram readings at home. Much of this equipment is still in the developmental phase but represents major change in the future of home care.
- Personal emergency response system (PERS), which is commonly worn by frail homebound elderly. This system uses a wireless transmitter to activate a receiving base that places a telephone call to a monitoring center that the patient has suffered a mishap, such as a fall. These devices typically send an alert signal without any additional information.
- Telephone triage and advice lines that have traditionally been used in emergency departments but now are coming under closer scrutiny for home care applications, especially for issues surrounding after hour and weekend coverage services.

Telecommunications are proving that geographical location and a lack of resources are no longer insurmountable obstacles to providing health care services. The widespread use of telecommunications in home care has yet to materialize, because technologies are primarily in the developmental phase. To date, the most common type of telehealth service occurs by a voice-only consultation.[38] This is probably related to the fact that the telephone system represents low cost and widespread connectivity, including its connectivity to home care nurses' pockets via cellular phones.

CRITICAL UNDERLYING ISSUES IN THE LITERATURE

When examining the literature on telehealth in home care, several critical issues emerge. All are important to consider because they have an impact on home care nursing practice.

Costs

At present, Medicare-certified home telephone visits are not reimbursed by the HCFA and they are not a standard reimbursement for most health maintenance organizations (HMOs). However, this may change in the near future as the nature of telehealth is better understood. It is clear that HCFA will consider reimbursement of telephone visits for the homebound public if it can be established that telehealth strategies substantially reduce costs of care, approximate the quality of in-person visits, and promote patient satisfaction.[2,3]

Government issues

The Federal Communications Commission (FCC) now allocates up to 400 million dollars annually to support improvements to rural telehealth networks.[2] Among other things, the Comprehensive Telehealth Act of 1997 makes telehealth services for the rural public eligible for Medicare reimbursement and provides grants and loans to rural hospitals, clinics, universities, libraries, and other organizations to develop local telehealth networks and foster rural economic development.[2,3,5] Home care nurses should take advantage of increasing federal interests in funding telehealth research to study the impact of such technologies on practice.

Standards

There are currently no uniform, professional standards to guide telehealth or telecare in the home other than those published by the American Academy of Ambulatory Care Nurses (AAACN) in 1997. Although a beginning step in defining telecare, these standards have several limitations. Standard IV: Using the Nursing Process in Telephone Nursing Practice lists all steps of the nursing process except that of nursing diagnosis.[1] As a profession, nurses must come to some diagnostic or problem-identification process as part of caring for the patient. If the AAACN is hesitant to cite nursing diagnosis as part of the phone visit because of perceived legal ramifications (e.g., making a nursing diagnosis without a face-to-face visit), perhaps they should have used the term *working nursing diagnosis.*[13,21] Also, the reference list at the end of the standards cites only six references, none of which appear to be research based.[1] The American Nurses Association (ANA) currently has formed the Nursing Organization Telehealth Committee to develop model guidelines and policies for professional nurses' participation in telehealth.[2] These guidelines are a work in progress.

Liability and malpractice issues

There appears to be two main grounds for liability when the nurse gives advice over the telephone: (1) the unauthorized practice of medicine and (2) exceeding the scope of nursing practice.[20] No cases involving telephone malpractice by nurses have been reported in the literature. However, analogies in the form of *physician* malpractice case studies, provide insights into the potential liability issues that nurses face when giving telephone advice.[13,20] Whether a nurse is liable or not depends on the role he or she played in the telephone consultation. The legal duty appears to begin when the provider begins to give advice over the phone. The provider cannot terminate the call midway in the conversation, because this action would constitute abandonment.[20,21] Another area of concern for liability has to do with nursing licensure regarding interstate and international contact with patients.[13,20] At present, all states require that nurses (and physicians) obtain a license from each state in which they practice (and practice may be viewed as one of consultation or direct care to the patient).[13] Inconsistencies with respect to practice acts and licensure pose a serious threat to the development of interstate telehealth networks. Several solutions have been proposed to these licensure problems, including a national or multinational license to practice telehealth.[13,20] The main criticism of a national telehealth licensure is that it undermines each state's ability to regulate the health, safety, and welfare of its own citizens.[13] Therefore getting Congress to enact such measures is another matter, indeed.

Confidentiality issues

Patients may be reluctant to receive telehealth if confidentiality is not maintained.[5,21] This is especially true because computer-educated patients know that databases can be infiltrated.[5] Moreover, home care nurses should be aware that cellular phone talk can be intercepted by anyone.

Ethics

Ethical dilemmas occur when the nurse is faced with incompatible action choices.[13] Home care nurses may be placed in ethically difficult positions if the emphasis on the telephone visit becomes one of costs and not on outcomes. Likewise, what happens if a telephone standard for care does not match the nurse's diagnostic reasoning or *gut feelings?*

RESEARCH ON TELEHEALTH

A literature search was done using Medline, CINANL, HealthStar, and Evidenced-Based Practice from 1990 to present. This search yielded over 140 articles, as well as website information sources on telehealth and telecare. Articles were screened to see if they were research based and then organized by topics. *Overall, there is a paucity of research on the impact of the telephone in home care. Moreover, there is no research that focuses on the constructs of telecaring in the home.* A review and critique of relevant research follows.

Community appraisel of telehealth

Siden used a qualitative research approach in the form of community-focused groups to determine the need for a telehealth link between a local community and tertiary-care medical center.[33] Participants were physicians, allied health professionals, and families and/or patients from the community. Data were analyzed for categories and themes using grounded theory approaches. Positive family/patient and health professional perceptions of telehealth included reduced travel burden for families/patients, the potential for professional education and learning resulting from consultations, and improved collaboration between professionals in different locales. Negative perceptions included issues of medical-legal liability, reimbursement of patient care, and families/patients' concerns about confidentiality, as well as potential decreased physical access to health care. All raised trust issues with telehealth, which indicates how important trust and confidence are in health care encounters for both patient and provider.[33] A primary limitation of this study was the small sample size of patients/families (N = 14), which restricts the generalizability of the findings.

Nurse-patient telecommunication and standards of care

Carlsson and others conducted a descriptive study to assess the experiences of a telephone help line for cancer patients.[8] The study was done over a 3-year period, and 735 calls were registered and documented on a standard report form by experienced oncology nurses. Most of the callers (77%) were women. An analysis of the calls indicated that issues addressed were medical or psychosocial. The medical questions asked were, in most cases, related to the person's illness or treatment. The psychosocial questions asked dealt with the caller's (patient or family's) own anxiety. Of interest, patients made more medical inquiries than family members, whereas family members were more concerned about psychosocial issues (P <0.01). As a critique, there was no indication that the nurses manning the telephone lines were given any protocols or training to document the standard report form. The reliability and validity of the findings in this study could be questioned if there was no consistency as to how the patient was interviewed or how the information was interpreted for documentation. However, to some extent these findings were supported by Edmond's descriptive analysis of 5 years of documented calls (N = 23, 142) to the emergency room.[11] The majority of calls (75.6%), taken by triage nurses, were about a physical medical problem with the second primary reason for the call being medication queries (8%). This study had policies for documenting patient calls, suggesting a consistency in data collection methods that promotes the reliability and validity of the findings.

Kiyak and others investigated the validity of patient/caregiver self reports of health.[18] They conducted a longitudinal 2-year study that compared self and family member's reports of physical and functional health among 40 patients with Alzheimer's disease and 53 age-matched non-demented healthy older persons. Elderly respondents and their families were interviewed twice yearly at home, for a total of five interviews, using a structured, multidimensional protocol that included cognitive, functional, and physical health status indicators. Of note, functional health was consistently rated as more impaired by family caregivers of demented patients than by the patients themselves, a discrepancy not observed in the cognitively intact comparison group. This research has significant implications for home care. Nurses must be careful when deciding whom to believe while making assessments over the telephone because the patient and caregiver may have totally different perceptions (and therefore relate different narratives) about what the problems really are.

Leggett-Frazier and others conducted a descriptive study to examine telephone communications between patients with diabetes and nurse educators.[19] A questionnaire was designed to examine the use of the telephone with diabetic patients from the perspective of diabetic nurse educators (DNE). Over 90% of the responders frequently reported discussing the following topics with patients: home blood glucose monitoring, hyperglycemia, hypoglycemia, insulin use, and diet. Most respondents (93%) agreed that the telephone contact helped in investigating problems that patients might be having in trying to follow their diabetes treatment regimes. The data indicated significant differences (P = 0.05) in how the nurses responded to patient queries regarding health topics about diabetes, such as usage of insulin. Of interest, analysis of telephone users showed that DNE experience and diabetes educator certification were significant factors in the differences observed in the reported topics discussed over the telephone. For example, significantly more respondents with more than 13 years of work experience in diabetes education included urine ketones as an acute-care intervention on the telephone compared with those respondents with less than 13 years experience (P <0.01). In addition, respondents with more than 3 years of experience were more likely to discuss sick-day guidelines (P <0.001) and hyperglycemia (P <0.05) over the telephone than were respondents with less than 3 years of experience. The researchers strongly recommended uniform guidelines for telephone contact with patients. This study was important in that it raised core issues regarding staff certification, training, and work experience when implementing telehealth.

Osborn and Townsend conducted a descriptive analysis of telephone communication between hospice nurses and a nurse practitioner (NP) group (N = 114).[25] The researchers identified the most common problems that prompt telephone calls from hospice regarding needs for assistance with patient care. Hospice nurses called about clinical problems (53.1%); medication and supply needs (29.4%); admission, discharge, and placement issues (14.7%); and other issues (2.8%). Analysis showed that NPs practiced in an advanced nursing role, such as adjusting medication. Findings supported the use of NPs for medical management of hospice patients by telephone. A limitation of this study was that the analysis reflected only a hospice population with its own unique needs. Hence, generalizability of findings to other home care populations may be questionable.

Morrison and Black cited three case studies of telephone care to people with HIV/AIDS in which basic reasons for the calls were of a medical and psychosocial nature.[22] Telephone advice was given by an experienced RN and physician working out of an AIDS clinic. In all three case studies, patients were given telephone advice that basically reassured them, preventing expensive and unnecessary trips to the clinic or emergency room. Based on these case studies, the researchers felt that a trained triage nurse could successfully handle the majority of such calls and suggested that physicians construct sound protocols for clinic personal to manage patient inquiries by telephone. A weakness of this study is its small sample size.

The recommendations for standardized protocols for telephone care are also reflected in works done by Keeling and Dennison and later Turner who conducted descriptive analyses of acute care nurses giving telephone advice to postdischarge patients.[17,37] Both studies conducted and evaluated nurse-initiated telephone follow-ups after hospital discharge for medical health problems. Perceived benefits of follow-up telephone calls cited flexible opportunities for the nurse to facilitate patient self-care, emotional support of patient transitions between the home and hospital, and improved patient satisfaction with care. Neither study employed standards or protocols for interviewing the patients, which could introduce bias in data collection. Also, findings in these studies are not generalizable as a result of convenience sampling and small sample sizes.

Nurses' perceptions of telehealth services

Dale interviewed 44 emergency room (ER) staff members and asked them to identify main skills and attributes necessary for effective telephone counseling.[9] The responses were then used to compile a questionnaire that was administered to 58 ER staff. A total of 37 staff members completed the survey (64% response rate) of whom 21 were staff nurses. The main skills and attributes noted (ranked in order of importance) were ability to extract the most important information from the caller's description of the problem, good communication skills, good listening skills, experience working in the ER, and a wide medical knowledge. Important attributes of a telephone nurse that were cited are confidence in what you are saying, patience in dealing with the caller, a good telephone manner, and a caring approach. Of interest, none of the staff reported having received any significant specific training in the provision of telephone advice at the undergraduate or postgraduate level. All staff members believed that training was an essential prerequisite for the advent of high-quality telephone care.

Hayes and others interviewed ER staff members and home care nurses who used a telecare system that transmitted voice and images to distant sites via a video link.[14] The evaluation team carried out a structured interview designed to assess the interviewees' perceptions of their experiences with technology and telehealth, the potential benefits of the system to their work, and the potential barriers to using the system effectively. After using the system, home health nurses (N = 2) predicted that the use of telehealth services could reduce unnecessary office visits and would ultimately reduce costs. Potential barriers to telehealth services expressed in this study included liability and logistic issues, including how to manage technical difficulties (also, nurses in both groups expressed skepticism that physicians would use telehealth services).

Telehealth outcome studies

Austin and others examined the effectiveness of two telephone intervention strategies for improving the health outcomes of patients with systemic lupus erythematosus (SLE).[4] Fifty-eight patients were randomly assigned to receive a 6-month telephone counseling intervention using either a treatment counseling (TC) or symptom monitoring (SM) strategy. Health outcomes were assessed using several scales that were internally consistent with alpha cronbach's approaching 0.70 or greater. Results suggest that telephone interventions, especially TC, can be effective for improving the functional status of persons with SLE. Findings also suggest that telephone interventions that focus on patient behaviors (e.g., self-care activities, communication skills, medication self-management, symptom monitoring, and stress control) can improve outcomes of care. This study's small sample size, convenience sampling, and narrowly defined patient population make generalizability of the findings to other patient populations questionable.

Davis conducted a pilot study involving 17 caregivers of patients with dementia in order to evaluate the effectiveness of telephone-based skill building for reducing caregiver stress and improving family caregiver coping.[10] A standardized telephone intervention by a trained nurse was given to the caregivers. Using a pre-test and post-test analysis, findings suggest that telephone-based skill building may increase dementia caregivers' sense of social support, reduce their depressive symptoms, and improve their lifestyle satisfaction. This study design can be used to research many issues in home care. For example, a pre-test and post-test analysis could be done to assess improvements in patient self-care (e.g., ability to manage medications and disease process) as fostered by telecare standards and interventions.

Naylor and others conducted an intervention study investigating the effects of a comprehensive discharge planning protocol.[23] What is important to note in this study is that a telephone visit, as part of a discharge planning protocol, provided cost-effective care and reduced patient hospital readmissions. For example, the mean length of time between the index hospital discharge and readmission for patients in the intervention group was 45.6 days as compared with 31.0 days for the control group. Also, total charges for health care services 2 weeks after discharge for the intervention group were $163,858 less than charges for the control group (P = 0.08). This study also supports the use of a clinical nurse specialist (CNS) in discharge planning. A limitation of the study is that the efficacy of the telephone visit could not be assessed on its own merit because it was part of a total discharge intervention program. In addition, although the researchers state that the CNS initiated a minimum of two telephone calls to the intervention group during the first 2 weeks after discharge to monitor the patient's progress and intervene as necessary, no standards for telephone interventions were given.

Racelis and others conducted a pilot study (N = 21) that compared two randomized groups of patients with peripheral arterial disease for a 1-year period for compliance with smoking cessation.[26] The control group received standardized teaching care, whereas the intervention group received the standardized teaching plan plus a quarterly telephone call to reinforce smoking cessation and diet information. The results of the pilot study reveal no significant differences between the control and experimental groups in compliance with smoking cessation. In this study telephone reinforcement was not sufficient to influence lifestyle changes. A particular weakness of this study is that the researchers did not obtain a baseline lifestyle evaluation at its beginning (the researchers observed that many lifestyle changes are made immediately at the time of diagnosis). Also, perhaps the telephone intervention would have improved had the calls been more frequent.

Sellors and others conducted a study to determine the predictors of noncompliance with a second dose of hepatitis B vaccine and the effectiveness of a compliance enhancement strategy.[31] Subjects who did not return for the second dose of the vaccine were randomly assigned to one of two intervention groups: an "enhanced" or a "regular" method of encouragement. The enhanced group received a mail and telephone reminder to come back for the second dose of the vaccine. The regular method group received only a mail reminder. The researchers concluded that hepatitis B vaccine recipients with lower educational levels are at increased risk of noncompliance with the second dose of the vaccine but are highly responsive to telephone reminders coupled with mail reminders. The enhanced group had both a mail and a telephone intervention. Perhaps a future study could evaluate the telephone intervention by itself instead of coupled with another intervention in order to better evaluate the efficacy of telephone visits. The relevance of this study to home care relates to issues of using the telephone to encourage patient participation with the plan of care.

Critique of research studies

Although the previous studies indicate that the telephone service is useful in patient care, most provide either no specific or poorly defined protocols as to how the nurses responded to patient calls. Very few of the researchers addressed issues of reliability or validity of their evaluation tools. Also, the descriptive studies were not able to track the results of the information furnished to the patients (callers) and whether the patients were satisfied with the information they received over the phone. Moreover, most of the studies had a small sample size with few outcome-based interventions. Hence, the generalizability of the findings are questioned.

Another significant gap in the research deals with a lack of theoretical framework from which to guide the study. Although telephone interventions seem like a good idea, very few of the researchers articulate *why* the research is important to nursing and *how* the research relates to fundamental concepts of caring. In addition, none of the research defines or identifies key concepts of telecaring that supports effective nursing interventions.

Lastly, virtually none of the telehealth research has been done by home care nurses. In that the telephone is such a part of home care service delivery, this absence seems odd. It will be important for home care nurses to bring their unique ways of knowing into telehealth research as a means to ensure authentic recommendations for care.[35]

IMPLICATIONS FOR HOME CARE NURSING PRACTICE, EDUCATION, AND RESEARCH

The implications of a home care telephone visit can be found within the domains of nursing. In terms of clinical practice, the research suggests potential benefits of telehealth to include early intervention and prevention of unnecessary rehospitalizations. It has the potential to enable the home care nurse access to hard to reach populations including rural patients. Moreover, telephone visits can be used as a means for patient education especially if the patient did not receive or understand teaching while undergoing hospitalization. Also, telephone visits have the potential to maintain a therapeutic relationship with the homebound patient in a cost-effective manner. That is not to say that telephone visits should totally replace direct visits but should become a part of services offered. For example, if the patient is to be seen 3 times a week, perhaps the nurse could actually visit the patient on a Monday and Friday and make a telephone visit in between actual physical visits. Key to this process is for

nurses to remember that when using telecommunications, most patients want (1) to be heard, (2) their problems or issues to be resolved, and (3) to be valued and respected as human beings.

Home care nurses should be aware that some people cannot use the telephone and plan accordingly.[15] Interstate licensure issues should be resolved. Lastly, the literature indicates that telephone calls should follow written standards and be clearly documented.[13,20] See Boxes 26-1, 26-2, and 26-3 for clinical recommendations for telecaring.

In terms of nursing education, it is clear that telecare should become a part of undergraduate nursing curriculum. Consequently, guidelines for making a telephone visit should be a part of every entry level nursing school communication course.[27]

In terms of nursing research, primary recommendations in this chapter stem from relevant studies done in acute care or outpatient settings. As federal funding for telecare is apparent, home care nurses should consider grant-writing (1) to support needed research in this area, (2) to develop applicable standards of care for homebound populations, and (3) to generate philosophical dialogues regarding ethics and implications for practice.

Box 26-1   USING THE TELEPHONE WITH THE INTENTIONALITY TO CARE FOR PATIENTS

You are going to use the telephone to communicate with your patient who is at home. This may include speaking with a caregiver or family member. Sit for a moment and clear your mind. What is it you wish to accomplish with this telephone call? How does this relate to your patient's health outcomes and goals of care? After you have answered the above questions, briefly picture your telephone interaction with the patient. During this moment, *know* yourself as patient educator, advocate, caregiver, spiritual-aesthetic communer, and case manager. *Know* the patient as the sum of all he or she is and wants to be. Recognize that a fundamental purpose of this interaction is to foster positive patient self-care strategies and optimal levels of health. Recognize that these interactions occur across many dimensions of being (e.g., time and space). Make the call . . .

Box 26-2   TELECARING TELEPHONE COMMUNICATION TIPS

Use active listening.
Speak clearly and directly into the telephone.
Eliminate or reduce background noise.
Focus conversation on patient outcomes of care.
Perform a complete assessment and avoid a premature nursing diagnosis or problem identification.
Verify elderly patients' understanding of information; ask them to repeat the information back to you.
Demonstrate sensitivity to and respect for cultural differences.
Provide warnings or state consequences regarding issues of patient noncompliance.
Provide telephone care with competence and discretion; adhere to state regulations regarding practice and licensure issues.
Practice basic telephone courtesy; avoid keeping patients on hold; always terminate the call in a professional manner.
Keep voice recordings short with simple instructions and include an option to contact a "real person."

Box 26-3   TELECARING TELEPHONE DOCUMENTATION TIPS

Nurse name and credentials
Caller identification
Date and time of the call
Reason for patient call
Name of standard, protocol, or outcome addressed
Teaching, medication review, or any advice or warnings given to the patient
As appropriate, instructions to seek ER evaluation or appropriate agency for acute health care concerns
Anyone else contacted or referred to with complete documentation of referral or multidisciplinary call(s), including response of caller

---

AREAS FOR FUTURE RESEARCH

A basic question to answer is, "Can a telephone visit promote outcomes of care for the homebound patient and provide satisfaction with care?" Research should be done in order to answer this question. Research methods should utilize both empirical and interpretative approaches because multiple paradigms in nursing encourage creativity, thinking, and innovative practice. The following systematic telecare research program is suggested:

1. *A generalized descriptive study of how home care nurses currently use the telephone in patient care.* What are the issues expressed on the phone? What kinds of services are provided on the phone? Is the conversation directed toward patient outcomes of care? How is this noted? Is there evidence of self-care interventions via the telephone, and if so, what are they and how do they affect the patient? This study is very important because it will provide direction for other telecare research in home care.

2. *An analysis of home care nurses' attitudes regarding telephone visits.* What do nurses think is important to do when talking to a patient on the phone? What kind of educational preparation do nurses think is needed for telecaring of the homebound public? What are the people, equipment, and environmental issues? How do nurses define telecaring? This study is important because it will provide pertinent information regarding student learning and staff development needs.

3. *An analysis of patients' and families' attitudes toward perceived uses and benefits of telehealth services.* When providing telehealth services, what are patient concerns and needs for care. This study is a basis for consumer-oriented care, as well as provides marketing strategies for the home care industry. It could also address service delivery, as well as technology issues.

4. *Identification of community self-perceived needs for telehealth services.* Studies of this nature will provide social and political support for public funding of telehealth services in the community.

5. *Outcome studies that test the quality and cost-effectiveness of telephone care itself.* For example, do telephone visits decrease costs of care for the homebound public? Furthermore, is the relationship one of quality caring? Such work should be expanded to population studies that analyze the effects of telehealth services on the postpartum patient, the dependent elderly patient, the mental health patient, the

hospice patient, and other groups of people as a basis for state and federal health care policy making.

6. *Epistomological studies that evaluate telecare as a construct for home care.* For example, what kinds of patient-nurse interactions emerge in telecare? Specifically, can telecare promote patient self-determination for self-care? If so, what is necessary or needed for this to occur, and how is it to be evaluated? Also, what are the philosophical dimensions of telecaring, and what does this mean for nursing?

This suggested research will be fundamental to understanding what telecaring really means for the public and for nursing. It will serve as a basis for telecommunication standards of care and delivery of telehealth services, as well as lay critical groundwork for multidimensional caring. Of importance, it will provide nurses with the knowledge to make informed decisions about how to provide telecaring, as well as to dialogue what it is and what it is not.

SUMMARY

The home represents a significant point of health care service delivery for nurses today and tomorrow. As telecommunication advances in home care and in the community, it is paramount that nurses understand its implications for benefice to the public and the profession. Today's age of technology offers the promise of a better future for all mankind. With thoughtful consideration, nursing can play a leadership role in this process.

REFERENCES

1. American Academy of Ambulatory Care Nurses: Telephone nursing practice administration and practice standards, *http://aaacn.inurse.com/,* 1997.
2. American Nurses Association: Nurses use telehealth to address rural healthcare needs, prevent hospitalizations, *Am Nurse,* p. 21, November/December, 1997. For more information about the Comprehensive Telehealth Act of 1997, go to *http://www.nursingworld.org/gova/index.htm*
3. American Operating Room Nurses: Telehealth—a complex issue being addressed by state and federal governments, *AORN* 66(4):709, 1997.
4. Austin JS and others: Health outcome improvements in patients with systemic lupus erythematosus using two telephone counseling interventions, *Arthritis Care Res* 9(5):391, 1996.
5. Braunstein M: Home care in cyperspace, *Comput Talk Homecare Providers,* p. 5, Fall 1995.
6. Brennan P: The future of clinical communication in an electronic environment, *Holistic Nurse Prac* 11(1):97, 1998.
7. Bruegel RB: The increasing importance of patient empowerment and its potential effects on home health care information systems and technology, *Home Health Care Manage Prac* 10(2):69, 1998.
8. Carlsson M and others: Telephone line help for cancer counseling and cancer information, *Cancer Pract* 4(6):319, 1996.
9. Dale J: Development of a telephone advice in A&E: establishing the view of staff, *Nurs Standard* 9(21):28, 1995.
10. Davis L: Telephone-based interventions with family caregivers: a feasibility study, *J Fam Nurs* 4(3):255, 1998.
11. Edmonds E: Telephone triage: 5 years experience, *Accid Emerg Nurs* 9:8, 1996.
12. Gadow S: Ethical narratives in practice, *Nurse Sci Q* 9(1):8, 1996.
13. Gobis LJ: Licensing and liability: crossing borders with telemedicine, *Caring* 16(7):18, 1997.
14. Hayes RP and others: Staff perceptions of emergency and home-care telemedicine, *J Telemed Telecare* 4(2):101, 1998.
15. Huges D: Telephone care for elders, *Gerontol Nurs* 12:27, 1995.
16. Keavey S: Using the telephone to give more and better care, *JAAPA* 9(9):41, 1996.
17. Keeling A, Dennison P: Nurse-initiated telephone follow-up after acute myocardial infarction: a pilot study, *Heart Lung* 24(1):45, 1999.
18. Kiyak H and others: Physical and functional health assessment in normal aging and in alzheimer's disease: self reports vs family reports, *Gerontologist* 34(3):324, 1994.
19. Leggett-Frazier N and others: Telephone communications between diabetes clients and nurse educators, *Diabetes Educ* 23(3):287, 1997.
20. McMichael MH: A point of law. Dialing for dollars? The risks of telephone triage nursing, *J Leg Nurse Consult* 9(1):16, 1998.
21. Michael J, Summers C: Telehealth: are you prepared to avoid the risks? *Home Healthcare Consult* 5(7):27, 1998.
22. Morrison RE, Black D: Telephone medical care of patients with HIV/AIDS, *AIDS Patient Care STDS* 12(2):131, 1998.
23. Naylor M and others: Comprehensive discharge planning for the hospitalized elderly: a randomized clinical trail, *Ann Intern Med* 120(12):999, 1994.
24. Neuman M: *Health as expanding consciousness,* St. Louis, 1986, Mosby.
25. Osborn CL, Townsend CH: Analysis of telephone communication between hospice nurses and a nurse practitioner group, *Home Health Care Manage Prac* 9(5):52, 1997.
26. Racelis MC and others: Impact of telephone reinforcement of risk reduction education on patient compliance, *J Vasc Nurs* 16(1):16, 1998.
27. Reed P: The ontology of the discipline, *Nurs Sci Q* 10(2):76, 1998.
28. Rice R: Ethics in home care: dollars for care, *J Geriatr Nurs* 12(1):46, 1999.
29. Rogers ME: Personal communication, October 1986.
30. Rogers ME: The science of unitary human beings: current perspectives, *Nurs Sci Q* 7:33, 1994.

31. Sellors J and others: Understanding and enhancing compliance with the second dose of hepatitis B vaccine: a cohort analysis and a randomized trail, *CMAJ* 157(2):143, 1997.

32. Shaughnessy P: Outcome-based quality improvement in the information age, *Home Health Care Manage Prac,* 10(2):11, 1998.

33. Siden HB: A qualitative approach to community and provider needs assessment in a telehealth project, *Telemed J* 4(3):225, 1998.

34. Smith M: Caring and the science of unitary human beings, *Adv Nurs Sci* 21(4):14, 1999.

35. Steel K and others: A home care annotated bibliography, *JAGS* 46:898, 1998.

36. Stulginsky M: Nurses' home health experience in telecaring, *Nurse Health Care* 14:402, 1993.

37. Turner D: Can telephone follow-up improve post-discharge outcomes? *Br J Nurs* 5(22):1361, 1997.

38. Warner I: Telemedicine in home health care: the current status of practice *Home Health Care Manage Prac* 10(2):62, 1998.

39. Watson J: *Human science and human care-a theory of nursing,* New York, 1988, National League for Nursing.

40. Wooten R and others: A joint US-UK study of home tele-nursing, *J Telemed Telecare* 4(1):83, 1999.

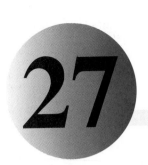

COMPLEMENTARY THERAPIES AND HOME CARE NURSING PRACTICE

Marlaine C. Smith

Complementary therapies are rapidly becoming part of mainstream health care. Eisenberg and his colleagues report that in a phone survey of 1539 adults throughout the United States, about a third had used some type of therapy considered "alternative" during the year prior to the survey.[17] Perhaps a more surprising finding is that 70% of those surveyed did not inform their physicians about this use. A 1998 follow-up study reveals that 42% of adults in the United States used at least one complementary therapy in the year before the survey.[18] In other studies of people with chronic diseases these percentages were the same or even higher.[2,11] Based on these trends, every home care nurse can expect that a substantial number of patients may be seeking alternative therapies for general health promotion, symptom management, or for treatment of disease. Home care nurses need to be knowledgeable about alternative therapies, open to exploring their use, and informed about resources for the safe and effective practice of these therapies.

The purpose of this chapter is to introduce home care nurses to the broad area of complementary therapies and to draw implications related to the use of these within the context of home care nursing. This chapter will provide an introduction to the array of therapies that are categorized as alternative or complementary. This is important for several reasons. First, with this overview, home care nurses may be better able to assess their patients' use of alternative therapies. Understanding the preferred healing practices of patients allows the nurse to incorporate these practices into the plan of care, to advise patients of any contraindications related to certain therapies, and to evaluate

patient response to the plan of care. Next, there is increasing evidence that many of these therapies influence patient health and quality of life. Both quality and cost outcomes of these therapies are being scrutinized; with demonstrated effectiveness and efficacy of alternative therapies we can expect to see more third party reimbursement, with patients exploring them as treatment options. Home care nurses should be aware of credentialed practitioners of a variety of popular alternative therapies so that they can refer their patients to reputable and competent providers. Finally, although most home care nurses may not have particular expertise in the practice of alternative therapies, some of these therapies may be easily integrated into home care nursing. This chapter will be organized in the following way: history and background of alternative health care, theoretical foundations, survey of alternative therapies with suggested applications to home care nursing practice, and implications for nursing and summary.

HISTORY AND BACKGROUND

The words *alternative therapies* have been used to differentiate a group of therapies from those used by conventional practitioners of Western medicine.[22] Alternative therapy is a broad spectrum of practices and beliefs that reflects the complex and holistic view of health and illness that is outside of the mainstream of biomedical practice.[17,37] It can be differentiated further in that alternative therapies are outside of the systems of standards and controls typical of traditional medicine. Most of these therapies have not been taught within schools of nursing or medicine, are not available through established delivery systems, and have not been reimbursable by most insurance companies. The term *alternative,* although still in use, is criticized by some because it connotes the idea that these therapies are substitutions for traditional medical care. The term *complementary therapies* has been suggested to represent the idea that these therapies can be used to *complement* or *supplement* the conventional plan of care. More recently Dr. Andrew Weil has recommended the use of the term *integrative therapies.*[43] Weil asserts that this language more accurately represents the idea that both traditional medicine and alternative practices have merit and can be synergistically combined for health and healing. The health care practitioner of the twenty-first century will integrate these practices into patient care.

Alternative therapies have a rich history in the healing traditions of many cultures. Chinese and Ayurvedic medicine are ancient and complex systems that incorporated acupuncture, herbs, meditation, and movement. Although these systems existed before the advent of conventional Western medicine, they are considered "alternative" within our culture. About a quarter of the world's population practices some form of traditional Chinese medicine.[5] Even in the early 1900s in the United States, individuals used a more natural approach to health care. At that time 1 in 5 doctors were homeopaths. The rise of biomedicine upset this balance.[5]

As discussed in Chapter 1, the roots of nursing are in the care of the sick by women in their homes. Women learned through practical wisdom and oral tradition, to use herbs, foods, water, and soothing presence to facilitate healing. The question of who controlled the province of healing was debated in the seventeenth century; clergy, lawyers, physicians, and women healers vied for their place in caring for the sick. The emergence of modern science and its myth of infallibility advanced physicians as the power brokers in health care. Unfortunately, the embodied practice wisdom of women healers was lost, in some cases burned at the stake with those convicted of witchcraft because of their remarkable results. With scientific and technological advancements, healing became entrenched within conventional medicine; pharmaceuticals and surgery rose as the primary legitimate therapies. All others, from physical manipulation to nutrition and herbal products, were marginalized, delegitimized, and relegated to the shadows. The powerful biomedical model overtook all approaches to the treatment of disease within the last half of the twentieth century.

Although this model still retains its power, the new focus on alternative therapy has emerged from several forces. First, the people, in grassroots movements, have created more humane, noninvasive, and participative delivery models. These movements, such as LaMaze childbirth education, family-centered care in hospitals, and hospice care for the dying, have successfully transformed some areas of health care. Many people want to take an active part in promoting their own health, and they are skeptical and distrusting of physicians and hospitals.[3] Concurrently, a critical mass of health care providers with philosophies and values inconsistent with the practice of health care in the biomedical model have emerged. Finally, the willingness of people to pay for alternative therapies has captured the attention of the payers, now eager to compete for these health care dollars.[17,18]

The spending for complementary health care is expanding exponentially in an era of shrinking resources. Right now in the United States, out-of-pocket expenditures for complementary therapies are approaching those for physician visits.[18] About 75% of the expenses for complementary therapies are paid out of pocket; this is about a billion more than what consumers paid for copayments for hospital care. There has been a 380% increase in the use of herbal remedies and a 130% increase in use of high dosage vitamins over the past decade.[5] The most intense interest in alternative therapies has been in oncology.[9] Oncology nurses and physicians adopted alternative therapies to relieve symptoms and promote comfort associated with the disease and the adverse effects of radiation and chemotherapy. But the general public is using alternative therapies for health promotion and disease prevention, as well as for the treatment of disease.

Within the literature, Donley reports that there are four reasons given for the use of alternative therapies by consumers: fear of harm and intrusion, a desire for a natural approach to treatment, access and lower costs, and a perceived apathy of providers to patient experiences. "Experience and the literature suggest that the traditional medical establishment has placed too much emphasis on high-technology medicine and has lost sight of human needs. Some physicians have become so enamored with science and evidence-based practice that symptoms, which are not easily quantified or are not coherent with diagnostic criteria, are not taken seriously."[13]

The health care system and the scientific community have awakened to their responsibilities to respond to the public's increasing use of alternative therapies. The public deserves the best information on which to base decisions related to their health care. Although it is true that most of these therapies do not harm patients, some in fact may be detrimental. For example, Gingko Biloba, because of its anticoagulant qualities, may be dangerous to patients who are undergoing surgery. Financial harm may be incurred through investing large amounts of money in therapies that will result in no benefit to the patient. Finally, because credentialing is not uniform in practitioners of alternative therapies, it is difficult to select qualified providers. Because of this lack of uniform regulation of practice, unscrupulous practitioners may be able to take advantage of the vulnerability and desperation of those who are ill.

In 1992 the National Institutes of Health established the Office of Alternative Medicine (OAM). Funds are provided through the OAM to support research in alternative therapies. Currently there are nine Office of Alternative Medicine sponsored centers with their own particular focus. This research is important to document the safety, efficacy, and effectiveness of alternative therapies. Health care systems and complementary practitioner groups are developing standards for credentialing and accreditation. These efforts support the responsible practice and informed utilization of complementary health care.

THEORETICAL FOUNDATIONS

Many of the therapies categorized as "alternative" have been an integral part of the practice of nursing since its inception. For example, the backrub was once a routine part of care in the hospital setting. These practices arose from our philosophy of care, and it is now time to reclaim our roots, to remember who we are and from whence we've come. Florence Nightingale was the first to articulate the philosophical traditions of nursing. Nightingale realized the inherent healing power of nature and defined the practice of nursing as "putting the patient in the best condition for nature to act . . ."

In other words, the nurse created an environment (e.g., fresh air, sound, color, beauty, warmth, and cleanliness) that facilitated innate healing processes.[32] Many alternative therapies are based on this premise.

The healing and caring tradition of nursing is nested within a relationship-centered ethic. Relationship is the essence of any healing. It may be what people are now seeking in their quest for alternative therapies. Donley notes, "The old texts of medicine and nursing spoke to a relationship with the patient that was in itself healing. Given the pace and the priorities of contemporary medicine, this human relationship may not develop. Lacking a meaningful encounter with their traditional doctor and nurse, the patient may seek support and healing from an alternative therapist."[13]

Watson, in her theory of human caring, articulates the interrelationship of caring and healing.[41,42] For Watson, caring is an energetic process that can potentiate health and healing. The nurse honors the person's uniqueness, preserves humanity, and inspires the other to appreciate and experience life fully. The engagement with the patient is an end in itself, not merely instrumental to the medical or technological goals.

What has been popularized as "holistic" practice has its origins within nursing. Rogers' conceptual system, describing the unity of the person and environment, is a perspective that has influenced nursing and provides a theoretical foundation for the integration of complementary therapies into nursing practice. According to Rogers, the nurse engages with the person in patterning toward maximizing well-being from the patient's perspective.[38,39]

Based on these nursing theories the following acronym, *CARE*, can provide a succinct theory-guided foundation for the use of complementary therapies in nursing practice. CARE represents: *Choice*, *Advocacy*, *Relationship*, and *Empowerment*. *Choice* means that each of us participates in our own healing journey. Each person has the right to decide the types of health care that are congruent with personal and cultural values. In any care decision each person participates knowingly in understanding personal health and in changing health patterning. *Advocacy* means that the nurse actively and accurately represents and supports the patient's point of view, both within the context of their relationship and with other providers in the health care system. Advocacy is removing barriers and providing access to information and services for the desired, safe, effective care. *Relationship* is central to all healing. The use of complementary modalities is not an instrumental process of selection and application. The patient's relationship to self, nature, significant others, the nurse, and a spiritual center form the ground from which the seeds of healing grow. The modalities in themselves are mere facilitators of this "right relationship" or harmony.[35] Finally, *empowerment* refers to the tenet that the nurse acknowledges, affirms, and supports the inherent responsibility and ability of the patient to be a full participant in her or his own health and healing.

SURVEY OF ALTERNATIVE/ COMPLEMENTARY THERAPIES

Although there are several frameworks for categorizing alternative therapies, the OAM's seven fields of practice will be used to organize this section. These fields of practice are (1) herbal medicine; (2) diet, nutrition, and lifestyle changes; (3) mind-body interventions; (4) manual healing; (5) alternative systems of medical practice; (6) bioelectromagnetic applications; and (7) pharmacological and biological treatments. Each of these will be described briefly for the purposes of providing an overview of information on the array of therapies that fall under the umbrella of "alternative." Some have greater relevance for nursing practice generally and home care practice specifically. Those will be elaborated more fully and some implications for home care nursing practice will be suggested.

Herbal medicine

The first field of practice identified by the OAM classification is herbal medicine. Herbal remedies are widely used by the general public in the United States. They are on the shelves of almost every grocery store and certainly within every health food store in the nation. The increasing use of herbal supplements has received national media attention. The World Health Organization estimates that 80% of the population of the world uses some forms of herbal medicine.[5] In a 1994 survey of 1653 adults conducted by the FDA, 8% reported the use of herbal supplements.[7] With the recent increase in attention and marketing, that percentage is certainly conservative.

Herbal medicine, also known as *botanical medicine* or *phytomedicine,* is the use of plant or plant parts to make a therapeutic product or supplement. Herbal remedies include those taken for cardiovascular health, cold or flu, detoxification, diet and weight loss, digestive aids, energy, immune boosting, laxatives, memory aids, depression or anxiety, sleep, stress reduction, PMS, and menopause. Herbal remedies are available in many forms: tinctures or extracts, capsules, tablets, teas, lozenges, vapor treatments, and topical products. The FDA regulates herbal products only as dietary supplements, not as drugs. Manufacturers cannot claim that a product cures a specific disease; however, they can make general claims about the common uses for the product.

Most people self-medicate with herbal remedies, selecting supplements based on the claims on their labels or from reports from the media or a personal network of friends. Some of the most popular herbs taken are listed in Table 27-1. Well-designed research on herbal remedies has supported many of the uses listed. Although nurses want to encourage self-care and can appreciate the important benefits derived from herbal remedies, it is critical to encourage people to take an informed, judicious approach to their use.

There is concern about the practice of self-medication with herbal remedies. Overuse and combination of herbs can have deleterious effects on the health of patients. Libster provides guidelines for selecting and consulting with medical herbalists.[31] She recommends evaluating the expertise of herbalists through appraising their education, experience, and ability to assess the patient thoroughly and understand the interactions between herbal and traditional medicines. In general, Libster recommends that the nurse consider referring a patient to a medical herbalist when he or she is using an herb for a particular health concern or when the patient will be using any herb for more than 30 days. Pregnant and lactating women and children should not be given herbs unless they are under the guidance of a knowledgeable practitioner of herbal medicine. Anyone taking a prescription medication should see a primary care provider and a medical herbalist before combining the two. Elderly patients are at a greater risk for experiencing sequelae from the combination of prescription drugs and herbs.

Table 27-1 Ten common herbal remedies[5,19]

Name	Common uses	Consideration
Chamomile	Antispasmodic for gastrointestinal (GI) and menstrual cramping, migraine Mild sedative as a tea To induce relaxation, sleep	Use cautiously in people with allergies to ragweed, pollen, asters, chrysanthemums Vomiting reported if dried flowers are ingested in large quantities Contraindicated during pregnancy or breast-feeding
Cranberry	Extract for preventing urinary tract infection	No adverse effects reported Available in capsules, juice
Echinacea	As antiviral, immunostimulant, for wound healing Treatment of colds, flu, sore throats	Available as liquid, powder, extract, tincture, tablets, tea Capsules relatively inactive Contraindicated for patients with HIV, collagen disease, MS, other autoimmune disorders Overuse can result in immune suppression Do not take longer than 8 weeks; 10-14 days is probably sufficient
Garlic	Antioxidant, antihypertensive To lower serum lipids To decrease platelet aggregation	Some heartburn, flatulence when taken in large quantities Equivalent of 5-10 cloves/day for the effects listed Prolonged and high dose may lead to decreased hemoglobin and lysis of RBCs Value of "odorless" garlic tablets is questionable
Kava Kava	To attenuate spinal seizures For antipsychotic properties For Anxiety disorders For Depression, insomnia For pain, muscle spasm, asthma	Changes in motor reflexes and judgment Visual disturbances Decreased platelet count with heavy, chronic use Contraindicated during pregnancy Avoid with psychotropic drugs Potentiated by alcohol
Gingko Biloba	For dilation of arteries, capillaries, veins For symptoms of Raynaud's disease, impotence and memory loss, overall brain function	GI upset possible May reduce clotting time; do not take at least 2 weeks before surgery or with prescription anticoagulants
Ginseng	To enhance ability to adapt to stress, improve performance and endurance To lower blood glucose To improve cognitive function	Diarrhea, skin eruption, nervousness, sleeplessness, and hypertension Adverse reactions: chest pain, headache, impotence, nausea, palpitations Avoid combining with stimulants like coffee or tea With any chronic condition consult with health professional before taking
Saw Palmetto	To manage prostate problem To increase sperm production, sexual response, breast size To promote diuresis	Contraindicated during pregnancy Take with morning and evening meal Get a baseline PSA before starting, false negatives after therapy

Table 27-1 Ten common herbal remedies[5,19]—cont'd

Name	Common uses	Consideration
Saw Palmetto—cont'd		
	For benign prostatic hypertrophy	Adverse reactions: abdominal and back pain, constipation, diarrhea, dysuria, headache hypertension, decreased libido
St. John's Wort	As antiinflammatory, diuretic For anxiety, depression As MAO inhibitor with antiviral activity As a treatment for HIV infection	Photosensitivity is common, resulting in rash; protection needed for fair-skinned people Contraindicated during pregnancy Avoid with prescription antidepressants Adverse reactions: constipation, dizziness, dry mouth, GI distress, restlessness, sleep disturbances
Valerian	As sedative	Can increase morning drowsiness Can have additive effects with other depressants Adverse reactions: headaches, excitability, cardiac disturbances

There are several implications related to the use of herbal medicines for the home care nurse. First is to incorporate questions about the use of herbal medicines as part of the overall health assessment. Because we know that many people are afraid to disclose these practices to "traditional health professionals," it may be best to frame the question in a way that invites a truthful response. For example, "We know that many people use over-the-counter remedies including vitamins, supplements and herbs. What kinds of these over-the-counter remedies do you take?" It is important to obtain a good history of when they are or were taken, the dosage, and the form or type. Inquire about how these remedies help the patient or how the patient believes they might help. Ask if the person has experienced any adverse reactions with the herbal remedies. Include questions about any consultations with herbal doctors (e.g., naturopath or doctor of Chinese medicine)? Finally, find out if this is information that has been revealed to the primary care provider. Have a resource and referral network available for your own use and for the patient. Identify a list of qualified medical herbalists. Several organizations that can help with the referral to reputable medical herbalists are listed at the end of this chapter.

The home care nurse should encourage the patient to seek education about any medication they take, including herbs. There are excellent books written for consumers on this topic. We can only anticipate that there will be a growing interest in the use of herbal remedies. Attending continuing education programs on herbal remedies, reading articles, and keeping pace with the latest research on the use of herbs will be important for the practice of home care nursing.

Diet, nutrition and lifestyle change

It may seem strange to think of diet, nutrition and lifestyle changes as "alternative" therapies; however, they are described as such in the OAM classification, probably because of the current popularity of vitamins, minerals, and dietary supplements. Food and water may be the most important supplements to healthy living; unfortunately they may also be the most neglected. For example, we know that adequate hydration in the elderly may be one of the most important elements for health. We know the importance of protein to tissue maintenance and wound healing. Nurses have cut their teeth on the "basic four" food groups and the mantra that eating a well-balanced diet is sufficient, countering the need for vitamin supplements.

Conventional wisdom is quite different now. Mainstream nutritionists teach the food pyramid;

however, other scientists refute this model, stating that it underrepresents the amount of protein needed and overrepresents the amount of carbohydrates. Furthermore, the pyramid does not differentiate between carbohydrates with a high glycemic index, that is, those that take longer to digest and metabolize, from those with a low glycemic index, those that are digested and metabolized quickly, producing a steep rise and drop in blood sugar.

Many nutritionists now believe that the "modern affluent diet" consisting of processed, refined, and high fat foods with a concomitant low intake of whole grains, fruits, and vegetables is responsible for the high prevalence of chronic degenerative disease in our population.[5] Fast foods and prepared and packaged convenience foods tend to be very high in fats, salt, sugar, refined carbohydrates, partially hydrogenated vegetable oils, and additives and preservatives, substances that are known to be harmful to health.[5]

There are many "diets" touted to provide the nutrition needed for maximum well-being. Rather than promote any one, it is more reasonable to follow a moderate approach that incorporates some of the most current wisdom on diet and nutrition. Some guidelines may be helpful in promoting healthful nutrition. These are listed in Box 27-1.

The first principle is to avoid ingesting food additives. This means eliminating foods and beverages that include aspartame, saccharin, food dyes, nitrites, sulfites, and monosodium glutamate. These substances are listed on the labels. The second principle is to avoid ingesting any foods with partially hydrogenated oils. Partially hydrogenated oils contain trans-fatty acids that may impair the metabolism of essential fatty acids. This may affect the synthesis of hormones and immune system function. Partially hydrogenated oils contain free radicals that promote aging, tissue damage, and the development of cancer.[5,44] The third principle is to avoid refined sugars and starches or the "white foods." The process of refining strips foods of their nutrients. Refined sugars and starches are linked to heart disease, dental decay, obesity, decreased immune functioning, and behavior and learning problems in children.[5] Fats are important in the diet; the next principle suggests decreasing the amount of saturated fat in the diet, using instead monounsaturated fats such as olive oil. Weil suggests the use of olive oil almost exclusively; canola

---

Box 27-1	10 PRINCIPLES OF HEALTHFUL NUTRITION

1. Avoid ingesting food additives including aspartame, saccharin, monosodium glutamate, nitrites, and sulfur dioxide, sodium bisulfate, and sulfites.
2. Avoid eating any foods containing partially hydrogenated oils.
3. Avoid foods that contain primarily refined sugars and starches.
4. Limit intake of saturated fat; use oils such as olive, grape, or sesame.
5. Increase intake of fresh yellow, red, and leafy green vegetables; cruciferous vegetables; fruits; onions; seeds; and nuts.
6. Ensure adequate protein intake including soy products such as soy milk, tofu, miso, or tempeh.
7. If allowed, enjoy a glass of red wine with one meal a day.
8. Increase intake of whole grains and legumes.
9. Take vitamin supplements daily.
10. Drink green tea.

Data from Belcher I and others: *Nurse's handbook of alternative and complementary therapies*, Springhouse, Penn, 1999, Springhouse; Weil A: *Eight weeks to optimum health*, New York, 1997, Fawcett.

---

oil only when the taste of olive oil is not appropriate for the dish.[44] Also, he emphasizes avoiding margarine or any hardened fat. Butter is preferable to margarine; however, because butter is a saturated fat, it should be limited. The fifth principle is to eat large amounts of colorful fruits and vegetables. These include green leafy, red, yellow, cruciferous (e.g., broccoli, cauliflower, brussel sprouts), onions, seeds, and nuts. These are the foods that contain the healing phytochemicals: antioxidants, carotenoids, some flavonoids, and polyphenols. The vegetables should be fresh. Ensuring adequate protein intake and adding soy protein to the diet is the sixth principle. Most of us rely on meat, eggs, and milk as sources for our protein. Fish, especially salmon, sardines, mackerel and kippers, are excellent sources of Omega-3 fatty acids, which are important for preventing heart disease, and promoting tissue repair and good immune functioning. Soy is an excellent source of flavonoids and phytoestrogens that are important in preventing cancer, minimizing collagen destruction, and enhancing immune functioning. We can introduce soy into our diets through protein drinks (many contain soy) and soy milk. Experiment with introducing tofu in favorite dishes.[5,44] The seventh principle is to enjoy a glass of red wine once a day if permitted. Obviously those who are alcoholic or are taking prescription medications that prohibit alcohol will forego this suggestion. Red wine contains flavonoids and polyphenols that may prevent heart disease and cancer. The eighth principle is to increase intake of whole grains and legumes. This includes whole grain breads and cereals, chick peas, lentils, and split peas. These are carbohydrates with a high glycemic index, and they contain healing phytoestrogens. Taking vitamin and mineral supplements is the ninth principle. Weil recommends the following formula: 1 to 2 grams of vitamin C taken 2 to 3 times a day; one capsule of mixed carotenes (25,000 IU of beta-carotene along with alpha-carotene, lutein, and zeaxanthin) with breakfast, 400 to 800 IU of vitamin E with lunch or the largest meal, and 200 to 300 micrograms of selenium.[43,44] A multivitamin can be taken in addition to the formula; the formula is adjusted by subtracting the amount in the multivitamin from Weil's recommended dosage. Many medications taken by patients will interfere with vitamin and mineral absorption, so it is important that supplements are part of their daily regimen. Elderly people who have difficulty preparing food, less of an appetite, depression, or difficulty chewing or swallowing need supplementation. They have higher requirements for certain nutrients such as vitamins D, B_6, B_{12}, and calcium. Smokers have a higher need for vitamin C, and people on a vegetarian diet need to be sure that they have adequate protein and vitamins and minerals. The tenth and final principle is the addition of green tea as a beverage to the diet. Green tea contains polyphenols that lower cholesterol and improve lipid metabolism. It also has anticancer and antibacterial properties.[44] It can be a refreshing and healthy substitute for coffee or black tea.

Diet and nutrition have profound implications for the practice of home care nursing. Patients recovering from surgery or living with symptoms and sequelae of chronic disease need special attention to their diet. Food and water should be viewed as life-giving, health-giving drugs. We need to instill in our patients the importance of what they eat. Following these principles of healthful nutrition can make a real difference in energy level, mood, functioning, and general health. Home care nurses already assess diet and nutrition. Including questions on a weekly diet history about all foods, amount of water, and supplements consumed can provide a snapshot of the quality of the patient's diet. Change in lifestyle related to diet is best made incrementally. Food has meaning to our patients, and it is important to preserve this meaning while promoting a more healthful diet. The home care nurse can encourage realistic goals and small steps toward incorporating changes in the diet. Encourage patient education on the use of the supplements, and suggest reading materials or accessing websites.

Mind-body interventions

Mind-body interventions include those activities that shift consciousness from the ordinary to the extraordinary, the mundane to the sublime, and an external to an internal level of awareness; these activities may result in physiological changes that may mediate symptoms or disease progression. The mind-body interventions underscore the inherent wholeness or irreducibility of the person to parts or aspects. The following interventions are included in this category: (1) dance, music, art, and narrative therapies; (2) relaxation, guided imagery, meditation, biofeedback, yoga, spiritual practice and prayer; (3) humor; and (4) aromatherapy.

The first group in this category are the therapies associated with aesthetic experience or creative expression. The premise underlying the healing potential of these therapies is that engagement in any form of art can shift our consciousness or awareness from our logical, linear processes to the receptive and creative processes. This shift can facilitate the expression of meanings of subjective experiences that may be related to our health. Gaining awareness of these experiences through engagement with art, music, poetry, narrative, or dance may provide insight that leads to opportunities to change and grow. The use of the creative arts may allow the person to express feelings, thoughts, and perceptions in forms beyond verbal language. The language of art is the language of the soul, the expression of our deepest hopes, dreams, fears, sorrows, and joys. The use of art therapies provides us an opening to allow the full expression of the self toward experiencing greater freedom and aliveness . . . To express and experience art is to be fully human.

Dance/movement therapy. The use of the body for expression as in dance or movement therapy has many benefits. First it may exercise the cardio-vascular-pulmonary systems; increase muscle tone, flexibility, and strength; and increase body awareness in space, thus preventing falls. As with all the mind-body interventions the "physical" benefits are not separate from the "psychological." Dance or movement may enhance energy, diminish lethargy and fatigue, increase concentration, and improve mood. Through dance we express our being in relation to our environment through rhythmic movement in space. Suggesting any form of movement is healthful.

Movement and dance are most effective when orchestrated in response to music. The tempo of the music may be altered to match the patient's abilities and preferences. Movement may be as limited as swaying arms and torso to the rhythms of music while sitting in a chair or as demanding as step aerobics or tap dancing. The key is to begin where the patient is and to increase movement gradually. Tai chi chiuan is a Chinese exercise program that may help the elderly patients experience greater awareness of their bodies in space. Research suggests that tai chi may reduce pain intensity for people with low back pain, improve general fitness, and enhance mobility of patients with osteoarthritis.[30] Expressive movement to music can make the boring routine of physical therapy or repetitive exercise more enjoyable.[5]

Music therapy. Music is a powerful therapeutic and has been used for patients with pain, depression, anxiety, stroke, and brain injuries and to communicate with people with Alzheimer's disease. It can promote connection, communication, introspection, and the release of emotion. Perhaps one of the greatest advantages of music therapy, especially for home care, is that it requires two ingredients: a comfortable environment and a source of music. Musical selections can be played on a tape or compact disc player, or favorite instruments can be used. The process may be receptive, such as listening, or expressive, such as playing or singing along. Studies have associated specific pieces of music with particular emotions. Generally, faster music is stimulating, whereas slower music has a calming effect. But these generalizations may not hold, because the response to music is highly individualized. It is best to ask patients for their preferences. Also try to "match" the tempo, tone, and qualities of a musical piece to the affect, rhythm, and tone of the person's pattern. For example, it is not a good idea to play a Sousa march to "cheer up" a person who seems sad or lethargic. It is best to find a mellow, slow piece that may move them to express outwardly what is within them. The use of music can be a stimulant for reminiscence and a catalyst for bringing groups of patients together. Family members can be encouraged to use music with their loved ones with Alzheimer's disease. Encouraging the person to tap in rhythm or sing along can be effective in shifting the pattern from restless or agitated to calmer and more harmonious.[5,24,25]

Art therapy. Art therapy can be used to facilitate expression of feelings, provide creative diversion, enhance sensory awareness, and facilitate communication with others. A variety of media such as watercolors, pastels, and clay; needlepoint; quilting; wood carving; and photography are expressive outlets. Encourage the patient to select a medium that is comfortable for him or her. Assess the patient's interest and past experience with arts or crafts. Even when fine motor control is lacking, there can be engagement with some form of artistic medium. The home care nurse might suggest arts or crafts as an activity that the family could do together. It provides more interaction than a passive activity such as watching television. Completing products or projects can provide an occasion to share work with others, which may engender a sense of productivity, worth, and belonging.

Narrative therapy. Writing can be an outlet for expression and healing. Writing encourages the reflection on and expression of the personal meanings of an illness. It can take the form of recording thoughts and feelings in a personal journal or expressing them in poetry. Through creative writing the person may chronicle the experience to share with others so that others might learn from the insights of those who have weathered the experience. For patients who cannot write or type, a tape recorder is useful. Providing patients with pathographies, others' personal stories of illness or health crises, can be a powerful path to the realization that they are not alone; others have endured similar experiences and have shared valuable lessons learned. Examples of these narratives are: *Elegy for Iris,*[4] a story written by the husband of a woman with Alzheimer's disease, and *At the Will of the Body,*[21] the story of a man who survived both cancer and a heart attack. The oral tradition of story-telling has similar effects and, as related to developmental age, is particularly useful when working with sick or dying children (see Chapter 7 and Chapter 24).

The next group of mind-body interventions employs a deliberate change in awareness of the body and inner space. These include relaxation response, breathing, guided imagery, biofeedback, meditation, prayer, and yoga.

Relaxation response. The relaxation response was identified by Benson as a way to mediate the dangerous effects of stress.[6] The stress response involves the activation of the sympathetic and parasympathetic nervous system with accompanying neuroendocrine responses that produce both immediate "fight-or-flight" symptoms and longer term manifestations of decreased immune response, increased blood platelets and glucose, protein catabolism, and sodium retention. These physiological changes can potentiate the development of heart disease, cancer, and autoimmune disorders. The role of stress in the development of disease is well-documented. The modulation of the stress response can occur with the relaxation response. Studies of the effects of progressive muscle relaxation have supported its benefits in reducing frequency of seizures, improving mood, decreasing pain, lowering blood pressure, decreasing anxiety, and increasing immune response.[22] The relaxation response is often experienced spontaneously but can be learned and practiced so that its benefits are experienced frequently. There are several different types of relaxation responses. One of the simplest to learn and practice is progressive muscle relaxation (PMR) (Box 27-2). Teaching patients the process of practicing PMR can be accomplished easily within the home. Home care nurses can demonstrate and practice the PMR with patients and/or family members. Commercial relaxation tapes are available for purchase at music stores, or home care nurses can make their own tape recording of a PMR exercise for their patients' use.

Breathing. The focus on breath is foundational to all of these mind-body therapies. In ancient times "breath" was associated with spirit and wind; it is our connection to the environment. Weil emphasizes the importance of attending to proper breathing.[44] He says, "I am often asked, 'If you could only tell people to do one thing that would give them greater access to spontaneous healing, what would it be?' I never hesitate in answering, 'Work with your breath!'"[44] Attention to breathing can produce the physiological changes of the relaxation response. Proper breathing is deep, diaphragmatic, and rhythmic. Breathing in this way is an excellent exercise to teach your patients. Box 27-3 provides examples. Encourage the patient to do breathing exercises at least 4 to 5 times a day. These simple exercises can make an amazing difference in the sense of well-being.

Guided imagery. Guided imagery begins with a relaxation induction exercise such as PMR. Following the experience of deep relaxation the patient is invited to imagine himself/herself in various situations or to imagine a goal to be achieved. These situations may be settling in at a favorite place, experiencing a favorite activity, or finding a guide who can share an important message. Simonton pioneered work with cancer patients applying imagery to potentiate the effects of chemotherapy and radiation.[40] For example, patients may be asked to visualize their cancer cells as pieces of ground meat and the chemotherapy as a ravenous dog racing through the body gobbling the meat. Research has supported the effectiveness of guided imagery in reducing pain, relieving nausea and vomiting, inducing relaxation, and helping patients to tolerate procedures. In 1994 a study group reported to the National Institutes of Health (NIH) that there was a relationship between imagined and actual bodily changes.[1,5]

Biofeedback. Biofeedback is learning to exercise control over ordinarily autonomic bodily functions through electronic monitoring. This is done through a process of relaxation, focus, and feedback on breathing, heart rate, blood pressure, or other physiological indicators. The perception of these physiological changes provides "feedback" to the participant so that the person knows when he or she is successful in producing these changes. Biofeedback is accomplished through the use of instruments that provide information on skin temper-

---

Box 27-2 PROGRESSIVE MUSCLE RELAXATION EXERCISE

Sit in a comfortable chair. Close your eyes and place your feet solidly on the floor. Relax into the back of the chair. Now turn your attention to the rhythm of your breathing. (Pause) Breathe at a rhythm that feels easy for you. (Pause) Now you are going to relax the muscles throughout your body. We'll begin at your head and move downward. Turn you attention to the muscles in your scalp, face, chin, and neck. Tense these muscles. Feel what it is like when you are holding tension in these muscles. Now release this tension. Relax the muscles in your scalp, then all your facial muscles; let your jaw drop; feel the muscles in your neck relax. Now turn your attention to your shoulders and back. Tense these muscles and feel what it is like to hold tension here. Now release this tension. Feel it flow out of your body. Your shoulder and back muscles are supported and relaxed. Now turn your attention to your chest and midriff area. Tense these muscles and hold that tension for a few seconds. Notice it. Now release it. Let every muscle empty itself of any hint of tension and let it flow down through your feet and into the ground. (Repeat this process for the arms, abdomen, buttocks and pelvis, and legs). Begin the exercise slowly at first, detailing each muscle group. With practice, eliminate the tensing and practice focusing on each muscle group, noticing tension and releasing it. Practice until the response can occur in seconds. The relaxation exercise can be done for 15 minutes 2 to 3 times a day.

Box 27-3 BREATHING

These exercises can be introduced progressively, beginning with the most simple.

1. Sit in a comfortable position, close your eyes, and loosen clothing. Place your hand gently on your abdomen. Focus your attention on your breathing, noticing each inhalation-exhalation cycle and the shift between the two. Your hand should be rising on your abdomen with each inhalation. Do not alter your natural breathing pattern in any way. Do this for 5 minutes.

2. Sit in a comfortable position, close eyes. Focus on your breathing imagining that the exhalation part of the cycle is the first phase instead of the inhalation cycle. Breathe in your normal pattern with this "reversed focus" for 5 minutes.

3. Begin this exercise in the same way as in 1 and 2. With your mouth closed, breathe through your nose to the count of 4; hold your breath to the count of 9; purse your lips slightly and exhale through your mouth to the count of 8. Continue the pattern for 4 cycles then breathe normally. Do not force yourself to hold your breath if it is uncomfortable. The ratio of the inhalation-hold-exhalation time is important, not the number of seconds. Practice this at least 2 times a day. As you get more experienced with this exercise, add another cycle 1 week at a time until you get up to 8 cycles each time you do the exercise.

Data from Weil A: *Eight weeks to optimum health,* New York, 1997, Fawcett.

---

ature (thermal biofeedback), blood pressure, pulse, respirations, EEG (electroencephalography) EMG (electromyography) or galvanic skin response (electrical conductivity from increased perspiration). Biofeedback has been used in more than 150 applications for migraine headaches, chronic pain syndromes, cardiac arrhythmias, hypertension, irritable bowel syndrome, Raynaud's disease and incontinence.[5] Because it is a specialized practice involving the use of instruments, it requires about 8 to 10 training sessions by a practitioner who is skilled in biofeedback. Once the person has learned the process, practice with the instruments can occur in the home.

Meditation. Meditation can be associated with spiritual traditions or can be practiced in a more secular manner. Meditation refers to the quieting of the mind from distracting thoughts through the focused repetition of a word, phrase, or sound. Distracting thoughts are noted; however, the person returns to the disciplined focus of the repetitive "mantra." Meditation begins with carving out space and time without distractions. Relaxing the body, breathing rhythmically, and focusing attention are all elements of meditation. Many tapes are available for patients who would like to practice forms of healing meditation. Meditation has usefulness for relieving pain, managing stress, anxiety, panic, headaches, insomnia, and immune deficiencies.[1]

Spiritual practice or prayer. At first glance it may seem strange to see spiritual practice or prayer listed as type of "therapy." But, it is! Prayer is based on the belief that a Higher Power exists who can intervene in the life of humans including healing. There are many forms of prayer from silent meditation to speaking aloud and from seeking help for self to seeking help for others.[15] Prayer may be an important part of the patient's life. Placing it in the realm of a "complementary therapy" supports the active participation of the nurse in praying with and for patients. Researchers have concluded that there are health benefits for those patients who have strong religious or spiritual beliefs.[5] A fascinating study by Byrd reveals that when intercessory prayer was offered for patients in the coronary care unit, the "prayed for" group had significantly fewer complications than those in the control group. Of course, the prayer tradition of any person is a deeply personal choice, so the home care nurse should respect this tradition when praying with the patient. The nurse's own intercessory prayer for the patient may be offered in the privacy of her or his own space.

Yoga. Yoga is situated within Ayurvedic medicine; however, many people practice yoga outside of the context of this system of medicine. Yoga literally means "to join"; it is the practice of joining mind-body-spirit. There are various schools of yoga. A popular form, hatha yoga, uses postures or *asanas,* breathing exercises or *pranayama,* and meditation to create peace, calm, and well-being. Yoga classes are often offered out of community recreation centers. If homebound patients are interested in yoga, several videotapes are available to guide people through the practice of yoga. Those who promote and practice yoga have described the benefits as providing greater flexibility, body awareness, calm, and increased concentration.

Humor. Humor is a way of altering our consciousness toward a generation of positive emotions and the neuroendocrine response that accompanies them. The cliché that "laughter is the best medicine" contains a profound truth. In *Anatomy of an Illness,* Norman Cousins chronicles how he healed himself of ankylosing spondylitis by injecting large intravenous doses of vitamin C and watching funny movies that provoked "belly laughs."[12] Laughter can raise endorphins and lower cortisol. Children laugh about 400 times a day, whereas adults laugh about 15 times a day. Perhaps that has something to do with the onset of chronic illnesses in middle age![22] Home care nurses can

suggest that their patients engage in some activities that will make them laugh, whether it is reminiscing with a friend or enjoying a favorite comedy on videotape.

Aromatherapy. Aromatherapy is placed in the category of mind-body interventions, although it doesn't seem to fit as well as many others. Aromatherapy is the inhalation or application of essential oils extracted from plants to promote relaxation and relieve various symptoms or prevent disease. Essential oils can be applied directly to the skin or pulse points, can be added to baths, or inhaled through diffusers. The smells of essential oils are hypothesized to stimulate the limbic system, which effects the emotions. Some believe that the vibrational energy of the essential oil acts as a tuning fork to promote resonance with a frequency of a particular emotion. The application of the oils directly to the skin are purported to be absorbed and result in hormonal and enzymatic changes. Aromatherapy is a popular healing art in Europe and is used to treat infections, headaches, premenstrual syndrome, skin disorders, arthritis and musculoskeletal pain, and to promote relaxation and well-being.[5] There is some empirical support that aromatherapy enhances relaxation and decreases anxiety.[22]

Manual healing

The category of manual healing includes an array of therapies that have in common touch or manipulation through the use of the hands. This includes the manipulative therapies of chiropractic and osteopathy; the touch therapies of massage and acupressure; the structural-functional-movement integration therapies of Trager, Alexander, Feldenkrais, and Rolfing; and the energy-based therapeutics of therapeutic touch.

Chiropractic. The first group of manual therapies consists of chiropractic and osteopathy. These involve the manipulation of the soft tissues, bones, and joints by trained doctors of chiropractic and osteopathy. Chiropractic was founded in the 1890s. This practice is based on the premise that the body has the ability to heal itself if it receives unobstructed flow of nerve impulses from the brain through the spinal cord to the peripheral nerves. The therapies involve hands-on spinal manipulation in order to free the spinal cord and spinal nerves from subluxations or pressure points. Chiro-

practic theory asserts that the spinal nerves enner-
vate all the vital tissues and organs and that this
proper ennervation is essential to organ and tissue
health. Pressure on the spinal nerves can result in
any number of symptoms or syndromes. There are
two types of chiropractic: the "straight" espouse
the philosophy that subluxation is the cause of all
disease; the "mixers" include a broader range of
philosophy of disease and approaches to treatment.
Chiropractic care is used for neuromusculoskeletal
conditions like back pain, whiplash, and headache.
Some scientific evidence suggests that chiropractic
care is useful for digestive disorders, dysmenorrhea, sprains and sports injuries, carpal tunnel syndrome, TMJ disorder, and tendonitis. The Agency
for Health Care Policy and Research (AHCPR) released a clinical practice guideline for acute low
back problems in adults, which endorsed spinal
manipulation "as an effective therapy for acute
lower back pain," adding that it "brought relief, as
well as functional improvement."[5] Cherkin and
MacCornack report that patients who had chiropractic treatment for low back pain were more satisfied with their treatment than those who received
their care from medical doctors. Many chiropractors practice a mixed model of care, that is, they
combine spinal manipulation with other therapies
such as nutrition, vitamin and mineral supplements, massage, electrical stimulation, ice, heat, ul-
trasound, and traction. For this reason chiropractors are often sought after because of their holistic
approach to care and philosophy that the treatment
is designed to support the body's own natural
healing capabilities. Home care nurses can develop
a referral network of chiropractors for those patients who want chiropractic care. In developing
this network it is important to inquire about education, type of practice, years of practice, and specialty therapies included in the practice. Talking
with patients of the chiropractor to determine their
satisfaction with outcomes of the therapies, number
of treatments, and cost of treatment can provide additional information for evaluating the quality of
the practitioner. Chiropractic care is now covered
by many insurance plans, usually for a limited
number of visits. Those patients interested in pursuing chiropractic care should examine the specific
limits of their coverage.

Osteopathy. Osteopathic medicine was founded
by Andrew Taylor Still in the 1874. Still developed
his process of manipulation to improve the existing
medical practice of the time. The principles of osteopathic medicine are (1) the interdependence of
structure and function and human behavior; (2) the
body's ability to heal itself; (3) the belief that
disease arises from disruptions in normal processes
of structure, function, and behavior; and (4) treatments include manual procedures that are used to
assess these disruptions and their origins in the
structure and function of internal organs or behavior.[5] Manual techniques are integrated into osteopathic practice. In 1993 the United States had over
32,000 doctors of osteopathy in practice. Osteopaths are doctors of Osteopathy (DO) who incorporate manipulation into their medical practice.
Today, it is often difficult to discern the differences
between the practices of medical doctors and osteopaths. Osteopaths can serve as primary care
providers and may provide a more holistic approach to health care. Those patients who want this
approach to care may have the option to select a
DO as their primary care provider.

Massage therapy. The second group of manual
therapies is the touch therapies such as massage
and acupressure. Massage is one of the oldest of
the identified "alternative" therapies. There are references to it in 4000-year-old Chinese medical
books, and Hippocrates, the Greek "father of medicine," described the importance of massage in the
healing arts. In the 1850s modern massage was
introduced by two physicians who studied it in
Sweden, thus the name "Swedish" massage.[1]
Massage became a part of nursing practice, and
nurses studied back massage within the nursing
arts curriculum. Recently this integration into hospital care has been lost because of greater attention
to completing medical-related procedures. Massage therapy has emerged as a specialized field of
practice, with schools of massage therapy preparing the therapists. "Massage therapy is the scientific manipulation of the soft tissues of the body to
normalize those tissues through application of the
hands to the body using fixed and moving pressure."[1] This technical definition loses the sense that
massage therapy, especially as integrated into
nursing practice, is a form of sensing and communicating with patients through touch. The nurse can
use hands to receive information about the pattern
held in the body and can express an intent to
care and be present through the hands. There are

over 80 different methods classified as massage. Swedish massage combines effleurage (gliding strokes), kneading and friction on the superficial layers of muscle, percussion or vibration. These techniques have been used in the back massage to promote relaxation, improve circulation, relieve muscle tension, and promote range of motion.[1] Deep-tissue massage releases patterns of muscular tension using pressure or friction. It is applied to deeper layers of muscle than is Swedish massage. Neuromuscular massage is a form of deep massage that is applied to a specific muscle. It is used to release trigger points, knots of muscle tension, and to release the tension place on nerves. Trigger point massage and myotherapy are similar. Manual lymph drainage is application of light strokes for the purposes of enhancing the lymphatic flow in conditions such as edema and neuropathies.[1] Research on massage therapy has been proliferating. Studies have documented the benefits of massage therapy for pain, inflammation, lymphedema, nausea, muscle spasm, soft tissue injury, anxiety, depression, insomnia, stress, and weight gain in low-birth-weight infants.[1,20]

Massage can be easily incorporated into the home care visit or can be taught to family members. Back, hand, and foot massage can be administered in a brief period of time and is one way to communicate caring with the patient. Learning to give a back massage to a family member can be beneficial to both the giver and receiver. It can enhance intimacy, communication, and a sense of satisfaction in comforting and being comforted by a loved one.

Acupressure. Acupressure is the use of the fingers to apply pressure to meridian points in order to stimulate them or sedate them. There are four systems of acupressure: shiatsu, tsubo, jin shin jyutsu, and jin shin do. All of these are based on the philosophy of Chinese medicine. Shiatsu and tsubo involves the use of the thumb to apply pressure and direct the flow of qi (energy). Jin shin jyutsu and jin shin do have developed specific protocols for the application of pressure to meridian points for specific illnesses. The treatments are similar to those of acupuncture in that pressure is applied to meridian points associated with specific organs and these are held in patterns that alter the flow of qi.[1]

Structural-functional integration therapies. The manual therapies characterized as structural-functional integration therapies include Alexander technique, Feldenkrais method, Trager, and Rolfing.

Alexander technique. Alexander technique is a set of movements that focus on the reeducation and alignment of the posture especially in the alignment of the head, neck, and shoulders. It involves simple movements to improve balance and pressure, which are applied to retrain the muscles. The technique is designed to help people use their bodies with greater awareness and less tension. It has been used for neck and back pain, postural misalignment, whiplash, myalgia, repetitive strain injury, anxiety, and other chronic conditions.[1]

Feldenkrais method. Feldenkrais is a method that focuses on movement patterns and consists of two branches: awareness through movement and functional movement. This method uses verbal cues and gentle deliberate touch to invite clients to explore alternatives in their patterns of moving.

Trager method. The Trager psychophysical integration method uses light, rhythmic rocking and shaking movements to release chronic patterns of tension held within the body. The goal is to promote freedom of movement. Anecdotal reports suggest that the method has been successful in treating movement dysfunction in multiple sclerosis and muscular dystrophy, muscle spasms, spinal cord injuries, TMJ, chronic pain, and headaches.

Rolfing technique. Rolfing is another structural integration technique that involves the stretching of the fascia sheaths by applying sliding pressure with the fingers, thumbs, and elbows. It has been used for stress and anxiety and for musculoskeletal pain and diminished function.

Therapeutic touch (TT). Energy-based therapies comprise the final group in the manual therapies category. These therapies are based on the world view that both the healer and the healed are vibrating fields of energy that are in process with the environmental fields.[26] TT is one therapy based on Rogers' Science of Unitary Human Beings.[38,39] Therapeutic touch is based on the assumption that people are energy fields, open systems engaged in continuous mutual process with the environmental field. The pattern of the human field can be sensed, in part, with the hands. Imbalances are perceived and the healer uses his or her intent to help or heal a person and may participate in the repatterning of the field. The practitioner of TT participates knowingly in this process of repatterning through a process of resonance.[36] The practitioner uses his or her hands as an instrument in this patterning of the energy field process.[39] The Krieger-Kunz method of therapeutic touch has received considerable attention in the nursing literature. It was specified by Dolores Krieger who learned the process from Dora Kunz, a healer.[28,29] This method of therapeutic touch involves five processes: The first is centering. Here, the practitioner takes the time to be still and focus intention through a purposeful, healing meditation. In this way, the practitioner can be fully present to the person and can be more awake and aware of the sensation and intuitive perceptions related to the field pattern. The second process is assessment. The practitioner places his or her hands several inches from the person and scans the field with his or her hands from head to toe. In this process the practitioner is noticing any differences in energetic sensation. This might be heat, cold, tingling, or variations in pressure. These variations are noted. The next process is unruffling the field. Here the practitioner is mobilizing the flow of the energy field through a gliding movement over the person. Next, there is the process of modulating the flow of energy through the practitioner's deliberate intentions to engage in patterning. The practitioner may focus intent on specific areas where the sensations of differences were noticed. Finally, the treatment continues until there is a sense of completion. Some studies on TT supported that it is effective in producing relaxation, wound healing, and relief of pain.[16] The results of a meta-analysis of the therapeutic touch research reveal that though a number of studies on TT had mixed or negative results, most studies supported the efficacy of the therapy.[23] Healing touch has some similarities to TT; it is different in that it is based on the belief in the chakras as energy centers. Anyone can learn therapeutic touch. There are thousands of TT practitioners throughout the country. Many classes in TT and healing touch are offered throughout the country. Home care nurses can learn TT and practice it with patients who are open to it.

Alternative systems of medical practice

The fifth category of alternative medicine is "alternative systems of medical practice." Included in this category are traditional Chinese medicine (TCM) including acupuncture and Ayurvedic,

homeopathic, and naturopathic medicine. These are developed systems with elaborated processes of diagnosis and specific therapies.

Traditional Chinese medicine and acupuncture. Traditional Chinese medicine (TCM) has been practiced for over 3000 years. It is based on the principle of balancing the flow of qi (chi) or the life force energy and harmonizing the opposing dynamics of this energy, *yin* and *yang*. According to TCM, all of life has this dual nature. Acupuncture, Chinese herbal therapy, Qi gong, and massage are used within TCM. Foods are classified according to their yin or yang properties, and the diet is regulated to promote balance. Qi gong is an integrated process of breathing, meditation, movement, and postures for self-healing and well-being.

Perhaps the most well-known modality of TCM is acupuncture. Acupuncture is the practice of diagnosis of imbalances in the flow of qi through 59 energy channels or meridians. The TCM practitioner uses pulse diagnosis to recognize these imbalances. Needles are inserted into particular acupuncture points to enhance and balance the flow of qi. Needles may be twirled, an electric current may be applied, or smoldering cones of an herb moxa (mugwort) may be placed on them. The most common effects of acupuncture are relaxation and a sense of well-being.[22] It is a very safe therapy in that adverse side effects are extremely rare. There are many schools teaching acupuncture within the United States, and a variety of practice patterns exist. The NIH Consensus Development Conference[33] on acupuncture issued a report concluding that there is evidence that acupuncture is effective for the relief of nausea and for dental pain. Also, there is evidence that it has been used successfully for the treatment of chronic pain, migraine headaches, nausea and vomiting, addiction, rehabilitation, dysmenorrhea, musculoskeletal injuries, fibromyalgia, and asthma.[22] Acupuncture is a covered benefit within many insurance plans.

Ayurvedic medicine. Ayurvedic medicine has its origins within the Vedas, the ancient Hindu writings; it has existed for over 2000 years. Ayurvedic is sanskrit for the "knowledge of life."[22] Ayurvedic medicine is based on the concept of three doshas (tridosha) or body humors called *vata, pitta,* and *kasha.* Prana is the vital life energy that enters the body through breath. Chakras are the energy centers of the body. Balance of these vital energies and purifying the mind, body, and spirit are corner-stones of this system. Ayurvedic medicine emphasizes the importance of diet, hatha yoga (breathing, postures, exercise, meditation), and cleansing or detoxification processes.

Naturopathic medicine. Naturopathy originated in the United States in the late 1800s. It is based on the principle that the body has an innate ability to maintain health. Naturopathic doctors (NDs) use the diagnostic procedures of allopathic (Western) medicine, but they approach treatment through supporting the body's healing capacities. There are eight tenets that form the foundation of naturopathic medicine. They include the following beliefs: the use of therapies that are least likely to result in complications; the doctor is a teacher; prevention is a focus of treatment; good nutrition is central to healing; optimum health, not just the eradication of disease, is a goal; and the importance of treating the whole person. Naturopaths use nutritional therapies, herbs, homeopathic remedies, hydrotherapy, acupuncture, manipulation, counseling, and teaching in their care of patients. There are more than 1000 naturopathic NDs practicing in the United States.[5]

Homeopathic medicine. Homeopathic medicine is based on the principles of the laws of similars, or that "like cures like." Hahnemann, a German physician, created homeopathy in the 1800s after he experimented with quinine, the cure for malaria. He found that the "cure" produced the "symptoms" of the disease. Homeopathy is an elaborate system that appreciates the intricate unity of body-mind-spirit. Hahnemann originated the term of allopathic medicine to delineate traditional medicine from homeopathy. In allopathic medicine, the approach is to prescribe a medicine that opposes the disease process. In homeopathic practice, a lengthy, detailed patient interview precedes any prescription. The purpose of the interview is to look at the underlying subtle "cause" of the disease. Homeopathic practitioners use large databases that link remedies with symptoms and temperamental profiles.[22] Homeopathic remedies are prescribed that contain an extremely diluted form of the same compound that is the hypothesized cause of the symptoms. Studies testing homeopathic remedies against a placebo have shown reduction of symptoms in asthmatics; reduction in pain and improvement in, function and mobility for

those with rheumatoid arthritis; reduction in the intensity of migraine headaches; shorter duration of influenza, and less severe diarrhea. Summaries of these studies appear in Fugh-Berman.[22] A meta-analysis reveals that 75% of the trials did show positive results for homeopathy.[25] Homeopathic remedies are available in most health food stores for the treatment of many common ailments. Although many persons use these remedies for self-care, it is worthwhile for a person who wants to try homeopathy to have a full evaluation from a skilled, reputable homeopathic practitioner, especially for the treatment of chronic disease.

Bioelectromagnetic applications

The next category in the OAM classification is bioelectromagnetic applications. These include light therapy, bioelectrical acupuncture, and electromagnetic field therapy.

Light therapy. Light therapy was popularized in the 1970s with the discovery that exposure to sunlight has an effect on mood. The condition of seasonal affective disorder (SAD) or depression that occurs during the winter months in northern climates without sufficient sunlight is described in the literature. The treatment for SAD began with exposing patients to full-spectrum lighting indoors.[34] Today other types of light therapies are used to treat disorders that range from psoriasis to forms of cancer. Some of these are ultraviolet (UV) light therapy, colored light therapy, photodynamic therapy, syntonic optometry, and cold laser therapy. There is no scientific evidence on the effectiveness of light therapy except for SAD and neonatal jaundice.[5]

Bioelectrical acupuncture. Bioelectrical acupuncture is the application of electrical stimulation to acupuncture needles or acupressure points for the purpose of stimulating the flow of energy or to stimulate currents into local nerves. Several devices are used by practitioners such as the dermatron, the locator-stimulator, or the SOLITENS device. These devices are used also to assess the flow of energy along meridian pathways.

Electromagnetic field therapy. Electromagnetic field therapy involves the use of a variety of devices that produce a magnetic field in the treatment of disease. One premise is that the device restores the magnetic equilibrium disrupted by the disease process. Another theory is that because of the magnetic nature of red blood cells, an applied field will draw red blood cells and thereby an increased oxygen and nutrient supply to an area of injury or disease. Electromagnetic field therapy has shown promising potential for accelerating the healing of fractures, bone grafts, cartilage, soft tissue tears, non-healing wounds, and pressure ulcers.[22] Electromagnetic field therapies may be used more frequently in the future for accelerating the healing of musculoskeletal injuries and in the slow healing wounds of diabetics and immobile patients.

Pharmacological and biological treatments

There are many therapies included in the category of pharmacological and biological treatments. Some of the more well-known of these are biological treatments for cancer such as antineoplastons, shark cartilage, immunoaugmentative therapy, induced remission therapy, and hyperoxygenation therapies. These therapies are administered by practitioners in clinics that are not supported by mainstream medicine. In fact, many have been attacked by the establishment, driving the practice of these therapies outside the United States.

Chelation. A more well-known therapy is chelation. Chelation is a process that removes metallic or mineral toxins from the body through binding them to ethylenediaminetetraacetic acid (EDTA), an amino acid. The EDTA is administered intravenously, and the toxic metals are excreted in urine. Although chelation is a standard treatment for lead poisoning, its primary use in the area of alternative therapy is for cardiovascular disease and autoimmune disorders. The rationale is that the EDTA can remove the calcium from arterial plaques, thereby reversing atherosclerosis. Others believe that it is an antioxidant that can reduce the damage and inflammation associated with free-radical damage. The treatment is available at clinics within the United States, and more than 1000 physicians support its use for cardiovascular disease.[5]

IMPLICATIONS FOR HOME CARE NURSING PRACTICE

Complementary therapies are moving into mainstream health care. These therapies can be integrated into the treatment plan of home care patients to improve their quality of care. Dossey and others provide detailed discussion and guidelines for the integration of complementary therapies into nursing practice.[14] The following are some general guidelines for the use of complementary therapies in home care practice:

- Assess the patient's values and wishes surrounding the types of therapies they are currently using and those they would like to explore.
- When the patient requests complementary therapies, the nurse should examine the evidence about the effectiveness of the therapies for the purpose that the patient has in mind. Share this knowledge or information sources such as articles or websites with the patient for the purpose of aiding in decision making.
- Evaluate the effectiveness of the complementary therapies that the patient is using.
- Encourage openness about the use of complementary therapies with the primary care provider.
- Develop a resource and referral file for information and lists of credentialed, well-qualified providers.
- Examine any contraindications for the use of selected complementary therapies such as herb-prescription drug interactions.
- Consider integrating complementary therapies such as breathing and relaxation, imagery, and massage into home care practice.
- Continue learning about complementary therapies, and share this with your patients and their families.
- For those with special interest in this area, the American Holistic Nurses Association offers a certification program. See Appendix XXVII-I.

SUMMARY

The home care nurses of the twenty-first century will be challenged to integrate the therapies of the biomedical model with those now referred to as alternative therapies. These therapies call us to the heart of nursing, to a practice that is relationship centered, focused on natural processes, and shows appreciation for the health and wholeness of those we serve.

REFERENCES

1. *Alternative medicine: expanding medical horizons:* Washington, DC, 1994, U.S. Government Printing Office.
2. Anderson W and others: Patient use and assessment of conventional and alternative therapies for HIV infection and AIDS, *AIDS* 7:561, 1993.
3. Astin J: Why patients use alternative medicine, *JAMA* 279:1555, 1998.
4. Bailey J: *Elegy for Iris.* New York, 1999, St. Martin's Press.
5. Belcher I and others: *Nurse's handbook of alternative and complementary therapies,* Springhouse, Pa, 1999, Springhouse.
6. Benson H: *The relaxation response.* New York, 1975, William Morrow.
7. Brevoort, P: The U.S. botanical market: an overview, *HerbalGram* 36:50, 1996.
8. Byrd RC: Positive therapeutic effects of intercessory prayer in a coronary careunit population *South Med J* 81(7):826, 1986.
9. Cassileth BR and others: Contemporary unorthodox treatments in cancer medicine, *Ann Intern Med* 01:105, 1984.
10. Cherkin DC, MacCornack FA: Patient evaluation of low back pain care from family physicians and chiropractors, *West J Med* 150:351, 1989.
11. Coleman LM and others: Use of unproven therapies by people with Alzheimer's disease, *J Am Geriatr Soc* 43:747, 1995.
12. Cousins N: *Anatomy of an illness as perceived by the patient,* New York, 1979, WW Norton.
13. Donley SR: The alternative health care revolution, *Nurs Econ* 16(6):298, 1998.
14. Dossey BM and others: *Holistic nursing: a handbook for practice,* Rockville, Md, 1999, Aspen.
15. Dossey L: *Healing words: the power of prayer and the practice of medicine,* New York, 1995, Harper Collins.
16. Easter A: The state of research on the effects of therapeutic touch, *J Holistic Nurs* 15(2):158, 1997.
17. Eisenberg DM and others: Unconventional medicine in the United States: prevalence, costs, and patterns of use, *N Engl J Med* 328:246, 1993.
18. Eisenberg DM and others: Trends in alternative medicine use in the United States, 1990-1997, *JAMA* 279:1569, 1998.
19. Fetrow CW, Avila JR: *Professional's handbook of complementary and alternative medicines,* Springhouse, Pa, 1999, Springhouse.
20. Field TM: Massage therapy effects, *Am Psychol* 53(12):1270, 1998.
21. Frank AW: *At the will of the body,* Boston, 1991, Houghton-Mifflin.
22. Fugh-Berman A: *Alternative medicine: what works,* Baltimore, Md, 1997, Williams & Wilkins.
23. Fry PW, Kijek J: An integrative review and meta-analysis of therapeutic touch research, *Altern Ther Health Med* 5(6):58, 1999.
24. Good M: Effects of relaxation and music on postoperative pain: a review, *J Adv Nurs* 24:905, 1999.
25. Hanser SB, Thompson LW: Effects of music therapy strategy on depressed older adults, *J Gerontol* 46:265, 1994.
26. Heidt P: Scientific research and therapeutic touch. In Borelli MD, Heidt P, editors: *Therapeutic touch,* New York, 1981, Springer.
27. Kleijnen J and others: Clinical trials of homeopathy, *Br Med J* 302:316, 1992.
28. Krieger D: *Accepting your power to heal: the personal practice of therapeutic touch,* Santa Fe, NM, 1993, Bear and Co.
29. Krieger D: Therapeutic touch: the imprimatur of nursing, *Am J Nurs* 7:767, 1975.
30. Kuhn MA: *Complementary therapies for health care providers,* Philadelphia, 1999, Lippincott William & Wilkins.
31. Libster M: Guidelines for selecting a medical herbalist for consultation and referral: consulting a medical herbalist, *J Altern Complement Ther* 5(5):457, 1999.
32. Nightingale F: *Notes on nursing: what it is and what it is not,* Philadelphia, 1895/1992, Lippincott-Raven.
33. *NIH consensus report on acupuncture,* Bethesda, Md, 1997, National Institutes of Health.
34. Ott J: *Health and light,* Old Greenwick, Conn, 1973, Devin-Adair.
35. Quinn J: On health, healing, and the haelen effect, *Nurs Health Care,* 1991.
36. Quinn J: Therapeutic touch as energy exchange: testing the theory, *Adv Nurs Sci* 6:42, 1983.
37. Rauckhorst L: Integration of complementary therapies in the nurse practitioner curriculum, *Clin Excellence Nurs Practitioners* 1(4):257, 1997.
38. Rogers ME: *An introduction to the theoretical basis of nursing,* Philadelphia, 1970, FA Davis.
39. Rogers ME: Nursing: science of unitary, irreducible, human beings: update—1990. In Barrett EM, editor: *Visions of Rogers' science-based nursing,* New York, 1990, National League for Nursing.
40. Simonton OC and others: *Getting well again,* Toronto, 1978, Bantam Books.
41. Watson J: *Nursing: human science and human care,* New York, 1988, National League for Nursing.
42. Watson J: *Postmodern nursing and beyond,* New York, 1999, Churchill-Livingstone.
43. Weil A: *Eight weeks to optimum health,* New York, 1997, Fawcett.
44. Weil A: *Spontaneous healing: how to discover and enhance your body's natural ability to maintain and heal itself,* New York, 1996, Fawcett.

Resources for Information
on Alternative Therapies

Academy for Guided Imagery
www.healthy.net/agi

Academy of Scientific Hypnotherapy
(619)427-6225

Acupressure Institute
www.healthy.net/acupressure

Alternative Care
www.sky.net/~ngt/welcome.html

Alternative Medicine Connection
www.Arxc.com/hotlinks.htm
Links to medical libraries and research center
pages

American Academy of Medical Acupuncture
www.medicalacupuncture.org

American Art Therapy Association, Inc.
www.arttherapy.org

American Association for Music Therapy
(610)265-4006

American Association of Oriental Medicine
www.aaom.org

American Board of Chelation Therapy
(800)356-2228

American Botanical Council
www.herbalgram.org

American Chiropractic Association
www.amerchiro.org

American College for Advancement in Medicine
www.ACAM.org

American Dance Therapy
adta@aol.com

American Holistic Nurses' Association
www.ahna.org

American Massage Therapy Association
www.amtamassage.org

American Osteopathic Association
www.am-osteo-assn.org

American School of Ayurvedic Sciences
(425)453-8022

Ask Dr. Weil
www.drweil.com/

Association for Applied Psychophysiology and
Biofeedback
aapb@resourcenter.com

Bastyr University
www.bastyr.edu
Natural health sciences

Bio-Electro-Magnetics Institute
johnz@scs.unr.edu

East-West Academy of Healing Arts
(800)824-2433
Qigong

Feldenkrais Guild of North America
www.feldenkrais.com

Healing Touch International
www.healingtouch.net

HealthWorld Online
www.healthy.net/library/journals/index.html
Consumer and professional information

Herb Research Foundation
www.herbs.org

Himalayan International Institute of Yoga Science
and Philosophy
Himalaya@epix.net

Institute of Noetic Sciences
www.noetic.org
Meditation

Maharishi International University
www.mum.edu
Meditation and Yoga

National Association for Holistic Aromatherapy
www.naha.org

National Center for Homeopathy
www.homeopathic.org

National College of Naturopathic Medicine
www.ncnm.edu

Natural Medicine and Alternative Therapy
www/amrta.org/~amrta

Oregon Health Sciences University
Complementary and Alternative Medicine
www.ohsu.edu/ohmig/cam.html

Rolf Institute of Structural Integration
www.rolf.org

Society for Light Treatment and Biological
Rhythms
www.websciences.org/sltbr
Light therapy

The Trager Institute
TragerD@aol.com

University of Pittsburgh Alternative Medicine
homepage
www.pitt.edu/~cbw/internet.html
Links to other alternative therapy resources

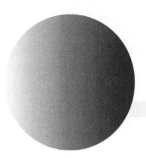

EPILOGUE: RECONSIDERING CARING IN THE HOME

Jean Watson

In reconsidering caring in the home, perhaps a case can be made for pure caring in that it is in noninstitutional, real-living situations, such as the home, that the most authentic and yet demanding aspects of personal-professional caring become manifest. This is true for the members of the family, as well as any professional care provider. The foundation for any professional home care approach becomes the authenticity and trusting relationship that the care provider brings to the situation; this includes creating and sustaining relationship-centered caring as the basis of all that occurs. What do we mean by this, and how does it become manifest?

RELATIONSHIP-CENTERED CARING AS A STARTING POINT AND BASIS FOR PROFESSIONAL NURSING IN THE HOME

First of all, the nurse, in this instance the professional care provider, brings his or her unique self into a relationship with the individual/family. This is done in such a way that the integrity and dignity of the individual and the family are honored within their own space with their own patterns and rhythms of living. The nurse and the nursing care are there to strengthen the existing relationships and patterns, not to alter, judge, or disrupt them, and to work within the individual's and family's frame of reference, rather than from the nurse's. In other words, we come to know the patient from his or her perspective.

What the nurse offers first, by way of establishing relationship-centered care as the focus of nursing in the home, is Self: by this I mean bring one's whole self into the present situation, the specific moments of caring, in such a way that the nurse is authentically present to other. He or she does this in such a way that silence is honored; the nurse is open to letting the situation come into being, rather than being there to control and manipulate outcomes and processes. The nurse seeks to hear, to listen to the patient's and family's story, to listen to the meaning and the moods and emotions behind the words in order to more fully grasp and connect with the lived reality of the situation, behind or beyond the words.

Being authentically present to another requires being centered, taking a reflective stance toward one's own behavior and responses, reflexively attending to self in relation to others and their responses. Often when entering into another's world, we are on guard, protecting ourselves, rather than being open to discover what is there to teach us from another's situation or condition. Authentic presence allows for a pause, an openness to enter into anothers' space and connect with them and their story in such a way that you too are invited to know what it is from the other side—to be open to your own compassion and to consciously, intentionally reflect and communicate caring back to others in the situation.

Once the trusting, caring relationship is established, the nurse of course seeks to sustain and deepen the connection, but it is from the relationship and the human-to-human connection that the care needs become more manifest, more honestly communicated. This relational orientation toward self and other in the home sets up caring condi-

500

tions, where the nurse can truly practice nursing. It is from the basis of relationship-centered caring that the medical treatment protocols are delivered and ministered, as well as the advanced nursing and caring-healing arts can more naturally flow. It is from this view and this philosophical orientation to caring in the home that professional caring can be witnessed and experienced at its best.

PROFESSIONAL HOME CARE NURSING IS NOT DEFINED AS DOING

To reconsider professional care in the home, with relationship as the center, one cannot restrict nursing to "doing care," or to "doing treatments," or to "doing nursing skills," or to "physical care alone." Indeed, nursing in the home cannot be defined or reduced to "doing" at all. However, caring in the home does not preclude these behaviors; indeed, in most instances home care includes "doing" some skills as one of the reasons for home care nursing.

Nevertheless, it is equally important to realize that professional nursing cannot be defined or limited by outdated views of nursing, especially so because home care nursing requires more independent and more professional views of practice, not less. Again, if in any setting it is perhaps caring in the home in which nursing calls forth and draws on the full use of self and the full actualization of a mature nursing paradigm.

SOME ELEMENTS OF A MATURE NURSING PARADIGM FOR HOME CARE NURSING

The following elements are at play in a mature professional nursing paradigm for home care:

- First of all, as already noted, the *full use of self in establishing and sustaining relationship-centered caring* is the basis for all care that occurs.
- Secondly, nursing in the home setting cannot be defined by what the nurse does, but rather by the *caring consciousness, intentionality, and relationship that combine to create a human-to-human connection. This connection is the link for sustaining care both in and out of the home.* Even when the nurse is not physically present, caring at a distance can be

sustained if the original conditions for meaningful relationship are created. Caring can be sustained because of the original starting point of professional care that was based on the nurse's full use of self in developing a trusting-helping-caring relationship. This foundation serves as the ground for all the caring that follows, whether the care is delivered in person and/or through technology or communication from a distance, such as E-mail, telephone, or other telehealth connections.

- The nurse practices mature nursing arts made manifest in the original Nightingale blueprint for nursing, as well as *contemporary advanced holistic caring-healing practices.* These practices include some of the original healing arts and the most effective mind-body-spirit medicine, also referred to as advanced caring healing practices. They are manifest in reconsidering aspects of care that are noninvasive, nonintrusive, and natural, such as environment as healing through more intentional attention to nature, sound, light, color, smells, form, shapes, variety—many of those basic "essentials" that Nightingale identified over 100 years ago as nursing! In more contemporary terms home care also brings into play the intentional use of touch, whether healing touch, therapeutic touch, or compassionate human touch for someone who is starved for touch. This extends to use of massage, reflexology, foot care, basic skin care, use of essential oils for skin care and also for calmative effect, comfort measures, and so on. The involvement of other members of the family in these and other "basic nursing arts," or "advanced caring-healing modalities" (depending on how one wishes to consider or reconsider such approaches to mature nursing care). These modalities and more are now considered part of professional clinical care practices within a mature nursing paradigm. Whenever home care nursing is redefined from the standpoint of a mature discipline of nursing, the nurse is invited to become part of the healing processes in a caring relationship that seeks to make whole the practitioner, as well as the family or patient. When nursing enters into this level of maturity, home care nursing becomes one of the purest exemplars of a model of caring-healing, as well as advanced professional practice.

This work by Robyn Rice takes nursing in the home to a new level of maturity that will help nursing to both clarify and sustain human caring, both at the human level and at the level of technology, or caring at a distance. These directions open nursing to both new and old territories, to practice a deeper level of caring than ever before thought possible.

BIBLIOGRAPHY

Tresolini CP, Pew-Fetzer Task Force: *Health professions education and relationship centered care:* report of Pew-Fetzer Task Force, San Francisco, 1994, Pew Health Professions Commission.

Watson J: *Postmodern nursing and beyond,* UK, 1999, Churchill-Livingstone/Harcourt-Brace. (Especially see pp 192-226.)

Appendix

LABORATORY VALUES

Test	Reference range	
	Conventional values	SI units*
Blood, plasma, or serum values		
Acetoacetate plus acetone	0.30-2.0 mg/dl	3-20 mg/l
Acetone	Negative	Negative
Acid phosphate	Adults: 0.10-0.63 U/ml (Bessey-Lowry)	28-175 nmol/s/L
	0.5-2.0 U/ml (Bodansky)	
	1.0-4.0 U/ml (King-Armstrong)	
	Children: 6.4-15.2 U/L	
Activated partial thromboplastin time (APTT)	30-40 sec	30-40 sec
Adrenocorticotropic hormone (ACTH)	6 AM 15-100 pg/ml	10-80 ng/L
	6 PM <50 pg/ml	<50 ng/L
Alanine aminotransferase (ALT)	5-35 IU/L	5-35 U/L
Albumin	3.2-4.5 g/dl	35-55 g/L
Alcohol	Negative	Negative
Aldolase	Adults: 3.0-8.2 Sibley-Lehninger U/dl	22-59 mU/L at 37° C
	Children: approximately 2 × adult values	
	Newborns: approximately 4 × adult values	
Aldosterone	Peripheral blood:	
	Supine: 7.4 ± 4.2 ng/dl	0.08-0.3 nmol/L
	Upright: 1-21 ng/dl	0.14-0.8 nmol/L
	Adrenal vein: 200-800 ng/dl	
Alkaline phosphatase	Adults: 30-85 ImU/ml	
	Children and adolescents:	
	<2 years: 85-235 ImU/ml	
	2-8 years: 65-210 ImU/ml	
	9-15 years: 60-300 ImU/ml	
	(active bone growth)	
	16-21 years: 30-200 ImU/ml	

Modified from Pagana KD, Pagana TJ: *Diagnostic testing and nursing implications,* ed 3, St. Louis, 1994, Mosby.
*The use of the System of International Units (SI) was recommended at the 30th World Health Assembly in 1977 to implement an international language of measurement. Because this system is being adopted by numberous laboratories, many of the common values are expressed in both conventional and SI units. SI units are calculated by multiplying the conventional unit by a number factor. The SI measurement system uses *moles* as the basic unit for the amount of a substance, *kilograms* for its mass, and *meter* for its length.

Continued

Test	Reference range	
	Conventional values	SI units*
Blood, plasma, or serum values—cont'd		
Alpha-aminonitrogen	3-6 mg/dl	2.1-3.9 mmol/L
Alpha-1-antitrypsin	>250 mg/dl	
Alpha fetoprotein (AFP)	<25 ng/ml	
Ammonia	Adults: 15-110 μg/dl	47-65 μmol/L
	Children: 40-80 μg/dl	
	Newborns: 90-150 μg/dl	
Amylase	56-190 IU/L	25-125 U/L
	80-150 Somogyi units/ml	
Angiotensin-converting enzyme (ACE)	23-57 U/ml	
Antinuclear antibodies (ANA)	Negative	
Antistreptolysin O (ASO)	Adults: ≤160 Todd units/ml	
	Children:	
	⠀⠀Newborns: similar to mother's value	
	⠀⠀6 months-2 years: ≤50 Todd units/ml	
	⠀⠀2-4 years: ≤160 Todd units/ml	
	⠀⠀5-12 years: ≤200 Todd units/ml	
Antithyroid microsomal antibody	Titer <1:100	
Antithyroglobulin antibody	Titer <1:100	
Ascorbic acid (vitamin C)	0.6-1.6 mg/dl	23-57 μmol/L
Aspartate aminotransferase (AST, SGOT)	12-36 U/ml	0.10-0.30 μmol/s/L
	5-40 IU/L	5-40 U/L
Australian antigen (hepatitis-associated antigen, HAA)	Negative	Negative
Barbiturates	Negative	Negative
Base excess	Men: −3.3 to +1.2	0 ± 2 mmol/L
	Women: −2.4 to +2.3	0 ± 2 mmol/L
Bicarbonate (HCO_3^-)	22-26 mEq/L	22-26 mmol/L
Bilirubin		
⠀⠀Direct (conjugated)	0.1-0.3 mg/dl	1.7-5.1 μmol/L
⠀⠀Indirect (unconjugated)	0.2-0.8 mg/dl	3.4-12.0 μmol/L
⠀⠀Total	Adults and children: 0.1-1.0 mg/dl	5.1-17.0 μmol/L
	Newborns: 1-12 mg/dl	
Bleeding time (Ivy method)	1-9 min	
Blood count (see complete blood count)		
Blood gases (arterial)		
⠀⠀pH	7.35-7.45	
⠀⠀Pco_2	35-45 mm Hg	4.7-6.0 kPa
⠀⠀HCO_3^-	22-26 mEq/L	21-28 nmol/L
⠀⠀Po_2	80-100 mm Hg	11-13 kPa
⠀⠀O_2 saturation	95%-100%	
Blood urea nitrogen (BUN)	5-20 mg/dl	3.6-7.1 mmol/L
Bromide	Up to 5 mg/dl	0-63 mmol/L
Bromosulfophthalein (BSP)	<5% retention after 45 min	
CA 15-3	<22 U/ml	
CA-125	0-35 U/ml	
CA 19-9	<37 U/ml	
C-reactive protein (CRP)	<6 μg/ml	

Test	Reference range	
	Conventional values	SI units*
Blood, plasma, or serum values—cont'd		
Calcitonin	<50 pg/ml	<50 pmol/L
Calcium (Ca)	9.0-10.5 mg/dl (total)	2.25-2.75 mmol/L
	3.9-4.6 mg/dl (ionized)	1.05-1.30 mmol/L
Carbon dioxide (CO_2) content	23-30 mEq/L	21-30 mmol/L
Carboxyhemoglobin (COHb)	3% of total hemoglobin	
Carcinoembryonic antigen (CEA)	<2 ng/ml	
Carotene	50-200 μg/dl	0.2-5 μg/L
Chloride (Cl)	90-110 mEq/L	0.74-3.72 μmol/L
Cholesterol	150-250 mg/dl	98-106 mmol/L
Clot retraction	50%-100% clot retraction in 1-2 hours, complete retraction within 24 hours	3.90-6.50 mmol/L
Complement	C_3: 70-176 mg/dl	0.55-1.20 g/L
	C_4: 16-45 mg/dl	0.20-0.50 g/L
Complete blood count (CBC)		
Red blood cell (RBC) count	Men: 4.7-6.1 million/mm^3	
	Women: 4.2-5.4 million/mm^3	
	Infants and children: 3.8-5.5 million/mm^3	
	Newborns: 4.8-7.1 million/mm^3	
Hemoglobin (Hgb)	Men: 14-18 g/dl	8.7-11.2 mmol/L
	Women: 12-16 g/dl (pregnancy: >11 g/dl)	7.4-9.9 mmol/L
	Children: 11-16 g/dl	1.74-2.56 mmol/L
	Infants: 10-15 g/dl	
	Newborns: 14-24 g/dl	2.56-3.02 mmol/L
Hematocrit (Hct)	Men: 42%-52%	
	Women: 37%-47% (pregnancy: $>33\%$)	
	Children: 31%-43%	
	Infants: 30%-40%	
	Newborns: 44%-64%	
Mean corpuscular volume (MCV)	Adults and children: 85-95 μ^3	80-95 fl
	Newborns: 96-108 μ^3	
Mean corpuscular hemoglobin (MCH)	Adults and children: 27-31 pg	0.42-0.48 fmol
	Newborns: 32-34 pg	
Mean corpuscular hemoglobin concentration (MCHC)	Adults and children: 32-36 g/dl	0.32-0.36
	Newborns: 32-33 g/dl	
White blood cell (WBC) count	Adults and children >2 years: 5000-10,000/mm^3	
	Children ≤2 years: 6200-17,000/mm^3	
	Newborns: 9000-30,000/mm^3	
Differential count		
Neutrophils	55%-70%	
Lymphocytes	20%-40%	
Monocytes	2%-8%	
Eosinophils	1%-4%	
Basophils	0.5%-1%	
Platelet count	150,000-400,000/mm^3	
Coombs' test		
Direct	Negative	Negative
Indirect	Negative	Negative
Copper (Cu)	70-140 μg/dl	11.0-24.3 μmol/L

Continued

Test	Reference range	
	Conventional values	**SI units***
Blood, plasma, or serum values—cont'd		
Cortisol	6-28 μg/dl (AM)	170-635 nmol/L
	2-12 μg/dl (PM)	82-413 nmol/L
CPK isoenzyme (MB)	<5% total	
Creatinine	0.7-1.5 mg/dl	<133 μmol/L
Creatinine clearance	Men: 95-104 ml/min	<133 μmol/L
	Women: 95-125 ml/min	
Creatinine phosphokinase (CPK)	5-75 mU/ml	12-80 units/L
Cryoglobulin	Negative	Negative
Differential (WBC) count (see CBC)		
Digoxin	Therapeutic level: 0.5-2.0 ng/ml	40-79 μmol/L
	Toxic level: >2.4 ng/ml	>119 μmol/L
Erythrocyte count (see Complete blood count)		
Erythrocyte sedimentation rate (ESR)	Men: up to 15 mm/hour	
	Women: up to 20 mm/hour	
	Children: up to 10 mm/hour	
Ethanol	80-200 mg/dl (mild to moderate intoxication)	17-43 mmol/L
	250-400 mg/dl (marked intoxication)	54-87 mmol/L
	>400 mg/dl (severe intoxication)	>87 mmol/L
Euglobulin lysis test	90 min-6 hours	
Fats	Up to 200 mg/dl	
Ferritin	15-200 ng/ml	15-200 μg/L
Fibrin degradation products (FDP)	<10 μg/ml	
Fibrinogen (factor I)	200-400 mg/dl	5.9-11.7 μmol/L
Fibrinolysis/euglobulin lysis test	90 min-6 hours	
Fluorescent treponemal antibody (FTA)	Negative	Negative
Fluoride	<0.05 mg/dl	<0.027 mmol/L
Folic acid (Folate)	5-20 μg/ml	14-34 mmol/L
Follicle-stimulating hormone (FSH)	Men: 0.1-15.0 ImU/ml	
	Women: 6-30 ImU/ml	
	Children: 0.1-12.0 ImU/ml	
	Castrate and postmenopausal: 30-200 ImU/ml	
Free thyroxine index (FTI)	0.9-2.3 ng/dl	
Galactose-1-phosphate uridyl transferase	18.5-28.5 U/g hemoglobin	
Gammaglobulin	0.5-1.6 g/dl	
Gamma-glutamyl transpeptidase (GGTP)	Men: 8-38 U/L	5-40 U/L at 37° C
	Women: <45 years: 5-27 U/L	
Gastrin	40-150 pg/ml	40-150 ng/L
Glucagon	50-200 pg/ml	14-56 pmol/L
Glucose, fasting (FBS)	Adults: 70-115 mg/dl	3.89-6.38 mmol/L
	Children: 60-100 mg/dl	
	Newborns: 30-80 mg/dl	
Glucose, 2-hour postprandial (2-hour PPG)	<140 mg/dl	
Glucose-6-phosphate dehydrogenase (G-6-PD)	8.6-18.6 IU/g of hemoglobin	

Test	Reference range	
	Conventional values	**SI units***

Blood, plasma, or serum values—cont'd

Test	Conventional values	SI units*
Glucose tolerance test (GTT)	Fasting: 70-115 mg/dl	
	30 min: <200 mg/dl	
	1 hour: <200 mg/dl	
	2 hours: <140 mg/dl	
	3 hours: 70-115 mg/dl	
	4 hours: 70-115 mg/dl	
Glycosylated hemoglobin	Adults: 2.2%-4.8%	
	Children: 1.8%-4.0%	
	Good diabetic control: 2.5%-6%	
	Fair diabetic control: 6.1%-8%	
	Poor diabetic control: >8%	
Growth hormone	<10 ng/ml	<10 μg/L
Haptoglobin	100-150 mg/dl	16-31 μmol/L
Hematocrit (Hct)	Men: 42%-52%	
	Women: 37%-47% (pregnancy: >33%)	
	Children: 31%-43%	
	Infants: 30%-40%	
	Newborns: 44%-64%	
Hemoglobin (Hgb)	Men: 14-18 g/dl	8.7-11.2 mmol/L
	Women: 12-16 g/dl (pregnancy: >11 g/dl)	7.4-9.9 mmol/L
	Children: 11-16 g/dl	
	Infants: 10-15 g/dl	
	Newborns: 14-24 g/dl	
Hemoglobin electrophoresis	Hgb A_1: 95%-98%	
	Hgb A_2: 2%-3%	
	Hgb F: 0.8%-2%	
	Hgb S: 0	
	Hgb C: 0	
Hepatitis B surface antigen (HB$_s$AG)	Nonreactive	Nonreactive
Heterophil antibody	Negative	Negative
HLA-B27	None	None
Human chorionic gonadotropin (HCG)	Negative	Negative
Human placental lactogen (HPL)	Rise during pregnancy	
5-Hydroxyindoleacetic acid (5-HIAA)	2.8-8.0 mg/24 hours	
Immunoglobulin quantification	IgG: 550-1900 mg/dl	5.5-19.0 g/L
	IgA: 60-333 mg/dl	0.6-3.3 g/L
	IgM: 45-145 mg/dl	0.45-1.5 g/L
Insulin	4-20 μU/ml	36-179 pmol/L
Iron (Fe)	60-190 μg/dl	13-31 μmol/L
Iron-binding capacity, total (TIBC)	250-420 μg/dl	45-73 μmol/L
Iron (transferrin) saturation	30%-40%	
Ketone bodies	Negative	Negative
Lactic acid	0.6-1.8 mEq/L	
Lactic dehydrogenase (LDH) isoenzymes	90-200 ImU/ml	0.4-1.7 μmol/s/L
	LDH-1: 17%-27%	
	LDH-2: 28%-38%	

Test	Reference range	
	Conventional values	SI units*

Blood, plasma, or serum values—cont'd

	LDH-3: 19%-27%	
	LDH-4: 5%-16%	
	LDH-5: 6%-16%	
Lead	120 μg/dl or less	<1.0 μmol/L
Leucine aminopeptidase (LAP)	Men: 80-200 U/ml	
	Women: 75-185 U/ml	
Leukocyte count (see Complete blood count)		
Lipase	Up to 1.5 U/ml	0-417 U/L
Lipids		
Total	400-1000 mg/dl	4-8 g/L
Cholesterol	150-250 mg/dl	3.9-6.5 mmol/L
Triglycerides	40-150 mg/dl	0.4-1.5 g/L
Phospholipids	150-380 mg/dl	1.9-3.9 mmol/L
Lithium	Therapeutic level: 0.8-1.2 mEq/L	
Long-acting thyroid-stimulating hormone (LATS)	Negative	Negative
Magnesium (Mg)	1.6-3.0 mEq/L	0.8-1.3 mm/L
Methanol	Negative	Negative
Mononucleosis spot test	Negative	Negative
Nitrogen, nonprotein	15-35 mg/dl	10.7-25.0 mmol/L
Nuclear antibody (ANA)	Negative	Negative
5'-Nucleotidase	Up to 1.6 units	27-233 nmol/s/L
Osmolality	275-300 mOsm/kg	
Oxygen saturation (arterial)	95%-100%	0.95-1.00 of capacity
Parathormone (PTH)	<2000 pg/ml	
Partial thromboplastin time, activated (APTT)	30-40 sec	
P_{CO_2}	35-45 mm Hg	
pH	7.35-7.45	7.35-7.45
Phenylalanine	Up to 2 mg/dl	<0.18 mmol/L
Phenylketonuria (PKU)	Negative	Negative
Phenytoin (Dilantin)	Therapeutic level: 10-20 μg/ml	
Phosphatase (acid)	0.10-0.63 U/ml (Bessey-Lowry)	0.11-0.60 U/L
	0.5-2.0 U/ml (Bodansky)	
	1.0-4.0 U/ml (King-Armstrong)	
Phosphatase (alkaline)	Adults: 30-85 ImU/ml	20-90 U/L
	Children and adolescents:	
	<2 years: 85-235 ImU/ml	
	2-8 years: 65-210 ImU/ml	
	9-15 years: 60-300 ImU/ml (active bone growth)	
	16-21 years: 30-200 ImU/ml	
Phospholipids (see Lipids)		
Phosphorus (P, PO_4)	Adults: 2.5-4.5 mg/dl	0.78-1.52 mmol/L
	Children: 3.5-5.8 mg/dl	1.29-2.26 mmol/L
Platelet count	150,000-400,000/mm^3	
P_{O_2}	80-100 mm Hg	

Test	Reference range	
	Conventional values	**SI units***

Blood, plasma, or serum values—cont'd

Test	Conventional values	SI units*
Potassium (K)	3.5-5.0 mEq/L	3.5-5.0 mmol/L
Progesterone	Men, prepubertal girls, and postmenopausal women: <2 ng/ml	6 nmol/L
	Women, luteal: peak >5 ng/ml	>16 nmol/L
Prolactin	2-15 ng/ml	2-15 µg/L
Prostate-specific antigen (PSA)	<4 ng/ml	
Protein (total)	6-8 g/dl	55-80 g/L
Albumin	3.2-4.5 g/dl	35-55 g/L
Globulin	2.3-3.4 g/dl	20-35 g/L
Prothrombin time (PT)	11.0-12.5 sec	11.0-12.5 sec
Pyruvate	0.3-0.9 mg/dl	34-103 µmol/L
Red blood cell count (see Complete blood count)		
Red blood cell indexes (see Complete blood count)		
Renin		
Reticulocyte count	Adults and children: 0.5%-2% of total erythrocytes	
	Infants: 0.5%-3.1% of total erythrocytes	
	Newborns: 2.5%-6.5% of total erythrocytes	
Rheumatoid factor	Negative	Negative
Rubella antibody test	HAI titer: >1:10-1:20	
Salicylates	Negative	
	Therapeutic: 20-25 mg/dl (to age 10 years: 25-30 mg/dl)	1.4-1.8 mmol/L
	Toxic: >30 mg/dl (after age 60 years: >20 mg/dl)	>2.2 mmol/L
Schilling test (vitamin B_{12} absorption)	8%-40% excretion/24 hours	
Serologic test for syphilis (STS)	Negative (nonreactive)	
Serum glutamic oxaloacetic transaminase (SGOT, AST)	12-36 U/ml	0.10-0.30 µmol/s/L
	5-40 IU/L	
Serum glutamic-pyruvic transaminase (SGPT, ALT)	5-35 IU/L	0.05-0.43 µmol/s/L
Sickle cell	Negative	
Sodium (Na^+)	136-145 mEq/L	136-145 mmol/L
Sugar (see Glucose)		
Syphilis (see Serologic test for syphilis, Fluorescent treponemal antibody, Venereal Disease Research Laboratory)		
Testosterone	Men: 300-1200 ng/dl	10-42 nmol/L
	Women: 30-95 ng/dl	1.1-3.3 nmol/L
	Prepubertal boys and girls: 5-20 ng/dl	0.165-0.170 nmol/L
Thymol flocculation	Up to 5 U	
Thyroglobulin antibody (see Antithyroglobulin antibody)		

Continued

Test	Reference range	
	Conventional values	SI units*

Blood, plasma, or serum values—cont'd

Test	Conventional values	SI units*
Thyroid-stimulating hormone (TSH)	1-4 µU/ml Neonates: <25 µIU/ml by 3 days	5 m U/L
Thyroxine (T₄)	Murphy-Pattee: neonates: 10.1-20.1 µg/dl 1-6 years: 5.6-12.6 µg/dl 7-10 years: 4.9-11.7 µg/dl >10 years: 4-11 µg/dl Radioimmunoassay: 5-10 µg/dl	50-154 nmol/L
Thyroxine-binding globulin (TBG)	12-28 µg/ml	129-335 nmol/L
Toxoplasmosis antibody titer	1:16-1:256 generally prevalent	
Transaminase (see Serum glutamic-oxaloacetic transaminase, Serum glutamic pyruvic transaminase)		
Triglycerides	40-150 mg/dl	0.4-1.5 g/L
Triiodothyronine (T₃)	110-230 ng/dl	1.2-1.5 nmol/L
Triiodothyronine (T₃) resin uptake	25%-35%	
Tubular phosphate reabsorption (TPR)	80%-90%	
Urea nitrogen (see Blood urea nitrogen)		
Uric acid	Men: 2.1-8.5 mg/dl Women: 2.0-6.6 mg/dl Children: 2.5-5.5 mg/dl	0.15-0.48 mmol/L 0.09-0.36 mmol/L
Venereal Disease Research Laboratory (VDRL)	Negative	Negative
Vitamin A	20-100 g/dl	0.7-3.5 µmol/L
Vitamin B₁₂	200-600 pg/ml	148-443 pmol/L
Vitamin C	0.6-1.6 mg/dl	23-57 µmol/L
Whole blood clot retraction (see Clot retraction)		
Zinc	50-150 µg/dl	

Urine values

Test	Conventional values	SI units*
Acetone plus acetoacetate (ketone bodies)	Negative	Negative
Addis count (12-hour)	Adults: WBCs and epithelial cells: 1.8 million/12 hours RBCs: 500,000/12 hours Hyaline casts: Up to 5000/12 hours Children: WBCs: <1 million/12 hours RBCs: <250,000/12 hours Casts: >5000/12 hours Protein: <20 mg/12 hours	
Albumin	Random: ≤8 mg/dl 24-hour: 10-100 mg/24 hours	Negative 10-100 mg/24 hr

Test	Reference range	
	Conventional values	**SI units***
Urine values—cont'd		
Aldosterone	2-16 µg/24 hours	5.5-72 nmol/24 hours
Alpha-aminonitrogen	0.4-1.0 g/24 hours	28-71 nmol/24 hours
Amino acid	50-200 mg/24 hours	
Ammonia (24-hour)	30-50 mEq/24 hours	30-50 nmol/24 hours
	500-1200 mg/24 hours	
Amylase	≤5000 Somogyi units/24 hours	6.5-48.1 U/hr
	3-35 IU/hour	
Arsenic (24-hour)	<50 µg/L	<0.65 mol/L
Ascorbic acid (vitamin C)	Random: 1-7 ng/dl	0.06-0.40 mmol/L
	24-hour: >50 mg/24 hours	>0.29 mmol/24 hours
Bacteria	None	None
Bence Jones protein	Negative	Negative
Bilirubin	Negative	Negative
Blood or hemoglobin	Negative	Negative
Borate (24-hour)	<2 mg/L	<32 µmol/L
Calcium	Random: 1 + turbidity	1 + turbidity
	24-hour: 1-300 mg (diet dependent)	
Catecholamines (24-hour)	Epinephrine: 5-40 µg/24 hours	<55 nmol/24 hours
	Norepinephrine: 10-80 µg/24 hours	
	Metanephrine: 24-96 µg/24 hours	<590 nmol/24 hours
	Normetanephrine: 75-375 µg/24 hours	0.5-8.1 µmol/24 hours
Chloride (24-hour)	140-250 mEq/24 hours	140-250 mmol/24 hours
Color	Amber-yellow	Amber-yellow
Concentration test	Specific gravity: >1.025	>1.025
(Fishberg test)	Osmolality: 850 mOsm/L	>850 mOsm/L
Copper (CU) (24-hour)	Up to 25 µg/24 hours	0-0.4 µmol/24 hours
Coproporphyrin (24-hour)	100-300 µg/24 hours	150-460 nmol/24 hours
Creatine	Adults: <100 mg/24 hours or <6% creatinine	
	Pregnant women: ≤12%	
	Infants <1 year: equal to creatinine	
	Older children: ≤30% of creatinine	
Creatinine (24-hour)	15-25 mg/kg body wt/24 hours	0.13-0.22 nmol/kg^{-1} body wt/24 hours
Creatinine clearance (24-hour)	Men: 90-140 ml/min	90-140 ml/min
	Women: 85-125 ml/min	85-125 ml/min
Crystals	Negative	Negative
Cystine or cysteine	Negative	Negative
Delta-aminolevulinic acid (ΔALA)	1-7 mg/24 hours	10-53 µmol/24 hours
Epinephrine (24-hour)	5-40 µg/24 hours	
Epithelial cells and casts	Occasional	Occasional
Estriol (24-hour)	>12 mg/24 hours	
Fat	Negative	Negative
Fluoride (24-hour)	<1 mg/24 hours	0.053 mmol/24 hours

Continued

Test	Reference range	
	Conventional values	**SI units***

Urine values—cont'd

Test	Conventional values	SI units*
Follicle-stimulating hormone (FSH) (24-hour)	Men: 2-12 IU/24 hours Women: During menses: 8-60 IU/24 hours During ovulation: 30-60 IU/24 hours During menopause: >50 IU/24 hours	
Glucose	Negative	Negative
Granular casts	Occasional	Occasional
Hemoglobin and myoglobin	Negative	Negative
Homogentisic acid	Negative	Negative
Human chorionic gonadotropin (HCG)	Negative	Negative
Human placental lactogen (HPL)	Levels rise progressively during pregnancy	
Hyaline casts	Occasional	Occasional
17-Hydroxycorticosteroids (17-OCHS) (24-hour)	Men: 5.5-15.0 mg/24 hours Women: 5.0-13.5 mg/24 hours Children: lower than adult values	8.3-25 μmol/24 hours 5.5-22 μmol/24 hours
5-Hydroxyindoleacetic acid (5-HIAA, serotonin) (24-hour)	Men: 2-9 mg/24 hours Women: lower than men	10-47 μmol/24 hours
Ketones (see Acetone plus acetoacetate)		
17-Ketosteroids (17-KS) (24-hour)	Men: 8-15 mg/24 hours Women: 6-12 mg/24 hours Children: 12-15 yr: 5-12 mg/24 hours <12 yr: <5 mg/24 hours	21-62 μmol/24 hours 14-45 μmol/24 hours
Lactose (24-hour)	14-40 mg/24 hours	
Lead	<0.08 g/ml or <120 g/24 hours	41-116 μm 0.39 μmol/L
Leucine aminopeptidase (LAP)	2-18 U/24 hours	
Magnesium (24-hour)	6.8-8.5 mEq/24 hours	3.0-4.3 mmol/24 hours
Melanin	Negative	Negative
Odor	Aromatic	Aromatic
Osmolality	500-800 mOsm/L	38-1400 mmol/kg water
pH	4.6-8.0	4.6-8.0
Phenolsulfonphthalein (PSP)	15 min: at least 25% 30 min: at least 40% 120 min: at least 60%	At least 0.25 At least 0.40 At least 0.60
Phenylketonuria (PKU)	Negative	Negative
Phenylpyruvic acid	Negative	Negative
Phosphorus (24-hour)	0.9-1.3 g/24 hours	29-42 mmol/24 hours
Porphobilinogen	Random: negative 24-hour: up to 2 mg/24 hours	Negative
Porphyrin (24-hour)	50-300 mg/24 hours	
Potassium (K⁺) (24-hour)	25-100 mEq/24 hours	25-100 nmol/24 hours
Pregnancy test	Positive in normal pregnancy or with tumors producing HCG	Positive in normal pregnancy or with tumors producing HCG

| | Reference range | |
Test	Conventional values	SI units*
Urine values—cont'd		
Pregnanediol	After ovulation: >1 mg/24 hours	
Protein (albumin)	Random: ≤8 mg/dl	
	10-100 mg/24 hours	>0.05 g/24 hours
Sodium (Na$^+$) (24-hour)	100-260 mEq/24 hours	100-260 nmol/24 hours
Specific gravity	1.010-1.025	1.010-1.025
Steroids (see 17-Hydroxycortico-		
steroids, 17-Ketosteroids)		
Sugar (see Glucose)		
Titratable acidity (24-hour)	20-50 mEq/24 hours	20-50 mmol/24 hours
Turbidity	Clear	Clear
Urea nitrogen (24-hour)	6-17 g/24 hours	0.21-0.60 mmol/24 hours
Uric acid (24-hour)	250-750 mg/24 hours	1.48-4.43 mmol/24 hours
Urobilinogen	0.1-1.0 Ehrlich U/dl	0.1-1.0 Ehrlich U/dl
Uroporphyrin	Negative	Negative
Vanillylmandelic acid (VMA) (24-hour)	1-9 mg/24 hours	<40 μmol/day
Zinc (24-hour)	0.20-0.75 mg/24 hours	

INDEX

A

Abdominal musculature assessment of mothers following birth, 385
Abducens, 338t
Absorbent products, for bladder dysfunction, 293
Absorption, insulin, 271
Abuse, defined, 128
ACCIDENTS, 424
Accidents, assessment of potential risks for home, 424
Acoustic nerves, 338t
Acquired immune deficiency syndrome; *see* AIDS
Active-assistive range of motion, 301
Active participation, patient's, in plan of care, 109
Active range of motion, 301
Activities of daily living (ADL)
  geriatric patients and, 426, 427
    mothers after child birth and, 386
  patients recovering from stroke and, 336
  patients with COPD and, 188
  patients with dementia and, 351
  patients with MS and, 346
Adaptive equipment, 309
ADL; *see* Activities of daily living
Administrative issues, with home infusion therapy, 311
Administrative law actions, health care providers and, 124-125

Adolescents, teaching strategies for, 120-121
Adult learning, principles of, 106
Advance directives, 133
Advanced practice nurses, 3
Aerosol therapy, 183, 185
Affective learning, 103
African-Americans, as population at risk for aids, 359
Afterload, 201
Agency
  health maintenance organization, 8
  home care, 6
  proprietary, 8
  public, 8
Agency for Health Care Policy (AHCPR), 247
Agency for Health Care Research and Quality (AHRQ), 247
Agent or proxy, health care, 133
Aging
  effects on bladder function, 280
  physiology, 418-420
AHCPR; *see* Agency for Health Care Policy and Research (AHCPR)
AHRQ; *see* Agency for Health Care Research and Quality (AHRQ)
AIDS
  CDC surveillance case definition of, 357
  chemical dependence and substance abuse, 361
  defined, 356
  epidemiology of, 359
  family coping with, 373

Tables are indicated by t following the page number.

AIDS—cont'd
  HIV presentation and clinical course of, 358
  intravenous pain management for, 370
  living at home with, 372-373
  medications to treat, 363-367t
  occupational and casual transmission of, 360
  pathophysiology of, 357-358
  patients with, 356-357
  populations at risk for, 359-360
  primary nursing diagnoses/patient problems,
    361
  primary themes of patient education, 361
  screening for, 360
Airborne infection, 88
  precautions against, 89
Air embolism, 324t
Air quality, for patients with COPD, 189
Airway clearance, ineffective, 186
Akathisia, 412
Akinesia, 412
Alcohol and substance abuse, 403-404
Alzheimer's Association, 352
Alzheimer's dementia, 348-352, 420
  incidence of, 348
  as neurological dysfunction, 330
  pathophysiology of, 349
  primary nursing diagnoses/patient problems,
    351
  primary themes of patient education, 351
  progression of, 349
  treatment of, 351
Ambu bag, 218
American Medical Association, 7
American Nurses Association, standards of care,
    12
American Nurse's Credentialing Center (ANCC),
    12
American Society of Parenteral and Enteral
    Nutrition, (ASPEN), 312
American Stroke Association, 344
Aminoglycosides, 325
Analgesic dosages, 437-438
ANCC; see American Nurse's Credentialing
    Center (ANCC)
Angiotensin-converting enzyme inhibitors, 207
Angiotension II receptor blockers, 207t

Ankle, range of motion exercises for, 304t
Anorexia, in hospice patients, 439
Antibacterials, for HIV infection and AIDS,
    366-367t
Antibiotics, for patients with COPD, 188
Antibiotic therapy, as type of home infusion
    therapy, 323
Anticoagulants, 325t
Antifungals, 325t
  for HIV infection and AIDS, 364
Antineoplastics, 325t
Antiprotozoals, for HIV infection and AIDS, 366t
Antivirals, for HIV infection and AIDS, 365t
Antiseptic solutions, for wound care, 262t
Antifungals, 325
Antineoplastics, 325
Antiviral drugs, 325
  for HIV infection and AIDS, 365t
Apical pulse, of infant, 388
Appropriateness of patient care, defined, 170
Aprons, OSHA bloodborne pathogen standard for
    wearing, 90
Art therapy, 488
Arterial blood gas values, normal, 216
Arterial ulcers, 242, 254
Aseptic solutions, for wound care, 262t
Assessing phase, of home visit, 58-60
Assessment; see Home Care Application in each
    clinical chapter
  nutritional, 60
  phase of home visit, 58-60
  physical, 60
  spiritual, 60
Assessment and evaluation skills, 25
Assessment interview, in assessing phase of home
    visit, 59
Assistive devices, for rehabilitation services, 279
Association of Women's Health, Obstetric, and
    Neonatal Nurses (AWHONN), 380
Asthma, 175
Atonic bladder, as micturition abnormality, 279
Audiocassette tapes, as home care teaching tool,
    112t
Automatic bladder, as micturition abnormality, 279
AWHONN; see Association of Women's Health,
    Obstetric, and Neonatal Nurses

B

Bacteriuria, 291
Bag technique, for infection control, 93
Bathroom and personal hygiene, guidelines for
    infection control, 95
Bedside cystometry procedure, 284
Behavioral learning theory, 104
Bennis, W., 141
Bereavement; *see* Death
Betadine solution, 249
Beta-lactum cephalosporins, 325t
Beta-blockers, 207
Biofeedback, 489
Bioelectromagnetic, applications of
    complementary therapies, 489
Bisexuals and homosexuals, as population at risk
    for AIDS, 359
Bladder
    assessments of habits associated with, 280
    atonic, 279
    automatic, 279
    effects of aging on, 279
    reflex, 279
    record, 283
    retraining of, 287
    uninhibited neurogenic, 279
Bladder
    bowel management for patients with, 294
    defined, 278
    dysfunction, 278-296
    essential elements of history, 281t
    patients with, 278-296
    primary nursing diagnoses/patient problems,
        285
    primary themes of patient education, 285
Bladder elimination
    after childbirth, 386
    infant's 391
    for patients recovering from stroke, 343
Bladder irrigation, 290
Bladder record, 283
Blood chemistries, pertinent to congestive heart
    failure, 205t
Blood glucose monitoring, self (SMBG), 275
Blood products, 325t
Blood transfusion; *see* Hemotransfusion

Body mechanics, awareness for rehabilitation
    services, 301
Boston Dispensary, 3
Bottle-feeding, infant, 393
Bowel elimination
    in patients with bladder dysfunction, 294
    in patients with MS, 347
    in patients recovering from stroke, 343
Breast-feeding, 393
Breathing
    diaphragmatic, 192
    ineffective pattern of, 186
    intermittent positive pressure, 183
    pursed-lip, 191
    techniques for pulmonary rehabilitation, 191
Breckinridge, Mary, 4,5
Brewster, Mary, 4
Bronchitis, as predisposing condition to
    respiratory failure, 216
Bronchodilator, for patients with COPD, 187
Bubonic plague, 81

C

Calendar, home visit planning using a, 146
Cancer, intravenous pain management for, 326
Cancer pain, drugs and routes of administration,
    437
Cannula
    inner, 219
    inner and out, 219, 220
Capitation, 11, 469
Cardiac assessment of patients with CHF, 203
Cardiac glycosides, 207
Cardiac output, pathophysiology of CHF and, 201
Cardiopulmonary assessment
    of patients with COPD, 187
    of patients with AIDS, 369
Cardiovascular assessment
    of infant during postpartum home care, 388
    of patients with diabetes, 268
Cardiovascular disease, as chronic complication of
    diabetes, 267
Cardiovascular functions, aging and, 418
Caregiver
    and active participation in plan of care, 109
    care path home guide for, 157

Caregiver—cont'd
  CP standard for home guide for, 158
  CP standards for discharge survey for, 160
  teaching strategies for, 121
Caregiver outcomes, progress toward meeting,
    154-155
Care paths
  defined, 148
  home guide for patient/caregiver, 157-160
  standard for skin/integumentary system, 153
  as tool of case manager, 148
Caring family; living with chronic mental illness,
    405
Caring in the home, 500-502
Cartoons, as home care teaching tool, 112t
Cartridge inhalers, 185
Caseload
  tips for organizing, 145
Case management
  clinical applications of, 143-149
  defined, 141
  home care definitions of, 141-142
  leadership strategies and, 149-151
Case managers
  home care definitions of, 141-142
  multidisciplinary resources and, 142
  National Association of, 142
Catatonic behavior, 410
Catheterization
  intermittent, 292
  suprapubic, 292
Catheters
  care of, 290
  for home infusion therapy, 313
  central venous (CVC), 314
  changing, 290
  dressing change and care, 315
  encrustation and obstruction of, 291
  epidural or intrathecal, 315-316
  external, 292
  Groshong, 314
  implantable access device, 314
  indwelling, 289
  inserting, 289
  leakage of, 263
  maintaining drainage systems and, 290

Catheters—cont'd
  odor of, 291
  for patients with bladder dysfunction, 288
  percutaneously inserted central catheter, 315
  routine care of, 290
  selecting the, 289
  severed intravenous, 324t
Cause and effect diagrams, as QI tool, 170
CDC; see Centers for Disease Control and
    Prevention (CDC)
Center for Health Policy Research, 11
Centers for Disease Control and Prevention
    (CDC), 82, 89, 312, 356
  definition of AIDS, 356
  standard precautions, 89-93
  suggestions for infection control procedures, 93
Central access devices, maintaining patency of,
    318-319t
Central nervous system (CNS)
  involvement in AIDS, 369
  multiple sclerosis effects on, 347
Central venous catheter (CVC), 313-315
Cerebrovascular accident (CVA), 330-344
  incidence of, 331
  primary nursing diagnoses/patient problems,
    336
  primary themes of patient education for, 336
  see Stroke
Cerebrovascular assessment, of patients with
    diabetes, 267
Cerebrovascular disease, as chronic complication
    of diabetes, 267
Cervical spine, range of motion exercises for, 302t
Chairbound patient, seating tips for, 307
Chemotherapy, as type of home infusion therapy,
    323
Chest physiotherapy, 198
CHF; see Congestive heart failure
Children, AIDS risk and, 359
Chronic bronchitis, 175
Chronic obstructive pulmonary disease (COPD),
    175-199
  diet, high fat with low carbohydrate, 194-197
  epidemiology of, 176
  etiology of, 176
  home oxygen therapy for, 178-180

Chronic obstructive pulmonary disease
(COPD)—cont'd
infection control issues for, 185-186
pathophysiology of, 176
physical assessment for patient with, 187
physiological relationship between lungs and, 177
primary nursing diagnoses/patient problems, 186
primary themes of patient education for, 190
screening for, 186
Chronic wounds, 239-264
classification of, 242
diet, 261
etiology and pathophysiology of, 239-242
infection control issues for, 245
primary nursing diagnoses/patient problems, 244
primary themes of patient education for, 245
specific therapies for, 252
see Wounds
Circulation
anterior and central, 333t
posterior, 334t
Circulatory overload, 324t
Civil actions, health care providers and, 125
Claims made policy, 127
Cleansing, of wounds, 249
Clindamycin, 325t
Clinical applications
of patient care, 175-465
of case management, 143
Clinical field staff
advanced practice nurses and, 28
role expectations of, 23-26
role preparation, referral, and implementation, 27-30
Clinical indicators, for multidisciplinary referrals, 28
Clinical issues, special, 379-465
Clinical pathway, term *care path* recommended, 148
Clinical practice, applying theory to, 15-23
Clinical practice guidelines on pressure ulcers in adults, 251-252
Clotting, of IV site, 322

CNS; *see* Central nervous system
Cognitive-developmental learning theory, 103
Cognitive learning, 102
Colony stimulating factors, 325t
Combination dressings, for wound care, 262t
Commission on Aging, 128
Commission on Insurance Rehabilitation Specialists, 142
Committees
administrative support for work in, 150
home care agency, 150-151
how to chair and run, 150
QI, 162
tips for chairing and conducting work in, 151
Communicable diseases
criteria for home care infections, 94
infection rate calculation for QI, 95
provision of infection control for patients with, 93
reporting, 129
unreported/unknown vs. identified cases of, 88
Communication devices, for ventilator-dependent patients, 219
Communication skills, 26
of patients with MS, 347
of patients recovering from stroke, 342-343
with families, 53-56
Community internet resources and services, national, 37-46
Community safety, instruction on map reading and, 30
Complementary therapies, 480-497
art therapy, 488
bioelectromagnetic applications of, 489
biofeedback in, 489
diet, nutrition, lifestyle changes in, 485-487
Feldenkrais method, 493
herbals, 483
history of, 480-482
humor, 491
implications for nursing practice, 496
manual healing, 491
mind-body interventions in, 487
narrative therapy, 488
relaxation response, 489
spiritual practice or prayer, 490
therapeutic touch, 493

Compression dressing, 255

Compression nebulizers, 185

Computer assisted instruction (CAI) programs, as home care teaching tool, 113t

Concentrators, oxygen, 182

Concrete operations, 120

Condom, how to use a latex, 371

Confusion, in elderly, 442

Congenital dislocation of hip, 390

Congestive heart failure (CHF), 200-214

  clinical manifestations of, 202

  diet, low sodium, 211

  mechanism of vasodilator action in therapy of chronic,   206-207

  medications for, 205-208

  New York Heart Association, classification of, 202

  physical assessment of, 203-204

  primary fluid and electrolyte imbalances in, 205t

  primary nursing diagnoses/patient problems, 205

  primary themes of patient education for, 209

  see Chronic congestive heart failure

Constipation, in hospice patients, 440

Contact infection transmission, 88

  precautions against, 89

Continence, medications that affect, 296t

Continuity, defined, 171

Continuous subcutaneous infusion, for pain therapy, 315

Contract, elements of learning, 117

Contractility, 201

Control

  infection, 81-101

  locus of, 104

Control charts, as QI tool, 165, 169

COPD; see Chronic obstructive pulmonary disease

Corticosteroids ,as medication for patients with COPD, 187

Cotton dressings, for wound care, 262t

Coughing, by hospice patients, 442

Cranberry juice, for patients with bladder dysfunction, 293

Cranial nerves, 337t

Credé's maneuver, 28

Criminal actions, against health care providers, 124

Crisis intervention theory, for mental health patients, 406

Critical pathway, "care path" recommended over, 148

Cultural care, 17, 106-107

CVC; see Central venous catheter

Cystic fibrosis, as predisposing condition to respiratory failure, 216

Cystometry procedure, bedside, 284t

D

Dakin's solution, 262

Dance therapy, 488

Death

  and bereavement, 445

  Kübler-Ross stages of, 442

  pediatric bereavement issues, 447

Debridement, of wounds, 249-250

Delusions, schizophrenic, 410

Dementia, 330

  Alzheimer's type, 348

  in elderly patients, 420-421

  signs and symptoms of stages of, 350

Deming, W.E., 161

Department of Health

  as investigator of complaints against nurses, 124

  regulation of service delivery by, 64

Department of Health Education and Welfare (DHEW), 6

Department of Health and Human Services (DHHS), 6

  organizational performance improvement process, 166

Depression

  behavioral signs of, 406

  drugs causing signs of, 404

  etiology and pathophysiology of, 405

  patient care plan for, 408t

  primary nursing diagnoses/patient problems, 402

  primary themes of patient education for, 408

Dermis, 240

Detergent solutions, for wound care, 262t

Developmental tasks, family, 395-396
DeVries, M., 151
DHEW; *see* Department of Health Education and Welfare
DHHS; *see* Department of Health and Human Services
Diabetes mellitus, 265-277
  acute complications of, 266
  chronic complications of, 267
  classification of, 265-266
  diet, 274
  foot care guidelines, 269
  management and patient education for, 268-276
  insulin action curves, 271
  insulin-dependent, 265
  sick-day management of, 276
  primary nursing diagnoses/patient problems, 270
  primary themes of patient education for, 270
Diabetic ketoacidosis (DKA), 266
Diabetic ulcers, 242-254
Diagnosing phase, of home visit, 60
Diagnostic-related groups (DRGs), 3
  arrival of, 8
  and Medicare, 141
Diagrams
  fishbone, 170
  flowcharts, 170
  as QI tool, 170
  scatter, 170
Diaphragmatic breathing, 192
Diet
  for complementary therapies, 485-487
  for patients with chronic wounds, 261
  for patients with COPD, 194
  for patients with CHF, 211
  for patients with diabetes, 273
  see Nutrition
Digitalis toxicity, 206
Dimensions of performance, definitions of, 167
Directives, advance, 133
Discharge
  criteria for patient, 147
  patient/caregiver checklist, for home mechanical ventilation, 224
  survey, CP standard for patient/caregiver, 160

Diseases
  communicable, 86
  infectious, 81-101
  notifiable, 84-85t
  patient education guidelines to reduce transmission of, 100
Disinfection, for home care, 91-92; *see* Infection control
Dislocation of hip, congenital, 390
District nurses, 3
Diuretics, 207t, 325t
DKA; *see* Diabetic ketoacidosis
Documentation
  corrections, additions, and late entries to, 130
  developing plan of, 58-80
  guidelines for homebound status, 67
  incident reports as, 131
  as legal issue, 129-130
  as outcomes of care, 63
  Medicare guidelines for, 64-68
  phase of home visit, 64
  skills, 26
  subjective vs. objective, 129t
  of treatment for wound care patients, 254
Domestic violence, safety plan for victim survivors of, 396
"Do not resuscitate" orders, 134
Dosage, analgesic, and comparative efficacy to standards,   451-452t
DPRV tracheostomy tube, 220
Drainage system, maintaining catheters and, 290
Dressings
  changing for home infusion therapy, 315
  wound care, 262-264t
DRGs; *see* Diagnostic-related groups
Droplet infection transmission, 88
  precautions against, 89
Drug classification, home infusion therapy, 325t
Dry mouth, in hospice patients, 441
Dynamic self-determination, Rice model of, 19-22
Dyskinesia, 412
Dysphagia, in hospice patients, 441
Dyspnea
  in hospice patients, 440
  paroxysmal nocturnal, 204
  in patients with COPD, 187
  in patients with CHF, 204

E

Ecomap, 51

Edema
   in hospice patients, 440
   insulin related, 273
   in ventilator-dependent patients, 226

Effectiveness, defined, 170

Efficacy, defined, 105

Efficiency, defined, 170

Elastomeric membrane pumps, 320

Elbow, range of motion exercises for, 302t

Elderly home care patients, 417-429
   demographics of, 417-418
   issues in home setting, 420-425
   primary nursing diagnoses/patient problems, 426
   primary themes of patient education for, 426
   support systems for, 428
   teaching the, 110-115

Electroconvulsive therapy (ECT), for patients with depression, 406

Electrolyte, imbalances associated with CHF, 205t

Embolism, air, 324

Emergency drug kit, for home infusion therapy, 327

Emphysema, 175
   as predisposing condition to respiratory failure, 215

Employment, information needed before accepting, 127-128

Empowerment, as leadership trend, 149-151

Encrustation, around catheter, 291

Energy conservation, tips for COPD patient in home setting for, 192

Enteral access, for home infusion therapy, 320

Enteral nutrition therapy, as type of home infusion therapy, 327

ENUFF, 55

Environmental assessment, for patients with bladder dysfunction, 285

Environment, as cause of COPD, 176

Environmental threats in the home, 457-463
   electric and magnetic fields, 489
   fine particulate matter, 458
   lead, 457
   pesticides, 459

Environmental threats in the home—cont'd
   radon, 458
   recommendations for care, 461
   volatile organic compounds, 457

Epidemiology
   defined, 83
   of AIDS, 359-360
   of chronic obstructive pulmonary disease (COPD), 176-177

Epidermis, 240

Epidural space catheter, for pain therapy, 319, 326

EPS; see Extrapyramidal symptoms

Erickson, E., 103

Ethical issues in home care, 30, 124-139
   of home care agency orientation, 30
   telehealth and, 472

Ethnicity, geographic, 106-107

Etiology
   of chronic obstructive pulmonary disease (COPD), 176, 178
   of chronic wounds, 239-240
   of depression, 405
   of schizophrenia, 407

Evaluating phase, of home visit, 63-64

Evidence-based practice, 166

Exercises
   for diabetic patients, 274
   Kegel, 287
   range of motion, 302-304

Exposure incident, OSHA bloodborne pathogen standard for, 92

External catheters, 292

Extrapyramidal symptoms (EPS), of schizophrenia, 411

Extravasation kits, 323

Exudate absorptive dressings, for wound care, 263t

F

Facial nerves, 338t

Facilitator, home care nurse as, 19

Fair Labor Standards Act, 127

Family
   adjustment to parental roles, 396
   assessment of, 52
   care of, 47-56
   defined, 47

Family systems theory, 48-50

Faulty equipment, guidelines to avoid liability for, 137

Feeding

breast-feeding, 393

bottle feeding, 393

parent-child interaction during, 384, 394

Feldenkrais method, 493

Fine particulate matter, environmental threats, 458

Fingers, range of motion exercises for, 303t

Fish-bone diagrams, as QI tool, 170

Flexibility and critical thinking skills, 26

Flip charts, as home care teaching tool, 113t

Flowcharts, as QI tool, 170

Fluid/electrolyte

blood chemistry levels and, 204

imbalances in patients with congestive heart failure, 205

Foam dressings, for wound care, 263t

FOME-CUF tracheostomy tube, 221

Fontanels, 388

Food diary, for adults, 79

Foot care, patient education guide for, 269

Forearm, range of motion exercises for, 302t

Formal operations, 120

Full thickness wound, therapy, 252

G

Gait training, 301

Gastrointestinal assessment

of patients with AIDS, 370

of patients with CHF, 204

of patients with diabetes, 268

of elderly patients, 419

Genitalia assessment, of infant during postpartum home care, 389-390

Genitourinary assessment

for patients with AIDS, 370

of patients with diabetes, 268

Genitourinary functions, aging and, 419

Genogram, 50

Geographical ethnicity, 105

Geriatric patients; *see* Elderly patients

Glossopharyngeal nerves, 338t

Gloves, OSHA bloodborne pathogen standard for wearing, 90

Glycated protein testing, 275

Glycemic control, assessment of, 275

Goggles, OSHA bloodborne pathogen standard for wearing, 91

Goldsmith, J., 141

Government regulations, impact on home care, 7

Gowns, OSHA bloodborne pathogen standard for wearing, 90

Grief, resolution of; *see* Bereavement

Groshong catheter, 314

Group teaching strategies, 111

Guthrie, E., 103

H

Habit training, for patients with bladder dysfunction, 288

Hair follicles, 240

Hallucinations, schizophrenic, 410

Handwashing

as home care application of infection control, 90

OSHA bloodborne pathogen standard for, 89

HBV, exposure of health care workers to, 96

Harris-Benedict equation, 78

HCFA form 485-488; *see* Health Care Financing Administration

Healing, wound assessment and evaluation of, 246-247

Health, defined and conceptualized, 18

Health beliefs, patient education and, 106-107

Health care, skyrocketing costs of, 140

Health care proxy or agent, 133

Health Care Financing Administration (HCFA), 6, 10, 166

home care certification and plan of treatment, 6,7

influence on home care agencies, 6-8

Health care providers, legal system and, 124-125

Health history

of geriatric patients, 426

of patients with bladder dysfunction, 280-281

Health Insurance Manual Publication Number 11 (HIM-11), 7

plan of care in, 7, 59, 64

Health maintenance organizations (HMOs), as private managed care system, 141

Heart failure, congestive, 200-214; *see* Congestive heart failure

Hematology panels, serum chemistry and, 503-513t

Hemophiliacs, as population at risk for AIDS, 359-360

Hemorrhagic stroke, 331

Hemotransfusions, 326

Henry Street Settlement House, 3

Hepatitis
    as changing disease, 82
    B infection, 87

Herbal therapies, 483

HHNS; *see* Hyperglycemic hyperosmolar nonketotic state

Hierarchy of needs, Maslow's, 104

High-pressure cylinders, of oxygen, 179

HIM-11
    conditions for coverage of home health care services in, 64
    coverage of services, 7
    teaching and training activities, 110

Hip
    range of motion exercises for, 303t
    signs of congenital dislocation of, 390

Historical database
    use in assessing phase of home visit, 59

Historical perspectives
    of home care nursing, 3
    of maternal-child nursing, 379

HIV infection
    as not synonymous with AIDS, 356
    exposure of health care workers to, 96
    fear of patients who have, 82
    home care workers with, 360
    mechanism of transmission of, 358
    presentation and clinical course of AIDS, 358

HMOs; *see* Health maintenance organizations

Home, patient education in the, 102-123

Homebound status, guidelines for documenting, 67

Home care
    advanced practice nurse and, 30
    application of standard precautions for infection control,   89-92
    applying theory to clinical practice, 15-23
    future trends, 469-502
    implementing student learning in, 33
    legal and ethical issues in, 124-139

Home care—cont'd
    record keeping in, 129
    teaching strategies for special patient groups in, 110-123
    theoretical framework for, 19
    using teaching tools in, 112t

Home care agency, 8
    field staff's orientation to, 27
    primary, 8
    responsibilities to patient, 128

Home care aide, clinical indicators for referral to, 28

Home care aide assignments, guidelines for, 72

Home care application
    for AIDS, 360
    for Alzheimer's patients, 349
    for bladder dysfunction, 280
    for COPD, 186
    for CHF, 202
    for chronic wounds, 244
    for CVA, 332
    for depression, 405
    for diabetes, 267
    for elderly patients, 425
    for home infusion therapy, 313
    of hospice goals, 434
    for multiple sclerosis, 346
    for schizophrenia, 409
    for postpartum home care, 381
    for rehabilitation services, 299
    for ventilator-dependent patients, 223

Home care nurse
    advanced practice nurses, 30
    case management and leadership strategies for, 140-160
    as advocate, 20, 25
    as educator, 20, 25
    as facilitator, 19, 20
    information needed before accepting employment, 127
    profile of, 24
    as spiritual-aesthetic communer, 20, 25
    role preparation and implementation of, 24-46
    see Clinical field staff, Home care nursing

Home care nursing
    concepts of, 1-172, 500-502
    historical perspectives of, 3-14

Home care nursing—cont'd
 philosophy of practice of, 13-14
 social perspectives of, 4-7
Home care services, guidelines for Medicare
  documentation to validate need for, 70t
Home discharge planning, for ventilator-
  dependent patients, 219, 221-223
Home Health Licensing Bureau, regulation of
  service delivery by, 64
Home care rehabilitation, conditions, and
  diagnoses appropriate for referrals for, 299
Home improvisation, instruction on, 30
Home infusion therapy, 310-329
 administrative issues with, 284
 complications of, 321
 extravasation or emergency drug kit for, 323
 troubleshooting in, 324
 types of
  antibiotic, 323
  chemotherapy, 323
  enteral nutrition, 327
  hemotransfusions, 326
  pain management, 326
  total parenteral nutrition, 327
Vascular access devices, 313-316
Home intravenous (IV) therapy; *see* Home
  infusion therapy
Home mechanical ventilation
 discharge patient/caregiver checklist for, 224
 equipment and supplies for, 217-222
Home mechanical ventilators
 common features of, 233-234
 management of, 232-237
 problem solving for alarms in, 229
Home mechanical ventilators; *see* also Ventilators
Home medical equipment, for rehabilitation
  services, 301, 309
Home milieu, introduction to, 30
Home oxygen therapy, for COPD, 179-185
Home remedies, common, 106
Home respiratory support, equipment used for,
  217-219
Home visits
 conducting, 58-80
  assessing phase, 59
  diagnosing phase, 60
  evaluating phase, 63

Home visits—cont'd
 conducting—cont'd
  implementing phase, 62
  planning phase, 61-62
 documentation guidelines, 64-69
 preparing for, 58
 using calendar to plan, 146
Homosexuals and bisexuals, as population at risk
  for AIDS, 359
Hospice and palliative care, 430-456
 bereavement adult, 422, 444-446
 bereavement pediatric, 422, 447
 clinical indicators for referral to, 28
 caregiver's concerns, 444
 pain management, 435
 pediatric issues, 446
  pain management, 447
 primary nursing diagnoses/patient problems,
  434
 primary themes of patient education, 435
 psychosocial aspects of care, 446
 symptom management, 439
Hospice program, admission to, 431
Hospice spiritual assessment, 61
Hospice team, 432-433
How to run a meeting and chair a committee, 151
Human caring, theory of, 18
Humanistic learning theories, 104
Humor therapy, 491
Hydrocolloid dressings
 transparent adhesive films and, 249
 for wound care, 263t
Hydrogel dressings, for wound care, 263t
Hydrogen peroxide, 249
Hydrophilic powder dressings, 263t
Hyperglycemia, 266, 275
Hyperglycemic hyperosmolar nonketotic state
  (HHNS), 266
Hyperkalemia, associated with CHF, 205t
Hypervolemia, associated with CHF, 205t
Hypochloremia, associated with CHF, 205t
Hypoglossal accessory nerves, 339t
Hypoglycemia, as complication of insulin therapy,
  272
Hypokalemia, associated with CHF, 205t
Hypovolemia, associated with CHF, 205t

I

IADL; *see* Instrumental activities of daily living
IDDM; *see* Insulin-dependent diabetes mellitus (IDDM)
Illiterate patient, teaching strategies for, 117
Immobility
    of elderly patients in home setting, 422
    hazards of, 423t
Implantable vascular access device (IVAD), 314
Implementing phase, of home visit, 62
Incident reports, 131
Incontinence
    drugs used to treat urinary, 296t
    medications that can affect, 282
    of patients with AIDS, 370
    types, causes, and treatment, 286
    urinary, 279
Indwelling catheters, 314
Infants
    assessment during postpartum home care, 388-395
    puncture sites for heelstick specimens of, 393
    selected reflexes of, 391t
    in sensorimotor period, 119
    stool patterns of, 391t
Infection
    as acute complication of diabetes, 266
    and catheterization, 291
    intravenous, 322
    control of, 81-101
    hepatitis B, 83, 86
    HIV, 83, 86
    IV therapy site, 313
    mechanism of, 88-89
        airborne transmission, 88
        contact transmission, 88
        droplet transmission, 88
        vector-borne transmission, 88-89
    risk for respiratory, in ventilator-dependent patients, 226
    urinary tract, 285
Infection control
    administrative considerations for, 96
    home, 93
    in homes of patients with chronic wounds, 245
    in homes of ventilator-dependent patients, 226

Infection control—cont'd
    for patients with AIDS, 362
    for respiratory equipment in home, 185
    surveillance report, 96
    understanding need for, 81-82
Infectious diseases, common, 86
Inflammatory phase, of wound healing, 243
Informed consent, 134
Infusion, devices and pump management for, 320
Infusion therapy, patients receiving home, 310-329
    practice guidelines for,
        CVC, 318
        epidural, 319
        implanted port access devices, 319
        peripheral, 319
        PICC, 318
Inhalers
    administration of, 185
    cartridge, 185
Injection sites, insulin, 271
Inner cannula care, 227
INS; *see* Intravenous Nurses Society
Insomnia, in hospice patients, 441
Instrumental activities of daily living (IADL), stroke patients and, 332
Insulin, 268
    absorption of, 270
    action curves, 271t
    administration of, 271
    complications of therapy, 272
    mixing, 270
    prefilled syringes, 272
    preparations, 270
    regimens for, 270
    storage and appearance of, 270
    time action profiles for, 271t
Insulin-dependent diabetes mellitus (IDDM), 265-266
Insurance, for nursing malpractice, 125
Integumentary assessment, for patients with AIDS, 370
Integumentary functions, aging and, 422
Intermediaries, 67
Intermittent catheterization, 292

Intermittent positive pressure breathing (IPPB), 183, 185

Internet resources for home care, 37-46

Intervention
for postpartum home care, 397
for ventilator-dependent patients, 225-227

Interview, assessment, 58-59

Intrathecal space catheter, for pain therapy, 315

Intravenous drug users and sex workers, as population at risk for AIDS, 359

Intravenous Nurses Society (INS), 312

Intravenous push (IVP) chemotherapeutic agents, 323

Intravenous therapy, in home as historical development, 8-9

IPPB; *see* Intermittent positive pressure breathing

IVAD; *see* Implantable vascular access device

IV therapy, 310
complications of, 321
dressing changes, 315
flushing protocols, 318
peripheral and central line, 313
see Home infusion therapy

J

Jaundice
in infants, 391
types and characteristics of neonatal, 392t

JCAHO; *see* Joint Commission on the Accreditation of Healthcare Organizations

Joint Commission on the Accreditation of Healthcare Organizations (JCAHO), 82, 312

Judgment skills, 26

Juvenile-onset diabetes; *see* Insulin-dependent diabetes mellitus (IDDM)

K

Kaposi's sarcoma, 369

Kegel exercises, 287

Keratinization, 240

Kitchen, guidelines for infection control in, 94

Knee, range of motion exercises for, 304t

Kübler-Ross stages of death and dying, 442

Kyphoscoliosis, as predisposing condition to respiratory failure, 216

L

Laptop computers, 69

Laundry, guidelines for infection control for, 94

Lead exposure, 457

Leadership
clinical applications of, 143
empowerment as trend in, 141

Leadership strategies, case management strategies and, 140-160

Leakage, of catheters, 291

Learning
affective, 103
behavioral theory for, 103
cognitive, 102
cognitive-developmental theory for, 103
defined, 102
humanistic theories of, 104
principles of adult, 106-107
psychomotor, 103
social-cognitive theories of, 104

Learning contract, elements of, 117

Left ventricular end-diastolic pressure (LVEDP), 200

Legal issues in home care, 124-139

Legal system, understanding our, 124-125

Leg ulcer wraps, 255t

Leininger, Madeline, 17

Length of stay (LOS)
historical changes in maternal, 379
maternal, 379

Liability
avoiding common areas of, 135-139
guidelines to avoid, 135-139
for communication and safety problems, 137
for faulty equipment, 137
for inadequate medical response, 138
for inappropriate admission into home care, 138
for medication errors, 136
for patient falls, 136
telehealth and care considerations, 135

Lipoatrophy, as complication of insulin therapy, 272

Liquid oxygen, 179, 182

Living will, 133

Locia progression, 386t

Locus of control, 104

Loop diuretics, 207t

Lower extremity assessment, of patients with diabetes, 268

Lower urinary tract, physiology of, 278-279

LPN; *see* Skilled nursing

Lungs, physiological relationship between COPD and, 177

LVEDP; *see* Left ventricular end-diastolic pressure

M

Macrovascular disease, as chronic complication of diabetes, 267

Make-believe play, as teaching strategy for children, 119

Malpractice, 125-127

  coverage for nurses, 127

Managed care, defined, 141

Manual healing, 491

Map reading, instruction, 30

Marker model, for QI, 164-166

Mask, Venturi, 182

Masks, OSHA bloodborne pathogen standard for, 90

Maslow's hierarchy of needs, 104

Maternal assessment, in postpartum home care, 382

Maternal-child nursing, postpartum home care and, 379-399

Maternal psychological adaptation, 387t

Medicaid

  guidelines for hospice patients, 431

  as public managed care system, 6, 141

  reimbursable home care services under, 8

  as Title XIX of Social Security system, 7

Medical health history, availability in assessing phase of home visit, 58

Medical records

  as public documents, 129

  right to confidentiality in, 135

Medicare

  benefits for rehabilitation services, 298-299

  comparison of standard and hospice benefits, 431t

  disbursement of monies to home care agencies, 6

Medicare—cont'd

  documentation

    guidelines for, 64-69

    importance for reimbursement, 64

    for patient education, 109

    for treatment of wound care patients in home, 256

    to validate home care services, 70

  emphasis of care prior to, 6,8

  guidelines for reimbursement of specialty services, 29

  guidelines for hospice patients, 431

  HCFA summary forms from, 6,8

  home care programs established under, 6

  payments for home infusion therapy, 311

  people receiving reimbursable home care services under, 8

  as public managed care system, 141

  as Title XVIII of Social Security Act, 7

Medications

  avoiding liability for errors with, 136

  for AIDS patients, 363-367t

  assessment in home visit, 59

  for bladder dysfunction, 281, 296

  for chronic wounds, 245

  for chronic obstructive pulmonary disease, 187-188

  for congestive heart failure, 205-208

  for depression, 407

  for patients recovering from stroke, 339

  responses of schizophrenic patients to, 410

  that affect continence, 282t

  to treat CHF in home, 207t

  use by elderly patients, 423

  used in treatment of HIV and AIDS patients, 363-367t

  for pain control, 452-456t

  for ventilator-dependent patients, 227

Meditation therapy, 490

Mental health patient, 401-416

  drug interactions with antipsychotic medications, 411

  teaching strategies for, 117

  Mini-Mental State Examination, 340-341, 407

  Short Portable Mental Status Questionnaire, 340, 407

Microvascular complications, as chronic complication of diabetes, 267

Micturition, abnormalities of, 279
  atonic bladder, 279
  automatic bladder, 279
  uninhibited neurogenic bladder, 279

Mini-Mental State Examination, 340-341, 407

Mobility
  aids, 309
  of patients with MS, 346
  of patients recovering from stroke, 342

Models
  as home care teaching tools, 109, 112-113t
  theoretical, 15-23

Motion, range of, 302-304

MS; *see* Multiple sclerosis

Multidisciplinary referrals, clinical indicators for, 28t

Multiple sclerosis (MS), 330, 344-348
  clinical manifestations of, 345t
  primary nursing diagnoses/patient problems, 348
  primary themes of patient education for, 348

Muscular dystrophy, as predisposing condition to respiratory failure, 216

Musculoskeletal function, of patients recovering from stroke, 342

Musculoskeletal system, aging and, 419

N

NAHC; *see* National Association for Home Care

Nail beds, signs of cardiac failure in, 204

Narcotics, intravenous administration of, 326

Narrative therapies, 488

Nasal cannula, 182

National Association of Case Managers, 142

National Association for Home Care (NAHC), 11

National Internet community resources and services, 37-46

National Multiple Sclerosis Society, 348

National Pressure Ulcer Advisory Panel (NPUAP), 247

National Stroke Association, 344

Nausea management, for patients with AIDS, 368

Nebulizers, compression, 185

Needles, OSHA bloodborne pathogen standard for, 91

Needs, Maslow's hierarchy of, 104

Neglect
  clinical indicators of elderly patient, 425
  defined, 128

Neonatal jaundice, types and characteristics of, 392t

Nephropathy, as chronic complication of diabetes, 267

Nerves, cranial, 337t

Neuman, M., 18

Neurological assessment of patients with AIDS, 369

Neurological diseases, intravenous pain management for, 326

Neurological dysfunction, patient with, 330-355

Neurological functions, aging and, 419-420

Neuromuscular assessment of infant during postpartum home care, 391

Neuropathy, as chronic complication of diabetes, 267

New York City Mission, Women's Branch of, 3

NIDDM; *see* Non-insulin-dependent diabetes

Nightingale, Florence, 3, 4, 16

Nitrates, 207t

NMS; *see* Neuroleptic malignant syndrome

Nonblanchable erythema of intact skin, therapy for, 247

Noncompliant patients, teaching strategies for, 110-111, 114-117

Non-insulin-dependent diabetes (NIDDM), 266

Nonprofit agency, defined, 8

Notes on Nursing, 16

Notifiable diseases, 84t

NPUAP; *see* National Pressure Ulcer Advisory Panel

Nurse manager role in home infusion therapy, 312

Nurses; *see* Home care nurses
  advanced practice, 30
  district, 3
  public health, 3
  skilled nurse, Medicare defined, 28, 65

Nursing health history, use in assessing phase of home visit, 58, 59

Nursing instructors, tips for field staff working
    with, 35
Nursing interventions
    for Alzheimer's patients, 350
    for patients with MS, 346
    for patients recovering from stroke, 336
Nursing management, for patients with AIDS, 362
Nursing process, patient education and, 108-109
Nursing theorists, 16-22
    Leininger, M., 17
    Neuman, M., 18
    Nightingale, F., 16
    Orem, D., 19-22
    Rice, R., 19-22
    Rogers, M., 16
    Watson, J. 18, 500
Nursing theory, 15-23, 500-502
    caring as human science, 18
    expanding consciousness, 18
    self-care, 17
    self-determination for self-care, 19-22
    unitary man, 16
Nutrition
    assessment, 75
    bladder and bowel dysfunction, 293-294
    for elderly patients in home setting, 421-422
    for patients with AIDS, 421
    for patients with chronic wounds, 244, 258-261
    for patients with COPD, 188-189, 194-197
    for patients with CHF, 208, 211-214
    for patients with diabetes, 273-274
    for patients recovering from stroke, 343
    for ventilator-dependent patients, 226
    see Diet
Nutritional therapist, clinical indicators for referral
    to, 27
Nutritional assessment
    of adults, 75
    of infant during postpartum home care, 393-394

O

Objects as home care teaching tool, 112t
OBRA; see Omnibus Budget Reconciliation Act
Obturator, 219
    tracheostomy tube and, 227

Occlusion, stroke syndromes secondary to, 333-
    335t
Occlusive stroke, 331
Occupational Safety and Health Administration
    (OSHA); see OSHA
Occupational therapist (OT), for patients
    recovering from stroke, 342
Occupational therapy, clinical indicators for
    referral for, 29
Occurrence policy, 127
Oculomotor nerves, 337t
Occupational therapist, for patients with COPD,
    191-192
Odor, catheter, 291
Olfactory nerves, 337t
Oncology Nursing Society (ONS), 312
Operational model, for service delivery, 147
Optic nerves, 337t
Oral blood glucose-lowering agents, 273
Orders, "do not resuscitate," 134
Orem, Dorothea, 17
Organizational performance improvement process,
    DHHS, 162-163
Orthopedic diseases, intravenous pain
    management for, 326
Orthopnea, in patients with CHF, 204
OSHA
    bloodborne pathogen standards, 89-93
    needleless IV systems and, 315
    recommended clinical policies for, 89
    recommended equipment for, 89
    regulations for infection control, 89-93
    suggestions for infection control procedures, 93
OT; see Occupational therapist
Out of bed (OOB) activities, for patients
    recovering from stroke, 343
Outcome failure analysis, 146
Outcome indicator threshold, 168
Outcome measures, 167-168
Outcomes of care, defined, 63
Outcome standards, 164, 166
Oxygen
    complications of, 179
    concentrators, 182
    conserving devices, 182
    liquid, 179

Oxygen—cont'd
    as medication for patients with COPD, 187
    as transtracheal therapy, 183
Oxygen equipment, home, 179
Oxygen therapy, for ventilator-dependent patients, 218

P

Pain
    after childbirth, 386
    of hospice patients, 435-437
    in patients with MS, 347
    pediatric, 447-448
    types of, 436
Pain assessment
    dimensions of, 435
    FACES pain rating scale for peds, 447
    guide for hospice patients, 435-437
    for patients with AIDS, 369
    WHO 3-step analgesic ladder, 438
Pain management, as type of home infusion therapy, 326
Pain therapy
    adjunct analgesics, 454-456t
    analgesics, 452-453t
    continuous subcutaneous infusion for, 315
    epidural space catheter for, 315-316
    intrathecal space catheter for, 315
Palliative care patient, 430-456; *see* Hospice patient
Pamphlets, as home care teaching tool, 112t
Parental roles, adjustment to, 396
Pareto charts, as QI tool, 170
Paroxysmal nocturnal dyspnea, in patients with CHF, 204
Partial thickness wound, therapy for, 252
Passive range of motion, 301
Pathophysiology
    of AIDS, 357-358
    of Alzheimer's dementia, 349
    of chronic obstructive pulmonary disease\E (COPD), 176
    of chronic wounds, 239-240
    of congestive heart failure (CHF), 200-202
    of depression, 405
    of diabetes, 265-267

Pathophysiology—cont'd
    of multiple sclerosis, 344
    of patients who are ventilator-dependent, 216
    of schizophrenia, 409
    of stroke, 331
Patient care, innovative approaches to, 140-160
Patient discharge, criteria, 147
Patient education
    about infection control, 93-95
    for AIDS, 360
    for cerebrovascular accident (CVA), 336
    for chronic wounds, 245
    for congestive heart failure, 208
    for diabetes, 268-276
    guide for foot care, 269
    guidelines for teaching and training activities in, 110
    guides as home care teaching tool, 112t
    in the home, 102-123
    for home infusion therapy, 328-329
    for hospice patients, 435
    on infection control, 93
    Medicare documentation guidelines for, 110
    nursing process and, 108-109
    for patients with bladder dysfunction, 284t
    for patients with COPD, 190
    for patients with depression, 408
    for rehabilitation services, 299
    for schizophrenic patient and care provider, 299
    sociocultural considerations and health beliefs and, 105-106
    teaching tools for, 109, 112t
    for ventilator-dependent patients, 223
Patient falls, liability guidelines, 136
Patient outcomes, progress toward meeting, 154-155
Patient responsibilities, 131, 133
Patient rights, 131, 132
Patients
    and active participation in plan of care, 109
    Alzheimer's, 122
    AIDS, 356-375
    bladder dysfunction, 278-296
    care path home guide for, 153
    care path standards for discharge survey for, 160

Patients—cont'd
  care path standards for home guide for, 157
  chronic obstructive pulmonary disease (COPD), 175-199
  chronic wounds, 239-264
  congestive heart failure (CHF), 202-214
  diabetic, 265-277
  documentation rights and responsibilities of, 131-133
  elderly home care, 417-429
  hospice, 430-456
  mental health, 401-416
  neurological dysfunction, 330-354
  quality care for, 161-172
  receiving home infusion therapy, 310-329
  receiving rehabilitation services, 297-309
  "right to know," 102
  seating tips for chairbound, 307
  teaching elderly, 110, 115
  teaching strategies for
    caregiver, 121
    elderly, 110
    illiterate, 117
    mental health, 117
    noncompliant, 110
    pediatric, 118
  ventilator dependence, 215-238
Patient's room, guidelines for infection control for, 95
Patient's Self-Determination Act, 133
Pediatric patient
  hospice and bereavement issues, 447
  pain management, 447-448
  postpartum care; see Postpartum care
  teaching strategies for, 118
  ventilator dependence, 230
Pelvic floor exercises, for patients with bladder dysfunction, 287
Penicillin, 325t
Percutaneous endoscropic gastrostomy (PEG)\E tubes, 343
Peripheral IV therapy, 313
Peripheral vascular disease, as chronic complication of diabetes, 267
Personal hygiene, guidelines for infection control and, 95

Persons with AIDS (PWA), 356
Pesticides, 459
Pets, guidelines for infection control and, 95
Pharmacological treatment, for patients with bladder dysfunction, 296
Phlebitis, as complication of IV therapy, 322
Photographs, as home care teaching tool, 112t
Physical assessment
  during home visit, 66
  for ventilator-dependent patients, 225
  of infant during postpartum home care, 388-393
  of mother during postpartum home care, 382-387
  of patients with AIDS, 362
  of patients with bladder dysfunction, 282
  of patients with CHF, 203
  of patients with COPD, 187
  of patients with diabetes, 268
  of wounds, 246
Physical therapy
  clinical indicators for referral for, 29t
  for patients recovering from stroke, 342
Physician
  as part of the multidisciplinary team, 142
  nursing implications of orders from, 130-131
  role in home infusion therapy, 312
Physiological solutions, for wound care, 262t
Physiology, of lower urinary tract, 278-279
Piaget, 103, 118-121
PICC line, 315
Plan of care (POC)
  developing plan of documentation and, 58-80
  for COPD patients, 186-190
  for dementia patient and home caregiver, 350, 420
  for home infusion therapy, 328
  for patients with AIDS, 360
  for patients with bladder dysfunction, 284t
  for patients with CHF, 205
  for patients with chronic wounds, 246
  for postpartum home care, 397
  for ventilator-dependent patients, 223
  goals and outcomes should reflect overall, 62-63
  Medicare documentation guidelines for, 64-69
  patient/caregiver active participation in, 109

Planning phase, of home visit, 60
POC; *see* Plan of care
Poliomyelitis, as predisposing condition to respiratory failure, 216
Positive pressure ventilators, 217
Posters, as home care teaching tool, 112t
Postpartum depression, 387
Postpartum Family Referral Form, 383
Postpartum home care
    equipment for, 385
    maternal-child nursing, 379-400
    practitioner competencies for, 381t
    primary nursing diagnoses/patient problems, 397
    primary themes of patient education for, 397
    scope of services for, 380-81
PPOs; *see* Preferred provider organizations
PPS; *see* Prospective payment system
Practice, rural vs. urban areas of, 32
Precautions, for safety in community, 31
Preferred provider organizations (PPOs) as private managed care system, 141
Preload, 200
Prenatal contact in postpartum home care, 381
Preschoolers, teaching strategies for, 119
Pressure management, trends in for wounds, 250
Pressure ulcer prevention recommendations for adult, 251
Pressure ulcers, 242
Primary nursing diagnoses/patient problems
    activity intolerance, 300
    AIDS, 361
    alteration in bowel elimination, 285
    alteration in urinary elimination, 285
    Alzheimer's dementia, 351
    cerebrovascular accident (CVA), 336
    decreased cardiac output, 205
    depression, 402
    diabetes mellitus, 270
    fluid volume excess, 205, 225
    impaired skin integrity, 244
    impaired verbal communication, 195
    ineffective airway clearance, 186
    ineffective breathing pattern, 186, 225
    intravenous therapy, 329
    multiple sclerosis (MS), 348

Primary nursing diagnoses/patient problems—cont'd
    infant, 397
    maternal, 397
    risk for respiratory infection, 226
    schizophrenia, 402
    stroke, 402
Process standards, 166, 168
Professional Consultation Committee, 150
Professional liability coverage, 127
Professional Research Committee, 128
Proprietary agency, 8
Prospective payment system (PPS), 8, 11
Proxy, health care, 133
Psychiatric home care, 401
Psychiatric home health nurse, clinical indicators for referral to, 28
Psychological assessment, of mother following childbirth, 387
Psychomotor learning, 103
Psychosocial conditions, for patients with COPD, 189-190
Psychosocial and spiritual assessment, of ventilator-dependent patients, 229-230
Public agency, defined, 6
Public health nurse, 4
Public policy, impact on home health care, 7
Pulmonary assessment, of patients with CHF, 203
Pulmonary disease, chronic obstructive, 175-199
Pulmonary rehabilitation, 191
Pumps, elastomeric membrane, 320
Pursed-lip breathing, 191
PWA; *see* Persons with AIDS
Pyrogenic reaction, in home infusion therapy, 324t

Q
QA; *see* Quality assurance
QI; *see* Quality improvement, Case management
Quality assurance (QA), 161
    comparing paradigms of QI and, 161t
    historical structure of, 161
    shifting paradigms to QI, 161
Quality improvement (QI), 161
    analysis and evaluation of, 170
    care standards, 164-165
    committee work for, 162-163

Quality improvement (QI)—cont'd
contemporary structure of, 165
cost vs. benefits of, 170-171
evidence-based practice, 166
future perspectives for, 170
OASIS, 161-162
programs, 27
tools for, 168-167
shifting paradigms from QA to, 161
theoretical framework for, 164
variation and trending, 170
Quality
concepts of, 162
measuring, 167
Quality care
concepts of, 161-162
for home infusion therapy, 312
Quality indicators, 167-168
threshold parameters or ranges of, 168
Quality patient care, 161-172
Questionnaire, Short Portable Mental Status
(SPMSQ), 340
Quinolones, 325t

R
Radon, as environmental threat, 458
Range of motion
active, 301
active-assistive, 301
exercises, 302-304
for patients recovering from stroke, 343
passive, 301
resistive, 301
REEDA scale, 386
Referral process, in postpartum home care, 382
Referrals
clinical indicators for multidisciplinary, 27t
for home infusion therapy, 312
Reflex bladder, 279
Reflexes, selected infant, 391t
Registered nurse (RN), as home care case
manager, 141-142
Rehabilitation care, 297-309
clinical indicators for referral to, 29t
adaptive equipment for home, 309

Rehabilitation care—cont'd
indications for, 298-299
primary nursing diagnoses/patient problems,
300
primary themes of patient education for, 300
Relaxation therapy, 489
Remodeling phase, of wound healing, 243-244
Renal assessment, of patients with diabetes, 268
Renal symptoms, in patients with CHF, 204
Report
aide visit, 72
skilled nursing clinical visit, 71, 73
Reproductive functions, aging and, 419
Reproductive tract, assessment of mother's
following birth, 385
Resistive range of motion, 301
Resources and services, national community,
37-46
Respiratory failure, predisposing conditions to,
216
Respiratory functions, aging and, 418
Restoration phase, of wound healing, 243
Retention, urinary, 278
Retinopathy, as chronic complication of diabetes,
267
Rice Model of Dynamic Self-Determination,
19-22
framework for questions during admission
planning, 144
Rights
to confidentiality in medical records, 135
patient, 131-132
RN; *see* Registered nurse
Robert's Rules of Order, 151
Rogers, M. 16
Rural vs. urban areas of practice, 32

S
Safe work environment, agency's provision of,
128
Safety precautions, 31
Saline, homemade sterile normal, 185
Sarcoma, Kaposi's, 357
Scatter diagrams, as QI tool, 170
Scheduling visits, for postpartum home care, 382

Schizophrenia, 409-415
    etiology and pathophysiology of, 409
    primary nursing diagnoses/patient problems,
        402
    primary themes of patient education for, 412
School-agers, teaching strategies for, 120
Select Committee on Aging, definition of
        negligence, 425
Self-care, assessment of motivational factors,
        19, 105
Self-efficacy, 105
Self-inflating manual ventilator (Ambu bag), 217
Self-monitoring of blood glucose (SMBG), 275
Sensorimotor period, infants in, 119
Sensory functions, aging and, 419
Sepsis, related to urinary tract infections in MS,
        345
Serum chemistry, hematology panels and,
        503-513t
Services, national community resources and,
        37-46
Sexual counseling
    for patients with AIDS, 371
    for patients with COPD, 190
    for patients with MS, 347
    for postpartum mother, 387-388
Sharps containers, OSHA bloodborne pathogen
        standard for, 91
Short Portable Mental Status Questionnaire
        (SPMSQ), 340
Shoulder, range of motion exercises for, 302t
Siblings, adjustment to infant, 396
Sick-day management, for patients with diabetes,
        275-276
Skeletal assessment, of infant during postpartum
        home care, 390
Skilled nursing (RN or LPN), clinical indicators
        for referral to, 28
Skin
    discussion of, 240
    infants', during postpartum home care, 391
Skin integrity
    impaired, 244
    in ventilator-dependent patients, 227
    of patients recovering from stroke, 344

Sleep apnea, as predisposing condition to
        respiratory failure, 217
Small vessel disease, 335t
SMBG; see Self-monitoring of blood glucose
        (SMBG)
Smoking, as cause of COPD, 176
Social-cognitive learning theories, 104
Social perspectives, of home health nursing, 4, 6-7
Social security
    payments (FICA), 127
    Title XVIII of Act, Medicare as, 6
    Title XIX of Act, Medicaid as, 7
Social services, clinical indicators for referral to,
        29t
Sociocultural considerations, patient education
        and, 106
Soiled dressings, disposal of as home care
        infection control precaution, 93
Solution, wound care, 262t
Special clinical issues, 379-465
Specimen collection, OSHA bloodborne pathogen
        standard for, 91
Speech language pathologist, clinical indicators
        for referral to, 29t
Spinal accessory nerves, 339t
Spiritual assessment
    in home visit, 60-61
    in hospice, 61
    of ventilator-dependent patients, 229
Spiritual practice or prayer, 490
Staffing, for home infusion therapy, 312
Standard precautions, CDC, 89-92
Staphylococcus, 87
Starling's Law, 200
State Board of Nursing
    as investigator of complaints against nurses, 124
    reporting professional misconduct to, 129
State Department of Public Health, reporting
        professional misconduct to, 129
Stoma, care of, 226, 228
Stool patterns, infant, 391t
Stress ulcers, in ventilator-dependent patients, 226
Stroke, 300; see Cerebrovascular accident (CVA)
    acute complications of, 332
    hemorrhagic, 331

Stroke—cont'd
occlusive, 331
prevention of, 344
risk screening for, 354-355
Stroke volume, pathophysiology of CHF and, 200-201
Structure standards, 164
Students
guidelines for working in home care sites with, 33
tips for field staff working with, 35
visits to home care sites, 33-35
Subcutaneous tissue, 240
Subcutaneous vascular access device, 315
Suctioning, of ventilator-dependent patients, 228
Sulfonamides, 325
Support systems, for elderly patients, 428
Suprapubic catheterization, 292
Sutures, 388
Sylfonylurea drugs, characteristics of commonly used, 273t
Sympathomemetics, 325t
Syringes
insulin, 268
mixing in, 270
prefilled insulin, 272
reuse of, 271

T

Tardive dyskinesia, 411
Teaching
age-related changes and alterations in techniques of, 114t
defined, 102
group strategies, 111
guidelines for activities, 110
tools
for patient education, 109
using pictures and symbols as, 111-112
Technology in home care, 12
Telecare; *see* Telehealth to telecare
Telehealth to telecare, 469-479
critical issues, 471
and the discipline of nursing, 470
ethical and legal issues, 135, 472
historical perspectives, 469

Telehealth to telecare—cont'd
implementation in home care, 470
implications for practice, 476
Telephone conversations, documentation of, 69
Theory; *see* Nursing theory and theorists
applying to clinical practice, 15-23
dynamic self-determination for self-care, 19-22
as environmental impact on health and healing, 16
as expanding consciousness, 18
as human caring, 18
as paradigm for home care nursing, 501
behavioral learning, 103
cognitive-developmental learning, 103
development of, 19-20
family systems, 48, 395
humanistic learning, 104
transcultural, 17
social-cognitive learning, 104
unitary man, 16-17
Therapy
aerosol, 183-185
complementary, 480-489
electroconvulsive, 409
home infusion, 310-329
insulin, 268
intermittent positive pressure breathing (IPPB), 183
oxygen, 179-182
transtracheal oxygen, 183
wound-specific, 252
Therapeutic touch, 493
Threshold parameters or ranges, quality indicators, 168
Thrombophlebitis
after childbirth, 386
as complication of IV therapy, 322
Thumb, range of motion exercises for, 303t
Ties, tracheostomy, 219
Time plots, as QI tool, 170
Tissue, subcutaneous, 240
Title XVIII of Social Security Act, Medicare as, 6-7
Title XIX of Social Security Act, Medicaid as, 6-7
Toddlers, teaching strategies for, 119
Toes, range of motion exercises for, 304t

Toilet access, for patients with bladder dysfunction, 292

Toileting, scheduled, for patients with bladder dysfunction, 260

Topical debriding dressings, 264t

Topical moisturizers, for wound care, 264t

Total parenteral nutrition, as type of home infusion therapy, 327-328

Toxins in the home, 462

Tracheostomal trauma, in ventilator-dependent patients, 227

Tracheostomy ties, 219

Tracheostomy tube, 219
  care of, 227
  cuffed, 220
  cuffed fenestrated, 220
  cuffless, 220
  DPRV, 220
  FOME-CUF, 219, 221
  neonatal and pediatric, 221
  obturator and, 221
  using Velcro collar to secure, 219

Tracheostomy tube cuff, management of, 227

Training
  gait, 301
  Medicare guidelines for, 110

Transcultural nursing theory, 17

Transfer training, 301

Transfusion, referral criteria for in-home, 312

Transmission categories, infection, 88

Transparent film
  adhesive, for wound care, 264t
  hydrocolloid dressings and, 263t
  nonadhesive, for wound care, 264t

Transtracheal oxygen therapy, 183

Trauma
  avoid for patients with peripheral vascular disease, 254
  as predisposing condition to respiratory failure, 216-217
  tracheostomal, 227

Trends, future home care, 469-502

Trigeminal nerves, 337t

Trochlear nerves, 337t

Tubes, tracheostomy, 219

U

Ulcers
  arterial, 242, 254
  diabetic, 242
  pressure, 242
  venous, 242
  venous stasis, 254

Uninhibited neurogenic bladder, as micturition abnormality, 279

Unitary man, 16-17

United Way, 4

Unna boot, application of, 255

Urinary incontinence, 278
  drugs used to treat, 269-270t
  prevalence of, 278
  types causes and treatment of persistent, 286t

Urinary problems, of hospice patients, 440

Urinary retention, defined, 278

Urinary tract, physiology of lower, 278-279

Urodynamic testing, bedside, 284

V

Vagus nerves, 339t

Vancomycin, 325t

Vasodilator action, in therapy of chronic congestive heart failure, 206-207

Variance tracking guide, 153

Vector-borne transmission, infection, 88

Venipuncture, student nurse performing in home, 34

Venous anatomy, 313

Venous stasis ulcers, 254

Venous ulcers, 242

Ventilation, equipment and supplies for home mechanical, 218

Ventilator
  assessment of, 199
  ventilator circuit, typical, 236
  communication devices for, 219
  infection control issues, 228
  management of, 232-237
  noninvasive support, 218
  patient care, 215-238
  positive pressure, 217
  primary nursing diagnoses/patient problems, 225

Ventilator—cont'd
    primary themes of patient education, 225
    pediatric issues, 230
    self-inflating manual, 217
Venturi mask, 184
Victory Secrets of Attila the Hun, 151
Video recording, as home care teaching tool, 112t
Vision assessment, of patients with diabetes, 268
Visit frequency
    extra visits, 147
    for patients with chronic wounds, 244
    for ventilator-dependent patients, 223
    research in home care, 145
Visiting Nurse Association (VNA), 3,6
Visit report; *see* Documentation guidelines
VNA; *see* Visiting Nurse Association
Volatile, organic compounds, as environmental
        threat, 457

W
Wald, Lillian, 3
Walkers, 304
Watson, Jean, 18, 500-502
Wellness, as consequence of nursing actions,
        15-16

Wheelchair, as mobility aid, 301
WHO; *see* World Health Organization
Will, living, 133
Women, AIDS risk for, 359
Working with managed care organizations, 147
World Health Organization (WHO), 437
Wounds and patient care, 239-264
    chemical irritants to, 241
    contamination of, 241
    current trends in care of, 249
    education guides for care of, 246
    mechanisms of healing in, 243-244
    nutritional considerations, 258
    patient/caregiver guidelines for care of, 245
    products for care of, 262-264t
    therapy for full thickness, 252, 254
    therapy for partial thickness, 252
    using zigzag method to culture, 247
Wrist, range of motion exercises for, 302t

Y
Yesavage Geriatric Depression Scale, 407

Z
Ziegler, Philip, 82